Clinical Pharmacology

Clinical Pharmacology

Edited by **Sean Boyd**

SYRAWOOD
PUBLISHING HOUSE

New York

Published by Syrawood Publishing House,
750 Third Avenue, 9th Floor,
New York, NY 10017, USA
www.syrawoodpublishinghouse.com

Clinical Pharmacology
Edited by Sean Boyd

© 2016 Syrawood Publishing House

International Standard Book Number: 978-1-68286-199-8 (Hardback)

Printed in the United States of America.

Contents

Preface

Clinical pharmacology is an applied field of study which focuses on the science and clinical applications of various drugs. The focus of this field is to understand the drug mechanism and side effects through clinical trials and experiments. This book unfolds the innovative aspects of this field by discussing topics such as pharmacokinetics and drug response, drug development, drug interactions, adverse effect of drugs, etc. It includes various researches and case studies contributed by internationally acclaimed scholars and aims to serve as a resource guide for students and clinical practitioners alike.

This book unites the global concepts and researches in an organized manner for a comprehensive understanding of the subject. It is a ripe text for all researchers, students, scientists or anyone else who is interested in acquiring a better knowledge of this dynamic field.

I extend my sincere thanks to the contributors for such eloquent research chapters. Finally, I thank my family for being a source of support and help.

Editor

Antibiotic sales in rural and urban pharmacies in northern Vietnam: an observational study

Do Thi Thuy Nga[1*], Nguyen Thi Kim Chuc[2], Nguyen Phuong Hoa[2], Nguyen Quynh Hoa[3], Nguyen Thi Thuy Nguyen[2], Hoang Thi Loan[2], Tran Khanh Toan[2], Ho Dang Phuc[4], Peter Horby[1,5], Nguyen Van Yen[6], Nguyen Van Kinh[7] and Heiman FL Wertheim[1,5]

Abstract

Background: The irrational overuse of antibiotics should be minimized as it drives the development of antibiotic resistance, but changing these practices is challenging. A better understanding is needed of practices and economic incentives for antibiotic dispensing in order to design effective interventions to reduce inappropriate antibiotic use. Here we report on both quantitative and qualitative aspects of antibiotic sales in private pharmacies in northern Vietnam.

Method: A cross-sectional study was conducted in which all drug sales were observed and recorded for three consecutive days at thirty private pharmacies, 15 urban and 15 rural, in the Hanoi region in 2010. The proportion of antibiotics to total drug sales was assessed and the revenue was calculated for rural and urban settings. Pharmacists and drug sellers were interviewed by a semi-structured questionnaire and in-depth interviews to understand the incentive structure of antibiotic dispensing.

Results: In total 2953 drug sale transactions (2083 urban and 870 rural) were observed. Antibiotics contributed 24% and 18% to the total revenue of pharmacies in urban and rural, respectively. Most antibiotics were sold without a prescription: 88% in urban and 91% in rural pharmacies. The most frequent reported reason for buying antibiotics was cough in the urban setting (32%) and fever in the rural area (22%). Consumers commonly requested antibiotics without having a prescription: 50% in urban and 28% in rural area. The qualitative data revealed that drug sellers and customer's knowledge of antibiotics and antibiotic resistance were low, particularly in rural area.

Conclusion: Over the counter sales of antibiotic without a prescription remains a major problem in Vietnam. Suggested areas of improvement are enforcement of regulations and pricing policies and educational programs to increase the knowledge of drug sellers as well as to increase community awareness to reduce demand-side pressure for drug sellers to dispense antibiotics inappropriately.

Keywords: Antibiotic, Dispensing, Prescription, Community, Practice, Vietnam, Pharmacy

Background

Both appropriate and inappropriate use of antibiotics is a key driver of antibiotic resistance development. However, overuse or misuse of antibiotics (e.g. low dose, too short duration, or treatment of self-limiting infections) provides an avoidable additional pressure leading to more antibiotic resistance [1-3]. In many countries inappropriate use of antibiotics is common practice in the community setting, where antibiotics are readily dispensed for self-limiting upper respiratory tract infections without a prescription [4-8]. To slow down the development of antibiotic resistance, an important control strategy is to reduce the inappropriate use of antibiotics in both community and hospital settings. The incentives behind inappropriate antibiotic dispensing need to be fully understood, so intervention strategies can be developed based on that knowledge.

In Vietnam, health seeking behavior has changed since market reforms that were initiated since 1980s. Despite a public health care system, patients often bypass the health

* Correspondence: ngadtt@oucru.org
[1]Wellcome Trust Major Overseas Programme, Oxford University Clinical Research Unit, Hanoi, Vietnam
Full list of author information is available at the end of the article

care system, and obtain medicines via self-medication or private pharmacies [9,10]. According to one study in 2002, the average household expenditure per episode of illness is 1.1 USD for self-treatment, 1.9 USD for private providers, and 5.2 USD for public providers. The relative higher costs of the health care system explain the preference for self-medication, which results in many cases of inappropriate drug use [10].

In Vietnam, legislation states that antibiotics can only be purchased with a medical prescription [11]. However, previous studies have shown that most antibiotics are sold without prescription. According to a community-based study undertaken in 1999, 78 percent of antibiotics were purchased in private pharmacies without a prescription. 67 percent of the participants consulted the pharmacist while 11 percent decided themselves about antibiotic use [12]. Only 27 percent of the pharmacy staff had correct knowledge about antibiotic use and resistance [8]. Reportedly, prevalence of self-medication with antibiotics through private pharmacies in rural Vietnam is 80%, and is even higher in children with 88% of the children receiving self-medication before hospital visit [13]. These results raised concerns about drugs being sold without prescriptions and the common practice of self-medication. Judicious use of antibiotics can decrease unnecessary adverse effects of antibiotics as well as out-of-pocket costs to the patient. But more importantly, decreased antibiotic usage will help delay the rise of drug resistant bacteria, which is now a growing world-wide public health problem [3].

The present study aims to understand the economic and behavioral incentives that support inappropriate dispensing of antibiotics at Vietnamese private pharmacies. This is crucial for designing effective interventions to reduce the inappropriate antibiotic use in the community.

Methods
Study sites and selection of pharmacies
The study was conducted at two well-established demographic surveillance sites (DSS) in the Hanoi region in 2010. The two study sites are: Bavi (site name: FilaBavi [14]) and Dong Da (site name: Dodalab [15]). Bavi is a rural community situated 60 km west of Hanoi. The basic health care system includes a district hospital with 150 beds, 3 regional polyclinics, 32 commune health stations, and 90 licensed private health facilities including private clinics, pharmacies, drug stores and drug outlets [16]. Dong Da is the biggest urban district of Hanoi with the public health care system including a district hospital with 300 beds, 3 regional polyclinics, 1 antenatal clinic, 21 commune health stations and 278 private pharmacies located in this district [15].

Private pharmacies in each site were randomly selected from a government pharmacy registry, using the Excel random number function for the rural and urban settings. The randomly selected pharmacies were approached sequentially based on ascending random number allocation to get permission to participate until 15 shops in each site were reached. All pharmacies that agreed to participate in the study allowed observers in their pharmacy during three days to observe and record drug sales and prices.

Sample size
One of the major areas of focus in this cross-sectional study was the selling of antibiotics without a prescription and the revenue of antibiotic sales as compared to all sales. Based on previous work we expected 80% of customers to buy antibiotics without a prescription [13]. With $\alpha = 0.05$, $Z_{1-\alpha} = 1.96$ and a precision of $d = 5\%$, we calculated that at least 246 drug transactions needed to be observed. In a pilot study, we observed that there were approximately five to six antibiotic transactions per pharmacy per day in a rural pharmacy. Hence, we estimated that we needed to observe at least 15 drug stores in 3 consecutive days in the rural area. We selected an equal number of urban and rural pharmacies to facilitate comparison although urban sales are expected to be considerably higher.

In-pharmacy observation
During three consecutive days from opening time to closing time of the pharmacy, investigators observed and recorded all information related to pharmacy and drug selling practices onto data capture forms. The forms captured the following basic pharmacy data: facilities, number of staff and education level, presence of Good Pharmacy Practice (GPP) certificates, and presence of pharmaceutical guidelines. Pharmacies that have a GPP certificate are required to ensure a supply of high quality healthcare products and deliver sufficient information and advice to the consumer. The GPP policy also requires pharmacies to have proper facilities (area, drug storage), and comply with prescription regulation.

For the observation of drug transactions, we captured the following information: gender, estimated age of customer, indication for buying drugs (coded according to the International Classification Primary Care – ICPC edition 2), presence of a prescription, compliance to prescription, and any advice provided by drug seller. In cases in which a prescription was provided we checked whether the drug on the prescription was substituted by another drug with a different generic name or a different content/concentration than on the prescription was dispensed or a different dosage/duration than on the prescription was dispensed. In case any of the above was done, we then determined that there was non-compliance with the prescription.

A "drug transaction" in this study included the purchase of any drug or other items present in the pharmacy (e.g. herbal medicine, cotton wools, band aid, etc.). Purchased drugs were recorded according to brand name which was subsequently recoded into the corresponding generic name and Anatomical Therapeutic Chemical (ATC) Classification System. For each drug we also recorded the origin, unit, dosage, and selling price.

The observers included pharmacists who recently graduated from Hanoi Pharmacy University, master pharmacy students, and trained field workers. They were trained in observation skills, interview skills and how to complete the capture forms by senior and experienced investigators. The training included presentation and explanation of the study, discussion, interaction and case practice by acting as drug sellers/owners and interviewers. Furthermore we performed a pilot in two pharmacies (one in urban, one in rural) to test the questionnaire and revise if needed. The pilot pharmacies were not selected for the real observation.

The pharmacist/seller was informed that the observation would be for all drug sales, and thus not antibiotics specifically, to reduce any potential biases by the observation. The observations were supervised and randomly checked by supervisors. At the end of each observing day, supervisors collected the forms and were checked for completeness. Bigger pharmacies had two observers present. Pharmacy customers were not interviewed by the study staff.

All data capture forms and questionnaires were designed in the English language and send for peer review to experts in the field. The revised version was then translated into Vietnamese and piloted in a rural and urban pharmacy.

Post-observation questionnaire and qualitative assessment

After the observation, one drug-seller and one pharmacy owner per pharmacy were asked to complete a semi-structured questionnaire which focused on antibiotic sales and their opinions about important causes for irrational antibiotics dispensing in their region. Answers were provided on a 5-point likert scale: "1 = strongly disagree" to "5 = strongly agree". To assess the reliability of survey responses, Cronbach's alpha was analyzed with respondents' scores for all questionnaire items by SPSS. It is a coefficient from 0–1, with values above 0.7 being acceptably consistent.

All forms were anonymous to encourage interviewees to frankly share information. In total, 43 informants attended this survey including 26 respondents in urban pharmacies and 17 in rural site. Among them, 4 respondents in urban and 13 in rural were both pharmacy owners and sellers.

Qualitative methods, focus group discussions (FGD) and in-depth interviews, were used to better explore experiences and opinions of the drug sellers and pharmacists, as well as their perceptions of the factors that impact on inappropriate antibiotic dispensing. One FGD was held in the rural area and a total of six individual in-depth interviews were performed in both sites due to difficulties in finding participants for the FGD, especially in urban area. The FGD included the following participants: two pharmacy owners, one drug seller and three commune health center workers. All of them had a primary degree on pharmacy and those working in commune health center (CHC) were also assistant doctors. The in-depth interviews were done with three rural (two pharmacy owners and one CHC staff) and three urban participants (two participants were both a pharmacy owner and drug sellers and one drug sellers, one owner is pharmacist and two other participants had a secondary degree on pharmacy). English guidelines were developed to cover general and specific issues for asking participants to discuss their own experiences and opinions.

Both discussion and in-depth interviews included the following themes: (1) financial incentives, (2) knowledge of government regulations and (3) potential solutions for controlling inappropriate antibiotic dispensing practices (see Additional file 1: Table S1). All discussions in both sites were led by NQH who had relevant training and experience. If needed, findings of the observation and questionnaire were presented during FGD and interviews to support the discussion. All contents of conversations were recorded and transcripts were made and translated into English. Data from transcripts were analyzed using qualitative content analysis by listening to the tapes and reading and re-reading the transcripts to become familiar with the data and to categorize information. We used both the Vietnamese transcript and the English translated version to identify common themes. Connections within and between themes were identified. The main themes and connections were used to identify important causes of inappropriate antibiotic dispensing in urban and rural pharmacies [17].

Ethical considerations

The Ethical Review Board of Hanoi Medical University approved the study (Decision No: 78/HDDD-YHN). Permission was obtained from the local health bureau for the study and verbal consent was obtained from the owner of each participating pharmacy. All pharmacy data was anonymized.

Data analysis

Collected data were cleaned and entered into a database and checked for quality by an independent data analyst. Antibiotic sales data was summarized using median and interquartile range (IQR) for skewed distributed data. Potential differences between urban versus rural pharmacies were compared by Mann–Whitney test for non-normal continuous data, Wilcoxon sign rank test for paired non-normal data and Chi-square test for categorical variables. P-values less than 0.05 were considered significant (2 tailed).

In term of revenue, the contribution of antibiotic sales to the total drug sales for each pharmacy was calculated. In addition, we calculated the retail mark-ups of the twenty most sold antibiotics. The mark up is the difference between the cost and selling price of a particular product. Here, we used the percentage mark up to assess the profit of antibiotics that was calculated as (selling price – purchasing price)/purchasing price × 100%. The purchase prices were obtained from major wholesalers and distributers in northern Vietnam. Data was analyzed by SPSS software, version 16 (SPSS Inc., USA). The currency exchange rate of Vietnam Dong (VND) to US dollar (USD) at the time of study was: 1 USD = 18,500 VND.

Results
Pharmacy characteristics
Among thirty randomly selected pharmacies, six urban pharmacies had a Good Pharmacy Practice (GPP) certificate, whilst none of the rural pharmacies had a GPP certificate.

None of the private pharmacy owners in the rural area were pharmacists, whereas 5 owners of urban pharmacies were pharmacists. Most urban pharmacies had two drug sellers working in each store while rural pharmacies usually had one seller per outlet. Drug sellers in the urban pharmacies had a higher level of education: 3/28 had a university degree on pharmacy, 21/28 were assistant pharmacists, and 4/28 had an elementary degree on pharmacy. In the rural pharmacies none were pharmacist, 9/17 were assistant pharmacists, 4 were elementary pharmacists and 4 were doctor assistants. Three urban pharmacies had a pharmacist on site in charge of managing and dispensing drugs. Only one pharmacy had up-to-date reference books available in the pharmacy and frequently used for consultation, the remaining did not (see Additional file 2: Table S2).

Observation of drug sales
In total 2953 drug sale transactions (2083 urban and 870 rural) were observed between the 30 pharmacies (Table 1). The proportion of transactions that included antibiotics was high: 24% (499/2083) in the urban sites and 30% (257/870) in the rural sites (p = 0.002). Most antibiotics were sold without a prescription: 88% (439/499) in urban and 91% (234/257) in rural area (p = 0.2 showing no significant difference between two areas). Compliance to regulations was better in the pharmacies

Table 1 Antibiotics dispensing practices according to prescription regulation

Outcomes	Urban (n = 2083)	Rural (n = 870)
Transaction with antibiotics	499 (24%)*	257 (30%)*
With prescription	60 (12%)	23 (9%)
Comply with prescription	49 (82%)	18 (78%)
Not comply with prescription	11 (18%)	5 (22%)
Without prescription	439 (88%)	234 (91%)
Client made decision	221 (50%)*	66 (28%)*
Drug seller made decision	218 (50%)	168 (72%)

*Significant different between urban and rural group using chi-square test (p < 0.05).

that had a pharmacist on site with 19% (21/112) of total antibiotics transactions having prescription versus only 10% (62/644) in the shops without pharmacist (p = 0.004).

There was no significant difference between GPP versus non-GPP pharmacies regarding antibiotics dispensing practices. Pharmacies with a GPP certificate sold antibiotics without prescription in 88% (196/224) of cases, similar to 90% (477/532) (p = 0.38) rate in pharmacies without such a certificate. In term of self-medication, 50% (221/439) of the urban pharmacy customers decided by themselves which antibiotics to buy, whereas the rural clients more often asked for advice from drug sellers, with only 28% self-prescribed (p < 0.0001).

It was observed that antibiotics were the most common drug sold at the pharmacies in both areas (17% in urban and 18% in rural, p = 0.15), followed by herbal medicines (15% in urban and 11% in rural, p < 0.0001). However, in term of monetary value, herbal medicines was the most important groups which mainly contributed to total sales of both urban and rural pharmacies with 24% in urban and 27% in rural, followed by antibiotics (24% in urban versus 18% in rural), analgesics group and vitamins (Figure 1). Average number of customers per pharmacy per day was 46 in urban and 19 in rural area. Among them, 11 clients in urban area had transactions that included antibiotics and the corresponding figure in rural area was 6 clients (Additional file 3: Figure S1). Other therapeutic groups, such as cardiovascular system, nervous system, or corticosteroid medications, were rarely dispensed in all observed pharmacies. Three most common sold antibiotics in the urban area were: amoxicillin (13%), azithromycin (12%), cephalexin (9%) while in rural pharmacies were amoxicillin (27%, p < 0.0001), cephalexin (20%, p < 0.0001) and ampicillin (12% versus 4% in urban setting, p < 0.0001). The main difference between the urban and rural pharmacies was that older antibiotics, such as chloramphenicol, and cotrimoxazole, were more commonly dispensed in the rural area. In the urban area more new and expensive

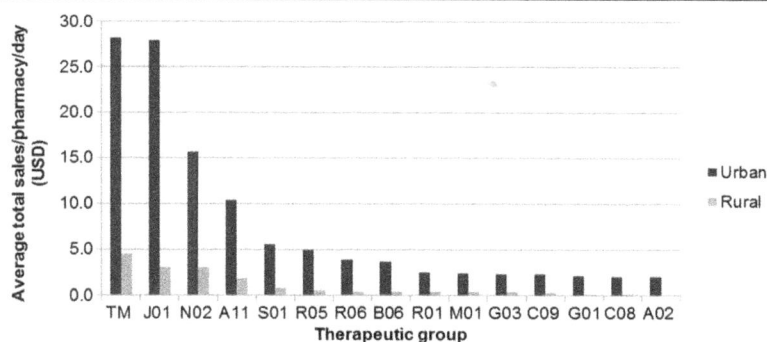

Figure 1 Average sales in USD per pharmacy per day by therapeutic groups in urban versus rural (in USD). TM: Herbal medicines, J01: Antibiotics, N02: Analgesic, A11: Vitamins, S01: Ophthalmological, R05: Cough and cold preparation, B06: Hematological agent, R06: Antihistamine, R01: Nasal preparations, M01: Anti-inflammatory and antirheumatic products, G03: genial system, C09: rennin-angiotensin, G01: Gynecological, C08: calcium channel blocker, A02: acid related disorders.

brands such as augmentin (amoxicillin-clavulanic acid), 3rd generation cephalosporins (cefuroxime, cefixime), and azithromycin were sold.

The most common reason for buying antibiotics in the urban sites was cough (32%), and in the rural sites this was fever (22%). Antibiotics were often sold in combination with other drugs: analgesics 17% (189/1122), cough and cold preparations 16% (182/1122), vitamins 9% (99/1122), corticosteroids 9% (98/1122), and herbal medicines 5% (54/1122).

Economic indicators of antibiotic sales

Antibiotics represented a considerable proportion of total revenues per day: 24% (27.9USD/115.8USD) in urban and 18% (3 USD/16.5 USD) in rural area (p = 0.59) (Figure 1). Urban pharmacies showed higher sales of imported antibiotics with median sale of 11.5 US dollars per pharmacy per day (IQR = 5.3 – 41.7) compared to domestic antibiotics (median = 5.1 US dollars, IQR = 4.2-6.6, P-value 0.003). The opposite was observed in the rural area where very little imported products were sold with median sales of zero US dollars per pharmacy per day compared to domestic products in term of total antibiotics monetary sales with median sale of 1.6 US dollars (IQR = 1.4-3.1), p value < 0.001). In the rural sites, available imported brands such as amoxicillin or cephalexin were mostly from India, with relatively low prices as compared to other brands. Meanwhile, more expensive imported brands were preferred by urban customers.

Retail mark-ups of twenty most common sold antibiotic generics across all pharmacies in each setting varied considerably. In the urban area, mark-ups ranged from 17-243% (median = 54%, IQR = 30-79%) and in the rural area from 21-186% (median = 58.5%, IQR = 39-67%). There was no significant difference between the mark ups between the two regions (p = 0.76). Several imported brands that were only dispensed in urban pharmacies

showed relatively high mark-ups such as: augmentin (amoxicillin – clavulanic acid), zinnat (cefuroxime), zithromax (azithromycin) as compared to domestic products (Table 2).

The semi structured questionnaire on antibiotic dispensing practices with drug sellers and drug store owners by semi-structured questionnaire, 41% (7/17) of rural respondents and 27% (7/26) of urban informants conceded that 20% to 40% of their total profit was due to antibiotic sales (p = 0.33). Meanwhile 53% (9/17) in rural and 23% (6/26) in urban site thought that profit from antibiotics accounted for less than 20% (p = 0.04). Only 6% (1/17) of rural respondents and 4% (1/26) in urban considered that profits from antibiotics accounted for 40-60% of their total profit.

Causes for inappropriate antibiotic selling

All rural pharmacy respondents thought that the fear of losing a customer leads to dispensing of antibiotics without prescription. This opinion was shared with 69% (18/26) of urban respondents. Pressure from patients that demand antibiotics was considered a significant driver of irrational dispensing practices in rural pharmacies according to 77% (13/17) of respondents, and 39% or urban respondents (p = 0.01). Only 27% (7/26) of the respondents in urban and 24% (4/17, p = 0.8) in rural area considered that knowledge of drug sellers was insufficient to dispense antibiotics appropriately. The majority of urban respondents (69%) thought that inappropriate prescription of doctors contributed to irrational antibiotic selling, whereas trust in doctors appeared stronger among respondents in rural setting (29%, p = 0.01). 31% in urban and 35% in rural sites conceded that inappropriate dispensing of antibiotics to be due to high profitability of antibiotic sales (p = 0.75). 71% (12/17) rural participants blamed inappropriate dispensing on other causes like quality of diagnostics and access to medical services versus 46%

Table 2 Mark-ups of 20 most common sold antibiotics according to generic names

Generic name	Origin	ATC code	Unit/Content	Unit price (USD) USD	% Mark-up	
					Urban	Rural
Amoxicillin	Vietnam	J01CA04	Tablet/500 mg	0.02	78	67
Amoxicillin	India	J01CA04	Tablet/500 mg	0.04	54	54
Amoxicillin	Austria	J01CA04	Tablet/500 mg	0.04	88	NA
Cephalexin	Vietnam	J01DA01	Tablet/500 mg	0.04	67	67
Cephalexin	India	J01DA01	Tablet/500 mg	0.05	58	58
Cephalexin	France	J01DA01	Tablet/500 mg	0.07	25	NA
Ampicillin	Vietnam	J01CA01	Tablet/500 mg	0.02	122	43
Ampicillin	India	J01CA01	Tablet/500 mg	0.03	100	40
Chloramphenicol	Vietnam	J01BA01	Tablet/250 mg	0.03	17	59
Cotrimoxazole	Vietnam	J01EC01	Tablet/480 mg	0.01	33	67
Metronidazole	Vietnam	J01XD01	Tablet/250 mg	0.01	82	150
Lincomycin	Vietnam	J01FF02	Tablet/500 mg	0.03	41	25
Penicillin	Vietnam	J01RA01	Tablet/1 MIU	0.02	60	50
Spiramycin	Vietnam	J01FA02	Tablet/0.75 MIU	0.04	43	29
Spiramycin	France	J01FA02	Tablet/0.75 MIU	0.14	68	21
Ciprofloxacin	Vietnam	J01MA02	Tablet/500 mg	0.02	233	186
Ciprofloxacin	German	J01MA02	Tablet/200 mg	0.65	33	NA
Erythromycin	Vietnam	J01FA01	Pack/250 mg	0.08	103	69
Erythromycin	France	J01FA01	Pack/250 mg	0.23	31	67
Azithromycin	German	J01FA10	Bottle/200 mg/5 ml	5.19	19	NA
Cefuroxime	UK	J01DA06	Tablet/500 mg	1.06	27	NA
Cefixime	Bangladesh	J01DA23	Pack/200 mg	0.20	49	NA
Amoxicillin+ Acid clavulanic	UK	J01CR02	Pack/250 mg	0.37	62	NA
Roxythromycin	India	J01FA06	Tablet/150 mg	0.06	81	NA
Klarithromycin	USA	J01FA09	Tablet/250 mg	0.43	31	NA
Tobramycin	Belgium	J01GB01	Vial/0.3%	2.05	18	NA
Cefpodoxim	India	J01DA33	Tablet/100 mg	0.04	19	NA
Clindamycin	India	J01FF01	Tablet/300 mg	0.05	117	NA

NA: Not available.

(12/26) in urban site (p = 0.12) (Table 3). Only a minority 8% of urban and 18% of rural respondents thought that the current situation of antibiotics dispensing was appropriate and does not need to be improved (p = 0.32).

Qualitative study
Incentives structure
Most interviewees in both the urban and rural setting did not think that profits from antibiotic sales predominated in comparison with other drugs. According to their opinion, vitamins, tonic drugs or functional foods are more profitable than the antibiotic group, which, however, is not confirmed by our quantitative data. "Antibiotics are commonly used items and customers know well

Table 3 Causes for irrational antibiotics dispensing

Reasons outcomes	Percentage of respondents within area agreed with given reasons	
	Urban (n = 26)	Rural (n = 17)
Fear of losing customers	18 (69%)	17 (100%)
Pressure from patient's demand	10 (38%)*	13 (76%)*
Insufficient knowledge of dispensers	7 (27%)	4 (23%)
Inappropriate prescribing of doctors	18 (69%)*	5 (29%)*
High profitability of antibiotics	8 (31%)	6 (35%)
Other (quality of diagnosis or health services)	12 (71%)	12 (46%)

*Significant different between groups using Chi-square test (p value <0.05).

their prices. That is why it not as profitable as less popular drugs like vitamins, tonics or functional foods" was the response of one rural seller. Nevertheless, they conceded that pharmacy's income would be affected if they comply with prescription regulation. "Not only antibiotics but also thirty other groups have to be dispensed with a prescription. If we wait for a prescription, we sell hardly anything and total sales would be definitely influenced" according to one urban seller.

All rural interviewees stated that patients' demand is a common factor affecting the sale of antibiotics. An example of this is described as: "I need to satisfy clients' demand. That's in the interest of our business!". According to their opinion, this factor can be changed if patients' awareness is improved and when the knowledge of sellers is strong enough to give professional advice. Meanwhile, fear of losing customers is common among urban sellers. "If I refuse to sell antibiotics without prescription, I will lose that customer for another pharmacy as they can easily buy anywhere".

Both urban and rural respondents reported that patients often avoided visiting doctors due to the inconvenience, and would rather go directly to a private pharmacy as the first choice for mild disease. "It's very annoying and time-consuming to be examined in a hospital. And private clinic are very costly, as they do many kinds of test. Our customers only go to see doctors in case of severe disease".

Knowledge on antibiotics/resistance and regulations

All urban and rural participants expressed that they will give antibiotics in case of suspected infection such as upper respiratory infections with fever, cough and sputum or even an injury to prevent infection. In addition, some rural interviewees noted that customers consider antibiotics to be a 'miracle drug' that can treat many kinds of diseases and sometimes they demand it simply for maintaining a private stock for self-medication. Meanwhile, all urban interviewees believed that misconceptions about antibiotic use changed among the urban population where there are better economic conditions and higher educational levels. "Recently, public awareness of drugs' side effects has been improved, so there is less abuse of antibiotics than before" according to an urban seller.

All interviewees stated that they had heard about antibiotic resistance. However, qualitative data also revealed insufficient knowledge of antibiotic resistance among drug sellers and pharmacy owners, especially in the rural area. Most urban drug sellers demonstrated reasonable knowledge regarding the possible effects of resistance on all populations, whereas some rural sellers did not. "Antibiotic resistance occurs in those overusing it. I do not abuse, so for me there is no need to worry" (Rural seller).

Most respondents believed that patient-related factors such as self-medication and poor adherence to antibiotic regimens contribute to the problems of antibiotic resistance. It has been reported in the rural setting that patients often buy antibiotics for an inappropriate duration. "I advised the customer to take antibiotics for at least 5 days, but they do not have enough money so they usually buy for just 2.5 days (10 tablets). When they recover, they will stop taking drugs, otherwise they would have bought more" (Rural seller).

It was also reported that there is not enough attention to antibiotics and resistance in the curriculum of pharmacists and drug sellers.

Regarding the knowledge of government regulations, most rural respondents did not know about GPP. "This is the first time I heard about GPP" said a rural seller. They also revealed misconception about prescription regulation by stating that: "Some kind of weak antibiotics such as amoxicillin or ampicillin can be sold without prescription" (Rural seller). In contrast, all urban interviewee understood clearly about GPP, but they conceded that there is little enforcement in dispensing practice. "There is no difference between GPP and non-GPP pharmacy in terms of regulation compliance. Over the counter dispensing of prescription only drugs is common in every pharmacy" (Urban seller).

Proposed solutions

Rural respondents did not think that GPP could be deployed broadly in the rural setting due to the poor conditions of the facilities and education level of the work force. However, if regulations are enforced they will shift their business to dispense over the counter drugs like vitamins, cough and cold preparation; tonics that are allowed by the law to compensate pharmacies for financial losses. The urban respondents believe that GPP brings improvement to infrastructure but not to dispensing practices. "To get a GPP certificate, we need to invest more in improving our infrastructure; as a result the pharmacy looks more spacious. However, quality of service and dispensing practices has not been much improved".

Pharmacy workers have the understanding that the GPP policy objective is to improve the quality of pharmacy services in terms of infrastructure and quality drug supply. However, the awareness about their own professional contribution in promoting rational medicine use and its role in public health is very limited.

Both urban and rural respondents considered that training for drug sellers and the general population was needed to improve their knowledge and awareness about antibiotics and resistance and thought that this would likely have a significant impact on controlling inappropriate antibiotic use in the community. "There will be less pressure to give customers antibiotics if their awareness is improved".

Discussion

The results of this study clearly illustrate the widespread inappropriate antibiotic dispensing at private pharmacies in the Hanoi region. With only about 10% complying with prescription regulations, the situation in Vietnam is worse than has been reported in Zimbabwe, where the proportion is 39% [18]. In a cross-sectional client simulation study in Syria, 87% of the pharmacies sold antibiotics without a prescription. This proportion increased up to 97% when the client simulators insisted on buying antibiotics [19]. Similar studies in Saudi Arabia and India had comparable results: 78% and 94% of visited pharmacies dispensed over the counter antibiotics [20,21]. The most frequent reason for buying antibiotics was acute upper respiratory tract infections, which are generally self-limiting [22,23].

There are several successful interventions in other countries that brought important reduction in antibiotic use. As reported in Chile, consumption of most oral antibiotic groups in the community pharmacies significantly decreased after fulfilling prescription-only regulations [24]. Similarly, inappropriate antibiotic prescribing in viral illness remarkable declined as in Korea by prohibiting prescribers from dispensing medications themselves [25]. In Vietnam, prescription-only regulation is embedded in the Drug Law that was issued in 2005 [26]. In spite of these regulations, there is no sanction for non-compliance. This may explain why, to this moment, no pharmacy has been penalized for antibiotic dispensing without a prescription. As there is a lack of enforcement of the regulations, self-medication is possible and is viewed as more economical and convenient than consulting a health professional [27,28]. Even if a pharmacy has a Good Pharmacy Practice registration, the results of this study revealed that the awareness of the concept of GPP among drug sellers was poor and they dispensed antibiotics without a prescription similar to pharmacies without a GPP standard. We also observed that more than 80% of the pharmacies rented pharmacist's licenses. According to Vietnamese regulations (Decree 79/2006/NĐ-CP), only pharmacists with at least 5 year experience can own a pharmacy [29]. However, pharmacists often rent out their license and work elsewhere, making it easier for non-pharmacists to own a pharmacy. Despite the limited number of pharmacies in our study, we did observe better practices in sites that had a pharmacist present. As health promoter in the situation of being the "front-line health worker", pharmacist should promote non-drug solutions for any health problems. Strengthening this role of pharmacist in distributing channel might have impact on reducing irrational antibiotics in community.

Antibiotics represented a considerable proportion of total revenues (24% in urban and 18% in rural pharmacies), illustrating that antibiotics sales contribute an important part of total sales of pharmacies. Imported brands were sold more in urban pharmacies, whereas rural pharmacies generally mostly sold domestically produced antibiotics. The study also found that in the urban area, patients' demands are a common factor affecting the sales of antibiotics, with half (50%) of urban clients self-prescribing. In contrast, clients in the rural sites more often asked for advice from drug sellers. However, lack of knowledge of drug dispensers is common and will not lead to better antibiotic dispensing practices. The qualitative study also disclosed that the government push to have all pharmacies comply with GPP standards is likely not a solution due to lack of enforcement and the shortage of a well-educated workforce [26]. According to the Vietnamese General Statistics Office, in 2010, there were only 0.4 pharmacists/10,000 inhabitants, and for assistant and elementary pharmacists this was about 2 and 0.6 per 10,000 inhabitants. Pharmacy staffs with a university degree mostly work in the big cities with 4.5 pharmacists/1000 inhabitants, despite a serious deficiency in remote areas with only 0.2 pharmacists/10,000 inhabitants [26].

Overuse of antibiotics in the community is caused by people buying antibiotics after self-diagnosis or diagnosis by, often poorly trained, health-care providers. The reasons for irrational antibiotic prescribing in Vietnam are the same as in other countries including perceived expectations of patients, time constraints, lack of knowledge, lack of diagnosis capability and financial benefits for the prescriber [26]. Identifying and modifying the incentives for inappropriate prescribing remains a major challenge.

In term of impact of implementing pricing policies, high prices of antibiotics and tendency to sell branded drugs rather than cheaper generics is one of the important factors affecting irrational use and inadequate treatment as people often cannot afford to buy a full treatment course. The current mechanism of drug price control is not able to achieve the desired objectives as the drug prices in Vietnam are higher as compared to international comparators [30]. The government has no leverage to negotiate on the wholesale prices even if those prices are higher than CIF prices (cost, insurance and freight). Retail prices are determined by the market, but there is a tendency to sell branded drugs rather than cheaper generics in urban areas. According to WHO's studies in private sector, there was a big variation in mark-ups along the Vietnam medicines supply chain [30]. Suppliers can easily increase prices and the government cannot control this. It is important to have a more structured and enforced price control mechanism, with strong generic policies, good procurement systems and single system leverage (such as health insurance and bulk procurements) to reduce drug prices.

Lastly, it was clearly revealed in both the quantitative and qualitative study that there is poor awareness of consumers. As shared experiences from several developed countries in Europe [31], education campaigns targeting on providers and consumers through mass media contributed to reduction of antibiotic overuse suggesting that public education campaigns can be effective.

There are some limitations to our study that needs to be discussed. Our study was conducted only in the Hanoi region, with a relative small sample size and can therefore not be generalized to the whole country. However, discussions with doctors and pharmacists from other regions, do confirm that the issues are similar elsewhere. In larger pharmacies, some transactions may have been missed when large numbers of customers come to shops simultaneously. However, we believe this was limited as in larger pharmacies, as two observers were present. Awareness of being observed might have influenced antibiotic dispensing practices (Hawthorne effect). To minimize this bias the sellers were unaware during the observation that the objective was to assess antibiotic sales. Questionnaires focusing on antibiotics were done after the observation. Some respondents were both drug seller and pharmacy shop owner, which might affect the results as the owner may mostly be interested in profit and their opinion about incentives driving irrational antibiotic dispensing might be different from a drug seller. There was limited participation for participants in the urban area to join focus group discussions which may account for the relative paucity of solutions. Only one focus group discussion could be performed in the rural setting and in the urban area we conducted in-depth interviews. With relatively few participants in the interview, we were not able to estimate where the saturation was reached. However, at the end of the discussion and interviews, little new ideas were recorded, so we do think we were close to saturation with our limited number of interviews. Furthermore, the study used wholesale prices to assess mark-ups of sold antibiotics as we were unable to obtain purchasing prices from the pharmacies. Finally, the limited observation time of three days in each pharmacy will not reflect the sales of antibiotics and dispensing practices fully as these may be subject to change due to diseases with seasonality (e.g. influenza season). However, we do think the observations nicely reveal the magnitude of inappropriate antibiotic dispensing.

Conclusion

The revenues from antibiotic sales are considerable for private pharmacies in both rural and urban northern Vietnam. Complying with drug regulations, to dispense antibiotics only with a prescription, would therefore lead to economic loss for pharmacies. This would make acceptance and compliance with regulations challenging. Increasing the requirement for pharmacies to be GPP certified may only help in case the regulation that a pharmacist should be on site is enforced. For non-GPP pharmacies, substituting antibiotic sales with sales of symptom relieving drugs or vitamins may be a strategy to compensate pharmacies for financial losses and to motivate them to comply with government regulations. Confronted with the situation of not enforcing regulations, continuing professional training for drug sellers will be helpful to increase their understanding of antibiotics, resistance and how to dispense it appropriately. As the consumers often demand antibiotics without a prescription, public awareness campaigns should also be a central component of future control strategies.

Additional files

Additional file 1: Table S1. Thermalized guideline for FGD and in-depth interview.

Additional file 2: Table S2. Pharmacy baseline information.

Additional file 3: Figure S1. Average number of clients per pharmacy per day.

Competing interests
We have no potential conflicts of interest to declare.

Authors' contribution
We are co-authors in this manuscript and have contributed sufficiently in the work as follow. DTTN: the first author who was responsible for and monitored the observation and in-depth interviews, performed statistical data analysis and drafted the manuscript. NTKC: The second author, who contributed in the planning of the study, supervised the observation period and took part in revising the manuscript. NPH: The third author, who was involved in supervising observation and revising manuscript. NQH: The fourth author, who performed in-depth interviews and revised manuscript. NTTN and HTL: The fifth and sixth authors, who have participated in data collection and statistical analysis. TKT and HDP: The seventh and eighth authors, who have contributed in statistical analysis and manuscript revision. PH: The ninth author, who was participated in designing of the study, NVY, NVK: The tenth and eleventh authors, who have took part in revising manuscript. HFLW: The last author, who was responsible for conception and designing study and manuscript revision. All authors have read and approved the final manuscript.

Acknowledgements
The project was funded by the Center for Disease Dynamics Economics and Policy (CDDEP), Washington DC, USA, as part of the Global Antibiotic Resistance Partnership (GARP), and the Wellcome Trust Major Overseas Program, United Kingdom. We would like to thank Professor Nguyen Duc Hinh, Rector of Hanoi Medical University for his agreement to participate in this study. We also would like to express our sincere thanks to the owners of thirty private pharmacies who well collaborated with us during this study as well as the Health Bureau of Hanoi. We highly appreciate the team of under graduated pharmacy students for their contribution in collecting data.

Author details
[1]Wellcome Trust Major Overseas Programme, Oxford University Clinical Research Unit, Hanoi, Vietnam. [2]Hanoi Medical University, Hanoi, Vietnam. [3]Vietnam National Cancer Hospital, Hanoi, Vietnam. [4]Department of

Probability and Statistics, Institute of Mathematics, VAST, Hanoi, Vietnam.
[5]Nuffield Department of Clinical Medicine, Centre for Tropical Diseases,
Oxford, UK. [6]Hanoi Department of Health, Hanoi, Vietnam. [7]National Hospital
for Tropical Diseases, Hanoi, Vietnam.

References

1. World Health Organization Report: *WHO Global Strategy for Containment Resistance to Antimicrobial Drugs.* Geneva: WHO report, WHO/CDS/CSR/DRS/2001.2; 2001.
2. Barbosa TM, Levy SB: **The impact of antibiotic use on resistance development and persistence.** *Drug Resist Update* 2000, **3**:303–311.
3. Tilak JD-M: **Bacterial resistance to antibiotics: a growing public health problem.** *McMaster Univ Med J* 2011, **8**:58–61.
4. Bi P, Tong S, Parton KA: **Family self-medication and antibiotics abuse for children and juveniles in a Chinese city.** *Soc Sci Med* 2000, **50**(10):1445–1450.
5. Llor C, Cots JM: **The sale of antibiotics without prescription in pharmacies in Catalonia Spain.** *Clin Infect Dis* 2009, **48**(10):1345–1349.
6. World Health Organization: *Medicines Use in Primary Care in Developing and Transitional Countries,* WHO Fact Book WHO/EMP/MAR/2009.3. Geneva: World Health Organization; 2009.
7. Landers TF, Ferng YH, McLoughlin JW, Barrett AE, Larson E: **Antibiotic identification, use, and self-medication for respiratory illnesses among urban Latinos.** *J Am Acad Nurse Pract* 2010, **22**(9):488–495.
8. Hoa NQ, Larson M, Kim Chuc NT, Eriksson B, Trung NV, Stalsby CL: **Antibiotics and paediatric acute respiratory infections in rural Vietnam: health-care providers' knowledge, practical competence and reported practice.** *Trop Med Int Health* 2009, **14**(5):546–555.
9. Okumura J, Wakai S, Umenai T: **Drug utilisation and self-medication in rural communities in Vietnam.** *Soc Sci Med* 2002, **54**(12):1875–1886.
10. Thuan NT, Lofgren C, Lindholm L, Chuc NT: **Choice of healthcare provider following reform in Vietnam.** *BMC Health Serv Res* 2008, **8**:162.
11. Vietnam Ministry of Health: *Vietnam Ministry of Health Decision No 1847/2003/QD-BYT about Regulation of Drug Prescribing and Selling Prescription Only.* Hanoi, Vietnam: Vietnam Ministry of Health; 2003.
12. Larsson M, Kronvall G, Chuc NT, Karlsson I, Lager F, Hanh HD, Tomson G, Falkenberg T: **Antibiotic medication and bacterial resistance to antibiotics: a survey of children in a Vietnamese community.** *Trop Med Int Health* 2000, **5**(10):711–721.
13. Larsson M: *Antibiotic Use and Resistance: Assessing and Improving Utilization and Provision of Antibiotics and Other Drugs in Vietnam,* PhD Thesis. Sweden: Karolinska Institutet; 2003.
14. Chuc NT, Diwan V: **FilaBavi, a demographic surveillance site, an epidemiological field laboratory in Vietnam.** *Scand J Public Health Suppl* 2003, **62**:3–7.
15. Tran TK, Eriksson B, Nguyen CT, Horby P, Bondjers G, Petzold M: **DodaLab: an urban health and demographic surveillance site, the first three years in Hanoi. Vietnam.** *Scand J Public Health* 2012, **40**(8):765–772.
16. Hoa NQ: *High Antibiotic Use and Resistance among Children Under Five,* PhD Thesis. Sweden: Department of Public Health Sciences, Karolinska Institutet; 2010.
17. Graneheim UH, Lundman B: **Qualitative content analysis in nursing research: concepts, procedures and measures to achieve trustworthiness.** *Nurse Educ Today* 2004, **24**(2):105–112.
18. Nyazema N, Viberg N, Khoza S, Vyas S, Kumaranayake L, Tomson G, Lundborg CS: **Low sale of antibiotics without prescription: a cross-sectional study in Zimbabwean private pharmacies.** *J Antimicrob Chemother* 2007, **59**(4):718–726.
19. Al-Faham Z, Habboub G, Takriti F: **The sale of antibiotics without prescription in pharmacies in Damascus. Syria.** *J Infect Dev Ctries* 2011, **5**(5):396–399.
20. Bin Abdulhak AA, Altannir MA, Almansor MA, Almohaya MS, Onazi AS, Marei MA, Aldossary OF, Obeidat SA, Obeidat MA, Riaz MS, Tleyjeh IM: **Non prescribed sale of antibiotics in Riyadh. Saudi Arabia: a cross sectional study.** *BMC Public Health* 2011, **11**:538.
21. Salunkhe SD, Pandit VA, Dawane JS, Sarda KD, More CS: **Study of over the counter sale of antimicrobials in pharmacy outlets in Pune, India: a cross sectional study.** *Int J Pharm Bio Sci* 2013, **4**(2):616–622.
22. Werner K, Deasy J: **Acute respiratory tract infections: when are antibiotics indicated?** *JAAPA* 2009, **22**(4):22–26.
23. Arroll B, Kenealy T, Falloon K: **Are antibiotics indicated as an initial treatment for patients with acute upper respiratory tract infections? A review.** *N Z Med J* 2008, **121**(1284):64–70.
24. Bavestrello L, Cabello A, Casanova D: **Impact of regulatory measures in the trends of community consumption of antibiotics in Chile.** *Revista medica de Chile* 2002, **130**(11):1265–1272.
25. Park S, Soumerai SB, Adams AS, Finkelstein JA, Jang S, Degnan DR: **Antibiotic use following a Korean national policy to prohibit medication dispensing by physicians.** *Health Policy Plann* 2005, **20**(5):302–309.
26. Nguyen KV, FL H, Wertheim & Group: *Situation Analysis: Antibiotic Use and Resistance in Vietnam,* Report from the GARP Vietnam National Working Group. Hanoi, Vietnam: GARP Vietnam; 2010.
27. Yi Wen EL, Dai W, Yuanhao Hong & Group: **A qualitative study about self-medication in the community among market vendors in Fuzhou. China.** *Health Soc Care Community* 2011, **19**:504–513.
28. Chandra S, DS B: **Evaluating medicines dispensing patterns at private community pharmacies in Tamilnadu, India.** *Southern Med Rev* 2010, **3**:27–31.
29. Vietnam Government Office: *Vietnam Government Decree No 79/2006/NĐ-CP on Implementing some articles of Drug Law.* Hanoi, Vietnam: Vietnam Government Office; 2006.
30. World Health Organization Report: *Medicines Prices: Make People Sicker and Poorer,* WHO Report, Country Office. Hanoi, Vietnam; 2011 [http://apps.who.int/medicinedocs/documents/s19220en/s19220en.pdf]
31. Huttner B, Goossens H, Verheij T, Harbarth S: **Characteristics and outcomes of public campaigns aimed at improving the use of antibiotics in out-patients in high-income contries.** *Lancet Infect Dis* 2010, **10**:17–31.

2

A cross-sectional investigation of the quality of selected medicines in Cambodia in 2010

Naoko Yoshida[1]*, Mohiuddin Hussain Khan[1], Hitomi Tabata[1], Eav Dararath[2], Tey Sovannarith[3], Heng Bun Kiet[2], Nam Nivanna[3], Manabu Akazawa[4], Hirohito Tsuboi[1], Tsuyoshi Tanimoto[5] and Kazuko Kimura[1]

Abstract

Background: Access to good-quality medicines in many countries is largely hindered by the rampant circulation of spurious/falsely labeled/falsified/counterfeit (SFFC) and substandard medicines. In 2006, the Ministry of Health of Cambodia, in collaboration with Kanazawa University, Japan, initiated a project to combat SFFC medicines.

Methods: To assess the quality of medicines and prevalence of SFFC medicines among selected products, a cross-sectional survey was carried out in Cambodia. Cefixime, omeprazole, co-trimoxazole, clarithromycin, and sildenafil were selected as candidate medicines. These medicines were purchased from private community drug outlets in the capital, Phnom Penh, and Svay Rieng and Kandal provinces through a stratified random sampling scheme in July 2010.

Results: In total, 325 medicine samples were collected from 111 drug outlets. Non-licensed outlets were more commonly encountered in rural than in urban areas ($p < 0.01$). Of all the samples, 93.5% were registered and 80% were foreign products. Samples without registration numbers were found more frequently among foreign-manufactured products than in domestic ones ($p < 0.01$). According to pharmacopeial analytical results, 14.5%, 4.6%, and 24.6% of the samples were unacceptable in quantity, content uniformity, and dissolution test, respectively. All the ultimately unacceptable samples in the content uniformity tests were of foreign origin. Following authenticity investigations conducted with the respective manufacturers and medicine regulatory authorities, an unregistered product of cefixime collected from a pharmacy was confirmed as an SFFC medicine. However, the sample was acceptable in quantity, content uniformity, and dissolution test.

Conclusions: The results of this survey indicate that medicine counterfeiting is not limited to essential medicines in Cambodia: newer-generation medicines are also targeted. Concerted efforts by both domestic and foreign manufacturers, wholesalers, retailers, and regulatory authorities should help improve the quality of medicines.

Keywords: Quality of medicine, Spurious/falsely labeled/falsified/counterfeit (SFFC) medicine, Authenticity, Essential medicine, Cambodia

Background

Spurious/falsely labeled/falsified/counterfeit (SFFC) medicines are deliberately and fraudulently mislabeled with respect to identity or source [1,2]. Falsifying is greatest in those regions where regulatory and legal oversight is weakest. Although precise, detailed data on SFFC medicines are difficult to obtain, estimates range from less than 1% of sales in developed countries to over 10% in developing countries, depending on the geographic area [3]. Several reports have documented adverse health consequences from consumption of SFFC medicines. More than 200 children died in a hospital in Bangladesh through ingesting SFFC paracetamol, which contained diethylene glycol, in 1990–93 [4]. In 1998, 30 infants died from SFFC paracetamol in India [5]. In Southeast Asia in 2001, 38% of 104 anti-malaria drugs were found to be SFFC [6]. In Cambodia in 1999, at least 30 people died through SFFC artesunate containing sulfadoxine-pyrimethamine, which is an older, less effective anti-malarial [5]. In 2005, a man aged 23 years treated with SFFC artesunate died in eastern

* Correspondence: naoko@p.kanazawa-u.ac.jp
[1]Drug Management and Policy, Faculty of Pharmacy, Institute of Medical, Pharmaceutical and Health Sciences, Kanazawa University, Kakuma-machi, Kanazawa, Ishikawa 920-1192, Japan
Full list of author information is available at the end of the article

Burma (Myanmar) [7]. In 1999, two people died through taking fake anti-diabetic medicines containing illegal quantities of glibenclamide in China; in 2008, four people died in Singapore after taking an SFFC phosphodiesterase type 5 inhibitor containing glibenclamide [8,9]. In addition to SFFC products, substandard and degraded medicines are classified as poor-quality medicines [10]. Substandard medicines are genuine medicines produced by legitimate manufacturers that do not meet the quality specifications declared by the producer [11]. Degraded products may result from exposure of good-quality medicines to light, heat, and humidity; however, it can be difficult to distinguish degraded medicines from those that left the factory as substandard [12]. Substandard and degraded medicines reduce the effectiveness of therapy.

In Cambodia, the Ministry of Health (MoH) reported in 2001 that 13% of medicines were SFFC, with 21% being substandard and 50% unregistered [13]; in the same country, 35 medicines were found to be SFFC among 142 products in 2004 [14]. Furthermore, in our previous study in Cambodia in 2006–09, we identified 19 SFFC products among life-saving essential medicines [15,16]. Evidence suggests that lack of awareness and inappropriate management in the supply chain could facilitate the distribution of SFFC medicines in the country [17].

To oppose the threat of SFFC medicines and prevent their spread, the Department of Drugs and Food (DDF) of the MoH has been conducting surveillance on the quality of medicines since 2006. In 2010, we selected some newer-generation medicines, including antibiotics, to assess falsifying trends in the context of this developing country. At the same time, we sought to identify the influential factors in falsifying practices and develop a cost-effective surveillance system to ensure the quality of medicines.

Methods
Sampling area
Samples were collected from the capital, Phnom Penh (urban area), and Svay Rieng and Kandal provinces (rural areas). The list of licensed outlets in Phnom Penh was obtained from the DDF, MoH of Cambodia, in June 2013. The calculated sample size was 193 pharmacies, 58 depot A outlets, and 79 depot B outlets, with an alpha value of 5 and power of 0.8. In Phnom Penh, as many private drug outlets as possible of the four types of private drug outlets (i.e., pharmacies, depot A, depot B, and non-licensed outlets) were visited within the period of sample collection. For sampling purposes, a stratified random scheme developed by means of random number tables was used. All the outlets found in Svay Rieng and all illegal outlets found in the sampling area were visited. Additionally, some samples were collected from wholesalers and drug outlets in Kandal province while the

sampling teams moved between Phnom Penh and Svay Rieng. In Cambodia, a pharmacy outlet is run by a registered pharmacist, a depot A outlet by an assistant pharmacist (with 4 years' pharmacy training), and a depot B outlet by a retired midwife or nurse [17]. The sampling areas were selected in consultation with the MoH, taking into account the degree of urbanization, population density, concentration of drug outlets, budgetary limitations, and geographic importance in sharing a border with another country.

Sample collection
Cefixime tablets, omeprazole capsules, co-trimoxazole (a combination of sulfamethoxazole and trimethoprim) tablets, clarithromycin tablets, and sildenafil tablets were selected as candidate medicines in consultation with the DDF. Cefixime, omeprazole, clarithromycin, and sildenafil were chosen in 2010 as newer-generation medicines; this was in contrast to selection from a list of essential medicines in our previous studies [15,16]. Sample information was collected using a sampling form that included the contents of the packages sold, price, and outlet information. Samples were collected between June 7 and 15, 2010 by two teams. Each team consisted of a research investigator, a locally recruited sampling officer, and a sampling assistant. The locally recruited members were provided with training before sampling and instructed to purchase medicines. The sampling officer purchased medicines in an outlet and completed a sampling form for each sample. Medicines collected from the same outlet and labeled with the same international non-proprietary name, brand name, strength, size, batch/lot number, and manufacturing and expiry dates were considered one sample. For authentication purposes, the teams collected containers or packages for most of the samples. Samples were preserved at 20–25°C until analysis.

Observation test
Details of the packaging condition and the label information of the samples were carefully noted. Compliance with the Association of Southeast Asian Nations Common Technical Dossier (ACTD) for the registration of pharmaceuticals for human use (to which drug registration in Cambodia conforms) was examined [18]. Bar codes were also recorded.

Materials for quality evaluation
United States Pharmacopeia (USP) reference standards of omeprazole, sulfamethoxazole, trimethoprim, and clarithromycin-related compound A (6,11-di-o-methyl erythromycin A) were purchased from the Reference Standard Center, Bureau of Drugs and Narcotics, Thailand (Nonthaburi, Thailand). Reference standards of cefixime, clarithromycin, and sildenafil citrate were

generously donated by Astellas Pharma Inc. (Tokyo, Japan), Taisho Toyama Pharmaceutical Co, Ltd. (Tokyo, Japan), and Pfizer Japan Inc. (Tokyo, Japan), respectively. Metronidazole and butyl *p*-hydroxy benzoate were purchased from Nacalai Tesque, Inc. (Kyoto, Japan). Primidone and sulfadoxine were purchased from Wako Pure Chemical Industries, Ltd. (Osaka, Japan). Lansoprazole was purchased from Sigma-Aldrich Co. LLC (St. Louis, MO, USA). Methanol and acetonitrile of high-performance liquid chromatography (HPLC) grade was purchased from Nacalai Tesque, Inc. (Kyoto, Japan). All other chemicals were commercially available and of analytical grade.

Quality evaluation

The Medicine Quality Assessment Reporting Guidelines (MEDQUARG) were followed when reporting in generally [10].

To assess the pharmaceutical quality of the samples, active ingredients of the samples were quantified by HPLC using ultraviolet detection (Shimadzu, Kyoto, Japan). The system suitability for analysis of each medicine was verified according to USP 30. A linear relationship between the peak area and concentration of each reference standard was observed within the range of 25–200% of the active ingredient ($r^2 = 0.999$–1.000), and the assay was performed within that range. The intra- and inter-day coefficient of variation was less than 3.0%. In addition, the methods were validated as being repeatable and accurate (n = 6). Metronidazole, butyl *p*-hydroxybenzoate, primidone, lansoprazole, and sulfadoxine were used as internal standards in the analysis of cefixime, clarithromycin, co-trimoxazole, omeprazole, and sildenafil, respectively. The samples were analyzed between July 2010 and March 2012 in Kanazawa University. The quality evaluation was completed within the expiry date for each sample.

For cefixime tablets, omeprazole capsules, co-trimoxazole tablets, and clarithromycin tablets, the assay, a content uniformity test, and dissolution test were performed with reference to USP 30, USP34, or British Pharmacopeia (BP) 2010 as indicated on the package insert or outer package.

For sildenafil tablets, the assay was performed according to the method described previously [19]. In each sample, three or six tablets were analyzed. The acceptable range was set as follows: in the quantity test, sildenafil tablets containing not less than 90% and not more than 110% on an average quantity taken from 10 units, and no unit less than 75% or more than 125% of the labeled amount of sildenafil; in the dissolution test, the acceptable range was an average dissolution rate in 3 or 6 units equal to or greater than 75% and no unit less than 50%, with a dissolution time of 15 minutes. The content uniformity test could not be conducted because of insufficient material.

Authenticity investigation

The methodology of the authenticity investigation and registration verification was adopted from the World Health Organization [15,16,20,21]. Label information on the packages and containers was cross-checked with a database prepared after collection. Photographs of each sample, its packaging, and package inserts were obtained for such purposes. These data were then catalogued. A database of manufacturer addresses was also prepared using printed information, Web searches, and e-mail and telephone communication. Portions of all samples were then sent to the respective manufacturers, requesting verification of their products. Information on the manufacturers and their medicines was requested from medicine regulatory authorities of the countries in which the manufacturing took place. Furthermore, each sample's registration was confirmed by the DDF.

Statistical analysis

Considering the limitations of the small sample size, descriptive analysis was performed using SPSS 19.0.0 (IBM SPSS Inc, Chicago, IL, USA). Where appropriate, Fisher's exact test was used to test the significance of categorical variables. Statistical significance was evaluated at the 5% level.

Results

Table 1 presents an outline of the samples. We collected a total of 325 samples from 111 drug outlets (including 14 wholesalers) in the study area. Of these, 60 (18.5%) were cefixime, 48 (14.8%) were clarithromycin, 91 (28.0%) were omeprazole, 44 (13.5%) were sildenafil, and 82 (25.2%) were co-trimoxazole. Of the samples, 237 (72.9%) were collected from Phnom Penh and 88 (27.1%) from the provinces: 81 (24.9%) from Svay Rieng and seven (2.2%) from Kandal. Foreign products constituted the majority (80%) of the total samples. Local manufacture was commonest for co-trimoxazole (48/82 samples).

Drug outlets

Of the 325 samples, we collected 108 (33.2%) from pharmacies, 62 (19.1%) from depot A outlets, 92 (28.3%) from depot B outlets, 32 (9.8%) from wholesalers, and 31 (9.5%) from non-licensed outlets. We found non-licensed outlets significantly more frequently in rural (33.0%, 29/88) than in urban areas (0.8%, 2/237) (Fisher's exact test: $p < 0.01$). Pharmacists were present in 72.4% (21/29) of the pharmacies. All 14 wholesalers but only one pharmacy had air conditioning.

Observations

We observed differences in package design (layout and/ or printed colors) in four products—one each of cefixime and clarithromycin and two kinds of omeprazole—

Table 1 Outline of the samples

	Sampling area		Shop category					Country of manufacturer	
	Urban	Rural	Pharmacy	Depot A	Depot B	Wholesaler	Non-licensed outlet	Domestic	Imported
Cefixime (n = 60)	42	18	20	10	19	6	5	4	56
Clarithromycin (n = 48)	36	12	17	10	15	4	2	10	38
Co-trimoxazole (n = 82)	58	24	21	16	28	7	10	48	34
Omeprazole (n = 91)	63	28	26	21	24	8	12	2	89
Sildenafil (n = 44)	38	6	24	5	6	7	2	0	44
Total (n = 325)	237	88	108	62	92	32	31	64	261

from the same lot number. With eight products—two kinds of cefixime, three kinds of clarithromycin, one co-trimoxazole, and two kinds of omeprazole—we observed a different package design with different lot numbers. Except for nine samples, ACTD requirements (which were fully implemented in early 2011) appeared in the information on the packaging. Six of those samples lacked lot numbers and manufacturing and expiry dates on their packaging. With three of those samples, the packaging did not include a manufacturing date. The registration number did not appear on the outer packaging with some samples (Table 2). One sample of cefixime bore a false lot number, had two spelling errors, and was confirmed as an SFFC medicine in the authenticity investigation.

About 80% (264/325) of the samples included a European Article Number code, which is a bar-code symbol used in supply chain management. However, 61 products had neither a European Article Number code nor a GS1 DataBar™ symbol (GS1, Brussels, Belgium), which can carry more information and be used to identify small items.

We observed varying degrees of discrepancies in compliance with ACTD in the information that appeared in package inserts (Tables 3 and 4). We collected package inserts from 106 products (284 samples, 87.4%). The package inserts of 102 products (87.2%) were written in English and/or Khmer and/or French: all these languages are officially accepted in Cambodia. However, four products were written in Vietnamese only (Table 3). Table 4 shows other discrepancies with the package inserts of 87 products, which were written in English. The indication,

dosage, and administration were described for all products (Table 4). One package insert failed to stipulate contraindications, two did not state precautions, and two did not indicate side effects; one product lacked all three of these items (Table 4). With over 10% of the products, information relating to clinical pharmacology (23 products), drug interactions (11 products), pregnancy and lactation (12 products), overdose and treatment (33 products), and storage conditions (20 products) was not provided (Table 4). The date of revision of the package insert was not given for 79 products (90.8%). Six (6.9%) products satisfied the items required by ACTD, whereas 55 (63.2%) products had missing data for multiple elements.

We collected products that were unregistered or lacked lot numbers, manufacturing dates, expiry dates, or registration numbers (in at least one item) from illegal outlets (7/24) more frequently than from legal ones (15/279) (Fisher's exact test: $p < 0.05$). However, the sampling area and origin of the samples were not statistically associated as acceptable findings.

Pharmaceutical quality

Among the 325 samples analyzed for their contents, 47 (14.5%) were of unacceptable quality (Table 5). Of 281 samples, we finally determined that 15 (4.6%) were unacceptable in content uniformity tests. In dissolution tests, which were not obligatory for registration in 2010 in Cambodia, 80 (24.6%) samples were unacceptable.

Table 2 Information on outer packaging

Items required by ACTD	Presence		Absence	
	n	(%)	n	(%)
Batch number	313	(98.1)	6	(1.9)
Manufacturing date	310	(97.2)	9	(2.8)
Expiration date	313	(98.1)	6	(1.9)
Registration number	304	(95.3)	15	(4.7)

n = 319 samples.

Table 3 Language of package inserts

Language	n	(%)
Khmer only	1	(0.9)
English only	74	(63.2)
English and Khmer	5	(4.3)
Khmer and other language	11	(9.4)
English and other language	8	(6.8)
French only	3	(2.6)
Vietnamese only	4	(3.4)
Unavailable	11	(9.4)
Total	117	(100.0)

Table 4 Information on package inserts

Items required by ACTD	Presence		Absence	
	n	(%)	n	(%)
Clinical pharmacology	64	(73.6)	23	(26.4)
Indications	87	(100.0)	0	(0.0)
Dosage and administration	87	(100.0)	0	(0.0)
Contraindications	86	(98.9)	1	(1.1)
Warnings and precautions	85	(97.7)	2	(2.3)
Drug interactions	76	(87.4)	11	(12.6)
Pregnancy and lactation	75	(86.2)	12	(13.8)
Side effects	85	(97.7)	2	(2.3)
Overdose and treatment	54	(62.1)	33	(37.9)
Storage conditions	67	(77.0)	20	(23.0)
Date of revision	8	(9.2)	79	(90.8)

n = 87 products, whose package inserts were written in English.

Interestingly, all the finally unacceptable samples (15 of 281 samples) in the content uniformity tests were of foreign origin and were registered products. Of the 64 domestic samples, 21 were unacceptable for one or more of the quality tests.

Authenticity

We received authentication reports from 49 of 75 (65.3%) manufacturers for 230 (71%) samples and 5 of 11 (45.5%) medicine regulatory authorities. On the basis of authenticity results, we confirmed one sample of cefixime as an SFFC medicine (Figure 1). The sample product was not registered in Cambodia; it was labeled with batch number 976213, manufactured date 11/2009, and expiry date 10/2011. The product was purchased from a pharmacy, and it came from an unknown wholesaler. The sample passed quantity, content uniformity, and dissolution test.

Of the 325 samples, 309 (95.1%) were registered by the DDF and 16 (4.9%) were not registered. Six samples of unregistered medicines were sold with labels indicating that they were registered. Two of these samples were supplied for use in the public sector (hospitals or health

centers) only; however, they were purchased from pharmacies. All 16 samples of such illegal medicines were imported products.

Discussion

The results of this survey indicate a number of problems in the manufacturing and distribution conditions, quality, and packaging of medicines in Cambodia. Among 111 drug outlets we visited, including wholesalers, only one pharmacy in Phnom Penh and all 14 wholesalers had air conditioning in their storage areas. Despite temperature rises above 40°C in the dry season in Cambodia, the other drug outlets did not have any temperature-control measures [22]. Storing medicines at high temperature and humidity could result in deterioration of quality and might facilitate the distribution of degraded medicines in the market [23-25]. In Cambodia, good pharmacy practice, distribution practice, and storage practice have not been implemented. Hence, the deterioration in quality may be due to storage or distribution. To prevent the distribution of degraded products, storage conditions at drug outlets need to be better controlled. To this end, good pharmacy practice will be introduced in Cambodia by the end of 2013.

Following quality evaluation of the collected samples, we found that some products had problems in their outer packaging, such as different colors and/or layout for the same product, spelling errors, and a lack of identification codes. These discrepancies may have resulted from insufficient awareness of the risks and countermeasures adopted by legitimate manufacturers against SFFC or substandard medicines. Such shortcomings could make it more difficult to distinguish SFFC medicines, and dealing with this problem should help prevent the entry of such products into the market. Additionally, the circulation of unregistered medicines and unauthorized distribution of publicly donated ones could affect the emergence of SFFC medicines in the supply chain. The SFFC medicine we detected in this survey—cefixime tablets bearing a false lot number—did not have Cambodian registration, bore spelling errors on the label, and was obtained at a pharmacy. Nevertheless, we found the sample to be

Table 5 Quality test results

	Number of collected samples	Quantity test			Content uniformity test			Dissolution test		
		Accepted	Unaccepted	Pending	Accepted	Unaccepted	Pending	Accepted	Unaccepted	Pending
Cefixime	60	56	3	1	55	0	5	51	3	6
Clarithromycin	48	44	4	0	42	1	5	27	11	10
Co-trimoxazole	82	73	9	0	81	0	1	65	15	2
Omeprazole	91	54	22	15	31	14	46	42	45	4
Sildenafil	44	32	9	3	-	-	-	28	6	10
Total	325	259	47	19	209	15	57	213	80	32

Pending: samples pending at time of decision because of insufficient material.

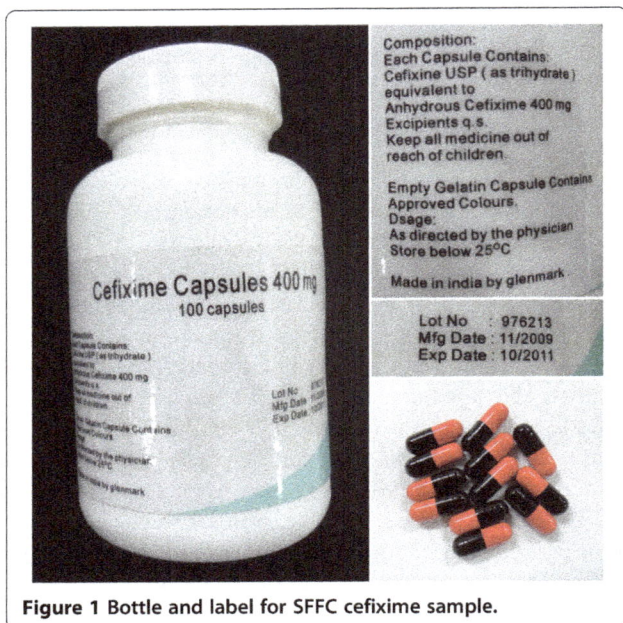

Figure 1 Bottle and label for SFFC cefixime sample.

acceptable in quantity, content uniformity, and dissolution tests according to USP 30. Cefixime, an oral third-generation cephalosporin, has excellent therapeutic action against infections caused by bacteria and is relatively high in price. Counterfeiters thus have an incentive in producing such antibiotics [26]. This is possibly the first report of SFFC cefixime in Cambodia. The findings of this survey indicate that not only are earlier-generation, commonly used essential medicines targeted by counterfeiters, newer-generation medicines are similarly falsified because of a better profit margin. Sildenafil, a newer-generation medicine, is a medicine that is more likely to be counterfeited in developed countries [27]. The present study shows that sildenafil had low distribution, and no counterfeit product was found. This finding suggests that the target medicine for counterfeiting may vary depending on the country.

In the pharmaceutical quality evaluation of the 325 samples we identified, 103 (31.7%) were unacceptable in one or more of the quantity, content uniformity, and dissolution tests. Most of those were enteric-coated omeprazole capsules, which especially showed an unacceptably high failure ratio in the dissolution test. Unacceptable samples in the dissolution test for omeprazole may have resulted from poor enteric coating, which could cause degradation of the omeprazole by gastric acid and lead to ineffectiveness after oral administration. Variables related to formulation or manufacturing processes of medicines can significantly affect dissolution and the expected medical effects. Consequently, some pharmaceutical manufacturers, mainly from overseas, may not have attained the

necessary technical level to produce enteric preparations. To maintain the quality of medicines, exporting countries should not allow substandard medicines to be exported to other developing countries. Furthermore, each manufacturer selects its specifications among existing pharmacopoeias and in-house specifications; thus, for some medicines, the conditions in dissolution testing are different between USP and BP standards. Indeed, it would be desirable for the MoH to define uniform requirements for dissolution testing. In early 2011, the MoH began implementing the dissolution test for registration; there was, however, no focus on this issue before 2011. Thus, samples collected in 2010 may have been particularly subject to problems with the dissolution test. Since dissolution testing has been added as a mandatory requirement for registering medicines in Cambodia, the situation may improve in the near future. Furthermore, the lack of information in package inserts and non-compliance with linguistic requirements of the ACTD could hinder the safe, proper use of medicines. Having adequate information on the packaging and inserts could minimize the misuse of medicines and reduce therapeutic failure [28,29]. For package inserts, three languages—French, English, and Khmer—are officially accepted in Cambodia. To encourage the proper use of medicines, some key words have been translated into Khmer by the MoH for products lacking Khmer instructions. Essentially, the contents of all package inserts need to be translated into Khmer from French or English. Furthermore, ACTD was implemented in Cambodia only at the end of 2010. Before 2008, there was no checking and verification of all registered products by design and brand name. Therefore, the MoH has carried out such checking and verification only since 2008. However, products registered before 2008 can be distributed and sold as usual until their licenses expires; it is not until the papers relating to such products are submitted for license renewal that the ACTD requirements come into effect. ACTD was fully implemented in early 2011.

Printing technology has improved and become widely available to the point where SFFC medicines are able to show very close similarity to original products [21,30]. Even medical practitioners may fail to spot SFFC medicines in their practices. Stopping SFFC medicines from entering the market is one way of preventing consumers being subjected to the health hazards associated with such medicines.

Toward creating a healthy, secure system for pharmaceutical distribution, it is likewise imperative to stop SFFC medicines from entering the market. Improved regulation of illegal medicines, revision and compliance of existing rules for pharmaceuticals, and introducing a pharmaceutical traceability system could help ensure the circulation of genuine medicines.

The collected samples in this study may not have been representative of conditions throughout Cambodia because of the limited area of sample collection, insufficient sample size in the stratified random sampling in Phnom Penh, and convenient sampling of some samples from selected drug outlets. Additionally, we did not receive responses relating to the authenticity investigation from 26 manufacturers; therefore, we were unable to confirm 95 samples as having been genuine or SFFC. Because of the insufficient number of samples, we could not verify the status of 43 medicines in our quality evaluation. These limitations make it difficult to assess the actual extent of SFFC and substandard medicines in the entire Cambodian supply chain.

Conclusions

In conclusion, the results of this survey indicate that medicine falsifying is not limited to essential medicines in Cambodia: newer-generation medicines are also targeted. Concerted efforts by manufacturers—both domestic and overseas—along with those by wholesalers, retailers, and regulatory authorities are necessary to ensure the quality of medicines.

Abbreviations
MoH: the Ministry of Health; DDF: the Department of Drugs and Food; ACTD: the Association of Southeast Asian Nations Common Technical Dossier; USP: United States Pharmacopeia; HPLC: high-performance liquid chromatography; BP: British Pharmacopeia.

Competing interests
The authors declare that they have no competing interests.

Authors' contributions
NY, HTa, HBK, NN, MA, and KK conceived and designed the experiments. NY, HTa, ED, TS, TT, and KK performed the experiments. NY, MHK, and HTa analyzed the data. TT and KK contributed reagents/materials/analysis tools. NY and MHK wrote the first draft of the manuscript. ED, HBK, NN, MA, HTs, TT, and KK contributed to the writing of the manuscript. All authors read and approved the final manuscript.

Acknowledgements
We are very grateful to Mr. Hironobu Shimizu, Ms. Miku Yuasa, Ms Mami Ishii, Mr. Koya Odaira, Ms. Yuka Kotsuji, and Mr. Jun Matsuo of Drug Management and Policy, Faculty of Pharmacy, Institute of Medical, Pharmaceutical and Health Sciences, Kanazawa University, Japan.
This work was supported by a Grant-in-Aid for Scientific Research (B) from the Japan Society for the Promotion of Science, KAKENHI 22406005. Cefixime and omeprazole were investigated with financial support from the Japan Pharmaceutical Manufacturers Association. The funders had no role in the study design, data collection and analysis, the decision to publish, or preparation of the manuscript.

Author details
[1]Drug Management and Policy, Faculty of Pharmacy, Institute of Medical, Pharmaceutical and Health Sciences, Kanazawa University, Kakuma-machi, Kanazawa, Ishikawa 920-1192, Japan. [2]Department of Drugs and Food, Ministry of Health, 151-153, Kampuchea Krom St, Khan 7 Makara, Phnom Penh, Cambodia. [3]National Health Product Quality Control Center, Ministry of Health, 151-153, Kampuchea Krom St, Khan 7 Makara, Phnom Penh, Cambodia. [4]Department of Public Health and Epidemiology, Meiji Pharmaceutical University, 2-522-1 Noshio, Kiyose, Tokyo 204-8588, Japan. [5]Faculty of Pharmaceutical Sciences, Doshisha Women's University, Kodo, Kyotanabe, Kyoto 610-0395, Japan.

References
1. World Health Organization: *Counterfeit drugs, report of a joint WHO/IFPMA Workshop, 1–3 April 1992.* Geneva, Switzerland: WHO; 1992.
2. World Health Organization: *Medicines: spurious/falsely-labelled/falsified/counterfeit (SFFC) medicines. Fact sheet N°275, May 2012.* [http://www.who.int/mediacentre/factsheets/fs275/en/]
3. World Health Organization: *Counterfeit medicines. Fact sheet revised on November 14, 2006.* [http://www.who.int/medicines/services/counterfeit/impact/ImpactF_S/en/]
4. Hanif M, Mobarak MR, Ronan A, Rahman D, Donovan JJ Jr, Bennish ML: **Fatal renal failure caused by diethylene glycol in paracetamol elixir: the Bangladesh epidemic.** *Br Med J* 1995, 311:88–91.
5. Rassool GH: **Substandard and counterfeit medicines.** *J Adv Nurs* 2004, 46:338–9.
6. Newton P, Proux S, Green M, Smithuis F, Rozendaal J, Prakongpan S, Chotivanich K, Mayxay M, Looareesuwan S, Farrar J, Nosten F, White NJ: **Fake artesunate in southeast Asia.** *Lancet* 2001, 357:1948–50.
7. Newton PN, McGready R, Fernandez F, Green MD, Sunjio M, Bruneton C, Phanouvong S, Millet P, Whitty CJ, Talisuna AO, Proux S, Christophel EM, Malenga G, Singhasivanon P, Bojang K, Kaur H, Palmer K, Day NP, Greenwood BM, Nosten F, White NJ: **Manslaughter by fake artesunate in Asia–will Africa be next?** *PLoS Med* 2006, 3:e197 [http://www.plosmedicine.org/article/info%3Adoi%2F10.1371%2Fjournal.pmed.0030197]
8. Cheng MM: **Is the drugstore safe? Counterfeit diabetes products on the shelves.** *J Diabetes Sci Technol* 2009, 3:1516–20.
9. Kao SL, Chan CL, Tan B, Lim CC, Dalan R, Gardner D, Pratt E, Lee M, Lee KO: **An unusual outbreak of hypoglycemia.** *N Engl J Med* 2009, 360:734–6.
10. Newton PN, Lee SJ, Goodman C, Fernández FM, Yeung S, Phanouvong S, Kaur H, Amin AA, Whitty CJ, Kokwaro GO, Lindegårdh N, Lukulay P, White LJ, Day NP, Green MD, White NJ: **Guidelines for field surveys of the quality of medicines: a proposal.** *PLoS Med* 2009, 6:e52 [http://www.plosmedicine.org/article/fetchObject.action?uri=info%3Adoi%2F10.1371%2Fjournal.pmed.1000052&representation=PDF]
11. Counterfeit medicines: *Some frequently asked questions-May 2005. Fact sheet, 5 May 2005.* [http://www.wpro.who.int/mediacentre/factsheets/fs_20050506/en/index.html]
12. Keoluangkhot V, Green M, Nyadong L, Fernández F, Mayxay M, Newton PN: **Impaired clinical response in a patient with uncomplicated falciparum malaria who received poor quality and underdosed intramuscular artemether.** *Am J Trop Med Hyg* 2008, 78:552–5 [http://www.ajtmh.org/content/78/4/552.full.pdf+html]
13. Ministry of Health: *Study report on counterfeit and substandard drugs in Cambodia 2001.* Phnom Penh, Cambodia: Ministry of Health; 2001.
14. Ministry of Health: *2nd study report on counterfeit and substandard drugs in Cambodia 2004.* Phnom Phenh, Cambodia: Ministry of Health; 2004.
15. Khan MH, Okumura J, Sovannarith T, Nivanna N, Akazawa M, Kimura K: **Prevalence of counterfeit anthelminthic medicines: a cross-sectional survey in Cambodia.** *Trop Med and Int Health* 2010, 15:639–44.
16. Khan MH, Okumura J, Sovannarith T, Nivanna N, Nagai H, Taga M, Yoshida N, Akazawa M, Tanimoto T, Kimura K: **Counterfeit medicines in Cambodia-possible causes.** *Pharm Res* 2011, 28:484–9.
17. Khan MH, Akazawa M, Dararath E, Kiet HB, Sovannarith T, Nivanna N, Yoshida N, Kimura K: **Perceptions and practices of pharmaceutical wholesalers surrounding counterfeit medicines in a developing country: a baseline survey.** *BMC Health Serv Res* 2011, 11:306 [http://www.biomedcentral.com/1472-6963/11/306]
18. Organization of the dossier: *The ASEAN common technical dossier (ACTD) for the registration of pharmaceuticals for human use;* 2002 [http://www.asean.org/archive/actr/7.doc]
19. Moriyasu T, Shigeoka S, Kishimoto K, Ishikawa F, Nakajima J, Kamimura H, Yasuda I: **Identification system for Sildenafil in health foods.** *Yakugaku Zasshi* 2001, 121:765–9. In Japanese.
20. Khan MH, Tanimoto T, Nakanishi Y, Yoshida N, Tsuboi H, Kimura K: **Public health concerns for anti-obesity medicines imported for personal use through the internet: a cross-sectional study.** *BMJ Open* 2012, 2:3 [http://bmjopen.bmj.com/content/2/3/e000854]
21. World Health Organization: **Growing threat from counterfeit medicines.** *Bull World Health Organ* 2010, 88:247–8.

22. Embassy of Japan in Cambodia: *Fact sheet revised on April, 2012*, In Japanese. [http://www.kh.emb-japan.go.jp/political/gaikyo.htm]

23. Kayumba PC, Risha PG, Shewiyo D, Msami A, Masuki G, Ameye D, Vergote G, Ntawukuliryayo JD, Remon JP, Vervaet C: **The quality of essential antimicrobial and antimalarial drugs marketed in Rwanda and Tanzania: influence of tropical storage conditions on in vitro dissolution.** *J Clin Pharm Ther* 2004, **29:**331–8.

24. Baratta F, Germano A, Brusa P: **Diffusion of counterfeit drugs in developing countries and stability of galenics stored for months under different conditions of temperature and relative humidity.** *Croat Med J* 2012, **53:**173–84.

25. Khan MH, Hatanaka K, Sovannarith T, Nivanna N, Casas LC, Yoshida N, Tsuboi H, Tanimoto T, Kimura K: **Effects of packaging and storage conditions on the quality of amoxicillin-clavulanic acid - an analysis of Cambodian samples.** *BMC Pharmacol Toxicol* 2013, **14:**33 [http://www.biomedcentral.com/2050-6511/14/33]

26. Singh BK, Parwate DV, Srivastava S, Shukla SK: **Selective and non-extractive spectrophotometric determination of cefdinir in formulations based on donor-acceptor complex formation.** *Quim Nova* 2010, **33:**1471–5.

27. Jackson G, Arver S, Banks J, Stecher VJ: **Counterfeit phosphodiesterase type 5 inhibitores pose significant safety risks.** *Int J Clin Prat* 2010, **64:**497–504.

28. Kachur SP, Black C, Abdulla S, Goodman C: **Putting the genie back in the bottle? Availability and presentation of oral artemisinin compounds at retail pharmacies in urban Dar-es-Salaam.** *Malar J* 2006, **5:**25.

29. Jackson Y, Chappuis F, Loutan L, Taylor W: **Malaria treatment failures after artemisinin-based therapy in three expatriates: could improved manufacturer information help to decrease the risk of treatment failure?** *Malar J* 2006, **5:**81.

30. Newton PN, Fernández FM, Plançon A, Mildenhall DC, Green MD, Ziyong L, Christophel EM, Phanouvong S, Howells S, McIntosh E, Laurin P, Blum N, Hampton CY, Faure K, Nyadong L, Soong CW, Santoso B, Zhiguang W, Newton J, Palmer K: **A collaborative epidemiological investigation into the criminal fake artesunate trade in South East Asia.** *PLoS Med* 2008, **5:**e32 [http://www.plosmedicine.org/article/info:doi/10.1371/journal.pmed.0050032]

3

An outpatient antibacterial stewardship intervention during the journey to JCI accreditation

Ping Song[1], Wei Li[2] and Quan Zhou[1*]

Abstract

Background: Antibacterial overuse, misuse and resistance have become a major global threat. The Joint Commission International (JCI) accreditation standards include quality improvement and patient safety, which is exemplified by antimicrobial stewardship. There are currently few reports on interventions to improve the quality of outpatient antibacterial prescribing.

Methods: A before-after intervention study, aiming at antibacterial use in outpatients, was performed in a university-affiliated hospital with 2.8 million outpatient visits annually during the journey to JCI accreditation (March of 2012 - March of 2013). Comprehensive intervention measures included formulary adjustment, classification management, motivational, information technological, educational and organizational measures. A defined daily dose (DDD) methodology was applied. Pharmacoeconomic data and drug-related problems (DRPs) were statistically compared between the two phases.

Results: The variety of antibacterials available in outpatient pharmacy decreased from 38 to 16. The proportion of antibacterial prescriptions significantly decreased (12.7% versus 9.9%, $P < 0.01$). The proportion of prescriptions containing the restricted antibacterials was 30.4% in the second phase, significantly lower than the value of 44.7% in the first phase ($P < 0.01$). The overall proportion of oral versus all antibacterial prescriptions increased (94.0% to 100%, $P < 0.01$) when measured as defined daily doses. Statistically significant increases in relative percentage of DDDs of oral antibacterials (i.e., DDDs of individual oral antibacterial divided by the sum of DDDs of all antibacterials) were observed with moxifloxacin, levofloxacin, cefuroxime axetil, ornidazole, clindamycin palmitate, cefaclor, amoxicillin and clarithromycin. Occurrence rate of DRPs decreased from 13.6% to 4.0% ($P < 0.01$), with a larger decrease seen in surgical clinics (surgical: 19.5% versus 5.6%; internal medicine: 8.4% versus 2.8%, $P < 0.01$). The total expenditure on antibacterials for outpatients decreased by 34.7% and the intervention program saved about 6 million Chinese Yuan Renminbi (CNY) annually.

Conclusion: The one-year intervention program on outpatient antibacterial use during the journey to JCI accreditation reduced the expenditure on antibacterials, improved the appropriateness of antibacterial prescriptions. Quality improvements need integrated multifaceted intervention measures and long-term adherence to the antibiotic stewardship. Approach of i.v. to oral antibacterial switch, classification management, and motivational measures may play the most efficient role in changing antibacterial prescription practices.

Keywords: Antibacterials, Continuous quality improvement, Drug utilization, Inappropriate prescribing, Outpatient health services, Pharmacoeconomics, Prescription auditing, Stewardship, Intervention

---

* Correspondence: zhouquan142602@zju.edu.cn
[1]Department of Pharmacy, the Second Affiliated Hospital, School of Medicine, Zhejiang University, Jiefang Road No. 88, Hangzhou, Zhejiang 310009, China
Full list of author information is available at the end of the article

Background

Over use or the improper use of antibiotics can result in drug resistant bacteria as well as considerable expense to health care system [1]. According to a new report *"Antibiotic Resistance Threats in the United States, 2013"* issued by the U.S. Centers for Disease Control and Prevention (CDC), antibiotic resistance in the United States adds $20 billion in excess direct health care costs, with additional costs to society for lost productivity as high as $35 billion a year. The use of antibiotics is the single most important factor leading to antibiotic resistance. Up to 50 percent of all the antibiotics prescribed for people are not needed or are not prescribed appropriately [2].

It is imperative to create a culture of safety and quality within an organization that strives to continually improve the quality of antibiotic prescribing. A systematic review showed that antibiotic prescribing is a complex process influenced by factors affecting all the actors involved, including physicians, other healthcare providers, healthcare system, patients and the general public [3]. Sumpradit et al. reported that prescription behavior could be influenced by the factors like knowledge, attitudes, subjective norms, peer pressure, patient expectations, drug promotion, physician's diagnostic skill and exposure to hospital formularies and standard therapeutic guidelines [4].

The benefits of antimicrobial stewardship have been well described and implemented in the inpatient setting [5-7]. Although studies of antimicrobial consumption in outpatient services have been conducted in countries like France, Jordan and the United States [8-10], there are very few intervention programs specially targeting the outpatient antibacterial use. A search of Medline between January 1 1993 and October 31 2013 revealed only two intervention studies when using the keywords: "antimicrobial stewardship and intervention and outpatient and prescribing". One study evaluated the effect of clinician education coupled with audit and feedback on broad-spectrum antibacterial prescribing for pediatric outpatients with acute respiratory infections [11], and the other study assessed the effect of a computerized clinical decision support system (CDSS) on preventing misuse of fluoroquinolone and azithromycin for acute respiratory infections [12]. Compared with these interventions confined to special type of infection or particular class of antibiotics, multifaceted interventions for quality improvement in outpatient antibiotic prescribing has not been reported.

The fourth edition of Joint Commission International (JCI) accreditation standard defined irrational drug use as inappropriate drug, dose, frequency and route of administration, real or potential drug-drug interactions (DDIs), ignorance of allergy history, therapeutic duplications, and variation from organization criteria for use [13]. Rational antibacterial use is one of key measurable elements in quality improvement required by JCI. The Second Affiliated Hospital of Zhejiang University, School of Medicine, Zhejiang University, China (SAHZU) successfully passed the JCI accreditation as an academic medical center hospital on Feb 24 of 2013. Rational antibacterial use was listed as one of the nine patient safety goals in SAHZU in 2012-2013. A working group composed of infectious disease physicians, pharmacists, microbiologists, and administrators was established. This group sought to implement multifaceted interventions at the individual, organizational and policy levels to change antibacterial prescription practices [4]. During the journey to JCI accreditation, the SAHZU group performed an outpatient antibacterial stewardship intervention. The aim of this article was to discuss the effectiveness of such stewardship intervention in the outpatient setting and provide some reference for international counterparts.

Methods

Data collection

A before-after intervention study, focusing on antibacterial use in outpatient service was performed in SAHZU, a 2200-bed hospital with 2.8 million outpatient visits annually in Zhejiang Province, which has a population of approximately 54.4 million. The first phase was March of 2012 and the second phase was March of 2013. The study was approved by Ethics Committee at SAHZU and it was in compliance with the Helsinki Declaration.

Types of departments included in this study were as follows: (1) Surgical clinics: Burn, Cardiovascular Surgery, General Surgery Gynaecology, Neurosurgery, Oral and Maxillofacial Surgery, Orthodontics, Orthopaedics, Otolaryngology, Plastic Surgery, Prosthodontics, Surgical Oncology, Thoracic Surgery and Urology; (2) Internal medicine clinics: Allergy and Clinical Immunology, Cardiology, Dermatology, Endocrinology, Gastroenterology, Haematology, Infectious Diseases, Medical Oncology, Nephrology, Neurology, Oral Medicine, Respiratory Medicine and Rheumatology.

The total number of prescriptions for outpatients and total number of prescriptions containing antibacterials (ATC code J01) were derived from the prescription evaluation software embedded in the pharmacy management information system. Antibacterial expenditure and cost of all medications were calculated respectively. Herb medicine prescriptions, compulsorily prescribed separately from western medicines in China, were excluded when to calculate the total number of prescriptions for outpatients. A subset of 5% of the antibacterial-containing prescriptions was selected to evaluate for drug-related problems (DRPs) through random sampling, and was retrospectively evaluated by clinical pharmacists. Antibacterial-associated DRPs included inappropriate drug combination, dose, dosing frequency and administration route, use beyond approved indications, discordance between diagnosis and purpose of medication use, mismatches between antibacterial spectrum and the patient's infection, abuse of intravenous (i.v.) medications instead of oral alternatives, ignorance of patient's concomitant diseased conditions and other miscellaneous problems.

Data on outpatient antibacterial use were collected using the Anatomical Therapeutic Chemical (ATC)/ defined daily dose (DDD) method (WHO, version 2013) [14,15]. Number of defined daily doses, also called DDDs, was calculated as total dose consumed divided by DDD. Relative percentage of DDDs of each oral antibacterial was calculated as DDDs of individual oral antibacterial divided by the sum of DDDs of all antibacterials. Daily expenditure is calculated as overall expenditure divided by DDDs. Occurrence rate of DRPs was calculated as the number of DRPs divided by the number of randomly selected antibacterial prescriptions.

The data presented in the study is available in the archives of Drug & Therapeutics Committee (DTC) of SAHZU. Access and use of these data need permission from the SAHZU DTC.

Comprehensive intervention measures
Formulary adjustment & classification management
Antibacterials were classified as non-restricted (also called "first line"), restricted ("second line"), or special-grade ("third line"). Non-restricted antibacterials refer to those with relatively low price, proven safety and clinical efficacy and little effect on bacterial resistance. Restricted antibacterials refer to those with proven safety and clinical efficacy, but relatively high price and greater impact on bacterial resistance. Special-grade antibacterials are those with common or serious adverse reactions, tendency of producing rapid bacterial resistance or inadequate clinical efficacy and safety data. Each grade of antibacterial matched corresponding prescribing privileges for physicians. The antibacterial formulary was updated (Table 1). i.v. antibacterials were deleted from the formulary of outpatient pharmacy. i.v. to oral antibacterial switch therapy was encouraged in outpatient services according to the principle of antimicrobial pharmacology (Table 2).

Motivational interventions
The director of each clinical department was asked to sign a goal-setting responsibility plan for antibacterial use with each director of clinical department. Reports of prescription-related near misses were encouraged through a voluntary online reporting system. Retrospective appropriateness evaluation of antibacterial-containing prescriptions was performed monthly by clinical pharmacists and the results were discussed in the meeting of the DTC and

published on the hospital local area network. "Dear doctor" letters were sent from the DTC to physicians. Physicians were given the opportunity to present evidence and argument against the results of audit-feedback during a seven-day public notice period. Physicians who wrote inappropriate prescriptions would generally face a fine according to the severity of the DRPs. The level of fine was divided into three grades [low-grade: 100 Chinese Yuan Renminbi (CNY); medium-grade: 200 CNY; high-grade: 300 CNY]. Prescribing privilege of the physician would be revoked if there was a second instance of a high-grade error.

Information technological interventions
Web-based prescription screening software and a CDSS for antibacterial prescribing, embedded in electronic medical records (EMRs), were implemented. Drug information resources were updated, specifying maximum dose, contraindications and special precautions. An improved interface was created between the pharmacy management information system for prescription auditing which displayed both medication information (i.e., medication name, dose, administration route, dose frequency and current medications) and patient's key information (e.g., patient name, identification number, age, diagnosis, allergy history, body weight, body surface area, nutrition status and clinical laboratory test results such as hepatic and renal function, blood routine examination, and serum drug levels).

Educational interventions
Physicians were instructed to follow the clinical guidelines. They also must record any real or potential allergies or sensitivities in the electronic medical record for outpatients and note the results of allergy skin tests when prescribing special medications for outpatients. Lectures were given, providing key opportunities for physicians to learn about the topics of medication management therapy, DDIs, medication errors, adverse drug reactions, therapeutic monitoring and typical cases of irrational physician orders. Physicians and pharmacists should receive specific training in antibacterial prescription before they are granted different levels of prescribing or dispensing privileges.

Outcome measures
The outcome measures included proportion of prescriptions containing antibacterials, proportion of prescriptions containing non-restricted antibacterials, proportion of prescriptions containing restricted antibacterials, proportion of prescriptions containing special-grade antibacterials, total expenditure on antibacterials for outpatients, proportion of expenditure on antibacterials relative to all medications, proportion of expenditure on i.v.

Table 1 Formulary adjustment & classification management

First phase (March, 2012)			Second phase (March, 2013)		
Category	Antibacterials	Level	Category	Antibacterials	Level
Macrolides	Oral clarithromycin, Oral azithromycin, Oral erythromycin, i.v. erythromycin	1	Macrolides	Oral clarithromycin, Oral azithromycin, Oral roxithromycin	1
	i.v. azithromycin	2	Cephalosporins		
Cephalosporins			The first generation	Oral cephradine	1
The first generation	Oral cephradine	1	The second generation	Oral cefuroxime axetil, Oral cefaclor	1
	i.v. cefathiamidine	2		Oral cefprozi	2
The second generation	Oral cefuroxime axetil, Oral cefaclor, i.v. cefuroxime sodium	1	The third generation	Oral cefdinir	2
	Oral cefprozi, i.v. cefotiam	2	Fluoroquinolones	Oral levofloxacin	1
The third generation	Oral cefetamet pivoxil hydrochloride, Oral cefdinir, i.v. ceftizoxime	2		Oral moxifloxacin	2
	i.v. ceftriaxone sodium	1	Penicillins	Oral amoxicillin	1
Cephamycins	i.v. cefmetazole sodium, i.v. cefminox sodium	2	Beta-lactam/beta-lactamase inhibitor combinations	Oral amoxicillin and clavulanate potassium	1
Monocyclic beta-lactam	i.v. aztreonam	3	Nitroimidazoles	Oral ornidazole	2
Fluoroquinolones	Oral levofloxacin, i.v. levofloxacin, i.v. ciprofloxacin	1	Tetracyclines	Oral minocycline	1
	Oral moxifloxacin, i.v. moxifloxacin	2	Lincosamides	Oral clindamycin palmitate	1
Aminoglycosides	i.v. etimicin	2	Miscellaneous	Oral sulfamethoxazole/ trimethoprim	1
	i.v. streptomycin sulfate	1			
Penicillins	i.v. benzylpenicillin sodium, Oral amoxicillin	1			
	i.v. sulbenicillin sodium	2			
Beta-lactam/beta-lactamase inhibitor combinations	Oral amoxicillin and clavulanate potassium	1			
	i.v. piperacillin/sulbactam, i.v. cefoperazone/sulbactam	2			
Nitroimidazoles	Oral ornidazole, i.v. ornidazole	2			
Tetracyclines	Oral minocycline	1			
Lincosamides	Oral clindamycin palmitate, i.v. clindamycin	1			
Miscellaneous	i.v. fosfomycin sodium	1			

Notes: Level 1: non-restricted (also called "first line") antibacterials; Level 2: restricted ("second line") antibacterials; Level 3: special-grade ("third line") antibacterials.

antibacterials relative to all antibacterials, sum of DDDs of antibacterials, proportion of DDDs of all oral antibacterials relative to all antibacterials, relative percentage of DDDs of each oral antibacterial, number of DRPs, occurrence rate of DRPs, occurrence rate of DRPs made by surgeons, occurrence rate of DRPs made by internal medicine physicians, occurrence rate of each DRP subtype and number of physicians who received fines during the study period.

Statistical analysis

A descriptive analysis was performed. Pearson's Chi-square test was used for testing percentage differences between two groups. Student's t-test was used for statistical comparisons between the means of two groups. A P value < 0.05 was considered to be statistically significant. A P value < 0.01 was considered to be highly significant.

Results

General information and pharmacoeconomic data on antibacterial prescriptions are presented in Table 3. During the first phase, average daily expenditure on i.v. antibacterials was approximately 12 times that of oral antibacterials [193.5 ± 172.2 CNY versus 16.1 ± 13.1 CNY, $P < 0.01$]. The changes in relative percentage of DDDs of

Table 2 Approach of i.v. to oral antibacterial switch therapy

i.v. antibacterials	Oral antibacterials	Daily expenditure ratio (oral to i.v.)
Fluoroquinolones		
i.v. moxifloxacin	Moxifloxacin tablets	0.10
i.v. levofloxacin	Levofloxacin tablets	0.13
Cephalosporins		
The first generation		
i.v. cefathiamidine	Cefradine capsules	0.056
	The second generation cephalosporins and macrolides	0.041-0.14 (median: 0.078)
The second generation		
i.v. cefotiam	Cefaclor capsules	0.092
i.v. cefuroxime sodium	Cefaclor SR tablets	0.99
	Cefprozi tablets	0.15
	Cefuroxime axetil tablets	0.061
The third generation		
i.v. ceftizoxime sodium	Cefdinir capsules	0.35
i.v. ceftriaxone sodium	Cefetamet pivoxil tablets	0.042
Macrolides		
i.v. azithromycin	Azithromycin tablets	0.29
	Roxithromycin tablets	0.13
	Clarithromycin SR tablets	0.088
	Clarithromycin tablets	0.21
Aminoglycosides		
i.v. etimicin	Levofloxacin tablets	0.097
	Cefdinir capsules	0.34
	Cefetamet pivoxil tablets	0.090
Nitroimidazoles		
i.v. ornidazole	Ornidazole tablets	0.017
Lincosamide		
i.v. clindamycin	Clindamycin palmitate tablets	1.11

Daily expenditure was expressed in Chinese Yuan Renminbi (CNY); i.v.: intravenous; SR: sustained release. Daily expenditure ratio (oral to i.v.) was calculated as daily expenditure of oral antibacterial divided by daily expenditure of the corresponding i.v. antibacterial.

oral antibacterials between the two phases are listed in Table 4. Statistically significant increases in relative percentage of DDDs of oral antibacterials were observed with moxifloxacin, levofloxacin, cefuroxime axetil, ornidazole, clindamycin palmitate, cefaclor, amoxicillin and clarithromycin. Cefaclor demonstrated the largest increase in utilization. Cefuroxime axetil was the most usually prescribed antibacterials during each phase. The total expenditure for outpatient antibacterials decreased by 34.7% and the intervention program saved 0.51 million CNY per month. It is estimated to save about 6 million CNY annually.

DRPs derived from randomly selected antibacterial prescriptions for outpatients are listed in Table 5. The proportion of injectable antibacterials prescribed dramatically decreased from 15.6% in the first phase to 0.2% in the second phase ($P < 0.01$). The occurrence rate of DRPs decreased from 13.6% in the first phase to 4.0% in the second phase ($P < 0.01$). In the first phase, surgeons demonstrated a significantly higher DRP rate than internal medicine physicians (19.5% versus 8.4%, $P < 0.01$); however, this difference was not seen in the second phase. Overall rates of DRPs decreased for both internal medicine physicians and surgeons when comparing the first and second phases (surgeons: 19.5% versus 5.6%; internal medicine physicians: 8.4% versus 2.8%, $P < 0.01$). The magnitude of decrease in occurrence of DRPs was more profound in surgeons. Significant differences between two phases were also observed with inappropriate co-medication with other antibacterials, mismatches between antibacterial spectrum and the patient's infection, and abuse of i.v. medications instead of oral alternatives ($P < 0.01$).

During the study period, sixty-one physicians were fined due to inappropriate prescribing. One surgeon received a fine of 13000 CNY at a monthly DTC meeting following audit-feedback. The inappropriateness of antibiotics prescribed by this surgeon was reflected in improper combination antibiotic treatment (19 prescriptions), lack of clear clinical features of infection plus improper combination antibiotic treatment (26 prescriptions), off-label use (2 prescriptions), inappropriate antibiotic choice (1 prescription), and inappropriate antibiotic choice plus improper combination antibiotic treatment (3 prescriptions). For example, he prescribed isepamicin sulfate-levofloxacin combination for a patient with enlarged axillary lymph nodes in the right axillary region, ceftizoxime-levofloxacin combination for treatment of lower extremity infection, and cefotiam-isepamicin sulfate-ornidazole combination for patient with acute appendicitis.

Discussion

The significant decrease in the proportion of antibacterial prescriptions was an interesting outcome, as outpatient turnover and total number of prescriptions for outpatients did not decrease between the two phases. The increased proportion of prescriptions containing non-restricted antibacterials and the decreased proportion of prescriptions containing restricted antibacterials indicated that the stewardship efforts were successful.

The i.v.-to-oral switch therapy may reduce length of hospital stay, healthcare costs and risk of complications related to i.v. access [16,17]. For outpatients, oral moxifloxacin is a superior choice versus the i.v. formulation, with the advantages including one-tenth of the daily expenditure of i.v. medication, convenient administration

Table 3 General information and pharmacoeconomic data on antibacterial prescriptions

Indicators	First phase (March, 2012)	Second phase (March, 2013)
Kinds of antibacterials in outpatient pharmacy	38	16
Kinds of the third line antibacterials	1	0
Kinds of the second line antibacterials	17	4
Kinds of the first line antibacterials	20	12
Kinds of i.v. antibacterials	22	0
Kinds of oral antibacterials	16	16
Total number of prescriptions for outpatients	88425	90459
Total number of prescriptions containing antibacterials	11194	8920
Proportion of prescriptions containing antibacterials[#]	12.7%	9.9%
Proportion of prescriptions containing non-restricted antibacterials[#]	55.1%	69.6%
Proportion of prescriptions containing restricted antibacterials[#]	44.7%	30.4%
Proportion of prescriptions containing special-grade antibacterials[#]	0.14%	0
Total expenditure on antibacterials for outpatients (million CNY)	1.4760	0.9644
Proportion of expenditure on antibacterials relative to all medications	6.9%	4.1%
Proportion of expenditure on i.v. antibacterials relative to all antibacterials	30.5%	0
Sum of DDDs of antibacterials for outpatients	65930	61403
Proportion of DDDs of oral antibacterials for outpatients relative to all antibacterials[#]	94.0%	100%

Notes: [#]$P < 0.01$ (first phase vs second phase). Differences between the two phases were tested for statistical significance using Pearson's Chi-square test. A P value < 0.05 was considered to be statistically significant. A P value < 0.01 was considered to be highly significant. CNY: Chinese Yuan Renminbi. DDDs: number of defined daily doses (total dose consumed/defined daily dose). Daily expenditure = overall expenditure/DDDs.

Table 4 Comparison in relative percentage of DDDs of oral antibacterials before and after intervention

Oral antibacterials	Relative percentage of DDDs	
	First phase (March, 2012)	Second phase (March, 2013)
Cefuroxime axetil tablets[#]	10.6%	13.2%
Levofloxacin tablets[#]	9.6%	12.6%
Moxifloxacin tablets[#]	8.6%	9.1%
Amoxicillin[#]	8.1%	11.4%
Cefdinir capsules	7.0%	7.2%
Clarithromycin tablets[#]	5.7%	7.4%
Cefradine capsules[#]	3.1%	1.8%
Ornidazole tablets[#]	2.3%	2.8%
Cefaclor SR tablets & Cefaclor capsules[#]	1.8%	9.3%
Cefprozi tablets[#]	1.72%	1.2%
Clindamycin palmitate tablets[#]	0.48%	1.2%

Notes: [#]$P < 0.01$ (first phase vs second phase). Differences between the two phases were tested for statistical significance using Pearson's Chi-square test. A P value < 0.01 was considered to be highly significant. DDDs: number of of defined daily doses (total dose consumed/defined daily dose). Relative percentage of DDDs: DDDs of individual antibacterial divided by the sum of DDDs of all antibacterials. SR: sustained release.

schedule (just one tablet ingestion once daily versus 90-min intravenous drip), lower occurrence rate of infusion-related side effects (e.g., thrombophlebitis), and omission of additional non-drug cost associated with infusion therapy (e.g., clinical work load, hospital waste and administration cost such as needles, syringes, dressings, antiseptics and administration set). Oral levofloxacin and ornidazole have near 100 percent bioavailability; therefore a comparable exposure to the i.v. regimen may be achieved after oral administration [18,19]. i.v. to oral switch programme for clindamycin and cefuroxime have been also proved with great economic advantages [20,21]. Clinicians should consider oral antibacterials as soon as possible for outpatients who need infection control. The DDDs value represents the tendency of drug use, with higher DDDs indicating more frequent utilization [22]. Sum of DDDs of antibacterials for outpatients in the second phase was lower than that in the first phase (61403 versus 65930). Moreover, in this program, statistically significant changes of proportion of DDDs of eight oral antibacterials between two phases indicated that i.v. to oral switch therapy approach was basically successful. A decrease in the relative percentage of DDDs for cefprozi tablets may have been due to the introduction of cefaclor sustained release formulation into SAHZU in July, 2012. A decrease in the relative percentage of DDDs for cefradine capsules may have been in part due to increased

Table 5 Drug-related problems derived from randomly selected antibacterial prescriptions for outpatients

Indicators	First phase (March, 2012)	Second phase (March, 2013)
Number of randomly selected antibacterial prescriptions for outpatients[*]	559	446
Number of DRPs	76	18
Occurrence rate of DRPS[#]	13.6%	4.0%
Occurrence rate of DRPs made by surgeons[Δ#]	19.5%	5.6%
Occurrence rate of DRPs made by internal medicine physicians[#]	8.4%	2.8%
Occurrence rate of each subtype of DRP		
(1) Inappropriate coadministration with non-antibacterials	4 (0.7%)	6 (1.3%)
(2) Inappropriate co-medication with other antibacterials[#]	17 (3.0%)	3 (0.7%)
(3) Inappropriate dosing frequency	8 (1.4%)	3 (0.7%)
(4) Inappropriate dose	1 (0.2%)	2 (0.4%)
(5) Inappropriate administration route	1 (0.2%)	0
(6) Use beyond approved indications	1 (0.2%)	2 (0.4%)
(7) Discordance between diagnosis and purpose of medication use	8 (1.4%)	2 (0.4%)
(8) Mismatches between antibacterial spectrum and the patient's infection[#]	15 (2.7%)	0
(9) Abuse of i.v. medications instead of oral alternatives[#]	16 (2.9%)	0
(10) No diluent for i.v. antibacterials	1 (0.2%)	0
(11) Ignorance of patient's other diseases	4 (0.7%)	0

Notes: [#]$P < 0.01$ (first phase *vs* second phase). [Δ]$P < 0.01$ (surgeons *vs* internal medicine physicians). Differences between two groups were tested for statistical significance using Pearson's Chi-square test. A *P* value < 0.05 was considered to be statistically significant. A *P* value < 0.01 was considered to be highly significant. DRPs: drug-related problems.

awareness of its potential renal toxicity (e.g. hematuresis) among physicians and pharmacists.

Occurrence rates of DRPs between surgical clinics and internal medicine clinics exhibited significant difference in the first phase, but not in the second phase, indicating that surgeons were previously less likely to appropriately prescribe outpatient antimicrobials than internal medicine physicians; however, upon intervention, surgeon prescribing practices improved greatly. A systematic review revealed that physicians' attitudes were the most influential intrinsic factor influencing antibacterial prescribing and healthcare system-related factors like time pressure and corresponding policies/guidelines implemented were the most common extrinsic factors [23]. A substantial number of surgeons were found to have suboptimal knowledge about antibacterial use and prescribing habits in the first phase. Besides of continuing education and training directed to them, fines were imposed on physicians who refused to mend their ways after repeated education. Furthermore, the outpatient service environment and treatment process were further improved. Such strenuous efforts improved the quality of antibacterial prescribing.

DRPs associated with "use beyond approved indications" were identified. Moxifloxacin tablet was prescribed for treatment of urinary tract infection in a prescription. However, package insert of moxifloxacin tablet specifies that the

formulation is only indicated for the treatment of adults (≥ 18 years of age) with infections caused by susceptible isolates of the designated microorganisms in the conditions listed below: acute bacterial sinusitis, acute bacterial exacerbation of chronic bronchitis, community acquired pneumonia, uncomplicated skin and skin structure infections and complicated intra-abdominal infections. Not all fluoroquinolones can be used for urinary tract infections based on their pharmacokinetic profiles [24]. Treatment of infections in the urine is a common misuse of moxifloxacin, and clinicians should be careful about use of this agent for these infections since moxifloxacin achieves considerably lower concentrations in the urine than other fluoroquinolones and it is not approved for this indication. This study showed that the use of 0.4% of antibacterial prescriptions in the second phase was still beyond approved indications. Although off-label manner of prescribing cannot always be avoided, physicians should only use unapproved drugs in cases when suitable alternatives are unavailable and there are scientific evidence regarding safety and effectiveness [25,26].

The incidence of DRPs such as bug-drug mismatches and abuse of i.v. medications rather than highly bioavailable oral alternatives were successfully reduced in the second phase (*P*<0.01). In the first phase, sulbenicillin, a penicillin antibiotic active against *P. aeruginosa*, was severely misused for treatment of infections which were not commonly caused by *P. aeruginosa*. For example, sulbenicillin was prescribed for outpatients who got tooth extraction. Finally, the DTC eliminated sulbenicillin from the antibiotic formulary for outpatient clinical practice. Special trainings sessions were directed toward dentists to prevent the overuse and misuse of antibacterials, which was successful.

With regard to the indicator "Inappropriate coadministration with non-antibacterials", no obvious improvement was observed. In China, antibacterials could be prescribed with other western medicines in the same prescription sheet. Coadministration of antibacterials and probiotics were observed in both phases. Spaced dosing was not specified when physicians wrote prescriptions. Since probiotics contain live microorganisms, concurrent administration of antibacterials could kill a large number of the organisms, reducing the efficacy of the *Lactobacillus* and *Bifidobacterium* species. However, all of patients in the two phases were instructed by pharmacists to separate administration of antibacterials from these bacteria-derived probiotics by at least two hours.

Although a significant reduction in occurrence of DRPs was observed after the intervention program, there still were 18 DRPs in the second phase. It indicated of further opportunities for improvement. In theory, the appropriateness of all prescriptions should be audited by pharmacists. In SAHZU, prospective prescription audit is a routine pharmaceutical service for inpatients. However, outpatient pharmacy has not yet established such working process due to big workload (5000 prescriptions each day). This hasn't been possible, due to the relatively insufficient personnel and the particularity of outpatient service medical treatment in comparison with inpatient service (about 10000 outpatients each day versus 2200 inpatients each day). In Mainland of China, there is hardly any hospital which practices prospective prescription audit promptly in outpatient service when physicians prescribe via electronic prescribing system. Some large hospitals in China take the following measures: (1) Install online prescription screening software embedded in electronic prescribing system and pharmacy administration system, allowing severe DRPs to be automatically intercepted when physicians are prescribing. (2) Pharmacists will contact the corresponding physicians if they detect DRPs when outpatients hand over the prescriptions to pharmacists. Such interventions bring potential problems, and are likely to cause the tension between the hospital and patients (i.e., a patient would be reluctant to go back to the physician's clinic for prescription revision because it will be perceived as a waste of time, and the physician's professional image might be damaged).

Suboptimal prescribing habits involving antibiotics in China is partly associated with economic incentives, driven by non-standardized drug-promotions by pharmaceutical companies. However, many medical disputes between patients and hospitals are associated with irrational drug use. Therefore, education is an essential element of an intervention program designed to influence prescribing behavior and can provide a knowledge basis that will enhance the acceptance of stewardship strategies. Communication is also important among physicians, pharmacists and administrators before initiating intervention programs. Consideration should be given to all staff involved (i.e., values, personality, perceptions, emotions and ability). The working mode of the DTC on outpatient antibacterial stewardship intervention, especially allowing physicians to present evidence and argument to the results of audit-feedback during a seven-day public notice period, was pivotal to the willing acceptance of punishment by physicians who made severe DRPs. Rational antibiotic use, to a certain extent, is a health administration issue more so than a professional issue.

A literature review of clinical and economic outcomes of pharmaceutical services related to antibacterial use showed that the most frequently observed outcomes with a positive impact were appropriateness of prescribing and cost savings [27]. Although the study in SAHZU showed some positive outcomes, it had some limitations which were shown as follows: (1) Follow-up of outpatients' therapeutic outcome was not conducted; (2) Patient adherence to treatment regimens were not monitored so that prescribing data may not accurately represent actual antibacterial consumption); (3) Multiple comparisons for the same dataset might increase type I error in showing the impact of interventions, and for these kind of studies interrupted time-series analysis would be more reliable method [28].

Conclusion

The effects of an outpatient antibacterial stewardship intervention were examined in an academic medical center hospital during the journey to JCI accreditation. The intervention program reduced the expenditure on antibacterials, improved the appropriateness of antibacterial prescriptions. Quality improvements need continuous efforts, integrated multifaceted intervention measures and long-term adherence to the antibiotic stewardship. Approach of i.v. to oral antibacterial switch therapy, classification management, and motivational measures may play the most direct and efficient role in changing antibacterial prescription practices.

Competing interests
The authors declare that they have no competing interests.

Authors' contributions
SP, LW and ZQ conceived and designed research; ZQ collected data and performed data analysis; and SP and ZQ wrote the paper. All authors' read and approved the final manuscript.

Acknowledgments

This work was supported by Zhejiang Provincial Bureau of Health (No.2012KYA090). The authors thank Professor Xuan-Ding Wang and Dr. Hai-bin Dai for their excellent work.

Author details

[1]Department of Pharmacy, the Second Affiliated Hospital, School of Medicine, Zhejiang University, Jiefang Road No. 88, Hangzhou, Zhejiang 310009, China. [2]Division of Medical Affairs, the Second Affiliated Hospital, School of Medicine, Zhejiang University, Hangzhou, Zhejiang 310009, Province, China.

References

1. Weiss K, Blais R, Fortin A, Lantin S, Gaudet M: Impact of a multipronged education strategy on antibiotic prescribing in Quebec, Canada. *Clin Infect Dis* 2011, **53**:433–439.
2. *Antibiotic resistance threats in the United States.* The U.S. Centers for Disease Control and Prevention; 2013. http://www.cdc.gov/drugresistance/threat-report-2013/.
3. Teixeira Rodrigues A, Roque F, Falcão A, Figueiras A, Herdeiro MT: Understanding physician antibiotic prescribing behaviour: a systematic review of qualitative studies. *Int J Antimicrob Agents* 2013, **41**:203–212.
4. Sumpradit N, Chongtrakul P, Anuwong K, Pumtong S, Kongsomboon K, Butdeemee P, Khonglormyati J, Chomyong S, Tongyoung P, Losiriwat S, Seesuk P, Suwanwaree P, Tangcharoensathien V: Antibiotics smart use: a workable model for promoting the rational use of medicines in Thailand. *Bull World Health Organ* 2012, **90**:905–913.
5. Davey P, Brown E, Charani E, Fenelon L, Gould IM, Holmes A, Ramsay CR, Wiffen PJ, Wilcox M: Interventions to improve antibiotic prescribing practices for hospital inpatients. *Cochrane Database Syst Rev* 2013, **4**, CD003543.
6. Nowak MA, Nelson RE, Breidenbach JL, Thompson PA, Carson PJ: Clinical and economic outcomes of a prospective antimicrobial stewardship program. *Am J Health Syst Pharm* 2012, **69**:1500–1508.
7. Ambroggio L, Thomson J, Murtagh Kurowski E, Courter J, Statile A, Graham C, Sheehan B, Iyer S, Shah SS, White CM: Quality improvement methods increase appropriate antibiotic prescribing for childhood pneumonia. *Pediatrics* 2013, **131**:e1623–e1631.
8. Al-Niemat SI, Bloukh DT, Al-Harasis MD, Al-Fanek AF, Salah RK: Drug use evaluation of antibiotics prescribed in a Jordanian hospital outpatient and emergency clinics using WHO prescribing indicators. *Saudi Med J* 2008, **29**:743–748.
9. Pulcini C, Lions C, Ventelou B, Verger P: Drug-specific quality indicators assessing outpatient antibiotic use among French general practitioners. *Eur J Public Health* 2013, **23**:262–264.
10. Hicks LA, Taylor TH Jr, Hunkler RJ: U.S. outpatient antibiotic prescribing, 2010. *N Engl J Med* 2013, **368**:1461–1462.
11. Gerber JS, Prasad PA, Fiks AG, Localio AR, Grundmeier RW, Bell LM, Wasserman RC, Keren R, Zaoutis TE: Effect of an outpatient antimicrobial stewardship intervention on broad-spectrum antibiotic prescribing by primary care pediatricians: a randomized trial. *JAMA* 2013, **309**:2345–2352.
12. Rattinger GB, Mullins CD, Zuckerman IH, Onukwugha E, Walker LD, Gundlapalli A, Samore M, Delisle S: A sustainable strategy to prevent misuse of antibiotics for acute respiratory infections. *PLoS One* 2012, **7**:e51147.
13. Joint Commission International: *JCI Accreditation Standards for Hospitals.* 4th edition. 2010. http://www.jointcommissioninternational.org/common/pdfs/jcia/IAS400_Standards_Lists_Only.pdf.
14. World Health Organization (WHO), Collaborating Center for Drug Statistics Methodology: *Guidelines for ATC classification and DDD assignment 2013.* 2013. http://www.whocc.no/filearchive/publications/1_2013guidelines.pdf.
15. Sözen H, Gönen I, Sözen A, Kutlucan A, Kalemci S, Sahan M: Application of ATC/DDD methodology to evaluate of antibiotic use in a general hospital in Turkey. *Ann Clin Microbiol Antimicrob* 2013, **12**:23.
16. van Niekerk AC, Venter DJ, Boschmans SA: Implementation of intravenous to oral antibiotic switch therapy guidelines in the general medical wards of a tertiary-level hospital in South Africa. *J Antimicrob Chemother* 2012, **67**:756–762.
17. Cunha BA: Intravenous to oral antibiotic switch therapy. *Drugs Today (Barc)* 2001, **37**:311–319.
18. Furlanut M, Brollo L, Lugatti E, Di Qual E, Dolcet F, Talmassons G, Pea F: Pharmacokinetic aspects of levofloxacin 500 mg once daily during sequential intravenous/oral therapy in patients with lower respiratory tract infections. *J Antimicrob Chemother* 2003, **51**:101–106.
19. Yen YH, Chen HY, Wuan-Jin L, Lin YM, Shen WC, Cheng KJ: Clinical and economic impact of a pharmacist-managed i.v.-to-p.o. conversion service for levofloxacin in Taiwan. *Int J Clin Pharmacol Ther* 2012, **50**:136–141.
20. Jewesson P: Cost-effectiveness and value of an IV switch. *Pharmacoeconomics* 1994, **5**:20–26.
21. Flamaing J, Knockaert D, Meijers B, Verhaegen J, Peetermans WE: Sequential therapy with cefuroxime and cefuroxime-axetil for community-acquired lower respiratory tract infection in the oldest old. *Aging Clin Exp Res* 2008, **20**:81–86.
22. Zhu XP, Zhu LL, Zhou Q: Prescribing practice and evaluation of appropriateness of enteral nutrition in a university teaching hospital. *Ther Clin Risk Manag* 2013, **9**:37–43.
23. Teixeira Rodrigues A, Roque F, Falcão A, Figueiras A, Herdeiro MT: Understanding physician antibiotic prescribing behaviour: a systematic review of qualitative studies. *Int J Antimicrob Agents* 2013, **41**:203–212.
24. Jancel T, Dudas V: Management of uncomplicated urinary tract infections. *West J Med* 2002, **176**:51–55.
25. Radley DC, Finkelstein SN, Stafford RS: Off-label prescribing among office-based physicians. *Arch Intern Med* 2006, **166**:1021–1026.
26. Tansarli GS, Rafailidis PI, Kapaskelis A, Falagas ME: Frequency of the off-label use of antibiotics in clinical practice: a systematic review. *Expert Rev Anti Infect Ther* 2012, **10**:1383–1392.
27. von Gunten V, Reymond JP, Beney J: Clinical and economic outcomes of pharmaceutical services related to antibiotic use: a literature review. *Pharm World Sci* 2007, **29**:146–163.
28. Wagner AK, Soumerai SB, Zhang F, Ross-Degnan D: Segmented regression analysis of interrupted time series studies in medication use research. *J Clin Pharm Ther* 2002, **27**:299–309.

4

Knowledge and beliefs on antimicrobial resistance among physicians and nurses in hospitals in Amhara Region, Ethiopia

Bayeh Abera[1*], Mulugeta Kibret[2] and Wondemagegn Mulu[1]

Abstract

Background: Antimicrobial resistance (AMR) is a major global public health problem both in hospital and community acquired infections. The present study assessed the knowledge and beliefs on AMR among physicians and nurses in 13 hospitals in Amhara region, Ethiopia, which is a low-income country.

Methods: A cross-sectional study using a self-administered questionnaire was applied.

Results: A total of 385 participants (175 physicians and 210 nurses) took part in the study. Sixty five percent of physicians and 98% of nurses replied that they need training on antimicrobial stewardship. Only 48% of physicians and 22.8% of nurses had exposures for local antibiogram data. Overall, 278 (72.2%) of participants were knowledgeable about AMR. Majority of participants agreed or strongly agreed AMR as worldwide and national problem but few considered AMR as problem in their own hospitals. The two most important factors mentioned for AMR development were patients' poor adherence to prescribed antimicrobials (86%) and overuse of antibiotics (80.5%). The most leading local factors identified for AMR development were: self-antibiotic prescription (53.5%), lack of access to local antibiogram data (12.3%) and prescriber poor awareness about AMR (9.2%). Factors perceived for excessive antibiotic prescriptions were: patient drive (56%), treatment failure (79%), unknown febrile illnesses (39.7%) and upper respiratory tract infections (33.4%).

Conclusion: Majority of physicians and nurses lack up to-date knowledge on AMR. Unavailability of local antibiogram data, self-prescription by patients and poor awareness on AMR are areas of interventions for prevention and control of AMR.

Keywords: Antimicrobial resistance, Knowledge, Belief, Ethiopia

Background

Antimicrobial resistance (AMR) is a growing serious worldwide public health problem in both hospital and community acquired infections [1]. Antimicrobial resistant bacteria have negative impact on treatment outcomes such as prolonged morbidity, hospital stay and increased risk of mortality [1,2]. Furthermore, patients infected with drug resistant bacteria demand more expensive therapy. Therefore, AMR results in increased health care costs and financial burden to families and societies [2,3]. Antimicrobial resistance problem is challenging in low-income countries because of high prevalence of infection, irrational uses of antimicrobials, over-the-counter availability of antibiotics and lack of clinical microbiology laboratories for antimicrobial susceptibility testing [4].

Development of AMR is accelerated by excessive antimicrobial prescription [5]. More than 50% of antibiotics worldwide are purchased without prescription [6]. The situation is more serious in developing countries because of antibiotic use without medical guidance and inadequate regulation of antibiotics [7]. Determinants for self-antibiotic prescription in low-income countries include over-the-counter sales of antibiotics, high cost of medical consultations and dissatisfaction with medical practitioners [8].

Containment of antimicrobial resistance requires change in the antimicrobial prescribing behavior of health workers.

* Correspondence: bayeabera15@gmail.com
[1]Department of Microbiology, Parasitology and Immunology, College of Medicine and Health Sciences, Bahir Dar University, P.O. Box 79, Bahir Dar, Ethiopia
Full list of author information is available at the end of the article

Changes in antimicrobial prescribing patterns will demand changes in physicians' behavior towards the magnitude of AMR problem. Nurses in hospitals play important role in prevention of transmissions of resistant bacteria and promoting awareness on AMR for patients and communities. Thus, information on physicians' and nurses' knowledge and belief on AMR will permit the development of more effective interventions on containment of AMR. Surveys have been conducted to assess physicians' knowledge and beliefs about antimicrobial use and resistance in USA and Europe [9-12]. However, these results are not necessarily applicable to the situation in low-income countries like Ethiopia.

The purpose of this study was to assess the knowledge and beliefs of physicians and nurses on AMR from 13 selected hospitals from public and private sectors in Amhara National Regional State (ANRS), Ethiopia. To our knowledge, this is the first study undertaken to assess the knowledge and beliefs about antimicrobial resistance among phycians and nurses in Ethiopia. The information generated in this study would be instrumental in planning and implementing preventive and control interventions on AMR at regional and national levels.

Methods
Study design, period and setting
A cross-sectional survey was conducted among eligible physicians and nurses working in hospitals in June 2013. Five in private and eight public hospitals were selected using systematic selection method by calculating the sampling interval. At the time of the survey, 235 physicians and 4,902 nurses were rendering services in a total of 26 hospitals (19= public and 7 private) in ANRS [13].

A sample size of 411 was calculated using the Epi info 7.0 soft ware (CDC, Atlanta, USA) considering a total population of 5,137 physicians and nurses. Expected maximum correct answer on the questions about knowledge of AMR (50%) was used. A 95% confidence level and 15% non-response were employed. Medical doctors from psychiatry, radiology, ophthalmology and anaesthesiology were excluded because they do not regularly prescribe antimicrobials. Participants, based on the number of physicians and nurses in each hospitals were selected by simple random sampling using lottery technique. However, in hospitals where the numbers of participants were less than five physicians, all participants were included.

Data collection instruments
Prior to data collection the questions were piloted at local hospital. A total of 34-item-questions were self-administered to survey professional profiles, knowledge and beliefs on antimicrobial resistance.

The seven-item questions were used to address professional profiles such as qualifications, speciality, working hospital departments, service years, sources of information on antimicrobial resistance, training on AMR, exposure of using antimicrobial susceptibility test (AST) results and working in public and private hospitals.

Participants' knowledge on AMR was surveyed by 13 item-questions. Lists of 7-item-questions addressing factors for development and spread of drug resistance. In addition, one open ended question was included to assess the perception of participants on factors promoting AMR at local and national levels. Three questions were used to assess their knowledge on scope of AMR problem from local to global levels. Two open ended questions were used to assess their knowledge about prevalence of drug resistant bacteria and hospital infections related to drug resistance.

Participants' beliefs on AMR were assessed by 14-item questions. A list of seven questions and one open ended question covering the potential interventions to reduce antimicrobial resistances had been used. Lists of five questions were applied to assess beliefs towards rational use of antibiotics. One open ended question was used to ask participants to mention the least effective antibiotic in their hospital practices.

Statistical analysis
The response alternatives for knowledge items were dichotomous. The questions on beliefs used Likert-style responses. Data was entered and analyzed using the Statistical Package for Social Sciences (SPSS® 20.0, USA). Chi-square test was used to assess the differences between physicians and nurses on knowledge and beliefs on AMR. P value of <0.05 (two sided) was taken as statistical significance.

Mean score
For knowledge assessment, each correct response was given a score of 1 while a wrong or doubtful response was scored as 0. For both study participants mean knowledge scores < 0.72 were considered as below the expected level of knowledge while average scores ≥0.72 were at the expected level of knowledge. Regarding beliefs, useful and very useful responses were considered as positive beliefs. Scores from 0.15 to 0.88 were interpreted as negative beliefs, and scores ranged from 0.88 to 1 were considered as positive beliefs.

Ethical consideration
Ethical clearance was obtained from the Research and Ethical Review Board of Bahir Dar University. Moreover, all patients gave written informed consent to participate in this study.

Results
Participants' profiles and sources of information on AMR
A total of 385 participants took part in this study; of whom, 37 (9.6%) were senior physicians, 138 (35.8%)

general practitioners and 210 (54.5%) nurses (Table 1). The overall response rate of participants was 91.4%. Of these, 175 (87%) physicians and 100% nurses filled the self-administered questionnaires. All study participants from private hospitals completed the questionnaires (response rate 100%). The overall mean service year was 7.2 (SD ± 8.2). The majority of the participants were from public hospitals (Table 1).

Participants' exposure of using antimicrobial susceptibility test (AST) result, training status on AMR and working departments are illustrated in (Table 1). Of the study participants, 13.5% of senior physicians, 29.7% general practitioners and 49.3% of nurses replied that they had no up-to-date information about AMR.

Participants were asked to mention their current sources of information about AMR. Overall, 19.7% respondents got information from relevant books, 3.4% from internet, 2.8% journals and 26.4% from other sources such as college or university courses and trainings. Regarding training need, 65% of physicians and 98% of nurses responded that they need further training on stewardship of antimicrobial resistance.

Knowledge on antimicrobial resistance

The overall mean knowledge score was 0.72 (SD ± 0.44). The mean knowledge score was 0.82 (SD ± 0.37) for physicians and 0.63 (SD ± 0.40) for nurses (p = 0.001).

Thus, 278 (72.2%) of participants were at the expected level of knowledge on AMR. Of these, 145 (82.8%) of physicians and 133 (63.5%) of nurses were knowledgeable (p = 0.001). Physicians' and nurses' knowledge about the scope of antimicrobial resistance problem at local, national and global levels are depicted in Table 2.

Knowledge on causes and prevalence of antimicrobial resistance

According to the respondents the most important perceived factors contributing for antimicrobial resistance development were: Patients' poor adherence to prescribed antibiotics (86% by respondents), widespread or overuse of antibiotics (80%) and broad spectrum antibiotics use (78.4%). Statistically significant difference was observed between physicians and nurses in rating factors for developing AMR (Table 3).

Furthermore, assessment of knowledge on local factors for spread of AMR was also augmented by open ended question. The most important local factors identified were: self-antibiotic prescription was responded by 53.5%, lack of access to local antibiograms was responded by 12.3% and prescribers and patients poor awareness on AMR was responded by 9.2%.

Participants were also asked to rate bacterial infections in which drug resistant bacteria would be a problem in hospitals. Pneumonia was rated by 29.3% and 57.6% of

Table 1 Profiles of participants in 13 selected hospitals in Amhara Region, Ethiopia

Variables	Senior physicians (n = 37)	GP (N = 138)	Nurses (n = 210)	Total (n = 385)
	N (%)	N (%)	N (%)	N (%)
Work place				
Public only	13 (35.2)	124 (89.9)	171 (81.4)	308 (80)
Private only	12 (32.4)	0	36 (17.1)	48 (12.5)
Both in Public and Private	12 (32.4)	14 (10.1)	3 (1.5)	29 (7.5)
Hospital department				
Medicine	11 (29.7)	58 (42)	75 (35.7)	144 (37.4)
Surgery	15 (40.5)	37 (26.8)	54 (25.7)	106 (27.5)
Paediatrics	3 (8.1)	20 (14.5)	45 (21.4)	71 (18.4)
Gynae-Obstatrics	7 (18.9)	13 (9.4)	15 (7.1)	35 (9.0)
Rotation (among wards)	0	10 (7.2)	21 (10)	31 (8.0)
Training attended on AMR	15 (40.5)	12 (8.7)	9 (4.3)	36 (9.3)
Exposure of using AST results	20 (53.1)	64 (46.4)	48 (22.8)	132 (34.3)
Source of information				
Books	15 (40.5)	46 (33.3)	15 (7.1)	76 (19.7)
Internet	6 (16.2)	7 (5)	0	13 (3.4)
Journals	7 (18.9)	4 (2.9)	0	11 (2.8)
School course and workshops	4 (10.8)	40 (28.9%)	51 (24.4)	95 (24.6)
Lack of up- to -date information	5 (13.5)	41 (29.7)	144 (68.5)	190 (49.3)

Key: GP: General Practitioner Medical Doctors.
Senior physicians: Medical doctors with specializations.

Table 2 Percentage of physicians and nurses rating the scope of AMR problem

Scope of antimicrobial resistance		Strongly agree	Agree	Disagree	Strongly disagree	Don't know
AMR is worldwide problem	Physicians	39	43.0	9.8	4.6	2.9
	Nurses	24.8	35.2	26.4	4.6	10
	Total	31.5	39.0	18.1	4.6	6.3
AMR is problem in Ethiopia	Physicians	51.3	36.8	3.9	0	8.9
	Nurses	37.1	52.8	7.1	1.4	1.4
	Total	42.0	49.3	4.9	0.5	3.3
AMR is a problem in your hospital	Physicians	25	50.0	18.4	1.3	6.5
	Nurses	22.3	53.8	17.1	2.8	4.3
	Total	23.6	52.0	17.8	1.9	4.6

physicians and nurses, respectively. Urinary tract infection was rated by 23.1% and 24.7% of physicians and nurses, respectively. Surgical site infection was rated by 19.5% and 20% of physicians and nurses, respectively. The interesting response was that 57.1% of nurses incorrectly perceived tuberculosis as the most prevalent hospital infections in which drug resistance is common but phycians rate tuberculosis by 2.3%.

Participants were asked to identify the most common drug resistant bacteria in hospitals they perceive from local to global levels by open question. Methicillin resistant *S.aureus* (MRSA) was mentioned by 22.3% and 2.4% of physicians and nurses, respectively. MDR-TB was listed by 40.4% of nurses and 4.1% physicians. *Pseudomonas aeruginosa* was rated by 5.7% of physicians (Table 3).

Beliefs on potential interventions for antimicrobial resistance

Considering the mean score of beliefs (0.88), 95 (54%) of physicians and 109 (52%) of nurses believed in the suggested potential solutions for preventing AMR. Antimicrobial usage policy and reduction of antimicrobial usage for outpatients were not important by 32.4% and 38% of respondents, respectively (Table 4). Furthermore, the most frequently considered interventions were local access for antimicrobial susceptibility data (31.4%) and providing education on antimicrobial stewardship (17.2%).

Beliefs on misuse of antimicrobials

Physicians' and nurses' beliefs towards the pushing factors for frequent prescription of antibiotics were significantly

Table 3 Physicians' and nurses' knowledge about the causes of antibiotic resistances and antibiotic resistant bacteria

Variables	Physicians (n = 175) Yes N (%)	Nurses (n = 210) Yes N (%)	Total Yes N (%)	P-value
Causes of AMR				
Widespread or over use of antibiotics promotes AMR	162 (92.5)	147 (70)	309 (80.5)	0.001
Usage of broad- spectrum antibiotics promote AMR	155 (88.5)	147 (70)	302 (78.4)	0. 001
Bacterial mutations cause of AMR	144 (82.3)	132 (62.8)	276 (71.6)	0.001
Poor hand washing practice in hospitals spread AMR	68 (38.8)	90 (42.8)	158 (41)	0.56
Poor infection control in hospitals spread AMR	104 (59.4)	114 (54.3)	218 (56.6)	0.40
Patient poor adherence promote AMR	160 (91.4)	171 (81.4)	331 (86)	0.002
Sub-standard quality of antibiotics	138 (78.8)	158 (75.2)	296 (76.8)	0.42
Examples of antibiotic resistant bacteria in hospitals				
Methicillin resistant *S. aureus* (MRSA)	39 (22.3)	5 (2.5)	44 (11.4)	0.001
MDR-TB	7 (4.1)	85 (40.4)	92 (23.9)	0.001
P. aeruginosa	10 (5.7)	0	10 (5.7)	
Local factors for development of AMR				
Self-prescription by patients	133 (76.0)	73 (34.7)	206 (53.5)	0.001
Lack of access to local antibiogram data	28 (16.0)	19 (9.0)	47 (12.3)	0.04
Prescribers' poor awareness on AMR	27 (15.4)	8 (3.8)	35 (9.2)	0.001

Key: AMR: Antimicrobial resistances and MDR-TB: multi-resistant drug resistant tuberculosis.

Table 4 Physicians' and nurses' beliefs on potential intervention to combat AMR

Variables		Very useful	Useful	Not useful	Not sure
Antimicrobial usage policy	Physicians	26.4	40	18.2	15.4
	Nurses	30.0	36.8	20.5	10.5
	Total	28.2	38.4	19.4	13
Reduction of antibiotic use for outpatient setting	Physicians	15.3	59.4	18.8	5.9
	Nurses	33.3	47.0	12.6	7.3
	Total	24.2	53.2	31.4	6.6
Establish national AMR surveillance	Physicians	66.4	31.7	1.1	0.6
	Nurses	56.8	37.3	3.6	2.1
	Total	61.6	34.5	2.5	1.3
Establish hospital infection control committee	Physicians	54.7	42.3	2.3	0.6
	Nurses	55.3	42.2	0	2.4
	Total	55.0	42.2	2.3	3
Develop institutional guideline for antimicrobial use	Physicians	73.0	25.8	1.1	0
	Nurses	63.1	31.5	0	5.2
	Total	68.0	28.6	1.1	5.2
Education on antimicrobial therapy for prescribers	Physicians	68.8	28.8	1.1	1.1
	Nurses	53.6	40.5	3.6	2.1
	Total	61.2	34.6	2.3	1.6
Establish microbiology diagnostic services	Physicians	67.6	24.1	0	4.7
	Nurses	57.3	33.1	0	9.4
	Total	62.4	28.6	0	7.0

different (Table 5). For both physicians and nurses, the most leading factors were: patients drive on prescribers to prescribe antibiotics, treatment failure and critically ill patients. Unknown febrile illness and upper respiratory infections were identified as important factors for excessive antibiotic prescriptions by 53.7% and 44.7% of respondents, respectively.

Participants' beliefs towards the least effect antibiotics due to resistant bacteria were: amoxicillin rated by 36.5%

of respondents, penicillin and cloxacillin by 22% each, chloramphenicol (16%) and cotrimoxazole (14%). Statistically significant difference was noted between physicians' and nurses' beliefs with regard to effectiveness of amoxicillin and cloxacillin ($p = 0.001$). Because, 28% of physicians and 8.5% of nurses mentioned amoxicillin as least effective antibiotics ($p = 0.001$). Cloxacillin was perceived as least effective by 14% of physicians and 8% of nurses ($p = 0.01$).

Table 5 Physicians' and nurses' belief on causes of unnecessary antibiotic prescriptions

Questions	Physicians (n = 175)	Nurses (n = 210)	Total	P value
	Yes (%)	Yes (%)	Yes (%)	
Patient push	61.0	53	56.7	0.04
Treatment failure	90.2	69.5	79.0	0.001
Critically ill or immune-compromised patient	52.3	67.1	60.4	0.01
Profit of hospitals	35.6	41	0.55	38.5
For which infections do you think unnecessary antibiotics would be prescribed?				
Upper respiratory tracts	44.7	24	33.4	0.001
Unknown febrile illness	53.7	28	39.7	0.001
Urinary tract infections	9.3	34.8	23.1	0.001
Diarrhoea	21.3	28	25.4	0.08

Discussion

Physicians and nurses are key stakeholders in prevention and control of AMR through prescribing antimicrobials wisely, controlling transmission of drug resistant bacteria and promoting awareness. Thus, the present study demonstrated the knowledge and beliefs of physicians and nurses about AMR from 13 selected hospitals in ANRS, Ethiopia.

Statistically significant difference was observed between physicians and nurses in some aspects of knowledge and beliefs on AMR (p = 0.001) (Table 3 and Table 5). Regarding to awareness on the scope of AMR problem, majority of respondents strongly agreed or agreed AMR as global and national public health problems. However, few participates recognized AMR as a problem in their won hospital. These findings are consistent with a study conducted in Sudan [14], India [15] and DR Congo [16]. In contrast, previous studies from Spain, Brazil and Peru showed that more than 90% of physicians perceived AMR as a global and national problem [17-19].

The majority of physicians and nurses did not mention the existence of antibiotic resistant bacteria. For instance, only 22.3% of physicians and 2.4% of nurses had information regards to MRSA. These are lower than physicians' knowledge of MRSA documented from India [15]. Although, MDR-TB is not a hospital pathogen, 40.4% of nurses mentioned it as one of the most prevalent drug resistant bacteria in hospitals. These knowledge gaps on local antibiotic resistant bacteria would be attributable to unavailability or lack of bacteriological culture and susceptibility testing in most hospitals [12]. Furthermore, only 9.3% of respondents have had training on antimicrobial stewardship education.

There was statistically significant difference between physicians and nurses with regard to the causes on development and spread of AMR (Table 3). The three leading causes of AMR were: patients' poor adherence to prescribed antibiotics, over use of antibiotics and frequent prescription of broad-spectrum antibiotics. Likewise, a study conducted in Scotland, France and Spain stated that too many antibiotic prescriptions, too many broad-spectrum antibiotics and inappropriate duration of antibiotic treatments were the leading factors [19,20]. Poor hand washing was not well recognized in this study as contributing factors to AMR in hospital settings similar to other studies [19,20]. Therefore, emphasis on proper hand washing and infection control measures must be implemented.

This study revealed that the most important local factors for spread and development of AMR were self-antibiotic prescription and patient poor adherence to prescribed antimicrobial agents. Moreover, lack of access to antibiotic susceptibility testing and prescribers' poor awareness on AMR were mentioned as local factors. Some other studies also supported this specified findings [6,7,14,16].

Regarding potential interventions to combat AMR, majority of participants believed in the most the favourite measures were: establishing national AMR surveillance program, avail clinical microbiology laboratory and local guidelines for rational use of antibiotics (Table 4). However, only 66.6% and 77.4% of respondents favoured antibiotic restriction policy and reduction of antibiotic use for outpatients, respectively. This finding is in agreement with a previous report on beliefs of physicians from USA [11]. Establishing local antimicrobial susceptibility tests and providing education on antimicrobials stewardship for health professional were identified as the most important interventions [14,19].

Physicians' and nurses' beliefs towards the pushing factors for frequent prescription of antibiotics were significantly different (p = 0.001). Treatment failure and critically ill patients were the most driving factors. Patients push to antibiotics was also mentioned by 56.7% of respondents [16]. More than half of physicians believed that unknown febrile illness was one of first factors for excessive antibiotic prescriptions.

According to the respondents, amoxicillin, penicillin and cloxacillin were perceived as the least effective antibiotics related to drug resistant bacteria. This perception could be considered as positive towards the recognition of drug resistance. Because, previous studies in the same region showed that bacterial isolates from clinical samples revealed high levels of resistance against these antimicrobials [21-23]. Furthermore, studies revealed that amoxicillin and cloxacilin are the most commonly prescribed antibiotics in different part of Ethiopia [24,25].

The major strength of this survey was large sample size and inclusion of 13 selected hospitals from public and private sectors. However, this study could not analyze the knowledge and belief differences among participants working in private and public hospitals because 32.4% of senior physicians and 10% general practitioners were working both in public and private-owned hospitals. Furthermore, participants' prescribing practices and knowledge on the exact prevalence of antimicrobial resistant bacteria was not assessed because there was no national antimicrobial surveillance program. As general limitation of knowledge and belief survey, study participants may have tendency to provide socially desirable responses.

Conclusion

This study revealed important information on knowledge and beliefs of physicians and nurses about AMR that would be implemented in a low-income country like, Ethiopia. In this survey, physicians and nurses working in hospitals had information gap on antimicrobial resistance. According to participants' response, unavailability of local antibiogram data linked with self- drug prescription by patients and poor awareness on AMR are an issue.

Competing interests
The authors declare that they have no competing interests.

Authors' contributions
AB designed the study, collected data, analyzed data and wrote the article. KM, reviewed the study plan, questionnaires and the article. MW analyzed data and reviewed the manuscript. All authors read and approved the final manuscript.

Acknowledgments
This study was funded by the College of Medicine and Health Sciences, Bahir Dar University. We would like to thank the study participants for providing responses.

Author details
[1]Department of Microbiology, Parasitology and Immunology, College of Medicine and Health Sciences, Bahir Dar University, P.O. Box 79, Bahir Dar, Ethiopia. [2]Department of Biology, Science College, Bahir Dar University, P.O. Box 79, Bahir Dar, Ethiopia.

References
1. World Health Organization: *Combat drug resistance.* WHO; 2011:1–2. http://www.who.int/world-health-day/2011/en/.
2. Coast J, Smith R, Miller M: **Superbugs: should antimicrobial resistance be included as a cost in economic evaluation?** *Health Economics* 1996, **5:**217–226.
3. Qavi A, Segal-Maurer S, Mariano N, Urban C, Rosenberg C, Burns J, Chiang T, Maurer J, Rahal JJ: **Increased mortality associated with a clonal outbreak of ceftazidime-resistant Klebsiella pneumoniae: a case–control study.** *Infect Control Hosp Epidemiol* 2005, **26:**63–68.
4. Vila J, Pal T: **Update on antimicrobial resistance in low-income countries: Factors favouring the Emergence of resistance.** *Open Infect Dis J* 2010, **4:**38–54.
5. World Health Organization: *Global strategy for the containment of antimicrobial resistance.* Geneva: WHO; 2001. Available from URL: http://www.who.int/drugresistance/WHO_Global_Strategy_English.pdf.
6. Cars O, Nordberg P: **Antibiotic resistance -The faceless threat.** *Int J Risk Saf Med* 2005, **17:**103–110.
7. Byarugaba DK: **A view on antimicrobial resistance in developing countries and responsible risk factors.** *Int J Antimicrob Agents* 2004, **24:**105–110.
8. Grigoryan L, Burgerhof JGM, Degener JE, Deschepper R, Lundborg CS, Monnet DL, Scicluna EA, Birkin J, Haaijer-Ruskamp FM: **Self-Medication with Antibiotics and Resistance (SAR) Consortium. Determinants of self-medication with antibiotics in Europe: the impact of beliefs, country wealth and the healthcare system.** *J Antimicrob Chemother* 2008, **61:**1172–1179.
9. Abbo L, Sinkowitz-Cochran R, Smith L, Ariza-Heredia E, Gómez-Marín O, Srinivasan A, Hooton TM: **Faculty and resident physicians' attitudes, perceptions and knowledge about antimicrobial use and resistance.** *Infect Control Hosp Epidemiol* 2011, **32:**714–728.
10. Srinivasan A, Song X, Richard A, Sinkowitz-Cochran R, Cardo D, Rand C: **A survey of knowledge, attitudes, and beliefs of house staff physicians from various specialties concerning antimicrobial use and resistance.** *Arch Intern Med* 2004, **164:**1451–1456.
11. Wester CW, Durairaj L, Evans AT, Schwartz DN, Husain S, Martinez E: **Antibiotic resistance: a survey of physician perceptions.** *Arch Intern Med* 2002, **162:**2210–2216.
12. Pulcini C, Williams F, Molinari N, Davey P, Nathwani D: **Junior doctors' knowledge and perceptions of antibiotic resistance and prescribing: a survey in France and Scotland.** *Clin Microbiol Infect* 2011, **17:**80–87.
13. Amhara National Regional State Health Bureau (ANRSHB): Annual Report. Bahir Dar: ARHB; 2012.
14. Kheder SI: **Physcians knowledge and perception of antimicrobial resistance: A survey in Khartoum Stata Hospital settings.** *Br J Pharmaceut Res* 2013, **3:**347–362.
15. Qavi A, Segal-Maurer S, Mariano N, Urban C, Rosenberg C, Burns J, Chiang T, Maurer J, Rahal JJ: **A survey of physicians' knowledge and attitudes** regarding antimicrobial resistance and antibiotic prescribing practices at the University Hospital of the West Indies. *West Indian Med J* 2010, **59:**165–170.
16. Thriemer K, Katuala Y, Batoko B, Alworonga JP, Devlier H, VanGeet C, Ngbonda D, Jacobs J: **Antibiotic Prescribing in DR Congo: A Knowledge. Attitude and Practice Survey among Medical Doctors and Students.** *PLoS One* 2013, **8:**e55495.
17. Guerra CM, Pereira CA, Neves Neto AR, Cardo DM, Correa L: **Physicians' perceptions, beliefs, attitudes and knowledge concerning antimicrobial resistance in a Brazilian teaching hospital.** *Infect Control Hosp Epidemiol* 2007, **28:**1411–1414.
18. Garcia C, Llamocca LP, Garcia K, Jimenez A, Samalvides F, Gotuzzo E, Jocob J: **Knowledge, attitudes and practice survey about antimicrobial resistance and prescribing among physicians in a hospital setting in Lima, Peru.** *BMC Clin Phar-macol* 2011, **11:**18.
19. San Francisco CN, Toro MD, Cobo J, de Ge-Garcia J, Vano-Galvan S, Moreno-Ramos F, Rodriguez ban J, Pano-parodo JR: **Knowledge and perceptions of junior and senior Spanish resident doctors about antibiotic use and resistance: Results of a multicenter survey.** *Enferm infecc Microbiol Clin* 2013, **31:**199–204.
20. Pulcini C, William F, Molinar N, Davey P, Nathwani D: **Junior doctors' knowledge and perceptions of antibiotic resistance and prescribing: a survey in France and Scotland.** *Clin Microbiol Infect* 2010, **17:**80–87.
21. Kibret M, Abera B: **Antimicrobial resistance trend of bacteria from clinical isolates: An 8-year retrospective study at Dessie Regional Laboratory, Northeast Ethiopia.** *Ethiop Pharm J* 2010, **28:**39–46.
22. Abera B, Biadglegne F: **Antimicrobial Resistance patterns of** *Staphylococcus aureus* and *Proteus* spp. from otitis media at Bahir Dar Regional Laboratory North West Ethiopia. *Ethiop Med J* 2009, **47:**271–276.
23. Abera B, Alem A, Bezabih B: **Methicillin-resistant strains of** *Staphylococcus aureus* and coagulase-negative staphylococus from clinical isolates at Felege Hiwot Refferal Hospital, North West Ethiopia. *Ethiop Med J* 2008, **46:**149–154.
24. Assefa AD: **Assessment of drug use pattern using WHO prescribing indicators at Hawassa University teaching and referral hospital, south Ethiopia: a cross-sectional study.** *BMC Health Serv Res* 2013, **13:**170.
25. Getachew E, Aragaw S, Adissie W, Agalu A: **Antibiotic prescribing pattern in refreal hospital in Ethiopia.** *J Pharm Pharmacol* 2013, **7:**2657–2661.

5

Predictive factors of self-medicated analgesic use in Spanish adults: a cross-sectional national study

Pilar Carrasco-Garrido[1*], Ana López de Andrés[1], Valentín Hernández Barrera[1], Isabel Jiménez-Trujillo[1], César Fernandez-de-las-Peñas[2], Domingo Palacios-Ceña[3], Soledad García-Gómez-Heras[4] and Rodrigo Jiménez-García[1]

Abstract

Background: Analgesics are among the most commonly consumed drugs by the world populations. Within the broader context of self-medication, pain relief occupies a prominent position. Our study was to ascertain the prevalence of self-medication with analgesics among the Spanish population and to identify predictors of self-medication, including psychological disorders, psychological dysfunction, mental health status, and sociodemographic and health-related variables.

Methods: We used individualized secondary data retrieved from the 2009 European Health Interview Survey (EHIS) for Spain to conduct a nationwide, descriptive, cross-sectional pharmacoepidemiology study on self-medication with analgesics among adults (individuals aged at least 16 years) of both genders living in Spain. A total of 7,606 interviews were analysed. The dichotomous dependent variables chosen were the answers "yes" or "no" to the question In the last 2 weeks have you taken the medicines not prescribed for you by a doctor for joint pain, headache, or low back pain?" Independent variables were sociodemographic, comorbidity, and healthcare resources.

Results: A total of 7,606 individuals reported pain in any of the locations (23.7%). In addition, analgesic consumption was self-prescribed in 23.7% (1,481) of these subjects. Forty percent (40.1%) of patients self-medicated for headache, 15.1% for low back pain, and 6.7% for joint pain. The variables significantly associated with a greater likelihood of self-medication of analgesics, independently of pain location, were: age 16–39 years (2.36 < AOR < 3.68), higher educational level (1.80 < AOR <2.21), psychological disorders (1.56 < AOR < 1.98), and excellent/good perception of health status (1.74 < AOR < 2.68). In subjects suffering headache, self-prescription was associated with male gender (AOR 2.13) and absence of other comorbid condition (AOR 4.65).

Conclusions: This pharmacoepidemiology study constitutes an adequate approach to analgesic self-medication use in the Spanish population, based on a representative nationwide sample. Self-prescribed analgesic consumption was higher in young people with higher educational level, higher income, smoker, and with psychological disorders and with a good perception of their health status independently of the location of pain.

Background

Pain is a common human experience that is explained through a complex study of people within everyday environments and social context [1,2]. It is one of the main causes of morbidity worldwide affecting 10% to 30% of the European adult population; however, some studies have reported prevalence up to 50% [3-7]. In North America, the prevalence rate is 31% [8].

Pain is studied from different viewpoints. Associated psychological aspects can affect the consumption of analgesics. In fact, depression, anxiety and personality traits should be taken into consideration when analyzing how pain is perceived [9,10]. Self-care is practiced daily throughout by several people around the world. Self-medication is viewed as responsible involvement by private individuals in caring for themselves or members of their family [11]. This circumstance has been accentuated by the growing replacement of prescribed medicines by over-the-counter (OTC) remedies [12,13].

Pain relief occupies a prominent position within the broader context of self-medication [14,15]. Analgesics

* Correspondence: pilar.carrasco@urjc.es
[1]Department of Preventive Medicine and Public Health, Rey Juan Carlos University, Avda. Atenas s/n., Alcorcón, Madrid, Spain
Full list of author information is available at the end of the article

are the most commonly consumed drugs in the world, and it is estimated that millions of people in the United States, Australia, and Europe use OTC analgesics on a daily basis [16-18]. A Spanish study using data from the 2003 Spanish National Health Survey showed that, among individuals consuming analgesics, 39.4% were self-medicating [19].

Pain interrupts attention and interferes with daily life. Both psychological and social factors have been shown to predict outcome in individuals with chronic pain. In fact, depression is a common comorbidity, yet it is undiagnosed in clinical practice [20,21]. Given that psychiatric disorders are better diagnosed by structured interviews as part of the clinical practice, it is difficult to obtain reliable results in population-based studies. Some authors have used the generic SF-36 quality of life questionnaire in order to differentiate between patients with and without psychological disorders [22]. Further, health surveys are significantly commended as they collect valuable information related to musculoskeletal pain, which is not available from most other sources of information.

Therefore, the aims of the current study were: first, to ascertain the prevalence of self-medication with analgesics among the Spanish population; second, to identify variables associated to self-medication, including psychological disorders, mental health status, and socio-demographic and health-related variables.

Methods

We conducted a nationwide, descriptive, cross-sectional epidemiologic study on self-medication among adults (individuals aged at least 16 years) of both genders living in Spain. This study was based on data obtained from the European Health Interview Survey for Spain (2009). As this study was conducted using de-identified public-use databases, it was not necessary to have the approval of an ethics committee.

The 2009 European Health Interview Survey for Spain (EHISS)

The European Health Interview Survey (EHIS) was proposed by the European Commission to European Union Member States to create a health information system through comprehensive and coordinated surveys conducted in the European Statistical System under the responsibility of "Eurostat". In such a way, all European Union States would share common guidelines for the survey modules (health determinants, health status, health care, background variables) and designs and based on a common questionnaire. The EHIS is implemented every five years, with the first wave completed between 2008 and 2009 [23].

In Spain, the EHIS was conducted by the National Statistics Institute (*Instituto Nacional de Estadística*, INE) under the aegis of the Spanish Ministry of Health and Social Affairs in 2009. This survey is a computer-aided home-based personal interview including nationwide representative sample of civilian, non-institutionalized population aged ≥ 16 years and residing in primary family dwellings (households) in Spain. Study subjects were selected by means of probabilistic multistage sampling, with the first-stage units being census sections and the second-stage units being primary family dwellings. Details of EHISS methodology are described elsewhere [24]. The data collection period ranged from April 2009 to March 2010. The analysis was performed in January 2013.

Analgesic consumption definition

The dependent variable of the current study was created using the following two questions: "In the last two weeks have you taken those medicines prescribed for you by a doctor for joint pain, headache, or low back pain?", or, "In the last two weeks have you taken the medicines not prescribed for you by a doctor for joint pain, headache, or low back pain?" An affirmative answer to the first question was considered as "prescribed analgesic use". An affirmative answer to the second question was classified as "self-medicated analgesic use". Total analgesic use included those with both prescribed and self-medicated drugs.

Socio-demographic variables, lifestyle habits and co-morbid conditions

The following independent variables were included in the analysis. Main socio-demographic features including sex, age, marital status (married or not married), educational level (classified as no formal education, junior school or high school), occupational status (unemployed, employed or inactive), and monthly income.

Within lifestyle habits, smoking habit differentiated between current smokers or non-smokers. The alcohol consumption was measured using the question "Have you consumed alcoholic drinks in the previous 2 weeks?" Individuals were also asked for: "Do you practice any leisure time physical activity for at least 3 day per week? (Answer: active or inactive) Finally, the body mass index (BMI) was calculated from the self-reported body weight and height. Individuals with a BMI ≥ 30 were classified as obese.

Self-perceived health status was assessed with the following question: "How did you self-perceive your health status over the previous 12 months?" Subjects described health status as excellent, good, fair, poor or very poor. This variable was dichotomized into two: excellent/good or fair/poor/very poor self-perceived health status. Mental health was assessed with 2 indicators extracted from the Short-Form SF-36 quality of life questionnaire: psychological dysfunction and mental health status. Both indicators are obtained through 9 items which are scored from 0 to 100 points, where higher scores represent better mental health [25].

To identify individuals with associated chronic conditions, we used self-reported affirmative answer to the presence of any physician diagnosed concomitant diseases including hypertension, hypercholesterolemia, respiratory disease (asthma and chronic bronchitis), heart disease, diabetes, and cancer. We recorded whether patients had none, 1–2, or > 2 diseases. The presence of depression or anxiety (psychological disorders) was assessed using the following 2 questions: "Have you suffered from depression and/or anxiety the previous 12 months?", and, "Has your medical doctor confirmed the diagnosis?"

Statistical analysis

Self-medication patterns were identified using descriptive statistics of the main study variables by calculating the prevalence of total use and self-medication with analgesics for joint pain, headache, low back pain, and any pain localization during the years 2009–2010. Pearson χ^2 test was used for the bivariate comparison of proportions.

Mean scores were also obtained for those variables from SF-36 (psychological dysfunction and mental health status) by calculating the difference in means between those who consume analgesics and those who did not for each of the pain localizations analyzed in the study, as well as the difference in means between those who consumed prescription analgesics and those who were self-medicated with analgesics for joint pain, headache, low back pain, and any localization.

To estimate the independent effect of the study variables on self-medication with analgesic drugs, we obtained the corresponding adjusted odds ratio (AOR) and the 95% Confidence Interval (95% CI) by means of multivariate logistic regression analysis. All variables showing a significant association in the bivariate analysis were included in the multivariate analysis, along with those variables that were considered relevant according to scientific literature. Four models were generated, as follows: one to identify factors associated with self-medication using analgesic drugs for joint pain; a second model to identify those factors predicting self-medication with analgesic drugs for headache; a third model for self-medication with analgesic drugs for low back pain; and a fourth logistic regression model to identify those factors associated with self-medication with analgesic drugs for pain at any pain localization. Estimates were made using the svy (survey commands) functions of the STATA program (STATA Corp, College Station, Texas, USA), which enabled us to incorporate the sampling design and weights into all statistical calculations (descriptive, χ^2, logistic regression). Statistical significance was set at a 2-tailed $\alpha < 0.05$.

Results and discussion

Our results were based on data obtained from 7,606 subjects who answered the questions regarding consumption of analgesic medication (prescribed or self-medicated) in the 2 weeks immediately preceding the survey for any of the localizations analyzed. The sample represented 31.8% of subjects interviewed in the EHISS. Table 1 shows data on total analgesic consumption (with or without medical prescription) for joint pain headache, and low back pain and for any localization, according to socio-demographic characteristics, lifestyle, and health-related study variables. The results showed that 19.9% of the population consumed analgesics for low back pain, 12.6% for joint pain, and 10.9% for headache. The prevalence of consumption for pain at any localization was 39.8% for women and 23.5% for men (P < 0.05). Values for the consumption of analgesics were significantly higher when subjects were aged >65 years, had >2 chronic conditions, a chronic mental illness (anxiety and depression) or worse self-rated health status (P < 0.05).

When pain location was analyzed, analgesic consumption was higher in women than men, individuals with >2 chronic conditions, subjects with psychological disorders, and those subjects reporting fair/poor/very poor health status (P < 0.05). It is noteworthy that consumption of analgesics was also higher in smokers and drinkers compared to non-smokers and no drinkers (P < 0.05). Table 1 summarizes the average scores for psychological dysfunction and mental health status. Subjects exhibiting joint pain who consume analgesics had the lowest scores in both domains of the SF-36.

Analgesic drug consumption was self-prescribed in 23.7% (1,481) of the sample. Table 2 shows the results of the 4 analyses performed to determine the proportion of analgesic self-medication for each of pain localizations according to socio-demographic characteristics, lifestyle and health-related variables. Men self-medicated their analgesic consumption than women (P < 0.05) and self-medication was significantly higher in the population aged 16–39 years than in remaining age groups (P < 0.05). Analgesic self-medication was more frequent in smokers and drinkers than in non-smokers and those subjects who not drinking. Additionally, more over-the-count medication was consumed by subjects reporting excellent/good health status and no chronic diseases (P < 0.05).

When analgesic self-medication was analyzed by location, those experiencing headaches exhibited higher self-prescription (40.1%) than those suffering low back pain (15.1%) or joint pain (6.7%). The frequency of self-medication was higher in men than in women, in those

Table 1 Prevalence of analgesic consumption (prescribed and self-medicated) for joint pain, headache, low back pain and any pain localization in Spanish adult according to socio-demographic variables, lifestyle, and health profile

		Analgesic consumption for joint pain		Analgesic consumption for headache		Analgesic consumption for low back pain		Any localization	
		N	%	N	%	N	%	N	%
Age*+†‡	16-39	176	2.3	738	10.6	1025	14.5	1662	23.4
	40-64	1232	12.8	1086	10.9	1963	20.7	3058	32.6
	>65	2009	33.5	590	9.6	1807	29.3	2886	47.4
Sex*+†	Male	820	7.2	688	7.2	1532	14.4	2445	23.5
	Female	2597	17.9	1726	14.5	3263	25.1	5161	39.8
Marital status*†‡	Not married	1641	10.8	1104	10.8	2224	18.8	3519	29.9
	Married	1776	14.0	1310	11.0	2571	20.7	4087	33.3
Educational level*+†‡	No formal education	1353	33.2	488	12.4	1306	32.1	1993	49.1
	Junior school	1158	17.7	549	9.6	1291	21.4	2093	34.8
	High school	906	6.2	1377	11.1	2198	16.6	3520	26.8
Occupational status*+†‡	Unemployed	209	8.44	269	11.58	446	18.80	671	27.97
	Employed	866	6.99	1205	10.91	1952	16.97	3155	27.59
	Inactive	2342	23.61	940	10.73	2397	25.15	3780	40.26
Monthly income*†‡	<850€	932	22.2	417	12.0	999	26.1	1540	40.3
	850-1400€	875	15.8	520	11.0	1180	22.6	1786	34.6
	>1400€	1094	9.6	1100	11.0	1935	18.5	3111	29.9
Smoking habit*+†‡	Non smoker	2935	14.9	1747	10.6	3683	20.8	5860	33.2
	Smoker	482	7.1	667	11.8	1112	17.7	1746	28.4
Alcohol consumption*+†‡	No	2552	12.9	1863	11.9	3572	20.6	5648	33.0
	Yes	610	9.6	434	8.2	931	16.1	1541	26.7
Physical activity*†‡	Inactive	2167	15.1	1340	10.9	2891	22.0	4484	34.3
	Moderate	1250	10.1	1074	10.9	1904	17.7	3122	29.3
Body Mass Index Kg/sq.m*†‡	<30	2148	10.3	1831	10.8	3392	18.4	5418	29.7
	≥30	850	22.1	407	12.1	952	26.4	1491	41.2
Self-assessment of health status*+†‡	Very good/Good	859	4.6	1302	8.8	2079	12.9	3632	22.7
	Fair/Poor/Very poor	2558	35.5	1112	17.1	2716	39.7	3974	57.7
Number of chronic conditions*+†‡	None	1839	9.0	1631	10.1	3035	17.3	4961	28.3
	1-2	1367	23.0	691	13.4	1550	27.1	2360	42.2
	>2	211	44.9	92	18.7	210	44.7	285	60.0
Psychological disorders*+†‡	No	2361	10.1	1784	9.6	3580	17.4	5911	28.8
	Yes	1056	31.8	630	21.3	1215	38.4	1695	54.1
Psychological dysfunction*+†‡ (mean. se) [mean difference]		64.3 (0.5)	[−14.4]	68.2 (0.6)	[−9.88]	67.9 (0.4)	[−11.4]	69.8 (0.3)	[−10.48]
Positive mental health*+†‡ (mean. se) [mean difference]		50.6 (0.5)	[−20.3]	57.5 (0.6)	[−2.18]	56.2 (0.4)	[−15.1]	58.6 (0.3)	[−14.18]
TOTAL		3417	12.6	2414	10.9	4795	19.9	7606	31.8

European Health Interview Survey (EHIS, 2009).
*Analgesic consumption for joint pain, +Analgesic consumption for headache.
†Analgesic consumption for low back pain, ‡Total analgesic consumption for any localization.

without other chronic condition or without psychological disorders, and in those subjects reporting excellent/good health status (P < 0.05). The highest values for self-medication were always recorded for individuals suffering from headaches.

Table 2 also shows the average scores obtained for psychological dysfunction and mental health status for use of analgesics without prescription. Self-medication with analgesics for joint pain was the variable with the lowest scores in both domains of the SF-36.

Table 2 Proportion of self-prescribed analgesic medication for joint pain, headache, low back pain and any localization in Spanish adult according to socio-demographic variables, lifestyle, health profile

		Self-medication for joint pain		Self-medication for headache		Self-medication for low back pain		Self-medication for any localization	
		N	%	N	%	N	%	N	%
Age*+‡‡	16-39	42	19.8	406	57.2	270	28.0	655	41.5
	40-64	106	8.8	370	37.2	253	13.7	664	23.6
	>65	61	3.2	49	8.1	68	4.1	162	5.7
Sex+‡‡	Male	58	7.5	349	55.2	225	17.0	587	27.8
	Female	151	6.4	476	32.8	366	14.1	894	21.3
Marital status+‡‡	Not married	96	6.7	382	45.2	289	19.0	697	28.1
	Married	113	6.7	443	36.2	302	12.4	784	20.6
Educational level*+‡‡	No formal education	38	2.9	47	11.3	52	4.6	115	6.4
	Junior school	59	5.4	135	29.5	84	7.6	255	14.4
	High school	112	12.7	643	50.7	455	23.2	1111	35.2
Occupational status*+‡‡	Unemployed	16	8.15	98	36.62	58	14.10	151	23.20
	Employed	95	10.05	548	49.85	393	21.39	948	32.76
	Inactive	98	4.83	179	24.54	140	8.26	382	13.32
Monthly income*+‡‡	<850€	28	3.1	69	21.2	53	6.4	139	11.4
	850-1400€	42	4.9	152	33.5	122	11.1	282	18.0
	>1400€	96	9.1	455	45.7	342	19.8	815	29.3
Smoking habit*+‡‡	Non smoker	159	5.8	506	34.3	370	12.9	946	19.8
	Smoker	50	11.3	319	53.0	221	21.7	535	34.9
Alcohol consumption+‡‡	No	146	6.2	605	39.0	428	15.1	1075	23.8
	Si	54	9.2	209	52.3	147	18.7	375	28.0
Physical activity*+‡‡	Inactive	108	5.1	408	37.0	287	12.7	736	20.3
	Moderate	101	9.1	417	43.2	304	18.2	745	27.8
Body Mass Index Kg/sq.m*+‡‡	<30	157	7.8	699	43.6	491	17.1	1238	27.0
	≥30	34	4.3	95	27.6	71	8.8	175	13.9
Self-assessment of health status*+‡‡	Very good/Good	106	12.8	690	56.7	466	25.3	1173	36.2
	Fair/Poor/Very poor	103	4.5	135	15.9	125	5.7	308	9.7
Number of chronic conditions*+‡‡	None	153	9.4	686	47.1	473	18.6	1206	28.7
	1-2	53	3.7	136	25.3	112	8.9	263	13.9
	>2	3	1.4	3	3.3	6	2.8	12	4.2
Psychological disorders t*+‡‡	No	168	7.9	751	47.9	521	17.6	1326	27.0
	Si	41	3.8	74	13.6	70	6.8	155	10.6
Psychological dysfunction+‡ (mean. se) [mean difference]		69.80 (2.1)	[5.8]	76.94 (0.8)	[14.6]	74.41 (1.0)	[7.7]	76.14 (0.6)	[8.3]
Positive mental health*+‡ (mean. se) [mean difference]		56.76 (2.5)	[6.6]	67.55 (0.8)	[16.9]	65.54 (1.1)	[11.0]	66.56 (0.6)	[10.4]
TOTAL		209	6.7	825	40.1	591	15.1	1481	23.7

European Health Interview Survey (EHIS, 2009).
*Self-medication for joint pain, +Self-medication for headache.
†Self-medication for low back pain, ‡Self-medication for any localization.

The results of the multivariate logistic regression analysis (adjusted odd ratio) to identify predictors of self-medication with analgesics are summarized in Table 3. The variables that were significantly associated with a greater likelihood of self-medication of analgesics for joint pain were age (aged 16–39 years, OR 3.16 95% CI 1.75-5.71), high educational level (OR 2.21, 95% CI 1.31-3.71), psychological disorders (OR 1.56, 95% CI 1.01-2.46), and excellent/good perception of health status (OR 1.74, 95% CI 1.74-2.49). In subjects suffering headache, analgesic self-prescription was associated with age (aged 16–39 years, OR 3.68, 95% CI 2.25-6.03), male

Table 3 Factors associated with analgesic self-medication among consumers with joint pain, headache, low back pain and any localization in Spanish adult

		Self-medication for joint pain AOR, 95% CI	Self-medication for headache AOR, 95% CI	Self-medication for low back pain AOR, 95% CI	Self-medication for any localization AOR, 95% CI
	>65	1	1	1	1
Age	40-64	1.78 (1.18-2.70)	2.55 (1.63-3.99)	1.67 (1.12-2.47)	2.38 (1.82-3.09)
	16-39	3.16 (1.75-5.71)	3.68 (2.25-6.03)	2.36 (1.54-3.62)	3.71 (2.77-4.97)
Sex	Female	1	1	1	
	Male	NS	2.13 (1.66-2.73)	NS	NS
	No formal education	1	1	1	1
Educational level	Junior school	1.37 (0.81-2.33)	1.46 (0.85-2.53)	1.01 (0.62-1.62)	1.29 (0.93-1.80)
	High school/University	2.21 (1.31-3.71)	1.87 (1.09-3.19)	1.80 (1.15-2.82)	1.89 (1.37-2.62)
Marital status	Married	1	1	1	
	Not married	NS	NS	1.44 (1.11-1.87)	NS
	<850€	1	1	1	1
Monthly income	850-1400€	NS	NS	1.24 (0.82-1.89)	1.03 (0.77-1.38)
	>1400€	NS	NS	1.70 (1.14-2.54)	1.33 (1.01-1.75)
Smoking habit	Non smoker	1	1	1	1
	Smoker	NS	NS	1.28 (1.01-1.66)	1.34 (1.12-1.60)
Self-assessment of health status	Fair/Poor/Very poor	1	1	1	1
	Very good/Good	1.74 (1.22-2.49)	2.38 (1.74-3.26)	2.68 (1.97-3.65)	2.24 (1.81-2.78)
	>2	1	1	1	1
Number of chronic conditions	1-2	NS	3.45 (1.05-11.32)	NS	NS
	None	NS	4.65 (1.43-15.06)	NS	NS
Psychological disorders	No	1	1	1	1
	Yes	1.56 (1.01-2.46)	1.98 (1.37-2.88)	1.61 (1.11-2.32)	1.62 (1.24-2.11)

European Health Interview Survey (EHISS, 2009) for Spain.
Data are expressed as adjusted odds ratio (AOR) and 95% confidence intervals (95% CI).
NS: non-significant association.

gender (OR 2.13, 95% CI 1.66-2.73) and higher educational level (OR 1.87, 95% CI 1.09-3.19), absence of other comorbid condition (OR 4.65, 95% CI 1.43-15.06), psychological disorders (OR 1.98, 95% CI 1.37-2.88), and excellent/good perception of health status (OR 2.38, 95% CI 1.74-3.26). Finally, the variables associated with a greater likelihood of self-medication for low back pain were age (aged 16–39 years OR 2.36, 95% CI 1.54-3.62), high educational level (OR 1.80, 95% CI 1.15-2.82), to be not married (OR 1.44, 95% CI 1.11-1.87), high monthly income (OR 1.70, 95% CI 1.14-2.54), smoking (OR 1.28, 95% CI 1.01-1.66), psychological disorders (OR 1.61, 95% CI 1.11-2.32) and excellent/good perception of health status (OR 2.68, 95% CI 1.97-3.65).

When analyzed the variables associated with self-prescription of consumption of analgesics for the presence of pain in any localization, 6 variables were present: aged 16–39 years (OR 3.71, 95% CI 2.77-4.97), high educational level (OR 1.89, 95% CI 1.37-2.62), high monthly income (OR 1.33, 95% CI 1.01-1.75), smoking (OR 1.34,

95% CI 1.12-1.60), psychological disorders (OR 2.24, 95% CI 1.81-2.78), and excellent/good perception of health status (OR 1.62, 95% CI 1.24-2.11).

Analgesic drugs are worldwide used and are justified and necessary in cases of intense and frequent pain [14]. The results of our study showed that 23.7% of Spanish adults who consume analgesic medication use OTC drugs. Our data is higher than the 13.6% found in Finland [26], substantially lower than the 55% use of OTC analgesics found in Australian adults [15] but similar than in American adults (33%) [18]. It seems that self-prescription of analgesic drugs, i.e., OTC use is highly prevalent in populations across the world.

A common denominator associated with OTC analgesic drug consumption is the influence of gender. Although some studies using similar methodology than our study reported a higher probability of self-prescribed analgesic drug consumption in women [18,27,28], gender differences could be related to a higher prevalence of headaches in women since headaches are associated with greater consumption of both prescribed and OTC analgesics [29,30]. Nevertheless, Krymchantowski et al. found that men suffering chronic daily headache exhibited higher medication use than women [31]. It is possible that gender differences in self-prescribed analgesic consumption are related to several factors including specific co-morbid conditions and socio-cultural factors.

We found that subjects aged 19 to 39 years were almost 4 times as likely to use OTC analgesics for any pain location as elderly people. Current results also agree with previous studies. Stosic et al. showed a higher self-prescribed analgesic consumption and use of OTC drugs in Australian adults younger than 54 years old compared to those older than 55 years [15]. Wilcox et al. reported that American adults in the forties had a higher OTC analgesic consumption [18]. Current and previous results suggest that OTC drugs seem to be self-prescribed in a greater manner in the mid-age of the life, probably related to higher prevalence of pain syndromes and higher educational level. In fact, our results revealed that individuals taking OTC analgesics were young and highly educated (university level). Spanish university graduates were twice as likely to take OTC drug consumption as those with lower educational level. Klemenc-Ketis et al. found that 92% of Slovenian university students reported the use of self-medication [28]. These results agree with several published studies where OTC consumption was also associated with higher educational level [19,32,33]. Self-medication is more common among healthcare professionals (e.g. physicians, nurses, and pharmacists) than in the general population [34,35]. This can be related to the fact that healthcare professionals have university studies in almost all countries.

Further, a higher level of education can be related to a higher monthly income. When variable monthly income was analyzed, the results showed that subjects earning more than €1400 per month were more likely to take OTC analgesics, especially for back pain. These data are consistent with those reported in a recent study conducted in American adults where individuals with lower income were less likely to consume OTC non-steroidal anti-inflammatory drugs than those subjects with a higher income [33]. It is possible that a higher educational level involves higher monetary income and both variables are related to greater self-prescription consumption for pain.

Our results showed that smokers were more likely to self-medicate than the non-smoker population. This finding was similar to that previously reported by Hagen et al. in Norwegian adults who observed that smokers exhibited double risk of suffering from medication overuse headache [36]. Although experimental studies support that nicotine has analgesic properties, epidemiological evidence suggests that smoking is a risk factor for chronic pain [37].

Other factors associated with self-prescription of analgesic consumption were the absence of com-morbid conditions, only for those subjects suffering from headaches and excellent/good perception of health status. Previous studies had shown that people with chronic diseases or poor perception of health status are more likely to use analgesic medication [14,26,38] which is in accordance with our results. This observation may be related to cultural attitudes to pain [1] or the fact that individuals who self-medicate visit their doctor less often since their pain is less severe. This would be of particular interest in head pain, since headaches of lower/mild intensity can be usually controlled with analgesics. In fact, analgesics are usually consumed by subjects with sporadic pain symptoms. However, unnecessary analgesic use should be avoided since some drugs imply specific risks and, in the case or headaches, can produce medication overuse headache. The biggest challenge for health care professionals remains the provision of adequate pain management on an individual basis [24].

It is well accepted that pain is associated with psychological factors, particularly depression. Anxiety and depression have received the main attention, mostly in relation to recurrence and chronic pain in individuals with low back pain due to its relationship with physical disability and work absenteeism [9,39]. Our results showed a statistically significant association between the presence of psychological disorders (assessed with the SF-36 questionnaire) and self-medication for all the types of pain analyzed, although the strongest association was found in individuals suffering from headaches. Our results are in line with those previously found in Swedish people in who chronic headache was more prevalent in subjects who overused analgesics (39.8%) than in those who did not (18%) [40]. This study also observed that depression was significantly associated factor for analgesic overuse in general (OR 3.52, 1.46-8.52) [40].

In this context, community pharmacists are important members of health-care team. The pharmacists are probably the health professionals who are closest and most accessible to the patients and the general population. Their opinions related to health education have an important impact on the health of the population [41,42].

Although strengths of our study include large sample size, a randomly selected population, the employment of standardized survey, and training of the data collectors; there are also a number of possible limitations. First, since we used data from a cross-sectional survey, we cannot determine cause and effect relationships between the variables associated with self-prescribed medication use. Second, the conclusions drawn are difficult to generalize, because the survey has not been validated for drug use. Third, information obtained on interviews is subjective and may be subject to recall errors or a tendency of subjects to give socially desirable responses in the interviews. In addition, several of the data obtained from the interviews were self-reported which can induce a bias and, therefore, the prevalence of self-medication may be underestimated. Another possible limitation is that the survey rather than identifying specific active ingredients, it identifies groups of medications for specific diseases. Nonetheless, health surveys are significantly commended as they collect valuable information related to musculoskeletal pain problems, which is not available from most other sources of information.

Conclusions

This pharmacoepidemiology study constitutes an adequate approach to analgesic self-medication use in the Spanish population, based on a representative nationwide sample. Our study found that 23.7% of Spanish adults use self-prescribed analgesic drug consumption to treat their pain with the highest incidence in headache (40.1%). We also observed that analgesic consumption without prescription seems to be higher in young people with higher educational level, higher monthly income, and smoker. In addition, subjects with psychological disorders and with a good perception of their health status also self-prescribed analgesic drugs. Further, self-prescribed analgesic consumption for headache was more frequent in men without co-morbid chronic diseases.

Competing interests

Financial competing interests
This study forms part of a project funded by the Fondo de Investigaciones Sanitarias (FIS) of the Carlos III Institute of Public Health.

Non-financial competing interests
All of the authors declare no financial political, personal, religious, ideological, academic, intellectual, commercial or any other conflicts of interest, and none related to study interpretation.

Authors' contributions

(CGP): Researched data, wrote the manuscript, contributed to the discussion and reviewed/edited the manuscript. (LAA): Contributed to the discussion and reviewed/edited the manuscript. (HBV): Researched data and reviewed/edited the manuscript. (JTI), (FPC), (PCD) and (GGS): Contributed to the discussion and reviewed/edited the manuscript (JGR): Researched data, contributed to the discussion, and reviewed/edited the manuscript. All authors reviewed and gave their final approval of the version to be submitted

Acknowledgments

This study forms part of a project funded by the Fondo de Investigaciones Sanitarias (FIS) of the Carlos III Institute of Public Health (reference PI13/00369).

Author details

[1]Department of Preventive Medicine and Public Health, Rey Juan Carlos University, Avda. Atenas s/n., Alcorcón, Madrid, Spain. [2]Department of Physical Therapy, Occupational Therapy, Rehabilitation and Physical Medicine, Rey Juan Carlos University, Alcorcón, Madrid, Spain. [3]Department of Nursing, Rey Juan Carlos University, Alcorcón, Madrid, Spain. [4]Department of Human Histology and Pathological Anatomy, Rey Juan Carlos University, Alcorcón, Madrid, Spain.

References

1. Eccleston C: A normal psychology of everyday pain. Int J Clin Pract Suppl 2013, 178:47–50.
2. Langford RM: Pain management today-what have we learned? Clin Rheumatol 2006, 25:S2–S8.
3. Langley P: The prevalence, correlates and treatment of pain in the European Union. Curr Med Res Opin 2011, 27:463–480.
4. Breivik H, Collett B, Ventafridda V, Cohen R, Gallacher D: Survey of chronic pain in Europe: prevalence, impact on daily life, and treatment. Eur J Pain 2006, 10:287–333.
5. Leijon O, Wahlström J, Mulder M: Prevalence of self-reported neck-shoulder-arm pain and concurrent low back pain or psychological distress: time-trends in a general population, 1990–2006. Spine 2009, 34:1863–1868.
6. Fricker J: Pain in Europe report. Research project by NFO Worldgroup, Mundipharma International Limited, Cambridge, UK. 2003, [available] http://www.paineurope.com/painsurveys/pain-in-europe-survey/publication-for-download.html.
7. Harker J, Reid KJ, Bekkering GE, Kellen E, Bala MM, Riemsma R, Worthy G, Misso K, Kleijnen J: Epidemiology of chronic pain in Denmark and Sweden. Pain Res Treat 2012, 2012:371248.
8. Strine TW, Hootman JM: US national prevalence and correlates of low back and neck pain among adults. Arthritis Rheum 2007, 57:656–665.
9. Mok LC, Lee IF: Anxiety, depression and pain intensity in patients with low back pain who are admitted to acute care hospitals. J Clin Nurs 2008, 17:1471–1480.
10. Haggman S, Maher CG, Refshauge KM: Screening for symptoms of depression by physical therapists managing low back pain. Phys Ther 2004, 84(12):1157–1166.
11. Ryan A, Wilson S, Taylor A, Greenfield S: Factors associated with self-care activities among adults in the United Kingdom: a systematic review. BMC Public Health 2009, 9:96.
12. Hanna LA, Hughes CM: Public's views on making decisions about over-the-counter medication and their attitudes towards evidence of effectiveness: a cross-sectional questionnaire study. Patient Educ Couns 2011, 83:345–351.
13. Häussinger C, Ruhl UE, Hach I: Health beliefs and over-the-counter product use. Ann Pharmacother 2009, 43:1122–1127.
14. Sawyer P, Bodner EV, Ritchie CS, Allman RM: Pain and pain medication use in community-dwelling older adults. Am J Geriatr Pharmacother 2006, 4:316–324.
15. Stosic R, Dunagan F, Palmer H, Fowler T, Adams I: Responsible self-medication: perceived risks and benefits of over-the-counter analgesic use. Int J Pharm Pract 2011, 19:236–245.
16. Hersh EV, Pinto A, Moore PA: Adverse drug interactions involving common prescription and over-the-counter analgesic agents. Clin Ther 2007, 29:2477–2497.
17. Roumie CL, Griffin MR: Over-the-counter analgesics in older adults: a call for improved labelling and consumer education Drugs Aging. 2004, 21:485–498.
18. Wilcox CM, Cryer B, Triadafilopoulos G: Patterns of use and public perception of over-the-counter pain relievers: focus on nonsteroidal antiinflammatory drugs. J Rheumatol 2005, 32:2218–2224.
19. Carrasco-Garrido P, Jiménez-García R, Barrera-Hernandez V, Gil de Miguel A: Predictive factors of self-medicated drug use among the Spanish adult population. Pharmacoepidemiol Drug Saf 2008, 17:193–199.
20. Walsh TL, Homa K, Hanscom B, Lurie J, Sepulveda MG, Abdu W: Screening for depressive symptoms in patients with chronic spinal pain using the SF-36 Health Survey. Spine J 2006, 6:316–320.
21. Keeley P, Creed F, Tomenson B, Todd C, Borglin G, Dickens C: Psychosocial predictors of health-related quality of life and health service utilisation in people with chronic low back pain. Pain 2008, 135:142–150.
22. Oswald J, Salemi S, Michel BA, Sprott H: Use of the short-form-36 health survey to detect a subgroup of fibromyalgia patients with psychological dysfunction. Clin Rheumatol 2008, 27:919–921.
23. European Commission: Eurostat. European health interview survey (EHIS). Accessed: April 5, 2013. Available at: http://epp.eurostat.ec.europa.eu/portal/page/portal/microdata/european_health_interview_survey.

24. Insituto Nacional de Estadistica: **Encuesta Europea de Salud para España.** Available at: http://www.ine.es/metodologia/t15/t153042009.pdf. Accessed: April 5, 2013.

25. Ware JE Jr, The SCD, MOS: **36-item short-form health survey (SF-36). I. Conceptual framework and item selection.** *Med Care* 1992, **30**:473–483.

26. Turunen JH, Mäntyselkä PT, Kumpusalo EA, Ahonen RS: **Frequent analgesic use at population level: prevalence and patterns of use.** *Pain* 2005, **115**:374–381.

27. Carrasco-Garrido P, Hernández-Barrera V, López de Andrés A, Jiménez-Trujillo I, Jiménez-García R: **Sex-differences on self-medication in Spain.** *Pharmacoepidemiol Drug Saf* 2010, **19**:1293–1299.

28. Klemenc-Ketis Z, Hladnik Z, Kersnik J: **A cross sectional study of sex differences in self-medication practices among university students in Slovenia.** *Coll Antropol* 2011, **35**:329–334.

29. Colás R, Muñoz P, Temprano R, Gómez C, Pascual J: **Chronic daily headache with analgesic overuse: epidemiology and impact on quality of life.** *Neurology* 2004, **62**:1338–1342.

30. Chilet-Rosell E, Ruiz-Cantero MT, Sáez JF, Alvarez-Dardet C: **Inequality in analgesic prescription in Spain. A gender development issue.** *Gac Sanit* 2013, **27**:135–142.

31. Krymchantowski AV, Moreira PF: **Clinical presentation of transformed migraine: possible differences among male and female patients.** *Cephalalgia* 2001, **21**:558–566.

32. Al-Windi A, Elmfeldt D, Svärdsudd K: **Determinants of drug utilisation in a Swedish municipality.** *Pharmacoepidemiol Drug Saf* 2004, **13**(2):97–103.

33. Delaney JA, Biggs ML, Kronmal RA, Psaty BM: **Demographic, medical, and behavioral characteristics associated with over the counter non-steroidal anti-inflammatory drug use in a population-based cohort: results from the Multi-Ethnic Study of Atherosclerosi.** *Pharmacoepidemiol Drug Saf* 2011, **20**:83–89.

34. Montgomery AJ, Bradley C, Rochfort A, Panagopoulou E: **A review of self-medication in physicians and medical students.** *Occup Med* 2011, **61**:490–497.

35. Klemenc-Ketis Z, Hladnik Z, Kersnik J: **Self-medication among healthcare and non-healthcare students at University of Ljubljana, Slovenia.** *Med Princ Pract* 2010, **19**:395–401.

36. Hagen K, Linde M, Steiner TJ, Stovner LJ, Zwart JA: **Risk factors for medication-overuse headache: an 11-year follow-up study. The Nord-Trøndelag Health Studies.** *Pain* 2012, **153**:56–61.

37. Weingarten TN, Podduturu VR, Hooten WM, Thompson JM, Luedtke CA, Oh TH: **Impact of tobacco use in patients presenting to a multidisciplinary outpatient treatment program for fibromyalgia.** *Clin J Pain* 2009, **25**:39–43.

38. Nielsen MW, Hansen EH, Rasmussen NK: **Prescription and non-prescription medicine use in Denmark: association with socio-economic position.** *Eur J Clin Pharmacol* 2003, **59**:677–684.

39. Schiphorst Preuper HR, Reneman MF, Boonstra AM, Dijkstra PU, Versteegen GJ, Geertzen JH, Brouwer S: **Relationship between psychological factors and performance-based and self-reported disability in chronic low back pain.** *Eur Spine J* 2008, **17**:1448–1456.

40. Schmid CW, Maurer K, Schmid DM, Alon E, Spahn DR, Gantenbein AR, Sandor PS: **Prevalence of medication overuse headache in an interdisciplinary pain clinic.** *J Headache Pain* 2013, **14**:4.

41. Caamaño F, Alvarez R, Khoury M: **The community pharmacists and their practice as health care providers.** *Gac Sanit* 2008, **22**(4):385.

42. Hanna LA, Hughes CM: **Pharmacists' attitudes towards an evidence-based approach for over-the-counter medication.** *Int J Clin Pharm* 2012, **34**(1):63–71.

6

Characterisation of an aerosol exposure system to evaluate the genotoxicity of whole mainstream cigarette smoke using the *in vitro* γH2AX assay by high content screening

Carolina Garcia-Canton[1,2]*, Graham Errington[1], Arturo Anadon[2] and Clive Meredith[1]

Abstract

Background: The genotoxic effect of cigarette smoke is routinely measured by treating cells with cigarette Particulate Matter (PM) at different dose levels in submerged cell cultures. However, PM exposure cannot be considered as a complete exposure as it does not contain the gas phase component of the cigarette smoke. The *in vitro* γH2AX assay by High Content Screening (HCS) has been suggested as a complementary tool to the standard battery of genotoxicity assays as it detects DNA double strand breaks in a high-throughput fashion. The aim of this study was to further optimise the *in vitro* γH2AX assay by HCS to enable aerosol exposure of human bronchial epithelial BEAS-2B cells at the air-liquid interface (ALI).

Methods: Whole mainstream cigarette smoke (WMCS) from two reference cigarettes (3R4F and M4A) were assessed for their genotoxic potential. During the study, a further characterisation of the Borgwaldt RM20S® aerosol exposure system to include single dilution assessment with a reference gas was also carried out.

Results: The results of the optimisation showed that both reference cigarettes produced a positive genotoxic response at all dilutions tested. However, the correlation between dose and response was low for both 3R4F and M4A (Pearson coefficient, r = −0.53 and −0.44 respectively). During the additional characterisation of the exposure system, it was observed that several pre-programmed dilutions did not perform as expected.

Conclusions: Overall, the *in vitro* γH2AX assay by HCS could be used to evaluate WMCS in cell cultures at the ALI. Additionally, the extended characterisation of the exposure system indicates that assessing the performance of the dilutions could improve the existing routine QC checks.

Keywords: GammaH2AX, DNA damage, *In vitro*, Cigarette smoke, Genotoxicity, High content screening

Background

Cigarette smoke is a complex aerosol mixture consisting of more than 6,000 identified compounds that can be divided between the particulate phase, accounting for 4.5% of the total aerosol mixture mass, and the gas phase, accounting for 95.5% of the total aerosol mixture mass [1].

Testing and understanding the toxicity of cigarette smoke *in vitro* is a key step in the characterisation of modified tobacco products with potentially reduced harm. Adopting such strategies are in line with recommendations published by the Institute of Medicine "Clearing the Smoke" [2] and the World Health Organisation Framework convention on Tobacco Control (WHO FCTC) "The scientific basis of tobacco product regulation" [3].

Johnson and colleagues published a thorough review on the *in vitro* systems used to evaluate the toxicity of cigarette smoke [4]. In this review, the authors highlighted that the majority of tobacco-related *in vitro* toxicology studies are carried out in non-human cell models which are poorly validated for tobacco product comparison. They also concluded that better methods are needed, especially

* Correspondence: Carolina_Garcia-Canton@bat.com
[1]British American Tobacco, Group Research and Development, Regents Park Road, Southampton, Hampshire SO15 8TL, UK
[2]Department of Toxicology and Pharmacology, Universidad Complutense de Madrid, Madrid, Spain

in relation to regulation and health claims. In the field of *in vitro* genotoxicity, the authors described that the evaluation of cigarette smoke has been carried out using mainly cigarette smoke condensate (CSC). However, CSC contains primarily particulate phase components compared to whole mainstream cigarette smoke (WMCS) which contains both particulate and gas phase components. We consider WMCS a more comprehensive exposure system to study toxicological effects *in vitro* (Table 1). Moreover, the *in vitro* genotoxicity data has been mainly obtained from animal-derived cell systems which are functionally very different from human-derived cells.

There are different *in vitro* genotoxicity assays that have been widely used in the assessment of tobacco products [4]. Some of the assays described such as the micronucleus or the mouse lymphoma assay focus on fixed DNA damage like chromosomal damage and mutations, their strengths and limitations have been previously summarised [7]. The comet assay is the only assay described by Johnson and colleagues that specifically detects DNA strand breaks. Although the assay is widely accepted and considered a mature method [8], it does not discriminate between single or double strand breaks and has shown high inter- and intra-experimental variation [9]. The *in vitro* γH2AX assay, on the other hand, is an emerging method for DNA damage detection. The phosphorylation of H2AX (named γH2AX) in response to DNA double strand breaks (DSB) was first described in 1998 [10] and has since been extensively investigated [11]. Some applications in which γH2AX has been used as a biomarker of DNA damage are pre-clinical drug development and clinical studies [12]. More recently, γH2AX has been suggested as a potential complement to the current battery of *in vitro* genotoxicity assays with applications in the assessment of cigarette smoke [7,13].

The aim of this study was to optimise the novel *in vitro* γH2AX assay by High Content Screening (HCS) that we had previously developed [14], in order to adapt it for the assessment of aerosols and to evaluate the genotoxic effect of two reference cigarettes in human lung-derived BEAS-2B cells at the air-liquid interface (ALI). The optimisation employs the Borgwaldt RM20S® smoking machine (RM20S®) as part of the exposure system that delivers WMCS to cells at the ALI [5].

The *in vitro* γH2AX assay has been previously used in the assessment of cigarette smoke using mainly CSC and indirect exposure to WMCS i.e. cell cultures that had a layer of media covering the cells continuously or intermittently during smoke exposure and therefore not considered true ALI exposure [15-19]. In general, flow cytometry has been the main method for γH2AX detection and analysis. In this study, we selected a microscopy-based automated scoring system known as HCS to acquire and quantify the γH2AX response after WMCS exposure to BEAS-2B cells at the ALI. WMCS was tested from two different cigarettes, 3R4F a reference cigarette from the University of Kentucky [20] and M4A a historical control used as internal reference in genotoxicity studies by British American Tobacco [21].

Overall, the results show that the *in vitro* γH2AX by HCS can be used as a high throughput tool to assess the genotoxic effect of WMCS in cultures exposed at the ALI. The results can be used to compare the genotoxic responses of different tobacco products. Furthermore, the optimised *in vitro* γH2AX assay for aerosol exposure could be a useful high content screening tool to assess the genotoxic potential of toxicants in gaseous form.

Methods

Cell culture

The human bronchial epithelial cell line BEAS-2B was purchased from ATCC (United States). Normal bronchial epithelium cells obtained from autopsy of non-cancerous individuals had been isolated, then infected with a replication-defective 12-SV40/adenovirus hybrid (Ad12SV40) and cloned to create an immortalised phenotype [22]. Cells were seeded into culture vessels that had been pre-coated with 0.03 mg/mL PureCol® bovine collagen solution (Nutacon, The Netherlands). Cells were then maintained in Bronchial Epithelial Growth Medium (BEGM®) at 37°C and 5% CO_2 in a humidified

Table 1 Physical forms of cigarette smoke used in *in vitro* testing

Name	Description
Cigarette smoke condensate (CSC)	Comprises the particulate phase along with some vapour phase components. Generated by cold-trapping and condensation of smoke at extremely low temperatures. The condensed 'tar' is then typically extracted and diluted using acetone.
Cigarette smoke particulate matter (PM)	Comprises the particulate phase only. Particulates are typically collected by passing cigarette smoke through a Cambridge filter pad and are subsequently eluted from the filter pad using a solvent such as dimethylsulphoxide.
Cigarette smoke extract (CSE)	Comprises the particulate phase along with some vapour phase components. Generated by bubbling smoke through a liquid (e.g. phosphate-buffered saline or cell culture medium).
Whole mainstream cigarette smoke (WMCS)	Cells are directly exposed to smoke at the air-liquid interface. This is more representative of human exposure conditions, as cells are exposed to the gas and vapour phase components in an aerosol [5].

Table adapted from [6].

incubator. BEGM® was prepared by supplementing Bronchial Epithelial Basal Medium with growth supplements provided in the manufacturer's BEGM® SingleQuot® kit (Lonza Group Ltd., Belgium) containing: bovine pituitary extract, hydrocortisone, human epidermal growth factor, epinephrine, insulin, triiodothyronine, transferrin, gentamicin /amphotericin-B and retinoic acid. BEAS-2B cells were cultured and expanded in-house, the cells were used between passages 3 and 12 only. All cultures were negative for mycoplasma. Additionally, the cells were authenticated using the short tandem repeat profiling to confirm the nature of the cell cultures (LGC Standards, United Kingdom) [23].

Smoking system

The selection of the RM20S® 8-syringe smoking machine as the WMCS exposure system was based on previous *in vitro* studies [5,24] and thorough evaluations of precision, accuracy, repeatability and reproducibility [25,26]. The smoking exposure system is schematically represented in Figure 1. The RM20S® employs a dilution system that mixes WMCS with different proportions of air to generate a dilution ratio represented as 1 : X (smoke volume : air volume). Cigarettes are automatically loaded into cigarette holders (Figure 1A) where WMCS is drawn directly into the glass syringe and diluted with air taken from the laboratory environment (Figure 1B) following a multi-step process operated by a plunger (Figure 1C). The diluted WMCS is then delivered to an exposure chamber (Figure 1D) containing four Transwell® inserts with BEAS-2B cells seeded on top of the insert's membrane (Figure 1E). At the time of the exposure the cells are directly exposed to WMCS at the air-liquid interface (ALI).

Dilution performance evaluation

A range of dilutions were selected for this study from 1:25 to 1:20000 (smoke volume : air volume) (Table 2). The methodology employed by Kaur and colleagues used methane (CH_4) as a reference gas standard with known parts per million (PPM) to compare syringe performance and has been adapted here to assess dilution performance [25]. For our experiments, three different methane reference standards in nitrogen were purchased from Air Products PLC (United Kingdom), 10% containing 100,000 PPM methane, 50% containing 500,000 PPM methane and 99.95% containing 1,000,000 PPM methane. The relevant reference gas was loaded into a sealed bag and connected directly to the smoking machine cigarette

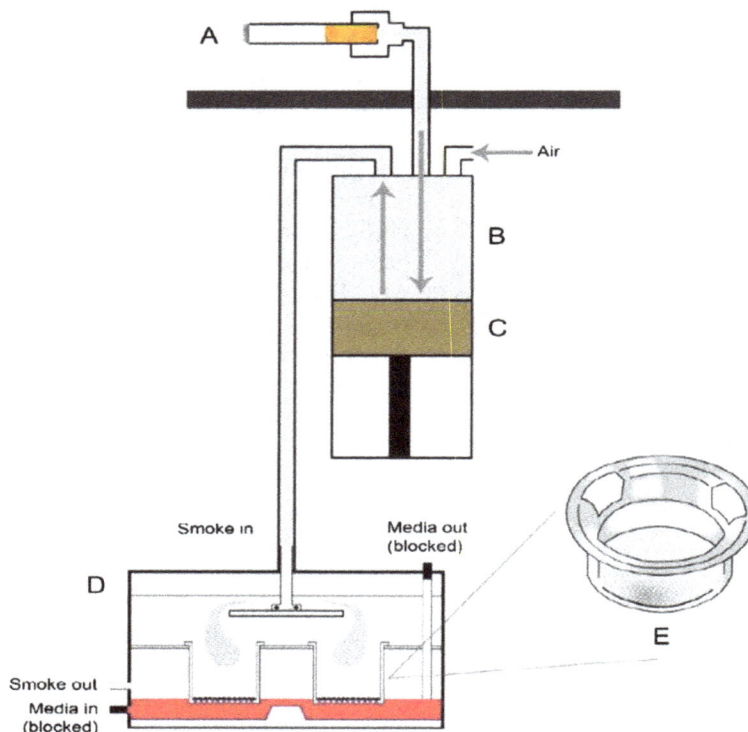

Figure 1 Schematic representation of a single RM20S® syringe combined with British American Tobacco's exposure chamber (UK patent publication WO 03/100417/ A1) (not to scale). The RM20S® can smoke up to eight cigarettes simultaneously. **[A]** Cigarette holder with cigarette in place; **[B]** 150 mL glass syringe where cigarette smoke dilution in air is prepared; **[C]** Plunger; **[D]** Exposure chamber containing porous membrane inserts with cells seeded on top at the ALI **[E]** Transwell® insert representation. Figure adapted from [26].

Table 2 Range of dilutions, details of methane reference gas and expected PPM

Dilutions	Expected PPM with 10% methane	Expected PPM with 50% methane	Expected PPM with 100% methane
1:25	4000		
1:50	2000		
1:100	1000		
1:250	400		
1:500	200		
1:1000	100		
1:1500	67		
1:2000		250	
1:3000		167	
1:4000		125	
1:6000		83	
1:8000		63	
1:16000			63
1:20000			50

holder (Figure 1A). The dilution to be tested was then programmed into the RM20S® and then gas diluted following International Standard Organization (ISO) 3308:2012 puffing profile consisting of 35 mL puff volume, 2 sec puff duration, and 60 sec puff interval [27]. A second empty sealed bag was connected to the exhaust position in the place of the exposure chamber to collect the diluted gas (Figure 1D). Quantification of methane in PPM was performed with a 3010 MINIFID portable heated flame ionization detector total hydrocarbon analyser (Signal Group Ltd, United Kingdom) as per manufacturer's instructions. Table 2 summarises details about dilutions, reference gas standard used per dilution and expected PPM. The laboratory environment was conditioned at $22 \pm 2°C$ and $60 \pm 5\%$ Relative Humidity (RH).

Smoke exposure

Cigarettes were conditioned for a minimum of 48 hours prior to use ($60 \pm 3\%$ relative humidity, $22 \pm 1°C$ according to ISO 3402:1999) [28] and smoked continuously throughout the exposure on a RM20S® smoking machine (Borgwaldt KC, Germany) using a 35 ml puff volume drawn over 2 seconds, once every minute according to ISO 3308:2012 [27]. The smoking environment was conditioned at $22 \pm 2°C$ and $60 \pm 5\%$ RH.

In this study two reference cigarettes were used to test whether the *in vitro* γH2AX assay by HCS could discriminate between products. The reference cigarette 3R4F supplied by the University of Kentucky, is a "US style" blended cigarette that delivers 9.4 mg tar and 0.7 mg nicotine under ISO conditions for cigarette smoking (ISO 3308:2012) [27]. Internal reference cigarette M4A is a flue

cured cigarette that delivers 10 mg of tar and 1.0 mg nicotine under ISO conditions for cigarette smoking (ISO 3308:2012) [27].

Controls

Etoposide (1 mM final) was used as a positive control during the experimentation (Sigma-Aldrich, United Kingdom). Etoposide is a well-known DNA-damaging compound and has previously been used in the *in vitro* γH2AX assay by HCS as a reference compound and positive control respectively [14,29]. Two different negative controls were used in this study; air control and incubator control. The air control was generated by the smoking machine to evaluate the quality of the air used to dilute the WMCS and mimic the exposure conditions. The incubator control evaluated the incubation conditions used to generate the positive controls.

WMCS treatment, γH2AX immunostaining and imaging analysis

The methodology used during this study to detect and quantify γH2AX by HCS was previously described [14] with variations for the ALI exposure. In this study, cells were seeded on top of the membrane of collagen precoated 24-Transwell® plate (Corning Incorporated Life Sciences, Unites States) at a concentration of 1.2×10^5 cells/mL and 500 μL of BEGM® were added underneath to keep the cells hydrated. The plates were then incubated overnight at 37°C in an atmosphere of 5% CO_2 in air. At the time of treatment, the culture media was removed from the Transwell® membrane so the cells could be exposed directly at the ALI. Then, four inserts were transferred to each exposure chamber containing 25 mL of Dulbecco's Modified Eagle Medium supplemented with 1% L-Glutamine and 0.5% penicillin/streptomycin (10000 IU/mL – 10000uG/mL). The exposure chambers were then placed in an incubator at 37°C and connected with plastic tubing to the smoking machine as represented in Figure 1D (smoke in/smoke out connectors). The smoking machine pre-programmed with the appropriate dilutions was set for a 3 hour exposure. We selected a 3 hour exposure as it is the minimum recommended in the International Conference on Harmonisation of Technical Requirements for Registration of Pharmaceuticals for Human Use (ICH guidelines) [30]. Following exposure, the inserts were placed in clean pre-labelled 24-well plates where the cells were fixed with 4% paraformaldehyde (100 μL/insert) and incubated for 15 minutes at room temperature. The fixed samples were processed for γH2AX immunostaining following manufacturer's recommendation (ThermoScientific, United States).

Image acquisition was performed using the Cellomics ArrayScan® VTI platform (ThermoScientific, USA). Image analysis used the Target Activation Bioapplication software v.6.6.1.4. The protocol was set to count a minimum of 500 cells per insert, giving a minimum of 2000 cells per concentration tested. Nuclear DNA staining (Hoechst dye) was used to identify viable cells nuclei. These nuclei were used as the target areas for the measurement of γH2AX specific fluorescence intensity represented as absolute intensity units. Viable cell counts from negative controls were defined as 100% cell viability. The viable cell counts in the WMCS and etoposide treated samples were then compared to those in the negative control, and the percentage cell viability was calculated and referred to as Relative Cell Counts (RCC).

Data analysis and criteria
Dilution performance evaluation
1-sample t-test was used to compare the results obtained in PPM for each dilution with the expected PPM. A variability of ±10% over the expected PPM was included afterwards as accepted measurement variation [31]. Repeatability and Reproducibility statistics were computed for all data points according to ISO 5725–2:1994 [32]. Experiments were replicated 3 times, with 6 repeats per dilution per experiment. Data analysis and graphical representations were performed with Minitab software v.16.

WMCS genotoxicity evaluation
The evaluation criteria used in this study (Table 3) was first described by Smart et al. for the analysis of γH2AX by flow cytometry [13] and recently applied by Garcia-Canton et al. for the analysis of γH2AX by HCS [14]. Experiments were replicated at least three times, with 4 repeats per dilution per experiment and graphical representation was performed using GraphPad Prism software v.6.01.

Results
The Borgwaldt RM20S® smoking machine combined with British American Tobacco's chamber were used as an exposure system during the optimisation of the novel in vitro γH2AX assay by HCS for the evaluation of aerosols.

The initial steps in this optimisation included extending the QC checks of the RM20S® to include 14 dilution performance evaluations (Table 2). From the 10 dilutions generating accurate deliveries, 6 smoke dilutions were

selected for further experiments based on range finder experiments (data not shown). The tested smoke dilutions covered a wide range of WMCS dilutions to assess the genotoxicity effect of two reference cigarettes (3R4F and M4A).

Dilution performance evaluation
An initial range of 14 dilutions from 1:25 to 1:20,000 were selected to evaluate the actual dilution delivery in PPM units using reference methane gases (Table 2). The data in Figure 2 graphically represents the results from the statistical 1-sample t-test analysis performed comparing PPM obtained per dilution (box plot) against the expected PPM (red dot), the analysis did not incorporate the ±10% tolerance accepted for machinery measurement variation and was, therefore, added to the expected PPM value afterwards [31]. Results indicate that in the majority of the cases (10 out of 14 dilutions) the dilution delivery was as expected when the ±10% tolerance was included in the analysis. There were four dilutions where the statistical analysis (1-sample t-test) showed a statistically significant difference between measured and expected PPM (including ±10% measurement variation), those dilutions are identified in Figure 2 with a hash (#) (1:1,000, 1:6,000, 1:8,000 and 1:20,000) and were not taken into consideration for the assessment of WMCS in the in vitro γH2AX assay.

Figure 3 represents the repeatability and reproducibility results indicating the precision of the smoking machine dilution performance within the same experiment and in different experiments respectively. The repeatability and reproducibility increased linearly with concentration as expected.

WMCS genotoxicity assessment
Initial range finder experiments showed that 3 hour exposures to WMCS from 3R4F cigarettes at dilutions more concentrated than 1:500 produced tar depositions, this effect was considered equivalent to precipitation. Only dilutions greater than 1:500 were included in further experiments. Both reference cigarettes 3R4F and M4A produced a significant increase in γH2AX frequency (above 1.5-fold increase) compared to the air-treated control in all the dilutions tested (Figure 4). In all experiments the positive control etoposide produced an increase greater than 1.5-fold compared to the air-treated control (Figure 4A and B). Relative Cell Counts (RCC) for all results presented were above the acceptance limit of toxicity (RCC > 25%) and therefore no cytotoxic-driven genotoxicity was observed (Table 3).

Figure 4A illustrates the response produced after 3 hour exposure to 3R4F WMCS. A variation in the response can be observed between the most concentrated WMCS (1:500) and the most diluted WMCS dilution (1:16,000).

Table 3 Genotoxicity evaluation criteria for the in vitro γH2AX assay by HCS

γH2AX response	Classification
> 1.5-fold γH2AX @ RCC > 25%	Genotoxic (+)
< 1.5-fold γH2AX @ RCC 100-0%	Non-genotoxic (−)
> 1.5-fold γH2AX @ RCC < 25%	"False" positive; Cytotoxic-driven genotoxicity (C)
1.5-fold γH2AX @ RCC ≥ 25%	Equivocal (±)

Table adapted from [13].

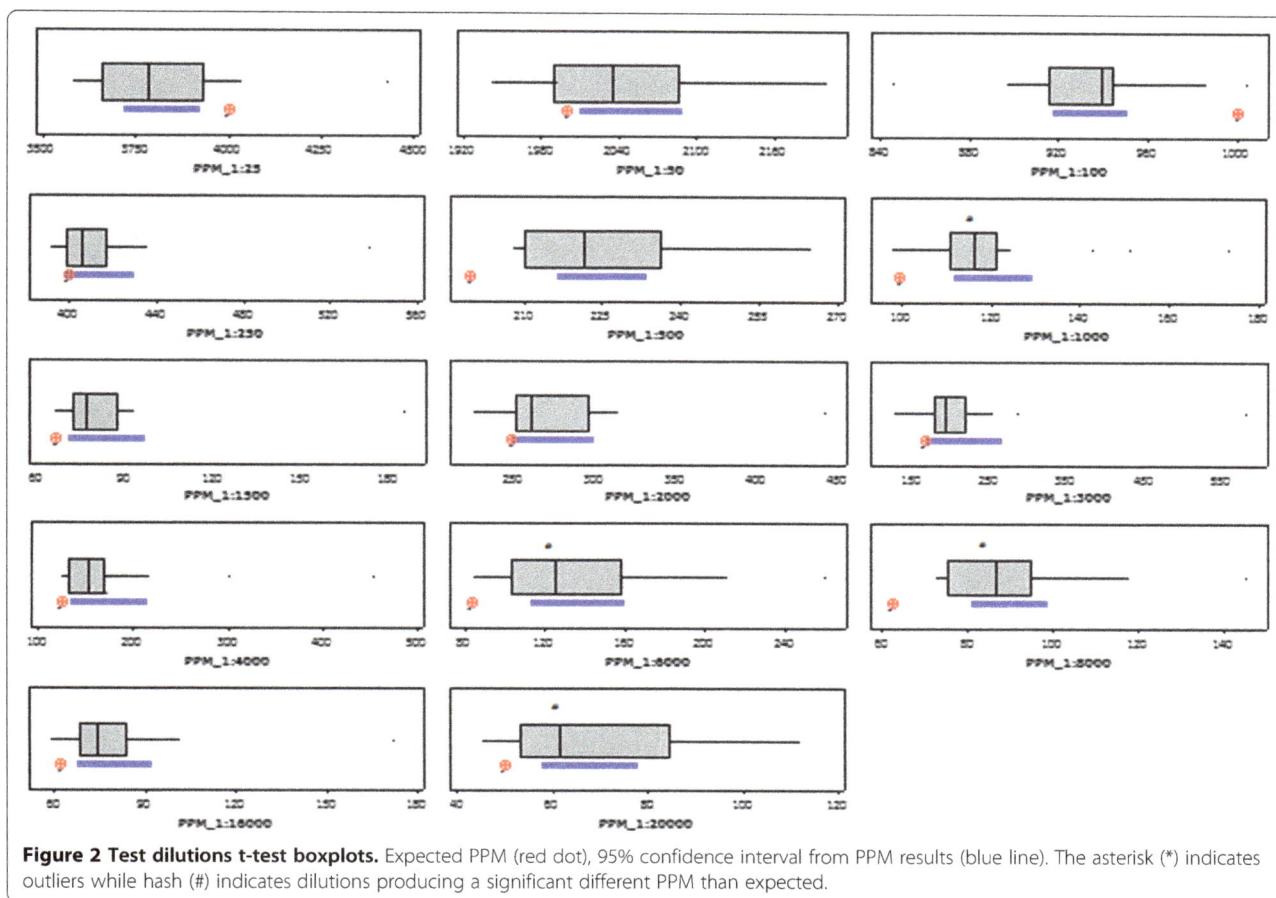

Figure 2 Test dilutions t-test boxplots. Expected PPM (red dot), 95% confidence interval from PPM results (blue line). The asterisk (*) indicates outliers while hash (#) indicates dilutions producing a significant different PPM than expected.

However, the linear regression model indicates a low correlation between the dose and the response (Pearson coefficient, r = –0.53). Figure 4B showed the results obtained after 3 hour exposure to M4A WMCS. In this case, a variation in the response can only be observed at the most diluted WMCS dilution tested (1:16,000). The linear regression model produced a low correlation between the dose and the response (Pearson coefficient r = –0.44).

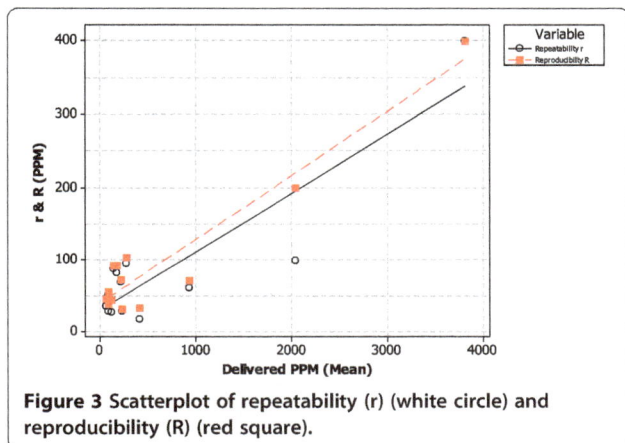

Figure 3 Scatterplot of repeatability (r) (white circle) and reproducibility (R) (red square).

Figure 4C graphically represents the fold-induction results from both reference cigarettes. In general, 3R4F WMCS exposure seems to have a more potent genotoxic effect compared to M4A WMCS exposure, especially at the most concentrated dilution 1:500.

Discussion

The main objective of this study was to optimise the novel *in vitro* γH2AX by HCS for the genotoxicity assessment of aerosols. During the optimisation, the genotoxic potential in the form of γH2AX induction from various dilutions of WMCS of two reference cigarettes were tested and differences in the response evaluated.

The cell system selected was the BEAS-2B cell line, a human-derived cell line from the lung, the first target tissue of inhaled aerosols. The non-tumorigenic human-derived BEAS-2B cell line was isolated from normal human epithelium and immortalised by virus infection [22]. The normal phenotype and wild-type p53 status support the use of this cell line in DNA damage studies [33-35]. BEAS-2B cells, however, lack normal metabolic activity for the majority of cytochrome P450 family, an essential factor for the phase I bioactivation of some cigarette smoke toxicants such as 4-(methylnitrosamino)-1-(3-

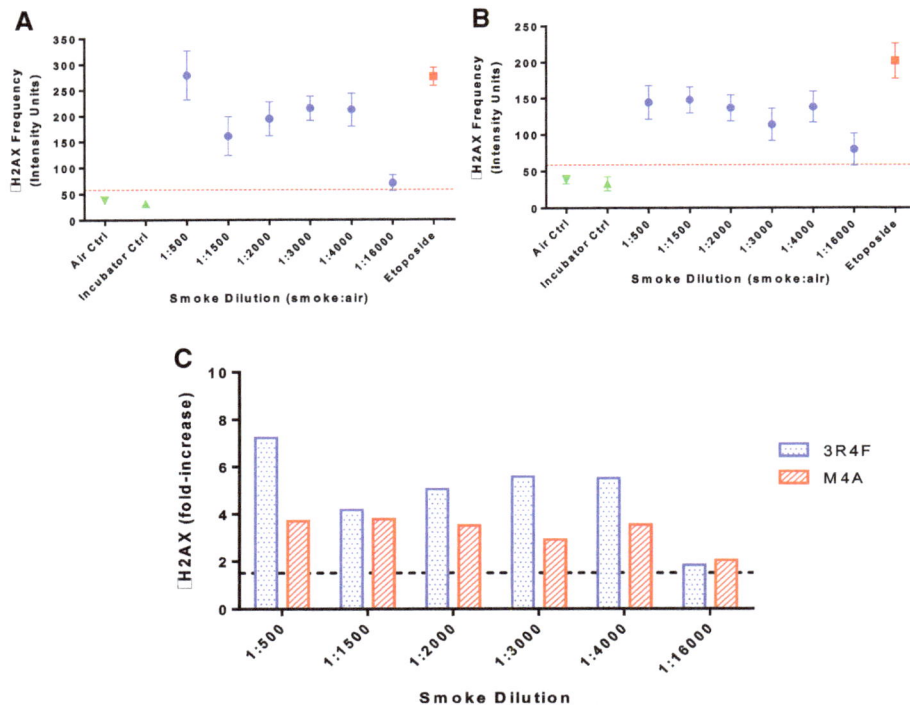

Figure 4 γH2AX frequency mean ± SD after 3 h exposure to WMCS from reference cigarette. **[A]** 3R4F, **[B]** M4A. Circle (−●-) represents WMCS results, square (−■-) represents positive control etoposide (1 mM final), triangles (−▼- and -▲-) represents negative controls, air and incubator controls respectively and dotted red line represents the 1.5-fold increase over the air control indicating the threshold of genotoxic response. **[C]** γH2AX fold-induction for both reference cigarettes 3R4F (blue) and M4A (red), dotted line indicates genotoxic level (>1.5-fold γH2AX response).

pyridyl)-1-butanone (NNK) [36]. The limitation in the metabolic capability of the cell line would need to be considered in future experimental designs i.e. including an external source of metabolic activation in part of the experiments to have a more comprehensive genotoxicity evaluation of the WMCS.

The Borgwaldt RM20S® smoking machine has been extensively used for the *in vitro* evaluation of WMCS [5,24,37]. Although, some QC analyses have been reported for the accurate performance of the syringes [25,26] further QC tests for the accurate performance of the programmed dilutions have proved necessary. Our results in this study indicate that not all of the programmed dilutions deliver the expected amount of reference gas in PPM (Figure 2). We have observed that more diluted dilutions seem to produce less accurate deliveries; this effect could be caused by the smoking machine dilution programming. The smoking machine performs a multistep process to dilute WMCS with laboratory conditioned air, the process requires the programming of more dilution steps for more diluted dilutions, hence, the potential for more variation. The discrepancy between expected and delivered aerosol could affect the exposure to the cell cultures and

ultimately the outcome of the assay. The same approach could be applied in the future to the particulate phase expected in the different dilutions employing Quartz Crystal Microbalances (QCM) previously described for this aerosol exposure system [38]. Nevertheless, the smoking machine performance has shown an overall good reproducibility and repeatability from dilutions delivering 50 PPM or above as can be seen in Figure 3. The performance of syringes and dilutions can be carried out using the same methodology and apparatus already in place for the standard QC checks. Moreover, the extended QC check could easily be incorporated into the routine service of the Borgwaldt RM20S® smoking machine.

The γH2AX results obtained during the assessment of two reference cigarettes seem to indicate that the *in vitro* γH2AX assay by HCS was able to detect the genotoxic potential of WMCS, however the correlation between the dose and the response was low for both reference cigarettes evaluated in this study across all the tested dilutions (Figure 4). Nevertheless, the γH2AX response obtained after BEAS-2B cells were exposed to a range of 3R4F WMCS dilutions for 3 hours was in general more potent than the response obtained for M4A

WMCS and can be visually observed in Figure 4C. If the genotoxicity response was primarily associated to the gas phase we would have expected a better γH2AX dose–response correlation with the different dilutions tested. Therefore, we have considered that the particulate phase may have a significant effect in driving the genotoxic potential. This could be further investigated by characterising the particulates deposited at different dilution levels with tools such as the QCM balance mentioned earlier in this discussion.

It is important to notice that 3 hour continuous exposure as recommended by ICH guidelines [30] could be the longest exposure time a submerged monolayer culture might be exposed at the ALI. In our experiments, the cell cultures were immediately fixed after the exposure to evaluate the DNA damage in the form of γH2AX. Pilot experiments were conducted where the cell cultures were left to recover for a further 24 hours submerged in media to evaluate potential DNA repair after the acute 3 hour exposure. The proliferation of the BEAS-2B cells was greatly affected in WMCS and air control samples. Interestingly, the same effect was not observed in incubator control cultures where the humidity is maintained at a higher level (data not shown). We concluded that for *in vitro* assays using submerged cultures as cell systems, 3 hour exposure at the current conditions of ALI exposure system would cause irreversible damage due to drying as opposed to aerosol exposure.

Following the optimisation described in this study, further investigations employing different exposure times, a larger number of products and an external source of metabolic activation would be necessary to support the applicability of the *in vitro* γH2AX assay for the evaluation of tobacco products in aerosol exposure. Future work could also carry out an in-depth characterisation on the effect that product variations such as different tobacco blends have in γH2AX induction to understand the differences in response.

Nevertheless, the optimisation performed here could also be applied to the genotoxicity evaluation of other aerosols such as aerosolised drugs, pollutants and cigarette smoke toxicants present in the gas phase (e.g. benzene).

Conclusions

Overall, the *in vitro* γH2AX assay by HCS could be used to evaluate WMCS in cell cultures at the ALI. Additionally, the extended characterisation of the exposure system indicates that assessing the performance of the dilutions could improve the existing routine QC checks.

Abbreviation

ALI: Air liquid interfase; BEGM: Bronchial epithelial growth medium; CSC: Cigarette smoke condensate; CSE: Cigarette smoke extract; DSB: Double strand break; HCS: High content screening; ISO: International standard organization; PM: Particulate matter; PPM: Parts per million; QCM: Quartz crystal microbalance; RCC: Relative cell count; RH: Relative humidity; SD: Standard deviation; WHO FCTC: World health organisation framework convention on tobacco control; WMCS: Whole mainstream cigarette smoke.

Competing interests

The authors declare that they have no competing interests.

Authors' contribution

CGC, GE and CM designed the study. CGC conducted all the experiments. Data analysis was performed by CGC and GE. CGC wrote the manuscript with GE and CM support. CM and AA provided scientific support. All authors approved the final manuscript.

Acknowledgements

This work was supported by Group Research and Development of British American Tobacco (Investments) Ltd as part of its research programme focusing on reducing the health impact of tobacco use. C. Garcia-Canton, G. Errington and C. Meredith are employees of British American Tobacco. A. Anadón is employee of the University Complutense of Madrid and has not received any funding for this research.
The authors thank Mr N. Asquith, Mr M. Barber and Mr D. Azzopardi for their technical help and support during the experimental phase; and Dr E Minet for his scientific advice while writing this manuscript.

References

1.　Rodgman A, Perfetti TA: **The Chemical Components of Tobacco and Tobacco Smoke**. 2nd edition. Edited by CRC Press. Florida (USA): 2013.
2.　Stratton K, Shetty P, Wallace R, Bondurant S: **Clearing the smoke: Assessing the science base for tobacco harm reduction**. Edited by National Academies Press. Washington, DC (USA): 2001.
3.　World Health Organization: *The Scientific Basis Of Tobacco Product Regulation*. WHO; 2008. technical report series; no. 951.http://www.who.int/tobacco/global_interaction/tobreg/publications/9789241209519.pdf.
4.　Johnson MD, Schilz J, Djordjevic MV, Rice JR, Shields PG: **Evaluation of in vitro assays for assessing the toxicity of cigarette smoke and smokeless tobacco**. *Cancer Epidem Biomar* 2009, **18**:3263–3304.
5.　Phillips J, Kluss B, Richter A, Massey E: **Exposure of bronchial epithelial cells to whole cigarette smoke: assessment of cellular responses**. *ATLA* 2005, **33**:239–248.
6.　Breheny D, Oke O, Faux SP: **The use of in vitro systems to assess cancer mechanisms and the carcinogenic potential of chemicals**. *ATLA* 2011, **39**:233–255.
7.　Garcia-Canton C, Anadon A, Meredith C: **GammaH2AX as a novel endpoint to detect DNA damage: applications for the assessment of the in vitro genotoxicity of cigarette smoke**. *Toxicol In Vitro* 2012, **26**:1075–1086.
8.　Lynch AM, Sasaki JC, Elespuru R, Jacobson-Kram D, Thybaud V, De Boeck M, Aardema MJ, Aubrecht J, Benz R, Dertinger SD, Douglas GR, White PA, Escobar PA, Fornace A Jr, Honma M, Naven RT, Rusling JF, Schiestl RH, Walmsley RM, Yamamura E, van Benthem J, Kim JH: **New and emerging technologies for genetic toxicity testing**. *Environ Mol Mutagen* 2011, **52**:205–223.
9.　Zainol M, Stoute J, Almeida GM, Rapp A, Bowman KJ, Jones GD: **Introducing a true internal standard for the comet assay to minimize intra- and inter-experiment variability in measures of DNA damage and repair**. *Nucleic Acids Res* 2009, **37**:e150.
10.　Rogakou EP, Pilch DR, Orr AH, Ivanova VS, Bonner WM: **DNA double-stranded breaks induce histone H2AX phosphorylation on serine 139**. *J Biol Chem* 1998, **273**:5858–5868.
11.　Fernandez-Capetillo O, Lee A, Nussenzweig M, Nussenzweig A: **H2AX: the histone guardian of the genome**. *DNA Repair (Amst)* 2004, **3**:959–967.
12.　Dickey JS, Redon CE, Nakamura AJ, Baird BJ, Sedelnikova OA, Bonner WM: **H2AX: functional roles and potential applications**. *Chromosoma* 2009, **118**:683–692.
13.　Smart DJ, Ahmedi KP, Harvey JS, Lynch AM: **Genotoxicity screening via the gammaH2AX by flow assay**. *Mutat Res* 2011, **715**:25–31.

14. Garcia-Canton C, Anadon A, Meredith C: **Assessment of the in vitro gammaH2AX assay by high content screening as a novel genotoxicity test.** *Mutat Res* 2013, **757:**158–166.

15. Albino AP, Huang X, Jorgensen E, Yang J, Gietl D, Traganos F, Darzynkiewicz Z: **Induction of H2AX phosphorylation in pulmonary cells by tobacco smoke: a new assay for carcinogens.** *Cell Cycle* 2004, **3:**1062–1068.

16. Albino AP, Huang X, Jorgensen ED, Gietl D, Traganos F, Darzynkiewicz Z: **Induction of DNA double-strand breaks in A549 and normal human pulmonary epithelial cells by cigarette smoke is mediated by free radicals.** *Int J Oncol* 2006, **28:**1491–1505.

17. Albino AP, Jorgensen ED, Rainey P, Gillman G, Clark TJ, Gietl D, Zhao H, Traganos F, Darzynkiewicz Z: **GammaH2AX: a potential DNA damage response biomarker for assessing toxicological risk of tobacco products.** *Mutat Res* 2009, **678:**43–52.

18. Tanaka T, Huang X, Jorgensen E, Gietl D, Traganos F, Darzynkiewicz Z, Albino AP: **ATM activation accompanies histone H2AX phosphorylation in A549 cells upon exposure to tobacco smoke.** *BMC Cell Biol* 2007, **8:**26.

19. Zhao H, Albino AP, Jorgensen E, Traganos F, Darzynkiewicz Z: **DNA damage response induced by tobacco smoke in normal human bronchial epithelial and A549 pulmonary adenocarcinoma cells assessed by laser scanning cytometry.** *Cytometry A* 2009, **75:**840–847.

20. University of Kentucky: **3R4F reference cigarette.** http://3r4f.com, (accessed September 2013).

21. Combes R, Scott K, Dillon D, Meredith C, McAdam K, Proctor C: **The effect of a novel tobacco process on the in vitro cytotoxicity and genotoxicity of cigarette smoke particulate matter.** *Toxicol In Vitro* 2012, **26:**1022–1029.

22. Reddel RR, Ke Y, Gerwin BI, McMenamin MG, Lechner JF, Su RT, Brash DE, Park JB, Rhim JS, Harris CC: **Transformation of human bronchial epithelial cells by infection with SV40 or adenovirus-12 SV40 hybrid virus, or transfection via strontium phosphate coprecipitation with a plasmid containing SV40 early region genes.** *Cancer Res* 1988, **48:**1904–1909.

23. Nims RW, Sykes G, Cottrill K, Ikonomi P, Elmore E: **Short tandem repeat profiling: part of an overall strategy for reducing the frequency of cell misidentification.** *In Vitro Cell Dev Biol Anim* 2010, **46:**811–819.

24. Massey E, Aufderheide M, Koch W, Lodding H, Pohlmann G, Windt H, Jarck P, Knebel JW: **Micronucleus induction in V79 cells after direct exposure to whole cigarette smoke.** *Mutagenesis* 1998, **13:**145–149.

25. Kaur N, Lacasse M, Roy JP, Cabral JL, Adamson J, Errington G, Waldron KC, Gaca M, Morin A: **Evaluation of precision and accuracy of the borgwaldt RM20S((R)) smoking machine designed for in vitro exposure.** *Inhal Toxicol* 2010, **22:**1174–1183.

26. Adamson J, Azzopardi D, Errington G, Dickens C, McAughey J, Gaca MD: **Assessment of an in vitro whole cigarette smoke exposure system: the borgwaldt RM20S 8-syringe smoking machine.** *Chem Cent J* 2011, **5:**50.

27. ISO: **ISO 3308: 2012 - routine analytical cigarette-smoking machine – definitions and standard conditions.** 2012.

28. ISO: **ISO 3402:1999 - tobacco and tobacco products – atmosphere for conditioning and testing.** 2010.

29. Garcia-Canton C, Anadon A, Meredith C: **Genotoxicity evaluation of individual cigarette smoke toxicants using the in vitro gammaH2AX assay by high content screening.** *Toxicol Lett* 2013, **223:**81–87.

30. ICH: **Guidance on genotoxicity testing and data interpretation for pharmaceuticals intended for human use S2(R1).** 2011. http://www.ich.org/fileadmin/Public_Web_Site/ICH_Products/Guidelines/Safety/S2_R1/Step4/S2R1_Step4.pdf.

31. Supplier Quality Requirements Taskforce, Daimler Chrysler Corporation, Ford Motor Company, General Motors Corporation: *Measurement Systems Analysis, Reference Manual.* Michigan, United States: General Motors; 2002.

32. ISO: **ISO 5725–2:1994 - accuracy (trueness and precision) of measurement methods and results – part 2: basic method for the determination of repeatability and reproducibility of a standard measurement method.** 2013.

33. Svetlova MP, Solovjeva LV, Tomilin NV: **Mechanism of elimination of phosphorylated histone H2AX from chromatin after repair of DNA double-strand breaks.** *Mutat Res* 2010, **685:**54–60.

34. Petitjean A, Mathe E, Kato S, Ishioka C, Tavtigian SV, Hainaut P, Olivier M: **Impact of mutant p53 functional properties on TP53 mutation patterns and tumor phenotype: lessons from recent developments in the IARC TP53 database.** *Hum Mutat* 2007, **28:**622–629.

35. IARC: **TP53 database.** http://p53.iarc.fr/, (accessed June 2013).

36. Garcia-Canton C, Minet E, Anadon A, Meredith C: **Metabolic characterization of cell systems used in in vitro toxicology testing: lung cell system BEAS-2B as a working example.** *Toxicol In Vitro* 2013, **27:**1719–1727.

37. Thorne D, Wilson J, Kumaravel TS, Massey ED, McEwan M: **Measurement of oxidative DNA damage induced by mainstream cigarette smoke in cultured NCI-H292 human pulmonary carcinoma cells.** *Mutat Res* 2009, **673:**3–8.

38. Adamson J, Hughes S, Azzopardi D, McAughey J, Gaca MD: **Real-time assessment of cigarette smoke particle deposition in vitro.** *Chem Cent J* 2012, **6:**98.

7

Pyrogen detection methods: Comparison of bovine whole blood assay (bWBA) and monocyte activation test (MAT)

Christian Wunderlich, Stephan Schumacher and Manfred Kietzmann[*]

Abstract

Background: Pyrogen detection is of utmost importance in pharmaceutical industry, laboratories and health care institutions. As an alternative to the animal-consuming rabbit pyrogen test or Limulus amoebocyte lysate test, the monocyte activation test was introduced as a gold standard method in the European Pharmacopoeia. However, the monocyte activation test has not gained wide acceptance in practice.

Methods: We stimulated bovine whole blood with different endotoxin preparations (lipopolysaccharide *E.coli* 0127: B8 and 0113:H10), as well as the non-endotoxin pyrogens peptidoglycan and lipoteichoic acid. Prostaglandin E_2 (PGE_2) served as read out.

Results: Employing PGE_2 as read out enabled detection limits of 0.04 EU/ml for lipopolysaccharide 0127:B8, 0.25 EU/ml for lipopolysaccharide 0113:H10 and 10 μg/ml of lipoteichoic acid as well as peptidoglycan. To evaluate the bWBA test system as a possible alternative to the MAT we performed a peer-to-peer comparison of the two methods and confirmed similar sensitivities.

Conclusions: In conclusion, the bovine whole blood assay (bWBA) reproducibly enabled sensitive detection of endotoxin and non-endotoxin pyrogens and may thus become a viable alternative for pyrogen testing.

Keywords: Endotoxin, Bovine whole blood, Prostaglandin E_2, Pyrogen, Monocyte activation test, Lipopolysaccharide, Lipoteichoic acid

Background

The detection of pyrogenic contamination is an essential part of drug safety testing in the pharmaceutical industry, reference laboratories as well as health care institutions. To guarantee patient safety, critical threshold levels of pyrogenic contamination have been determined and must not be exceeded. Therefore the European Pharmacopoeia (EP) promotes the monocyte activation test (MAT) as most suitable test for pyrogen testing [1]. Former methods, the rabbit pyrogen test (RPT) [2] and the Limulus amoebocyte lysate (LAL) test [3] are limited by inherent disadvantages since the RPT has a comparably low sensitivity for pyrogens [4] and the LAL is unable to detect non-endotoxin pyrogens [5]. Moreover, both are animal-consuming tests

which, according to the 3 R concept – replacement, reduction, refinement –, should be avoided [6-8].

Nevertheless, product safety has to remain the first priority of medical product legislation, while economic considerations are also important to the industry and suitable methods need to offer a reasonable cost-benefit ratio. The MAT utilizes human blood [9,10] and is characterized by a high sensitivity for detecting endotoxin and non-endotoxin pyrogens. However, apparently it did not satisfy the needs of the pharmaceutical industry because it has not been widely used since its introduction in 2010. This might be partly due to the fact that accessing fresh human whole blood or producing large amounts of cryoblood of uniform quality for use in the MAT is certainly a logistic challenge. According to the European Pharmacopoeia, blood donors must confirm that they have been free of signs of infection and have not taken anti-inflammatory medications for one week before

* Correspondence: Manfred.Kietzmann@tiho-hannover.de
University of Veterinary Medicine Hannover, Foundation, Institute of Pharmacology, Toxicology and Pharmacy, Bünteweg 17, Hannover 30559, Germany

donation [1]. Additionally, commercialized cryoblood is routinely tested for sterility and HIV, HAV, HCV and HBV [11]. However, there remain several potentially influencing factors that cannot be standardized in a human-based test system since lifestyle and genetic background certainly differ significantly between donors.

In principal, if blood from a large animal species and a designated breed would be used for pyrogen detection most of these limitations could be overcome, because the animals can be housed under standardized specific pathogen-free conditions. Several aspects favor the use of bovine blood, for instance the fact that the Toll-like receptor equipment of bovine leukocytes is comparable to humans [12] as well as reports suggesting the suitability of bovine blood for the detection of lipopolysaccharides (LPS) [13].

In a previous study we reported that bovine whole blood can be used for a sensitive detection of LPS 0111:B4 from *E.coli* by using Prostaglandin E_2 as readout [14]. In the present study we investigated whether the system we established was also capable of detecting other endotoxins and gram-positive cell wall components. Additionally, we compared our method with the commercially available PyroDetect System (MAT) in a peer-to-peer setup.

Methods
Used stimulants
Endotoxin derived from *Escherichia coli* 0127:B8 (L3129, Sigma-Aldrich, Steinheim, Germany; stock ≥ 500000 EU/mg), WHO standard endotoxin from *Escherichia coli* 0113:H10:K (10 000 IU per vial, Merck, Darmstadt, Germany), peptidoglycan from *Bacillus subtilis* (low endotoxin, ≤ 1 EU/mg, InvivoGen, Toulouse, France) and lipoteichoic acid from *Staphylococcus aureus* (low endotoxin, ≤ 1 EU/mg, InvivoGen) were used as stimulants. Solutions were prepared with LAL-water or pyrogen-free saline. Aliqouts were stored at −20°C, except for the WHO Endotoxin, which was stored at −80°C. Immediately prior to use the aliquots were thawed, sonicated and diluted with pyrogen-free saline into different concentrations. Concentrations used for LPS 0127:B8 were 0.039, 0.078, 0.156, 0.313, 0.625 and 1.25 EU/ml, for LPS 0113: H10 0.063, 0.125, 0.25, 0.5, 1 and 2 EU/ml. Peptidoglycan and lipoteichoic acid were diluted to 1, 10, 50, 100 and 1000 µg/ml.

Blood collection and ethical statement
Blood was obtained via venipuncture from healthy cattle (mainly Holsteins except two crossbreds and one red Holstein) into 7.5 ml heparinized tubes (Li-Heparin, 19 IU/ml, SARSTEDT Monovette, Nümbrecht, Germany). The animals were owned by and stabled in the Clinic for Cattle of the University of Veterinary Medicine Hannover, Foundation. All blood donors were female, non-lactating

cows and were fed with hay ad libitum. The age ranged from 2.5 to 13 years.

This study received ethical approval by the Lower Saxony State Office for Consumer Protection and Food Safety (LAVES), Oldenburg (Az. 33.9-42502-05-13A361). All procedures involving animals were carried out in accordance with German legislation on animal welfare.

In vitro assay using bovine peripheral blood
225 µl lithium heparin blood from different donors were pipetted into 96-well cell culture plates (SARSTEDT, Nümbrecht, Germany) and stimulated for 24 hours with 25 µl pyrogen solution or vehicle. After incubation at 37°C and 5% CO_2, the 96-well plates were centrifuged at 2272 × g for 10 minutes, the supernatants were collected and frozen at −80°C until analysis. PGE_2 concentration was determined using the Cayman Prostaglandin E_2 Express EIA Kit (Cayman Chemical Company, Ann Arbor, MI, USA) following the manufacturer's instructions.

Comparison with the PyroDetect system
The PyroDetect System (Merck, Darmstadt, Germany) was used according to the manufacturer's instructions as a quantitative test with the exception that samples were not tested at different dilutions. The quantitative test is described by the producers as method A. By using method A, a quantitative comparison of the samples with the standard endotoxin is possible. In summary, the stimulating agents were pipetted as 20 µl portions into the 96-well plate (included in the kit) under a horizontal flow bench. Apart from the spike and blank wells – the former was filled with stimulant and spiked RPMI medium, the latter with a total of 40 µl RPMI – 20 µl RPMI were added to each well. The two cryo blood vials (included in the kit) were thawed in a water bath for 1 minute and diluted immediately with 8 ml RPMI 1640 cell culture medium each (included in the kit). Afterwards the cryopreserved blood mixture was pipetted into the plate at a volume of 200 µl per well. After incubation for 16 hours at 37°C with 5% CO_2 the mixture in the wells was resuspended five times and transferred to the ELISA plate (included in the kit). The IL-1β ELISA was performed following the manufacturer's instructions. To compare this test system with the bovine whole blood assay the same stimulants (diluted in RPMI) were tested simultaneously using the blood of 6 animals (separately) following the method described before.

Statistical analysis
Statistical analysis was carried out using the software SAS 9.3 (SAS, Cary, NC, USA). Data were checked for normal distribution by visual inspection and the Kolmogorov-Smirnov test. Some data sets showed a left-skewed distribution and failed the normality test. Therefore a permutation test (10000 permutations) was

used for calculating a randomized complete block design (equivalent to exact Friedmann Test) and P values smaller 0.05 were considered significant. Calculations were done with the SAS macro RIBDPERM.MAC (provided by Erich Schumacher, Institut für Angewandte Mathematik und Statistik, Universität Hohenheim). Data are represented as box-plot with median and min to max whiskers.

Results

Pyrogen stimulation

LPS from E.coli 0127:B8 was used as a stimulating agent and we found a dose-dependent increase of PGE_2 starting at a dose of 0.08 EU/ml and reaching a plateau at 0.16 EU/ml (Figure 1). Using the WHO standard endotoxin (LPS E.coli 0113:H10) we discovered a dose-dependent increase of PGE_2 release starting at 0.25 EU/ml (Figure 2). Peptidoglycan (PGN) from *Bacillus subtilis* induced a dose-dependent increase of PGE_2 in concentrations of more than 10 μg/ml (Figure 3). Likewise, lipoteichoic acid (LTA) from *Staphylococcus aureus* provoked a significant increase of PGE_2 at concentrations of 10 μg/ml and above (1 μg/ml provoked an increase as well, but fell just short of the level of significance, p = 0.056). The maximum PGE_2 production was seen at 50 μg/ml, but although eicosanoid release elicited by higher LTA concentrations declined, it remained significantly higher compared to unstimulated blood (Figure 4).

Bovine whole blood assay compared to PyroDetect system

After 16 hours of stimulation – analogously to the manufacturer's lab procedure – the PyroDetect System ELISA detected the presence of 0.25 EU/ml standard

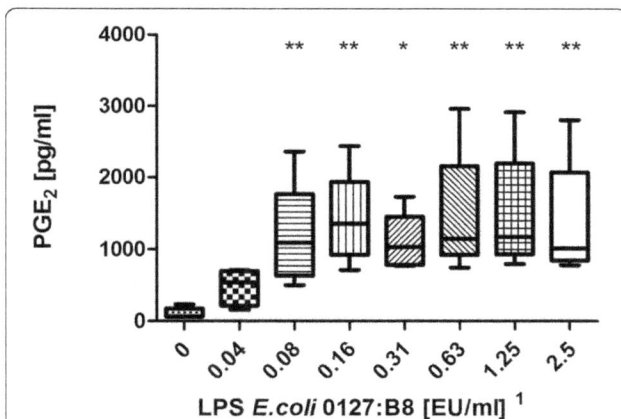

Figure 2 Stimulation with WHO standard endotoxin.
Prostaglandin E_2 concentration after LPS stimulation of fresh (stored < 2 h) bovine whole blood. Box-plot with median and min to max whiskers of n = 5, permutation test, *p ≤ 0.05, **p ≤ 0.01 compared to unstimulated blood. Result is representative of three independent experiments[1].

endotoxin (Figure 5), whereas 0.0625 EU/ml and 0.125 EU/ml did not induce measurable cytokine production. Importantly, the PyroDetect System also detected the presence of all other pyrogens at all concentrations used. Unfortunately, the color reaction of the ELISA was so intense that we were unable to quantify it thus precluding the specification of EU equivalents.

The simultaneous stimulation of bovine blood from 6 animals with the same pyrogens resulted in detection limits comparable to those obtained from the previous experiments. Results of one animal were excluded from analysis because of preexisting PGE_2 release from the

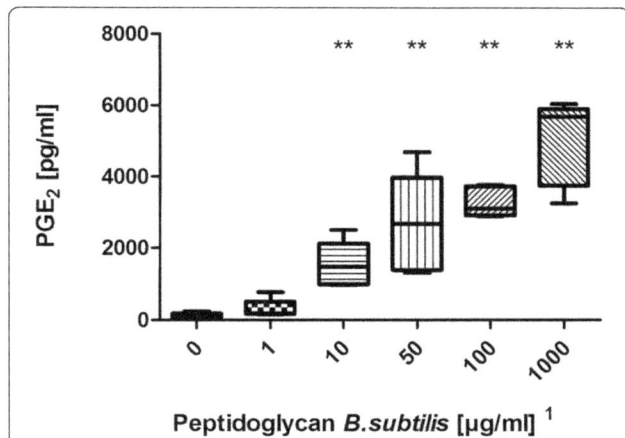

Figure 1 Stimulation with LPS from E.coli 0127:B8. Prostaglandin E_2 concentration after LPS stimulation of fresh (stored < 2 h) bovine whole blood. Box-plot with median and min to max whiskers of n = 9, permutation test, *p ≤ 0.05, **p ≤ 0.01 compared to unstimulated blood. Result is representative of three independent experiments[1].

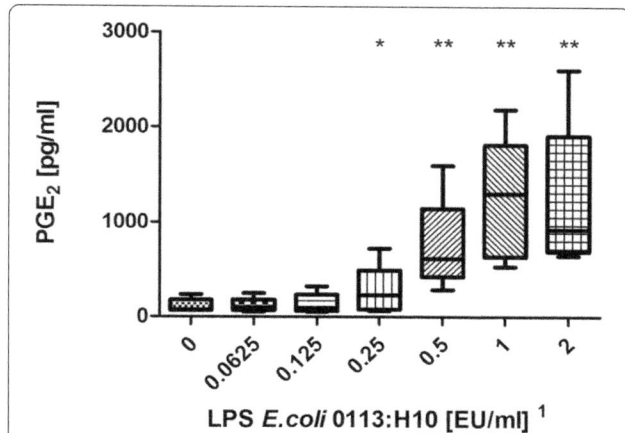

Figure 3 Stimulation with peptidoglycan from Bacillus subtilis. Prostaglandin E_2 concentration after PGN stimulation of fresh (stored < 2 h) bovine whole blood. Box-plot with median and min to max whiskers of n = 5, permutation test, **p ≤ 0.01 compared to unstimulated blood. Result is representative of three independent experiments[1].

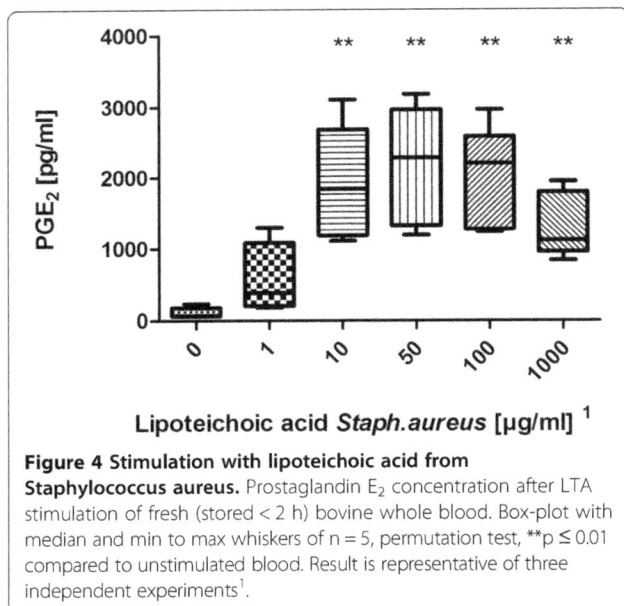

**Figure 4 Stimulation with lipoteichoic acid from
Staphylococcus aureus.** Prostaglandin E_2 concentration after LTA
stimulation of fresh (stored < 2 h) bovine whole blood. Box-plot with
median and min to max whiskers of n = 5, permutation test, **p ≤ 0.01
compared to unstimulated blood. Result is representative of three
independent experiments[1].

unstimulated blood. The comparative detection limits of
the two test methods are given in Table 1.

Discussion

We have previously shown that LPS 0111:B4 from *E.coli*
can be reliably detected using a bovine whole blood
assay and PGE_2 as readout [14]. Hartung and Wendel
[15] reported the suitability of a test method utilizing
human whole blood for the detection of endotoxin as
well as non-endotoxin pyrogens. The quite similar toll-
like receptor (TLR) equipment of human and bovine
leukocytes [12] gave reason to expect the same would be

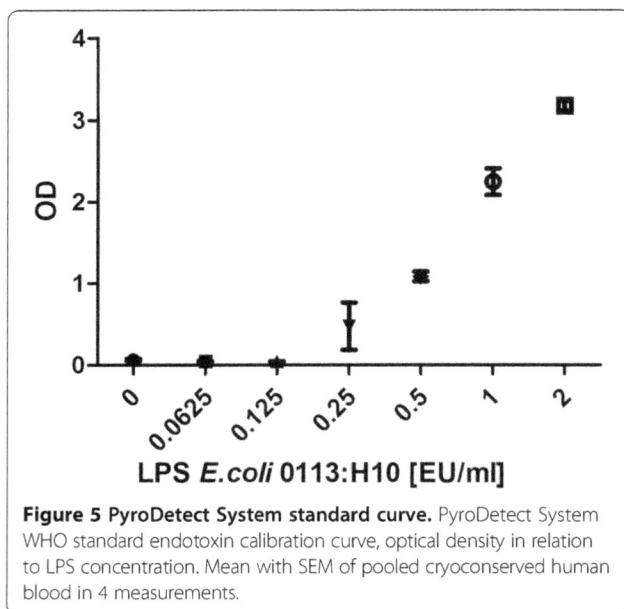

Figure 5 PyroDetect System standard curve. PyroDetect System
WHO standard endotoxin calibration curve, optical density in relation
to LPS concentration. Mean with SEM of pooled cryoconserved human
blood in 4 measurements.

possible using our test system. Thus, we decided to investigate whether the bovine whole blood assay was capable of detecting a broad range of pyrogens with the
required sensitivity.

Detection of LPS

The bWBA was capable of detecting the presence of two
different kinds of endotoxins. Remarkably, the detection
of LPS 0127:B8 was 3 – 6 fold more sensitive than the
detection of LPS 0113:H10 (0.04 – 0.08 EU/ml vs. 0.25 –
0.5 EU/ml) which was confirmed using the PyroDetect
System. Similar findings were reported by others who
showed an up to 1000-fold difference in potency of different endotoxins [16,17]. However, the observed detection limits of both test systems for the WHO standard
endotoxin (LPS *E.coli* 0113:H10) still complied with the
specifications of the MAT and the required sensitivity of
pyrogen testing of 0.5 EU/ml [1].

Detection of PGN

The bWBA was capable of detecting 10 – 50 µg/ml PGN.
It is still a matter of controversy how the stimulatory potency of PGN is conveyed. Although it has long been
thought to be an agonist of the TLR2, PGN is probably
sensed by the nucleotide-binding oligomerization domain-
containing proteins (NOD) 1 and 2 [18]. Moreover, it has
been reported that commercial PGN preparations are
often contaminated with endotoxin [19] and highly purified PGN was unable to stimulate cytokine release in a human whole blood test system [20,21]. This issue was also
discussed in a meta-analysis of Rockel and Hartung [22]
and to date there is no evidence that highly purified PGN
is an immune stimulant. In order to prevent the effects of
a potential endotoxin contamination we used a PGN preparation from Invivogen. This manufacturer guarantees an
endotoxin content of less than 1 EU per milligram. Regarding that in our study detectable LPS concentrations
were in the pg/ml range, whereas non-endotoxin pyrogens
could be detected in the µg/ml range a falsification of the
results due to LPS contamination should be unlikely
although it cannot be completely excluded.

Detection of LTA

The bWBA was capable of detecting 10 µg/ml LTA.
Interestingly, we observed a decrease of PGE_2 release at
the highest concentrations of LTA, a finding which has
not been reported in the literature so far. A possible explanation could be a complex formation of LTA at high
concentrations [23], a phenomenon that seems to occur
because of the intermolecular interactions of LTA molecules. Another explanation could be an enhanced binding by the bovine scavenger receptor type 1 [24], which
has the ability to interact with or bind, for example,

Table 1 Detection limits of the different stimulants

	Detection limits			
	Experiment 1 n = 6 – 9	Experiment 2 n = 6	Experiment 3 n = 5	PyroDetect System Poolblood
LPS *E.coli* 0127:B8	0.08 EU/ml	0.04 EU/ml	0.08 EU/ml	0.04 EU/ml ‡
LPS *E.coli* 0113:H10	not tested	0.5 EU/ml	0.25 EU/ml	0.25 EU/ml
Peptidoglycan *Bac. subtilis*	10 µg/ml	50 µg/ml	10 µg/ml	1 µg/ml ‡
Lipoteichoic acid *Staph. aureus*	10 µg/ml	10 µg/ml	10 µg/ml	1 µg/ml ‡

Different animals were used, permutation test, compared to unstimulated blood. Experiment 3 was the comparison with the PyroDetect System. ‡ = lowest concentration tested.

pyrogens. However, it remains unclear why this did not seem to apply to PGN. Yet, despite the decline of PGE_2, the high concentrations of LTA still remained detectable and concentrations above 100 µg/ml are very unlikely to occur in pyrogen-contaminated medicinal products.

A meta-analysis by Rockel and Hartung discussed LTA as a possible reference stimulant for grampositive bacteria, analogous to endotoxin for gramnegative bacteria [22]. Similar to PGN some commercial LTA preparation have been reported to be contaminated by LPS [25], so again we used a preparation from Invivogen to reduce the risk of false positive results. Nevertheless, it is not clear whether LTA itself is a pyrogen or not. Zähringer et al. [18] elegantly elucidated how contaminating lipopetides like MALP-2 likely explain the TLR2-stimulating effects of LTA and PGN preparations. A TLR2-agonistic activity of natural and synthetic lipopeptides has also been confirmed by others [26].

Comparison of the MAT and bWBA

In order to compare the sensitivity of the bovine whole blood assay with the commercially available PyroDetect System we decided to perform a peer-to-peer comparison with the same stimulants. The comparison of the two methods resulted in the same detection level of WHO standard endotoxin, 0.25 EU/ml – sufficing the postulated allowed level of 0.5 EU/ml in pharmaceutical products [1]. With regard to PGN, LTA and LPS 0127:B8 the PyroDetect System appeared to be more sensitive. It was capable of identifying the presence of 1 µg/ml PGN or LTA (the lowest concentrations used in our experiments) and other studies suggest that the MAT can detect concentrations as low as 100 ng/ml LTA [25,27]. The human blood-based MAT has been validated for endotoxin detection but there was no formal evaluation study with respect to non-endotoxin pyrogen detection [22]. However, Hasiwa et al. [28] strongly suggested that the MAT is able to detect non-endotoxin pyrogens and whether a

formal validation is necessary is beyond the scope of this discussion.

The inferior performance of the bovine assay in terms of non-endotoxin pyrogens may indicate a shortcoming. The difference in sensitivity of the two methods may partly be due to the different endpoints used. As an acute phase protein IL-1β is produced by blood cells only in response to potentially dangerous exogenous stimuli, e.g. pyrogens [29] resulting in a strong increase of its concentration. In contrast, certain endogenous levels of PGE_2 are physiologically present in (bovine) blood. Therefore, interindividual differences in basal plasma levels demanded a quite distinct increase of eicosanoid production in order to be statistically significant. Unfortunately, we were unable to obtain a commercial kit suitable for the determination of cytokines in bovine whole blood [14]. Future investigations will need to clarify whether the bWBA can be optimized in order to increase its sensitivity, but the fact that the level of significance was just barely missed after stimulation with 1 µg/ml LTA seems promising.

Some medicinal products like vaccines may benefit from in vitro pyrogen testing in the target species. Bacterial vaccines contain bacterial components by definition and different species may display differing sensitivities towards certain bacteria [30]. Thus, testing vaccines in the target species may increase product safety. Considering the diversity of veterinary species it will, however, be very difficult to test every product in the target species, especially because many human medicinal products (with the exception of vaccines) are used off-label in veterinary medicine. With that said, pyrogen testing using quality-controlled blood from cattle housed under standardized conditions may be an option with favorable risk/benefit-ratio.

Conclusions

With regard to the aim of reduction, refinement and replacement (3R) of animal experiments the introduction of the MAT seemed promising for the reduction of the use of RPT and LAL [31]. However, this objective does not seem to have been achieved because the MAT is not widely used yet. Here we show the potential of detecting endotoxin and non-endotoxin pyrogens using a bovine whole blood assay. Further efforts are indispensable to improve the method's functionality, detection limits and robustness as well as to verify whether it can detect further pyrogens including lipopeptides. If the bWBA meets these requirements it should be possible to produce large standardized batches of bovine blood in reference laboratories which could then offer pyrogen testing services using the bWBA as an alternative to the RPT.

Endnote

[1]Notably, concentrations in the figures refer to the stimulant solutions used. These were diluted tenfold in the final setup (using 225 µl whole blood and 25 µl stimulant). Results depicted in the figures are representative of repeated experiments. The detection limits from all experiments are presented in Table 1.

Abbreviations

bWBA: Bovine whole blood assay; MAT: Monocyte activation test; RPT: Rabbit pyrogen test; LAL: Limulus amoebocyte lysast test; EP: European pharmacopoeia; LPS: Lipopolysaccharid; PGN: Peptidoglycan; LTA: Lipoteichoic acid; PGE$_2$: Prostaglandin E$_2$; E.coli: Escherichia coli; WHO: World health organization; TLR: Toll-like receptor; EU: Endotoxin unit; NOD: Nucleotide oligomerization domain; MALP-2: Macrophage-activating lipopeptide 2.

Competing interests

The authors declare that they have no competing interests.

Authors' contributions

CW, SS and MK conceived and designed the study. CW performed the experiments, CW and SS analysed the data and wrote the manuscript, MK contributed valuable discussion and critically revised the article. MK had full access to the data and is the guarantor of the study. All authors read and approved the final manuscript.

Acknowledgments

We thank the Clinic for Cattle, University of Veterinary Medicine Hannover, Foundation, especially to Dr. Kathrin Herzog and Prof. Dr. Jürgen Rehage for their excellent support in obtaining the bovine blood samples. We also gratefully acknowledge the help of Dr. Karl Rohn who provided assistance with the statistical analysis (Institute for Biometry, Epidemiology and Information Processing (IBEI), University of Veterinary Medicine Hannover, Foundation).

References

1. EDQM: *Europäisches Arzneibuch*. Stuttgart: 7. Aufl., Deutscher Apotheker Verlag; 2011.
2. Weary M, Wallin R: The rabbit pyrogen test. *Lab Anim Sci* 1973, **23:**677–681.
3. Levin J, Bang FB: The role of endotoxin in the extracellular coagulation of limulus blood. *Bull Johns Hopkins Hosp* 1964, **115:**265–274.
4. Weigandt M: *Der Humane Vollblut-Pyrogentest-Optimierung, Validierung und Vergleich mit den Arzneibuchmethoden*. Diss: Univ. Heidelberg, Med.Fak; 2001.
5. Fennrich S, Fischer M, Hartung T, Lexa P, Montag-Lessing T, Sonntag HG, Weigandt M, Wendel A: Detection of endotoxins and other pyrogens using human whole blood. *Dev Biol Stand* 1999, **101:**131–139.
6. Russell W, Burch R: *The Principles of Humane Experimental Technique*. London, UK: Methuen; 1959.
7. Guhad F: Introduction to the 3Rs (Refinement, Reduction and Replacement). *J Am Assoc Lab Anim Sci* 2005, **44:**58–59.
8. Gruber FP, Hartung T: Alternatives to animal experimentation in basic research. *ALTEX* 2004, **21**(Suppl 1):3–31.
9. Schindler S, Asmus S, Von Aulock S, Wendel A, Hartung T, Fennrich S: Cryopreservation of human whole blood for pyrogenicity testing. *J Immunol Methods* 2004, **294:**89–100.
10. Charton E, Brügger P, Spreitzer I, Golding B: Alternatives to animal testing. In *EDQM Symposium; 16.09.2011*. Strasbourg, France: EDQM, Council of Europe; 2011.
11. MERCK: *PyroDetect Cryoblood Artikel-Nr. 1.44155.0001*. Darmstadt, Germany: Merck KGaA; 2014.
12. McGuire K, Jones M, Werling D, Williams JL, Glass EJ, Jann O: Radiation hybrid mapping of all 10 characterized bovine Toll-like receptors. *Anim Genet* 2006, **37:**47–50.
13. Imamura S, Nakamizo M, Kawanishi M, Nakajima N, Yamamoto K, Uchiyama M, Hirano F, Nagai H, Kijima M, Ikebuchi R, Mekata H, Murata S, Konnai S, Ohashi K: Bovine whole-blood culture as a tool for the measurement of endotoxin activities in Gram-negative bacterial vaccines. *Vet Immunol Immunopathol* 2013, **153:**153–158.
14. Wunderlich C, Schumacher S, Kietzmann M: Prostaglandin E2 as a read out for endotoxin detection in a bovine whole blood assay. *J Vet Pharmacol Ther* 2014, ePub ahead of print.
15. Hartung T, Wendel A: Die Erfassung von Pyrogenen in einem humanen Vollblutmodell. *ALTEX* 1995, **12:**70–75.
16. Dehus O, Hartung T, Hermann C: Endotoxin evaluation of eleven lipopolysaccharides by whole blood assay does not always correlate with Limulus amebocyte lysate assay. *J Endotoxin Res* 2006, **12:**171–180.
17. Hasiwa M, Kullmann K, Von Aulock S, Klein C, Hartung T: An in vitro pyrogen safety test for immune-stimulating components on surfaces. *Biomaterials* 2007, **28:**1367–1375.
18. Zähringer U, Lindner B, Inamura S, Heine H, Alexander C: TLR2–promiscuous or specific? A critical re-evaluation of a receptor expressing apparent broad specificity. *Immunobiology* 2008, **213:**205–224.
19. Li H, Nooh MM, Kotb M, Re F: Commercial peptidoglycan preparations are contaminated with superantigen-like activity that stimulates IL-17 production. *J Leukoc Biol* 2008, **83:**409–418.
20. Travassos LH, Girardin SE, Philpott DJ, Blanot D, Nahori M-A, Werts C, Boneca IG: Toll-like receptor 2-dependent bacterial sensing does not occur via peptidoglycan recognition. *EMBO Rep* 2004, **5:**1000–1006.
21. Rockel C, Hartung T, Hermann C: Different Staphylococcus aureus whole bacteria mutated in putative pro-inflammatory membrane components have similar cytokine inducing activity. *Immunobiology* 2011, **216:**316–321.
22. Rockel C, Hartung T: Systematic review of membrane components of Gram-positive bacteria responsible as pyrogens for inducing human monocyte/macrophage cytokine release. *Front Pharmacol* 2012, **3:**56.
23. Ofek I, Simpson WA, Beachey EH: Formation of molecular complexes between a structurally defined M protein and acylated or deacylated lipoteichoic acid of streptococcus pyogenes. *J Bacteriol* 1982, **149:**426–433.
24. Dunne DW, Resnick D, Greenberg J, Krieger M, Joiner KA: The type I macrophage scavenger receptor binds to gram-positive bacteria and recognizes lipoteichoic acid. *Proc Natl Acad Sci U S A* 1994, **91:**1863–1867.
25. Kimbrell MR, Warshakoon H, Cromer JR, Malladi S, Hood JD, Balakrishna R, Scholdberg TA, David SA: Comparison of the immunostimulatory and proinflammatory activities of candidate Gram-positive endotoxins, lipoteichoic acid, peptidoglycan, and lipopeptides, in murine and human cells. *Immunol Lett* 2008, **118:**132–141.
26. Barrenschee M, Lex D, Uhlig S: Effects of the TLR2 agonists MALP-2 and Pam3Cys in isolated mouse lungs. *PloS one* 2010, **5:**e13889.
27. Holtkamp B, Schmitz G, Hartung T: In vitro Pyrogentest Nachweis eines breiten Pyrogenspektrums im Monozyten-Aktivierungstest. *BIOspektrum* 2010, 07/10, 16. Jahrgang: 779–782.
28. Hasiwa N, Daneshian M, Bruegger P, Fennrich S, Hochadel A, Hoffmann S, Rivera-Mariani FE, Rockel C, Schindler S, Spreitzer I, Stoppelkamp S, Vysyaraju K, Hartung T: Evidence for the detection of non-endotoxin pyrogens by the whole blood monocyte activation test. *ALTEX* 2013, **30:**169–208.
29. Daneshian M, Von Aulock S, Hartung T: Assessment of pyrogenic contaminations with validated human whole-blood assay. *Nat Protoc* 2009, **4:**1709–1721.

30. Usui M, Nagai H, Tamura Y: **An in vitro method for evaluating endotoxic activity using prostaglandin E(2) induction in bovine peripheral blood.** *Biologicals* 2013, **41**:158–161.

31. Fennrich S, Fischer M, Hartung T, Lexa P, Montag-Lessing T, Sonntag HG, Weigandt M, Wendel A: **[Evaluation and further development of a pyrogenicity assay based on human whole blood].** *ALTEX* 1998, **15**:123–128.

8

A meta-analysis of the proportion of antimicrobial resistant human *Salmonella* isolates in Ethiopia

Getachew Tadesse

Abstract

Background: Antimicrobial resistant *Salmonella* is a global problem and recently, a strain on the verge of pan-resistance was reported. In Ethiopia, the therapeutic management of Salmonellosis is difficult because drug sensitivity tests are not routinely carried out and treatment alternatives are not available in most health care facilities. The objectives of this study were to estimate the temporal changes and proportions of drug resistant isolates in Ethiopia.

Methods: Published studies on drug resistant *Salmonella* isolates were searched in Medline, Google Scholar and the lists of references of articles. Eligible studies were selected by using inclusion and exclusion criteria. Generic, methodological and statistical information were extracted from the eligible studies. The extracted data included the proportions of ampicillin, co-trimoxazole, chloramphenicol, ceftriaxone, ciprofloxacin and multi-drug resistant isolates. Pooled proportions were estimated by a random effects model.

Results: The odds of multi-drug resistant isolates in the 2000s was higher than before the 1990s (OR = 18.86, 95% CI = 13.08, 27.19). The pooled proportions of ampicillin, co-trimoxazole, chloramphenicol, ciprofloxacin and multi-drug resistant isolates in the 2000s were 86.01%, 68.01%, 62.08%, 3.61% and 79.56% respectively. *S.* Concord (>97%) was resistant to ampicillin, co-trimoxazole, chloramphenicol and ceftriaxone.

Conclusion: The proportion of drug resistant isolates has increased since the 1970s. All drugs currently used for the treatment of Salmonellosis but ciprofloxacin are not reliable for an empirical therapy. Alternative drugs should be included in the essential drug list and measures should be taken to re-enforce the drug use policy.

Keywords: Antimicrobial resistance, Ethiopia, Humans, *Salmonella*

Background

The emergence of drug resistant pathogens is associated with a variety of biological, pharmacological and societal variables with the worst combinations in developing countries [1]. Antimicrobial resistant *Salmonella* is one of the global problems in present day clinical practices and recently, a strain on the verge of pan-resistance was reported [2]. In sub-Saharan Africa (SSA), the prevalence of MDR *Salmonella* has increased and outbreaks due to MDR strains were recorded [3-5]. Infections with MDR pathogens are associated with excess morbidity and mortality probably because of the co-selection of traits of drug resistance and virulence [6]. In developing countries like Ethiopia, the therapeutic management of the disease is difficult because drug sensitivity tests are not routinely carried out and treatment alternatives are not available in most health care facilities.

Salmonella is one of the major causes of gastroenteritis and fever in Ethiopia. The bacterium was isolated from a number of patients including pediatrics [7] and malnourished children [8]. *S.* Concord, *S.* Typhi, *S.* Typhimurium and *S.* Paratyphi were the dominant serotypes that accounted for 82.1% of the isolates from patients [9]. *S.* Concord was isolated from a bone processing plant [10], an immigrant in Ireland [11], diarrheal and/or febrile patients [12,13] and Ethiopian adoptees in Europe and the USA [14-16] but its occurrence in other countries in SSA is reportedly low [17]. Typhoidal *Salmonella* was the second common isolate [9] and a case fatality rate of 15.7% was recorded in hospital admitted children [18]. In 2006, typhoid fever was diagnosed in 37(6.7%) febrile children

Correspondence: getadesse1@yahoo.com
Department of Biomedical Sciences, College of Veterinary Medicine and Agriculture, Addis Ababa University, P.O. Box 34, Debre Zeit, Ethiopia

aged 3-14 years [19]. _S._ Typhimurium is prevalent in SSA [17-19], highly invasive [20-22] and causes high mortality in AIDS patients [23].

Despite the importance of the disease, surveillance and monitoring systems are not in place and the pharmaco-epidemiology of the bacteria is not adequately described. However, integration of previous estimates could provide an insight into the temporal changes and the proportions of drug resistant isolates. The objectives of this study were to quantify the temporal changes and estimate the proportions of drug resistant isolates by using meta-analytical methods.

Methods

The study was conducted according to the guideline of the PRISMA group (Preferred Reporting Items for Systematic Reviews and Meta-Analyses) [24]. The PRISMA check list was used to ensure inclusion of relevant information (Additional file 1). The outcomes of interest were the proportions of ampicillin, co-trimoxazole, chloramphenicol, ceftriaxone, ciprofloxacin and multi-drug resistant isolates. MDR was defined as resistance to three or more drugs.

Literature search and eligibility criteria

The literature search strategy is described in a previous report [9]. Briefly, studies were searched in Medline, Google scholar and the lists of references of articles. The last search was done on March 30, 2014. To be eligible, a study had to be (i) published, (ii) written in English and (iii) cross sectional or retrospective. Initially, studies with titles and abstracts that are not relevant to the outcomes of interest were excluded. Of the screened articles, duplicates and studies that reported small number of isolates (1-22) were excluded.

Data extraction

The first author, year of study, location, study design, antimicrobial test methods and interpretative standards, numbers of isolates and numbers of drug resistant isolates were extracted. If the proportion of drug sensitive isolates (q) was reported, the number of resistant isolates was calculated by multiplying the number of isolates (n) by one minus the proportion of drug sensitive isolates (1-q). The study level proportions were derived from the extracted data. The data was abstracted by TG.

Data analysis

A zero reported for the numbers of drug resistant or sensitive isolates was imputed as 0.5 [25]. The proportions and standard errors were calculated by the following formulae: $p = r/n$ and s. e. $= \sqrt{p\,(1-p)/n}$, where r = number of resistant isolates and n = number of isolates. To normalize the distribution of the data, the proportions were transformed to logit event estimates [26,27]: $lp = \ln\,[p/(1-p)]$, where lp = logit event estimate; $\ln$ = natural logarithm; p = study level estimate. The variances were calculated by the following formula: $v\,(lp) = 1/\,(np) + 1/[n\,(1-p)]$, where v = variance and n = sample size.

Bias and heterogeneity analyses

The antimicrobial test methods and the interpretative standards (break point levels) were examined to assess the within study biases. Funnel plots were used to get visual impressions of the across study biases (small study effects). The Begg and Mazumdar adjusted rank correlation and the Egger's regression asymmetry tests were used to test the significance of funnel plots' asymmetries.

Heterogeneities were assessed by the Galbraith plot and the Cochran's Q test. The percentage of the variation attributable to heterogeneity was quantified by the inverse variance index (I^2) [28]. As the power of the Cochran's Q test is low in small number of studies, studies were considered heterogeneous if the ratio of Q and the degree of freedom was greater than one. I^2 values of 25% 50% and 75% were considered as low, moderate and high heterogeneity respectively.

Temporal change and trend analyses

The average temporal changes were estimated by using a meta-regression model: $y = a + bx + u + e$; where a = constant, b = regression coefficient, x = year of study, u = error term with known standard deviation and e = error term of the additive component of the variance (tau^2). If two or more calendar years were reported, the median was considered as year of study. Tau^2 was estimated by the methods of moments. The Knapp-Hartung variance modification factor was used to calculate the probability values and confidence intervals of the coefficients. The Mantel extension Chi Square for trend was used to assess the changes in the proportion of MDR isolates across decades (1970s/80s, 1990s and 2000s).

Pooling and sensitivity tests

The DerSimonian and Laird random effects model was used to pool logit event estimates [29]. Pooled logit estimates were back-transformed to proportions by the following formula: $p = e^{lp}/(e^{lp} + 1)$, where p = proportion and e = the base of the natural logarithm. Single study omitted influence analyses were done to assess the sensitivities of pooled estimates. A study was considered to be influential if the pooled estimate without it was not within the 95% confidence bounds of the overall mean. The statistical significance of a difference between proportions was assessed by the Yates corrected Chi Square test [30,31]. Alpha was set at 0.05.

Microsoft Office Excel 2007 was used to calculate study level proportions, logit event estimates, standard errors and to back-transform logit event estimates to proportions. Epi info™ (Version 3.5.1, Center for Disease Control, CDC, USA) was used to assess the trend and compare proportions. All other analyses were done by using Stata (Version 11.1, Stata Corp, College Station, Texas).

Results and discussion
Literature search and eligible studies
Figure 1 presents the search results. The search yielded 140 studies. The titles and abstracts of 112 studies were not relevant to the outcomes of interest. Of the articles screened for eligibility, 14 were excluded: one study was not available; three were duplicates and ten reported small numbers of isolates. Fourteen studies were eligible for quantitative syntheses. Eleven studies were used to estimate the temporal changes and trends [12,13,32-40]. Five studies [13,37-40] were used to estimate the proportions of drug resistant isolates in the 2000s. Four studies were used to estimate the proportions of drug resistant *S. Concord* in the 2000s [13-15,41]. In the 2000s, only two studies reported the drug resistance features of 15 *S. Typhi*, two *S. Paratyphi* and seven *S. Typhimurium* [13,37]. The search was comprehensive and most, if not all published reports were considered in the analysis. With the exception of one review on *S. Typhi* [42], a review on the antimicrobial resistance features of human *Salmonella* isolates in Ethiopia was not found.

Characteristics of the eligible studies
The studies were carried out between 1974 and 2009 in Central, Northern, Southern and Eastern Ethiopia (Table 1). Three studies were on *S. Concord* isolated from Ethiopian adoptees in Europe and the USA. A total of 1030 isolates were tested with a variety of antimicrobials that included the penicillins, cephalosporins, phenicols, quinolones, aminoglycosides, tetracyclines, macrolides and peptides.

Risks of bias and heterogeneity
The disk diffusion method was reported in 11 studies [12,13,32-40]. The micro-broth dilution method [14,41] and the Episilon test (E-test) were used to determine minimum inhibitory concentrations (MIC) [13]. Five studies [12,32,33,35,36] used the breakpoint levels of Bauer *et al.* 1966 [43] and nine studies used the standards of NCCLS (National Committee for Clinical and Laboratory Standards) or CLISI (Clinical and Laboratory Standards Institute) [13-15,34,37-41]. The DTU (Technical University of Denmark) food defined resistance break point levels were used to assess resistance to ceftiofur, florfenicol and aminoglycosides [14]. In five studies carried out before 2000, the proportions of ampicillin resistant isolates were underestimated because the breakpoint level (11 mm or less) was lower than the level (13 mm or less) in the modified versions. Similarly, differences in the break point levels of drugs such as tetracycline (14 mm or less in Bauer *et al.* 1966 [43]

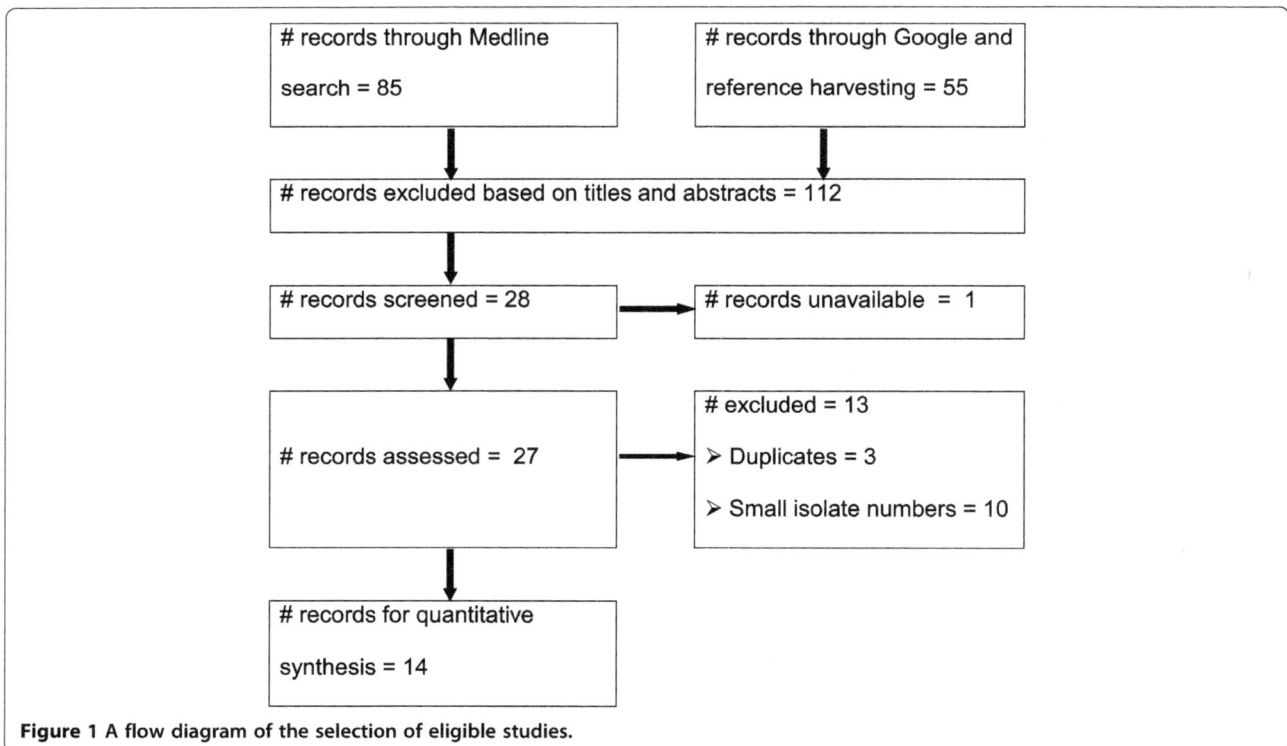

Figure 1 A flow diagram of the selection of eligible studies.

Table 1 Characteristics of the eligible studies

Author	Location	Ys	n	Number of resistant isolates (%)					
				Amp	Sxt	Chl	Cro	Cip	MDR
[12]	AA	1974-1981	216	nr	0(0)	nr	nt	nt	39(18.1)
[32]	AA	1975-1980	165	22(13.3)	0(0)	19(11.5)	nt	nt	23(13.9)
[33][a]	AA	1982-1983	45	12(26.7)	0(0)	8(17.8)	nt	nt	10(22.2)
[34][b]	AA	1992-1993	37	30(81.1)	28(75.7)	31(83.8)	nt	nt	30(81.1)
[35]	AA	1993-1996	110	40(36.4)	57(51.8)	39(35.5)	nt	nt	41(37.3)
[36][b]	AA	1995	45	31(68.9)	26(57.8)	21(46.7)	nt	nt	26(57.8)
[37]	JM	2000	59	35(59.3)	24(40.7)	21(35.6)	nt	nt	45(76.3)
[38][b]	GD	2003-2005	59	54(91.5)	38(64.4)	46(78.0)	nt	6(10.2)	46(78)
[13][b]	AA/JM	2004-2006	113	93(82.3)	91(80.5)	92(81.4)	89(78.8)	1(0.9)	91(80.5)
[39]	BD	2003-2008	84	77(91.7)	67(79.8)	37(44.1)	nt	nt	72(85.7)
[40][c]	HR	2007	28	28(100)	nt	18(64.3)	nt	nt	20(71.4)
[41][d,e]	DM	2007-2009	8	8(100)	8(100)	8(100)	8 (100)	0(0)	8(100)
[14][d,e,]	EU/USA	2003-2007	35	34(97.1)	35(100)	35(100)	34(97.1)	0(0)	35(100)
[15][d,e]	BL	2006-2009	26	26 (100)	26(100)	26(100)	26(100)	0(0)	26(100)

AA = Addis Ababa; AA/JM = Addis Ababa and Jimma; Amp = ampicillin; BD = Bahirdar; BL = Belgium; Chl = chloramphenicol; Cip = ciprofloxacin; Cro = ceftriaxone; DM = Denmark; ET = Ethiopia; EU/USA = Europe and the United States of America; HR = Harar; JM = Jimma; GD = Gondar; n = number of isolates; nr = not reported; nt = not tested; Sxt = co-trimoxazole; Ys = Year of study.
[a]The numbers of chloramphenicol and ampicillin resistant isolates were derived from the proportions of sensitive isolates.
[b]The third highest mono-drug resistant isolates number was considered as the number of MDR isolates assuming that the prevalence of MDR isolates is mainly a reflection of the highly resisted drugs.
[c]Data on amoxicillin was substituted to ampicillin assuming that the mechanism of resistance could be similar.
[d]The data show the proportions of drug resistant S. Concord.
[e]The exact origin of the adoptees was not reported.

vs. 11 mm or less in the modified versions) might have affected the proportions of MDR isolates. However, as the occurrence of drug resistant isolates in the earlier years was comparatively lower than in the 2000s, the risks of underestimation or overestimation of the study level proportions are negligible.

Figure 2 presents funnel plots of the estimates. The plots demonstrate different patterns. The Egger's bias coefficients for ampicillin, co-trimoxazole, chloramphenicol and MDR estimates were 7.04 (95%CI = -1.67, 15.76), $p > 0.05$; -4.12 (95% CI = -8.32, 0.08), $p > 0.05$; 4.54 (95% CI = -8.72, 17.81), $p > 0.05$ and 11.06 (95% CI = 0.09, 22.04), $p > 0.05$ respectively and the probability values calculated by the Begg and Mazmudar test were greater than 5%. The plots and tests did not suggest the presence of bias.

Figure 3 depicts forest plots of the proportions of drug resistant isolates. The percentages of the variations of the logit event estimates attributable to heterogeneities are presented in Tables 2 and 3. The heterogeneities could be mainly due to increases in the proportions of resistant isolates across years.

Temporal changes and trend

Figure 4 presents regression plots of the logit event estimates of drug resistant isolates against years of studies. The plots demonstrate increasing patterns. The percentages of

the explained variances were more than 41% (Table 2). The proportions of MDR isolates differ by decade (X^2 for trend = 301.82; $p < 001$). Compared to the 1970/80s, MDR isolates occurred more frequently in the 1990s (OR = 6.92, 95% CI = 4.73, 10.11) and 2000s (OR =18.86, 95% CI = 13.08, 27.19). The pooled proportion of MDR isolates in the 2000s was higher than the proportion in the 1990s [X^2 = 25.32; $p < 0.001$; OR = 2.73 (95% CI = 1.81, 4.1)].

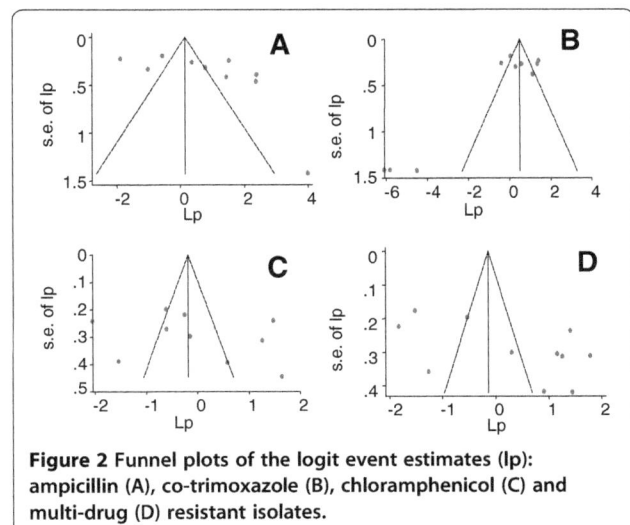

Figure 2 Funnel plots of the logit event estimates (lp): ampicillin (A), co-trimoxazole (B), chloramphenicol (C) and multi-drug (D) resistant isolates.

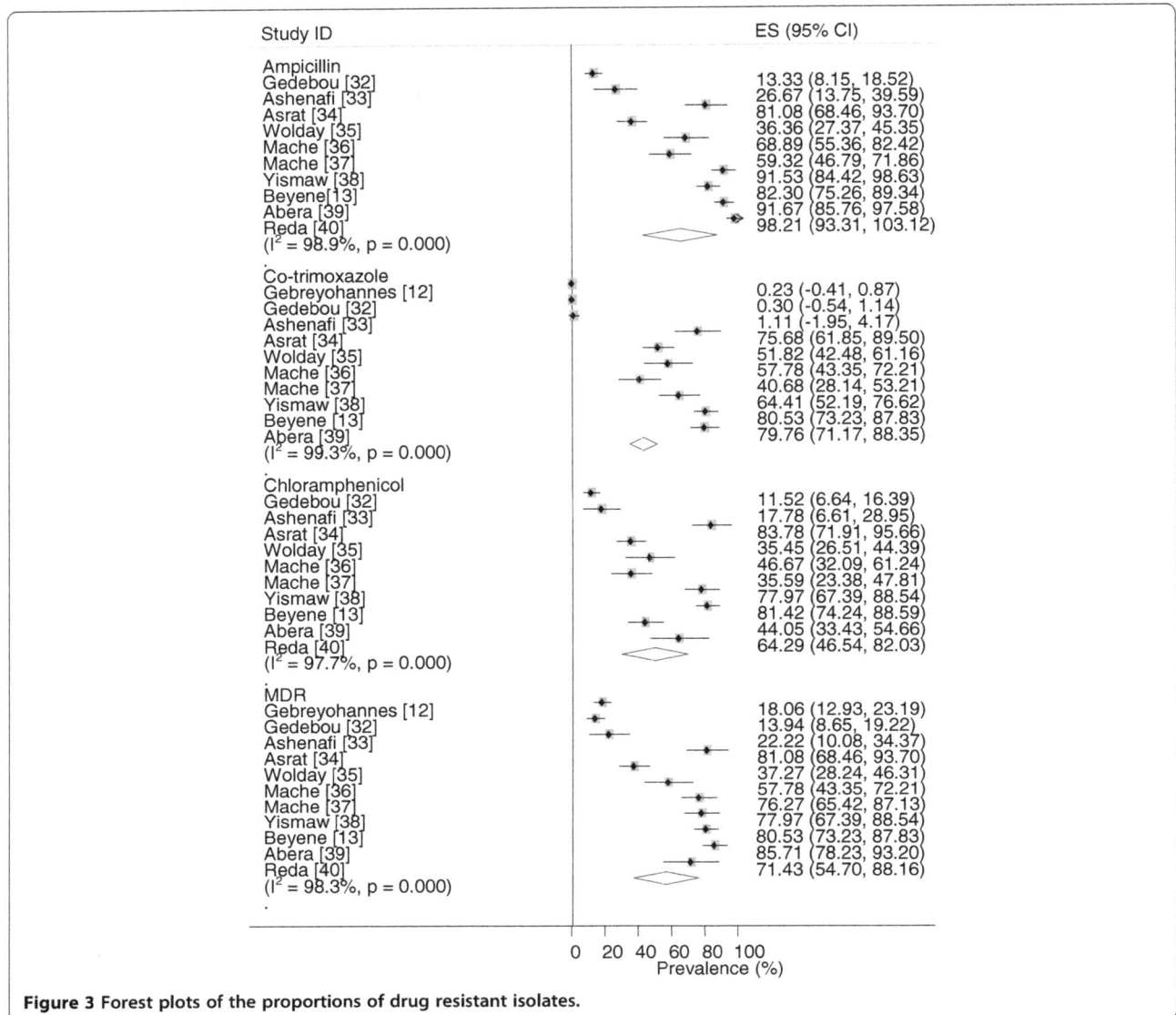

Study ID   ES (95% CI)

Ampicillin
Gedebou [32]   13.33 (8.15, 18.52)
Ashenafi [33]   26.67 (13.75, 39.59)
Asrat [34]   81.08 (68.46, 93.70)
Wolday [35]   36.36 (27.37, 45.35)
Mache [36]   68.89 (55.36, 82.42)
Mache [37]   59.32 (46.79, 71.86)
Yismaw [38]   91.53 (84.42, 98.63)
Beyene [13]   82.30 (75.26, 89.34)
Abera [39]   91.67 (85.76, 97.58)
Reda [40]   98.21 (93.31, 103.12)
(I^2 = 98.9%, p = 0.000)

Co-trimoxazole
Gebreyohannes [12]   0.23 (-0.41, 0.87)
Gedebou [32]   0.30 (-0.54, 1.14)
Ashenafi [33]   1.11 (-1.95, 4.17)
Asrat [34]   75.68 (61.85, 89.50)
Wolday [35]   51.82 (42.48, 61.16)
Mache [36]   57.78 (43.35, 72.21)
Mache [37]   40.68 (28.14, 53.21)
Yismaw [38]   64.41 (52.19, 76.62)
Beyene [13]   80.53 (73.23, 87.83)
Abera [39]   79.76 (71.17, 88.35)
(I^2 = 99.3%, p = 0.000)

Chloramphenicol
Gedebou [32]   11.52 (6.64, 16.39)
Ashenafi [33]   17.78 (6.61, 28.95)
Asrat [34]   83.78 (71.91, 95.66)
Wolday [35]   35.45 (26.51, 44.39)
Mache [36]   46.67 (32.09, 61.24)
Mache [37]   35.59 (23.38, 47.81)
Yismaw [38]   77.97 (67.39, 88.54)
Beyene [13]   81.42 (74.24, 88.59)
Abera [39]   44.05 (33.43, 54.66)
Reda [40]   64.29 (46.54, 82.03)
(I^2 = 97.7%, p = 0.000)

MDR
Gebreyohannes [12]   18.06 (12.93, 23.19)
Gedebou [32]   13.94 (8.65, 19.22)
Ashenafi [33]   22.22 (10.08, 34.37)
Asrat [34]   81.08 (68.46, 93.70)
Wolday [35]   37.27 (28.24, 46.31)
Mache [36]   57.78 (43.35, 72.21)
Mache [37]   76.27 (65.42, 87.13)
Yismaw [38]   77.97 (67.39, 88.54)
Beyene [13]   80.53 (73.23, 87.83)
Abera [39]   85.71 (78.23, 93.20)
Reda [40]   71.43 (54.70, 88.16)
(I^2 = 98.3%, p = 0.000)

0   20 40 60 80 100
Prevalence (%)

Figure 3 Forest plots of the proportions of drug resistant isolates.

Table 2 Temporal changes of the proportions of drug resistant isolates

Drug	I^2 residuals	Adjusted R^2	b(95% CI)	p
Amp[a]	82.62	77.58	0.54(0.52, 0.55)	0.001
Sxt[b]	72.31	89.52	0.53(0.52, 0.54)	0.000
Chl[a]	84.73	41.05	0.55(0.52, 0.58)	0.003
MDR[b]	88.37	55.32	0.52(0.50, 0.54)	0.021

Amp = ampicillin; b = coefficient of year of study; Chl = chloramphenicol; I^2 = inverse variance index; MDR = multi-drug resistance; R^2 = proportion of explained variance; Sxt = co-trimoxazole.
[a]The estimates were derived from data extracted from 10 studies [13,32-40].
[b]The estimates were derived from data extracted from 10 studies [12,13,32-39].

Table 3 Pooled proportions of drug resistant *Salmonella* isolated between 2000 and 2008

Drug	Pooled estimate		Heterogeneity			
	p(95% CI)	Z-p	Q	Q-p	Q/df	I^2
Amp	86.01(70.77, 93.98)	0.000	29.32	0.000	7.3	86.4
Sxt	68.01(48.13, 82.98)	0.075	31.54	0.000	10.5	90.5
Chl	62.08(41.05,79.38)	0.258	49.38	0.000	12.4	91.9
Cip	3.61(0.32, 30.62)	0.009	5.7	0.02	5.7	81.5
MDR	79.56(74.90, 83.54)	0.000	3.60	0.464	0.9	0.0

Amp = ampicillin; Chl = chloramphenicol; Cip = ciprofloxacin; df = degree of freedom; I^2 = inverse variance index; Q = Cochran's X^2; Q-p = probability value of Cochran's Q test; Sxt = co-trimoxazole; Z-p = probability value of Z test.

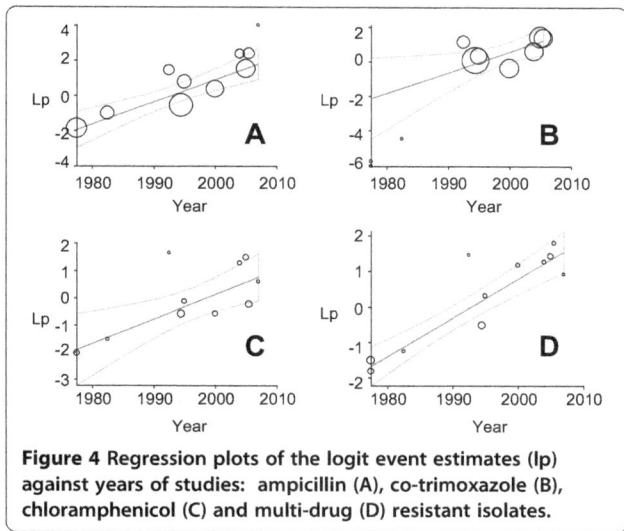

Figure 4 Regression plots of the logit event estimates (lp) against years of studies: ampicillin (A), co-trimoxazole (B), chloramphenicol (C) and multi-drug (D) resistant isolates.

The increase in the proportion of drug resistant isolates could be due to the irrational use of antimicrobials. Several studies have reported the inappropriateness of the prescription and dispensing methods in both the public and private health set-ups. For instance, in Northern Ethiopia, Gondar, ampicillin and penicillin G were two of the three commonly dispensed antimicrobials and most drugs were prescribed by young interns and dispensed by less qualified personnel [44]. In Southern Ethiopia, Hawassa, amoxicillin, ampicillin, chloramphenicol, penicillin G and ceftriaxone were the most commonly prescribed antibacterials [45]. Moreover, the prescriptions had little justifications [46] and the proportion of patients exposed to antimicrobials (>58%) [45-49] was comparatively higher than the standard (20.0%-26.8%) [50]. The pediatric age group was more exposed to antimicrobials than adults and the differences between the prescription behaviors of personnel with shorter and longer pre-service trainings and between public and private health facilities were not significant [47]. Furthermore, prescription-only medications were dispensed without a medical prescription; verbal instructions (87%) were practiced in both pharmacies and rural drug vendors [51] and several patients medicate themselves [52]. Essential drug lists, standard treatment guidelines and drug formulary were available in some but not in all health care settings [53]. In general, the prescription and dispensing practices are not consistent with the rational antimicrobial use guideline and could have favored the selection of antimicrobial resistant microbes.

Pooled proportions

Table 3 presents the pooled estimates of drug resistant isolates in the 2000s. More than half of the isolates were resistant to ampicillin, co-trimoxazole and chloramphenicol. All single study omitted pooled estimates were within the 95% confidence limits of the respective overall means. The pooled estimates show the magnitude of the problem and the unreliability of ampicillin, co-trimoxazole and chloramphenicol as empirical therapeutic agents. Moreover, the occurrences of isolates resistant to ceftriaxone, 89(78.8%) [13] and norfloxacin, 13(15.5%) [39] were reported.

The higher prevalence of MDR isolates could be associated with the presence of Class I integrons in several isolates. Class I integrons were identified in 52 (53.1%) MDR *Salmonella* predominantly of animal origin [54] and in *S.* Concord with extended spectrum β-lactamase genes (*bla*CTX-M-15) [16]. As data on the genetic features of isolates of human origin is limited, further genetic characterization of isolates is important to understand evolving and epidemic prone strains.

Dominant serotypes

Table 4 presents pooled proportions of drug resistant *S.* Concord. The MDR profiles are shown in Table 5. Before the 1990s, more than 81% of the isolates were resistant to ampicillin, co-trimoxazole and chloramphenicol [12]. However, in the 2000s more than 97% of the isolates were resistant to the older antimicrobials including the cephalosporins. Furthermore, resistance to aztreonam [14], nalidixic acid [13,15] and intermediate resistance to ciprofloxacin were recorded [14,15,41]. As is the case of *S.* Kentucky [2], *S.* Concord appears to have taken several steps to become pan-resistant and given its higher occurrence and invasiveness (30.6%) [13], it might have caused considerable morbidities and mortalities in Ethiopian children.

Data on the sensitivities of *S.* Typhi, *S.* Paratyphi and *S.* Typhimurium are limited. However, there are evidences on the occurrence of isolates that are resistant to the older drugs [13,37] and norfloxacin [55]. In addition, *S.* Typhimurium isolates of animal origin were shown to be resistant to several drugs including ceftiofur and ciprofloxacin [56-61]. Furthermore, MDR genes located on

Table 4 Pooled proportions of drug resistant S. Concord

Drug	Pooled proportion[a]		Hetetrogeneity			
	p(95% CI)	Z-*p*	Q	Q-*p*	Q/df	I²
Amp	98.68(94.85,99.67)	0.000	0.09	0.954	0.05	0.0
Sxt	98.68(94.85,99.67)	0.000	0.09	0.954	0.05	0.0
Chl	97.98(93.92,99.35)	0.000	0.20	0.903	0.1	0.0
Cro	97.98(93.92,99.35)	0.000	0.20	0.903	0.1	0.0
MDR	98.68(94.85,99.67)	0.000	0.09	0.954	0.05	0.0

Amp = ampicillin; Chl = Chloramphenicol; Cro = ceftriaxone; df = degrees of freedom; Q = Cochran's X²; Q-*p* = probability value of the Cochran's Q test; Sxt = co-trimoxazole; Z-*p* = probability value of the Z test.
[a]The estimates were based on four studies [13-15,41]. Data from two studies [14,41] were combined before pooling. Intermediate resistance to ciprofloxacin was recorded in twelve isolates [14,41].

Table 5 MDR features of S. Concord

Author	MDR profiles	No. (%)
[13][a]	Amp Chl Cro Gen Sxt	41(48.8)
	Amp Chl Cro Gen Sxt Tet	29(34.5)
	Amp Chl Cro Gen Nal Sxt Tet	5(6.0)
[14][b]	Amp Azt Chl (Cep Cfp Cfr Cft Cfz Cpo Cro Ctz) Str SulTmp	34(97.1)
	Amp Azt Chl (Cep Cfp Cfr Cft Cfz Cpo Ctz) Str SulTmp	1(2.9)
[15][c]	Amp Chl Cro Gen Str Sul Sxt Tmp	3(11.5)
	Amp Chl Cro Gen Sul Str Sxt Tet Tmp	19(73.1)
	Amp Chl Cro Gen Nal Str Sul Sxt Tet Tmp	4(15.4)
[41][d]	Amp Chl Cfo Cro Gen Str Sul Tet Tmp	8 (100)

Amp = ampicillin; Azt = aztreonam; Cep = cephalothin; Cfo = cefotaxime; Cfp = cefepime; Cfr = cefuroxime; Cft = ceftiofur; Cfz = cefazolin; Cpo = cefpodoxime; Cro = ceftriaxone; Ctz = ceftazidime; Chl = chloramphenicol; Gen = gentamicin; Nal = nalidixic acid; Sul = sulfamethoxazole; Str = streptomycin; Sxt = co-trimoxazole; Tet = tetracycline; Tmp = trimethoprim.
[a]Each profile was recorded in more than 5% of the MDR isolates. One isolate was resistant to ofloxacin.
[b]Resistance to gentamicin (97%), tetracycline (69%) and intermediate resistance to ciprofloxacin (14%) were recorded.
[c]Seven isolates showed intermediate resistance to ciprofloxacin.
[d]Resistance to florfenicol (6/8), colistin (1/8) and intermediate resistance to ciprofloxacin (6/8) were recorded.

a virulence-associated plasmid of S. Typhimurium were identified [62] and ST313 appears to have occupied a niche provided by HIV, malaria, and malnutrition in SSA [63].

Implications and limitations
The results of this study have several implications in clinical practices and in policy and research issues. The comparatively lower proportion of ciprofloxacin resistant isolates suggests the potential use of ciprofloxacin as an empirical therapeutic agent. However, as there are evidences of intermediate resistance to ciprofloxacin, alternative drugs should be included in the essential drug list of the country so as to manage severe and life threatening infections. The fluoroquinolones were used to treat children suffering from MDR Gram negative bacterial infections [64] and azithromycin is an attractive alternative against MDR *Salmonella* [65,66]. An association between mass oral azithromycin treatment and a reduction in all-cause and infectious mortalities in rural children was recorded [67].

Policy and decision makers could make use of the evidences as inputs to re-enforce the drug use policy and to devise strategies and measures that could help reduce the rates of emergence of drug resistant pathogens. Apart from the active involvement of the regulatory bodies and the long-arm of the law on drug smuggling and over- the-counter sells of prescription-only drugs, educational initiatives could be of practical significance to reduce the rates of emergence of drug resistant pathogens

in the country. Educational programs were reported to be effective in improving the diagnostic qualities of health workers and reducing unjustified prescriptions [68]. Although information sources offer a framework to base educational intervention measures, a regular training is more effective than guidelines alone [69].

The reservoirs and host ranges of the NTS isolates are unknown and the factors associated with the emergence of drug resistant strains are not adequately described. Some of the strains (e.g. *S.* Concord) are becoming international concerns and containment of the problem needs an international approach [15]. To this effect, a large scale investigation into the pharmaco-epidemiology of *Salmonella* is needed and research efforts should be directed towards hypothesis driven preventive measures.

Apart from the small number of eligible studies, the exact origins of the study subjects were not reported. The pooled estimates were also derived from data collected between 2000 and 2009. Therefore, as most patients could be from the urban areas where access to health care facilities is relatively better than the rural areas, the estimates are more applicable to the urban than the rural population and the current proportions of drug resistant isolates may be higher than the present estimates.

Conclusion
The proportion of drug resistant *Salmonella* has increased since the 1970s and a considerable proportion of the isolates are multi-drug resistant. Ciprofloxacin could be used as an empirical therapeutic agent. The third generation cephalosporins are not useful against *S.* Concord infections. Alternative drugs should be included in the essential drug list and intervention measures should be taken to re-enforce the drug use policy. Further large scale studies are required to describe the pharmaco-epidemiology of *Salmonella* in Ethiopia.

Additional file

Additional file 1: PRISMA Checklist.

Competing interests
The author declares no competing interests.

Author's contribution
TG conceived the design, searched the literature, extracted and analyzed the data, interpreted the results and drafted the manuscript.

Acknowledgements
I thank Dr. Byleyegne Molla, Dr. Endrias Zewdu, Dr. Sefinew Alemu and Mr. Bayeh Abera for providing me with their articles and Dr. Tesfaye Sisay for his help in literature search.

References

1. Amábile-Cuevas CF: **Global Perspectives of Antibiotic Resistance**. In *Antimicrobial Resistance in Developing Countries*. Edited by Sosa AJ, Byarugaba DK, Amábile-Cuevas CF, Hsueh P, Kariuki S, Okeke IN. New York: Springer Science + Business Media; 2010:3–13.

2. Le Hello S, Harrois D, Bouchrif B, Sontag L, Elhani L, Guibert V, Zerouali K, Weill FX: **Highly drug-resistant *Salmonella* enterica serotype Kentucky ST198-X1: a microbiological study**. *Lancet Infect Dis* 2013, 13:672–679.

3. Kariuki S, Revathi G, Kariuki N, Kiiru J, Mwituria J, Hart CA: **Increasing prevalence of multidrug-resistant non-typhoidal *Salmonellae*, Kenya, 1994-2003**. *Int J Antimicrob Agents* 2005, 25:38–43.

4. Coovadia YM, Gathiram V, Bhamjee A, Garratt RM, Mlisana K, Pillay N, Madlalose T, Short M: **An outbreak of multiresistant *Salmonella* typhi in South Africa**. *Q J Med* 1992, 82:91–100.

5. Niehaus AJ, Apalata T, Coovadia YM, Smith AM, Moodley P: **An outbreak of foodborne salmonellosis in rural KwaZulu-Natal, South Africa**. *Foodborne Pathog Dis* 2011, 8:693–697.

6. Mølbak K: **Human Health Consequences of Antimicrobial Drug-Resistant *Salmonella* and Other Foodborne Pathogens**. *Clin Infect Dis* 2005, 41:1613–1620.

7. Shimelis D, Tadesse Y: **Clinical profile of acute renal failure in children admitted to the department of pediatrics, Tikur Anbessa Hospital**. *Ethiop Med J* 2004, 42:17–22.

8. Shimeles D, Lulseged S: **Clinical profile and pattern of infection in Ethiopian children with severe protein-energy malnutrition**. *East Afr Med J* 1994, 71:264–267.

9. Tadesse G: **Prevalence of human Salmonellosis in Ethiopia: a systematic review and meta-analysis**. *BMC Infect Dis* 2014, 14:88.

10. Pegram RG, Roeder PL, Hall ML, Rowe B: **Salmonella in livestock and animal by-products in Ethiopia**. *Trop Anim Health Prod* 1981, 13:203–207.

11. Morris D, Whelan M, Corbett-Feeney G, Cormican M, Hawkey P, Li X, Doran G: **First report of extended-spectrum-beta-lactamase-producing Salmonella enterica isolates in Ireland**. *Antimicrob Agents Chemother* 2006, 50:1608–1609.

12. Gebre-Yohannes A: ***Salmonella* from Ethiopia: prevalent species and their susceptibility to drugs**. *Ethiop Med J* 1985, 23:97–102.

13. Beyene G, Nair S, Asrat D, Mengistu Y, Engers H, Wain J: **Multidrug resistant *Salmonella* Concord is a major cause of Salmonellosis in children in Ethiopia**. *J Infect Dev Ctries* 2011, 5:23–33.

14. Hendriksen RS, Mikoleit M, Kornschober C, Rickert RL, Duyne SV, Kjelsø C, Hasman H, Cormican M, Mevius D, Threlfall J, Angulo FJ, Aarestrup FM: **Emergence of multidrug-resistant *Salmonella* Concord infections in Europe and the United States in children adopted from Ethiopia 2003-2007**. *Pediatr Infect Dis J* 2009, 28:814–818.

15. Vanhoof R, Gillis P, Stévart O, Boland C, Vandenberg O, Fux F, Collard J, Bertrand S: **Transmission of multiple resistant *Salmonella* Concord from internationally adopted children to their adoptive families and social environment: proposition of guidelines**. *Eur J Clin Microbiol Infect Dis* 2012, 31:491–497.

16. Fabre L, Delauné A, Espié E, Nygard K, Pardos M, Polomack L, Guesnier F, Galimand M, Lassen J, Weill FX: **Chromosomal integration of the extended-spectrum beta-lactamase gene blaCTX-M-15 in *Salmonella* enterica serotype Concord isolates from internationally adopted children**. *Antimicrob Agents Chemother* 2009, 53:1808–1816.

17. Galanis E, Lo Fo Wong DM, Patrick ME, Binsztein N, Cieslik A, Chalermchikit T, Aidara-Kane A, Ellis A, Angulo FJ, Wegener HC: **Web-based surveillance and global Salmonella distribution, 2000-2002**. *Emerg Infect Dis* 2006, 12:381–388.

18. Worku B: **Typhoid fever in an Ethiopian children's hospital: 1984-1995**. *Ethiop J health Dev* 2000, 14:311–315.

19. Animut A, Mekonnen Y, Shimelis D, Ephraim E: **Febrile illnesses of different etiology among outpatients in four health centers in Northwestern Ethiopia**. *Jpn J Infect Dis* 2009, 62:107–110.

20. Ley B, Le Hello S, Lunguya O, Lejon V, Muyembe JJ, Weill FX, Jacobs J: **Invasive *Salmonella* enterica Serotype Typhimurium Infections, Democratic Republic of the Congo, 2007-2011**. *Emerg Infect Dis* 2014, 20.

21. Berkley JA, Lowe BS, Mwangi I, Williams T, Bauni E, Mwarumba S, Ngetsa C, Slack MP, Njenga S, Hart CA: **Bacteremia among children admitted to a rural hospital in Kenya**. *N Engl J Med* 2005, 352:39–47.

22. Gordon MA, Graham SM, Walsh AL, Phiri LW, Molyneux E, Zijlstra EE, Heyderman RS, Hart CA, Molyneux ME: **Epidemics of invasive *Salmonella* enterica serovar Enteritidis and *S. enterica* serovar Typhimurium infection associated with multidrug resistance among adults and children in Malawi**. *Clin Infect Dis* 2008, 46:963–969.

23. Fisk TL, Lundberg BE, Guest JL, Ray S, Barrett TJ, Holland B, Stamey K, Angulo FJ, Farley MM: **Invasive infection with multidrug-resistant *Salmonella* enterica serotype Typhimurium definitive type 104 among HIV-infected adults**. *Clin Infect Dis* 2005, 40:1016–1021.

24. Moher D, Liberati A, Tetzlaff J, Altman DG, The PRISMA Group: **Preferred Reporting Items for Systematic Reviews and Meta-Analyses: The PRISMA Statement**. *PLoS Med* 2009, 6:e1000097.

25. Tricco AC, Ng CH, Gilca V, Anonychuk A, Pham B, Berliner S: **Canadian oncogenic human papillomavirus cervical infection prevalence: Systematic review and meta-analysis**. *BMC Infect Dis* 2011, 11:235.

26. Calvo-Muñoz I, Gómez-Conesa A, Sánchez-Meca J: **Prevalence of low back pain in children and adolescents: a meta-analysis**. *BMC Pediatr* 2013, 13:14.

27. Hurley JC: **Lack of impact of Selective Digestive Decontamination on Pseudomonas aeruginosa ventilator associated pneumonia: benchmarking the evidence base**. *J Antimicrob Chemother* 2011, 66:1365–1373.

28. Higgins JP, Thompson SG: **Quantifying heterogeneity in a meta-analysis**. *Stat Med* 2002, 21:1539–1558.

29. DerSimonian R, Laird N: **Meta-analysis in clinical trials**. *Control Clin Trials* 1986, 7:177–188.

30. Yang Y, Li X, Zhou F, Jin Q, Gao L: **Prevalence of Drug-Resistant Tuberculosis in Mainland China: Systematic Review and Meta-Analysis**. *PLoS One* 2011, 6:e20343.

31. Gao L, Zhang L, Jin Q: **Meta-analysis: prevalence of HIV infection and syphilis among MSM in China**. *Sex Transm Infect* 2009, 85:354–358.

32. Gedebou M, Tassew A: **Antimicrobial resistance and R factor of *Salmonella* isolates from Addis Ababa**. *Ethiop Med J* 1981, 19:77–85.

33. Ashenafi M, Gedebou M: ***Salmonella* and *Shigella* in adult diarrhoea in Addis Ababa- prevalence and antibiograms**. *Trans R Soc Trop Med Hyg* 1985, 79:719–721.

34. Asrat D: ***Shigella* and *Salmonella* serogroups and their antibiotic susceptibility patterns in Ethiopia**. *East Mediterr Health J* 2008, 14:760–767.

35. Wolday D: **Increase in the incidence of multidrug-resistant *Salmonellae* in Ethiopia**. *J Antimicrob Chemother* 1998, 41:421–423.

36. Mache A, Mengistu Y, Cowley C: ***Salmonella* serogroups identified from adult diarrhoeal out-patients in Addis Ababa Ethiopia: antibiotic resistance and plasmid profile analysis**. *East Afr Med J* 1997, 74:183–186.

37. Mache A: ***Salmonella* serogroup and their antibiotic resistance patterns isolated from diarrhoeal stools of pediatric out patients in Jimma Hospital and Jimma Health Center, South West Ethiopia**. *Ethiop J Health Sci* 2002, 37:37–45.

38. Yismaw G, Negeri C, Kassu A, Tiruneh M, Mulu A: **Antimicrobial Resistance Pattern of *Salmonella* Isolates from Gondar University Hospital, Northwest Ethiopia**. *Ethiop Pharm J* 2007, 25:85–90.

39. Abera B, Biadglegne F: **Antimicrobial resistance of fecal isolates of *Salmonella* and *Shigella* spp. at Bahir Dar regional health research laboratory, Northwest Ethiopia**. *Ethiop Pharm J* 2009, 27:55–60.

40. Reda AA, Seyoum B, Yimam J, Andualem G, Fiseha S, Vandeweerd JM: **Antibiotic susceptibility patterns of *Salmonella* and *Shigella* isolates in Harar, Eastern Ethiopia**. *J Infect Dis Immun* 2011, 3:134–139.

41. Hendriksen RS, Kjelsø C, Torpdahl M, Ethelberg S, Mølbak K, Aarestrup FM: **Upsurge of infections caused by *Salmonella* Concord among Ethiopian adoptees in Denmark**. *Euro Surveill* 2010, 15:pii=19587.

42. Beyene G, Asrat D, Mengistu Y, Sofa A, Wain J: **Typhoid fever in Ethiopia: Review**. *J Infect Dev Ctries* 2008, 2:448–453.

43. Bauer AW, Kirby WM, Sherris JC, Turck M: **Antibiotic Susceptibility Testing by a Standardized Single Disk Method**. *Am J Clin Pathol* 1966, 45:493–496.

44. Desta Z, Abdulwhab M: **Prescription writing in Gondar outpatient teaching hospital, Ethiopia**. *East Afr Med J* 1996, 73:115–119.

45. Desalegn AA: **Assessment of drug use pattern using WHO prescribing indicators at Hawassa University teaching and referral hospital, South Ethiopia: a cross-sectional study**. *BMC Health Serv Res* 2013, 13:170.

46. Desta Z, Abula T, Beyene L, Fantahun M, Yohannes AG, Ayalew S: Assessment of rational drug use and prescribing in primary health care facilities in north west Ethiopia. *East Afr Med J* 1997, **74**:758–763.

47. Fenta A, Belay M, Mekonnen E: Assessment of antibacterial drug exposure patterns of patient encounters seen by different categories of prescribers at health institutions in Bahir Dar, Ethiopia. *Ethiop Med J* 2013, **51**:33–39.

48. Assessment of the Pharmaceutical Sector in Ethiopia. In [http://www.who.int/medicines/areas/coordination/Ethiopia-pharmaceutical.pdf]

49. Tsega B, Hailu W, Ergetie Z: Measuring quality of drug use in primary healthcare facilities: a yearlong assessment of WHO prescribing indicators, Wolkite town, South West Ethiopia. *Int J Pharm & Ind Res* 2012, **2**:485–491.

50. Isah AO, Ross-Degnan D, Quick J, Laing R, Mabadeje AFB: The development of standard values for the WHO drug use prescribing indicators. In [http://archives.who.int/prduc2004/rducd/ICIUM_Posters/1a2_txt.htm]

51. Abula T, Worku A, Thomas K: Assessment of the dispensing practices of drug retail outlets in selected towns, North West Ethiopia. *Ethiop Med J* 2006, **44**:145–150.

52. Suleman S, Ketsela A, Mekonnen Z: Assessment of self-medication practices in Assendabo Town Jimma zone, Southwestern Ethiopia. *Res Soc Adm Pharm* 2009, **5**:76–81.

53. Angamo MT, Wabe NT, Raju NJ: Assessment of Patterns of Drug use by using World Health Organization's Prescribing Patient Care and Health facility indicators in Selected Health Facilities in Southwest Ethiopia. *JAPS* 2011, **1**:62–66.

54. Molla B, Miko A, Pries K, Hildebrandt G, Klee J, Schroeter A, Helmuth R: Class 1 integrons and resistance gene cassettes among multidrug resistant *Salmonella* serovars isolated from slaughter animals and foods of animal origin in Ethiopia. *Acta Trop* 2007, **103**:142–149.

55. Abera B, Biadegelgen F, Bezabih B: Prevalence of *Salmonella typhi* and intestinal parasites among food handlers in Bahir Dar Town, North West Ethiopia. *Ethiop J Health Dev* 2010, **24**:46–50.

56. Aragaw K, Molla B, Muckle A, Cole L, Wilkie E, Poppe C, Kleer J, Hildebrandt G: The characterization of *Salmonella* serovars isolated from apparently healthy slaughtered pigs at Addis Ababa abattoir, Ethiopia. *Prev Vet Med* 2007, **82**:252–261.

57. Alemayehu D, Molla B, Muckle A: Prevalence and antimicrobial resistance pattern of *Salmonella* isolates from apparently healthy slaughtered cattle in Ethiopia. *Trop Anim Health Prod* 2003, **35**:309–319.

58. Molla B, Salah W, Alemayehu D, Mohammed A: Antimicrobial resistance pattern of *Salmonella* serotypes isolated from apparently healthy slaughtered camels (*Camelus dromedarius*) in Eastern Ethiopia. *Berl Münch Tierärztl Wschr* 2004, **117**:39–45.

59. Molla W, Molla B, Alemayehu D, Muckle A, Cole L, Wilkie E: Occurrence and antimicrobial resistance of *Salmonella* serovars in apparently healthy slaughtered sheep and goats of central Ethiopia. *Trop Anim Health Prod* 2006, **38**:455–462.

60. Sibhat B, Zewde BM, Zerihun A, Muckle A, Cole L, Boerlin P, Wilkie E, Perets A, Mistry K, Gebreyes WA: *Salmonella* serovars and antimicrobial resistance profiles in beef cattle, slaughterhouse personnel and slaughterhouse environment in Ethiopia. *Zoonoses Public Hlth* 2011, **58**:102–109.

61. Alemu S, Zewde BM: Prevalence and antimicrobial resistance profiles of *Salmonella enterica* serovars isolated from slaughtered cattle in Bahir Dar, Ethiopia. *Trop Anim Health Prod* 2012, **44**:595–600.

62. Kingsley RA, Msefula CL, Thomson NR: Epidemic multiple drug resistant *Salmonella typhimurium* causing invasive disease in sub-Saharan Africa have a distinct genotype. *Genome Res* 2009, **19**:2279–2287.

63. Feasey NA, Dougan G, Kingsley RA, Heyderman RS, Gordon MA: Invasive non-typhoidal salmonella disease: an emerging and neglected tropical disease in Africa. *Lancet* 2012, **379**:2489–2499.

64. Leibovitz E: The use of fluoroquinolones in children. *Curr Opin Pediatr* 2006, **18**:64–70.

65. Ferrera KP, Bomasang ES: Azithromycin versus First Line Antibiotics in the Therapeutic Management of Documented Cases of Typhoid Fever: A Meta-analysis. *Phil J Microbiol Infect Dis* 2004, **33**:163–168.

66. Frenck RW, Nakhla I, Sultan Y, Bassily SB, Girgis YF, David J, Butler TC, Girgis NI, Morsy M: Azithromycin versus Ceftriaxone for the Treatment of Uncomplicated Typhoid Fever in Children. *Clin Infect Dis* 2000, **31**:1134–1138.

67. Keenan JD, Ayele B, Gebre T, Zerihun M, Zhou Z, House JI, Gaynor BD, Porco TC, Emerson PM, Lietman TM: Childhood mortality in a cohort treated with mass azithromycin for trachoma. *Clin Infect Dis* 2011, **52**:883–888.

68. Chuc NT, Larsson M, Do NT, Diwan VK, Tomson GB, Falkenberg T: Improving private pharmacy practice: a multi-intervention experiment in Hanoi Vietnam. *J Clinic Epidemiol* 2002, **55**:1148–1155.

69. Laing R, Hogerzeil H, Ross-Degnan D: Ten recommendations to improve use of medicines in developing countries. *Health Policy Plan* 2001, **16**:13–20.

9

Underuse of medication for circulatory disorders among unmarried women and men in Norway?

Øystein Kravdal[1,2,4*] and Emily Grundy[3]

Abstract

Background: It is well established that unmarried people have higher mortality from circulatory diseases and higher all-cause mortality than the married, and these marital status differences seem to be increasing. However, much remains to be known about the underlying mechanisms. Our objective was to examine marital status differences in the purchase of medication for circulatory diseases, and risk factors for them, which may indicate underuse of such medication by some marital status groups.

Methods: Using data from registers covering the entire Norwegian population, we analysed marital status differences in the purchase of medicine for eight circulatory disorders by people aged 50-79 in 2004-2008. These differences were compared with those in circulatory disease mortality during 2004-2007, considered as indicating probable differences in disease burden.

Results: The unmarried had 1.4-2.8 times higher mortality from the four types of circulatory diseases considered. However, the never-married in particular purchased less medicine for these diseases, or precursor risk factors of these diseases, primarily because of a low chance of making a first purchase. The picture was more mixed for the divorced and widowed. Both groups purchased less of some of these medicines than the married, but, especially in the case of the widowed, relatively more of other types of medicine. In contrast to the never-married, divorced and widowed people were as least as likely as the married to make a first purchase, but adherence rates thereafter, indicated by continuing purchases, were lower.

Conclusion: The most plausible interpretation of the findings is that compared with married people, especially the never-married more often have circulatory disorders that are undiagnosed or for which they for other reasons underuse medication. Inadequate use of these potentially very efficient medicines in such a large population group is a serious public health challenge which needs further investigation. It is possible that marital status differences in use of medicines for circulatory disorders combined with an increasing importance of these medicines have contributed to the widening marital status gap in mortality observed in several countries. This also requires further investigation.

Keywords: Norway, Circulatory disorders, Marital status, Medication, Underuse, Register data

Background

Numerous studies from many different countries have shown that married people have lower all-cause mortality than the unmarried and lower mortality from several specific causes and cause groups, including circulatory diseases [1-3]. Health-related and other types of selection to and from marriage are known to play a role in this differentiation [4], but marriage is also considered to have health protective effects. These include economic benefits [5], social support, social control by a spouse [6,7] and, partly because of this social control, a lower propensity for risky behaviours [8-10]. These factors may affect health partly through differences in health-related behaviours more generally, including participation in screening programmes, medical consultation rates and adherence to medication, all of which would potentially lead to differences in medication use.

Our aim in this paper is to see whether there are differences by marital status in the purchase (encashment)

* Correspondence: okravdal@econ.uio.no
[1]Norwegian Institute of Public Health, Oslo, Norway
[2]Department of Economics, University of Oslo, Oslo, Norway
Full list of author information is available at the end of the article

of prescribed drugs for eight types of circulatory disorders. We also consider incident and continuing purchase of these medicines. These marital status differences in medication purchase (assumed to be indicative of medication use) are compared with marital status differences in mortality from four specific circulatory causes, used as an indicator of probable differences in disease burden. We use data from registers that cover the entire Norwegian population, and in particular the Norwegian Prescription Database, which includes all purchases of prescription medicine since 2004. The analysis covers the years 2004-2008.

Circulatory diseases are the most common group of causes of death in high income countries, so such an analysis of marital status differentials in the use of medicines for these diseases and their risk factors is potentially very important from a public health perspective. This is particularly the case in the context of improvements in the efficacy of therapeutic treatments for circulatory diseases. Advances in drug-based and surgical treatments have been found to matter greatly at the population level [11,12] and perhaps explain ¼ to ½ of the reduction in the mortality from circulatory diseases over a couple of decades from about 1980 [13-15], and an American study showed that many years of life are lost because a large proportion of the population receive inadequate treatment for coronary heart diseases [16]. Analyses of differentials in medication use by marital status may thus also shed light on recent increases in marital status differentials in circulatory disease mortality, which have contributed strongly to the increases in the corresponding all-cause mortality differentials observed in a number of countries [17-19]. In Norway, especially the never-married have experienced a rising excess mortality compared to the married [17].

Previous research on marital status differentials in medication use is sparse and inconclusive. Delayed diagnosis or treatment for cardiovascular problems among unmarried groups has been reported in some studies [20,21], which accords with studies showing that unmarried people are often diagnosed later with cancer [22,23] and have lower participation rates in screening for various diseases [24]. Differences in adherence to treatments for various diseases by marital status and availability of social support have also been reported. For example, some studies have shown that unmarried people are less likely to follow doctors' advice about medication after diagnosed coronary diseases [25-28] or hypertension [29], and adverse changes in health care utilisation among recently widowed chronically ill men have been reported as well [30]. However, other recent studies of adherence to treatment for circulatory diseases or conditions (risk factors) have not found marital status differences [31,32]. Moreover, the evidence – in either direction - is generally relatively weak because of small sample sizes

[28,29,31] and possible bias arising from use of self-reported measures of medication adherence [25,29,31], rather than measures from prescription registers [32] or electronic monitoring [28].

Methods
Data
The study is based on analysis of two data files, constructed (in 2009-2012) from various Norwegian population registers. Both include, for everyone who has lived in Norway since 1960, year of death, immigration and emigration (if any) and marital status and educational level at the beginning of each year (since 1980, though only the information for the years after 2004 was used in the analysis). These variables were taken from the Central Population Register and the Educational Database (operated by Statistics Norway). Additionally, one of the files includes information from the Cause-of-death Register (up to 2007), while the other includes information from the Norwegian Prescription Database (NorPD) for 2004-2008. NorPD covers all purchases of prescription medicine (defined by Anatomical Therapeutic Chemical (ATC) classification) since 2004 by Norwegian residents, except individuals living in institutions [33]. Because of the latter exclusion, we restricted our analysis to persons younger than 80 during the period under study. The lowest age considered is 50. While circulatory diseases occur among younger individuals, and are treated medically, there are few deaths from this cause group at these lower ages.

Separate analyses were undertaken for women and men, as several studies have suggested that some of the health benefits of partnership may be sex-specific, especially in older age groups [34,35]. In all models, we controlled for level of education, which is an important determinant of marriage and divorce [36,37] as well as health [38] and health care use [39]. Age was, of course, also controlled for.

The use of register data for this research purpose has been approved by the Regional Committees for Medical and Health Research Ethics and the Norwegian Data Protection Authority.

Mortality analysis
Discrete time hazard models for all-cause and cause-specific mortality were estimated for the period 2004-2007, following standard procedures [40]. A series of one-year observations was constructed, starting in January 2004, for all those then aged 49-78 and living in the country. The last observation was the year of death, the year the person turned 79, the year of emigration, or 2007, whichever came first. Those who became 50 or immigrated during the observation period were added from January of the year of their 50th birthday or the

year after immigration, respectively. Observations were excluded if the person lived temporarily abroad at the beginning of the year. Logistic models were estimated from all remaining observations. In total, there were 35,174 deaths within 2,602,246 person-years of observation among men and 23,970 deaths within 2,693,670 person-years of observation among women. Table 1 shows the distribution of these by marital status.

The specific causes of death considered are ischemic heart diseases (ICD-10 codes I00-I25), other heart diseases (I26-I52), cerebrovascular diseases (I60-I69) and all other circulatory diseases (other I00-I99).

Analyses of medicine purchases: prevalence, incidence and discontinuation

In the analysis of drug purchases we considered eight groups of drugs, defined by Kuo et al. [41] as indicating treatment for specific disorders. These disorders were (ATC codes shown in notes to Table 2): i) coronary and peripheral vascular diseases treated with platelet aggregation inhibitors, ii) coronary and peripheral vascular diseases treated with anticoagulants, iii) hypertension without any diagnosed heart disease, iv) hyperlipedemia, v) arrhythmic cardiac diseases, vi) angina, vii) congestive heart failure (usually in combination with hypertension), and viii) other ischemic heart diseases (usually in combination with hypertension). The analysis included three steps. First, logistic models for the chance of purchasing certain drugs at least once during 2004-2008 (i.e. prevalence of medication purchase and, presumably, use) were estimated, conditional on living in the country at the beginning and end of that period. There were 579,218 observations for men and 620,911 for women.

In the second step, discrete-time hazard models for the chance of starting to purchase the specific type of drug (i.e. incidence) were estimated for those who did not use it in 2004. More specifically, one-year observations from 2005 were created conditioned on the individual being of age 50-79 that year, being alive both at the start and the end of the year and not yet having

started to purchase the medicine by the beginning of the year. The outcome variable was whether the drug was purchased at least once during the year.

Similarly, in the third step, discrete-time hazard models for discontinuing the purchase of the medicine were estimated. One-year observations from 2005 were created conditioned on the individual being of age 50-79 that year, being alive both at the start and the end of the year, having purchased the medicine at least once during the preceding year, but having had no earlier discontinuation of the purchase of that medicine (i.e. the individual has either purchased the medicine in every year from 2004 to the preceding year, or started in 2005 or later and kept purchasing until at least the previous year). The outcome variable was whether the drug was purchased at least once during the year. For simplicity, the signs of the effects are reversed in the tables and can thus be interpreted as effects on continuation rather than discontinuation.

Results
Marital status differences in mortality from circulatory diseases

Mortality from circulatory disease was more than twice as high among the never-married as among the married for both men and women. For all circulatory diseases combined the odds ratio for men was 2.11 (95% CI 1.99-2.23) and that for women 2.37 (2.15-2.61). Odds ratios for men and women varied between 1.94 and 2.84 across the four main sub-categories of circulatory diseases considered (Table 2). For men the estimates were 1.93-2.52 for the divorced and 1.51-1.75 for the widowed. Similar results were seen for women, with odds ratios of 1.63-2.14 for the divorced, and 1.44-1.66 for the widowed.

Associations between marital status and purchase of medication 2004-2008

Never-married men and women were generally less likely than the married to purchase medicine for circulatory disorders (Table 2 and signs shown in Panel A of Table 3). The only exceptions were that there was no significant

Table 1 Number of deaths and person-years of exposure in the mortality analysis of women and men aged 50-79 in 2004-2007, by marital status

	Never-married	Married	Widowed	Divorced/separated
Men				
Number of deaths from all causes	5325	19995	3321	6533
Number of deaths from all circulatory diseases	1679	6031	1145	2025
Person-years of exposure	277508	1818415	99705	406618
Women				
Number of deaths from all causes	2027	10515	7490	3938
Number of deaths from all circulatory diseases	509	2248	2262	829
Person-years of exposure	175001	1670393	400626	447650

Table 2 Effects of marital status on all-cause and cause-specific mortality (ICD-10 codes in parentheses) 2004-2007[a] and the chance of purchasing various types of medicines for circulatory disorders 2004-2008 among women and men aged 50-79[b]

		Effects of marital status (with 95% confidence intervals)			Number of deaths or persons purchasing the medicines
		Never-married	Widowed	Divorced/ separated	
Men					
Mortality from	All causes	2.05*** (1.98-2.11)	1.56*** (1.50-1.62)	1.96*** (1.91-2.02)	35174
	All circulatory diseases (I00-I99)	2.11*** (1.99-2.23)	1.65*** (1.54-1.75)	2.08*** (1.97-2.18)	10880
	Ischemic heart diseases (I20-I25)	1.94*** (1.80-2.10)	1.67*** (1.52-1.82)	1.93*** (1.80-2.07)	5737
	Other heart diseases (I26-I52)	2.71*** (2.39-3.08)	1.63*** (1.52-1.82)	2.52*** (2.24-2.85)	1809
	Cerebrovascular diseases (I60-I69)	1.99*** (1.75-2.26)	1.51*** (1.31-1.74)	2.07*** (1.84-2.33)	2066
	Other circulatory diseases	2.13*** (1.81-2.50)	1.75*** (1.46-2.10)	2.11*** (1.82-2.10)	1268
Purchase of medication for	Coronary and peripheral vascular diseases, antiplatelet[c]	0.70*** (0.68-0.73)	1.00 (0.95-1.05)	1.02 (0.99-1.05)	42780
	Coronary and peripheral vascular diseases, anticoagulant[d]	0.88*** (0.85-0.91)	1.04* (1.00-1.08)	1.03** (1.00-1.06)	59898
	Hypertension[e]	0.98 (0.95-1.01)	1.10*** (1.06-1.15)	0.97*** (0.94-0.99)	56019
	Hyperlipedemia[f]	0.69*** (0.68-0.71)	0.95*** (0.93-0.98)	0.89*** (0.87-0.90)	185023
	Anti-arrhythmic cardiac diseases[g]	1.02 (0.97-1.08)	1.09*** (1.03-1.16)	1.09*** (1.04-1.14)	18204
	Ischemic heart diseases/angina[h]	0.75*** (0.73-0.78)	0.98 (0.94-1.02)	0.99 (0.97-1.02)	65918
	Congestive heart failure/hypertension[i]	0.92*** (0.90-0.94)	1.10*** (1.07-1.32)	0.96*** (0.95-0.98)	195657
	Other ischemic heart diseases/hypertension[j]	0.88*** (0.86-0.90)	1.08*** (1.05-1.11)	0.96*** (0.94-0.97)	198133
Women					
Mortality from	All causes	2.05*** (1.95-2.15)	1.40*** (1.35-1.44)	1.70*** (1.64-1.77)	23970
	All circulatory diseases (I00-I99)	2.37*** (2.15-2.61)	1.53*** (1.44-1.62)	1.83*** (1.69-1.98)	5848
	Ischemic heart diseases (I20-I25)	2.38*** (2.05-2.77)	1.44*** (1.31-1.59)	1.80*** (1.59-2.04)	2323
	Other heart diseases (I26-I52)	2.84*** (2.30-3.50)	1.66*** (1.44-1.90)	2.14*** (1.79-2.56)	1163
	Cerebrovascular diseases (I60-I69)	2.18*** (1.82-2.61)	1.51*** (1.35-1.69)	1.63*** (1.40-1.91)	1678
	Other circulatory diseases	1.94*** (1.43-2.64)	1.63*** (1.36-1.95)	1.91*** (1.36-1.95)	684
Purchase of medication for	Coronary and peripheral vascular diseases, antiplatelet[c]	0.84*** (0.78-0.90)	1.12*** (1.08-1.16)	1.24*** (1.19-1.29)	22058
	Coronary and peripheral vascular diseases, anticoagulant[d]	0.92*** (0.88-0.96)	1.07*** (1.04-1.10)	1.08*** (1.05-1.11)	51264
	Hypertension[e]	0.96* (0.93-1.00)	1.03*** (1.01-1.06)	0.94*** (0.92-0.97)	58882
	Hyperlipedemia[f]	0.78*** (0.77-0.81)	0.95*** (0.94-0.97)	0.92*** (0.91-0.94)	175477
	Anti-arrhythmic cardiac diseases[g]	1.00 (0.92-1.09)	1.08*** (1.03-1.13)	1.07** (1.01-1.14)	11746
	Ischemic heart diseases/angina[h]	0.85*** (0.82-0.89)	1.11*** (1.08-1.13)	1.20*** (1.16-1.23)	52641
	Congestive heart failure/hypertension[i]	0.95*** (0.93-0.97)	1.07*** (1.06-1.09)	0.99 (0.97-1.01)	203305
	Other ischemic heart diseases/hypertension[j]	0.87*** (0.85-0.89)	1.03*** (1.01-1.04)	0.94*** (0.92-0.95)	187899

[a]Discrete-time hazard models are estimated. The models also include age (in five-year groups), year (in one-year groups), and educational level (in five categories). *p < 0.10; **p < 0.05; ***p < 0.01.
[b]Logistic models for the chance of purchasing the medicines are estimated. The models also include age (in five-year groups) and educational level (in five categories). Medicines are grouped as in Kuo et al. [41]. See details in notes c-j.
[c]ATC codes B01AC, C04AD03 (except B01AC06, B01AC08, B01AC09, B01AC11, B01AC15, B01AC19, B01AC21).
[d]ATC codes B01AA, B01AB, B01AD, B01AX.
[e]ATC codes C02AA02, C02AB02, C02AC, C02BA, C02BB, C02CA, C02CC, C02DA, C02DB, C02DD, C02DG, C03AA, C03AB, C03AX, C03DA, C03DB, C02L.
[f]ATC codes C10AA, C10AB, C10AC, C10AD, C10AX, C10BA, C10BX.
[g]ATC codes C01AA, C01BA, C01BB, C01BC, C01BD, C01BG, C01EB10.
[h]ATC codes C01DA, C01DX16.
[i]ATC codes C01CA07, C01CE01, C01CE02, C01EB09, C03CA, C03CB, C03CC, C09AA, C09BA, C09BB, C09CA, C09DA, C09DB.
[j]ATC codes C07AA, C07AB, C07AG, C07BA, C07BB, C07BG, C07CA, C07CB, C07CG, C07DA, C07DB, C07EA, C07EB, C07FA, C07FB, C08CA, C08CX, C08DA, C08DB, C08EA, C08EX, C08GA.

Table 3 Sign and significance (+ and - meaning p <0.10; ++ and - - meaning p <0.05; +++ and - - - meaning p <0.01) of effects of marital status on the chance of purchasing medicine in 2004-2008, the chance of starting to purchase medicine 2005-2008, and the chance of continuing with the medicine purchases 2005-2008

		Men Never-married	Widowed	Divorced/separated	Women Never-married	Widowed	Divorced/separated
Panel A: Purchase of medicine in 2004-2008 (signs as in estimates in Table 2)							
Coronary and peripheral vascular diseases, antiplatelet		- - -			- - -	+ + +	+ + +
Coronary and peripheral vascular diseases, anticoagulant		- - -	+	+ +	- - -	+ + +	+ + +
Hypertension			+ + +	- - -	-	+ + +	- - -
Hyperlipedemia		- - -	- - -	- - -	- - -	- - -	- - -
Anti-arrhythmic cardiac diseases			+ +	+ +		+ + +	+ +
IHD/Angina		- - -			- - -	+ + +	+ + +
Congestive heart failure/hypertension		- - -	+ + +	- - -	- - -	+ + +	
Other IHD/hypertension		- - -	+ + +	- - -	- - -	+ + +	- - -
Panel B: Starting and continuing purchase of medicine 2005-2008[a]							
Coronary and peripheral vascular diseases, antiplatelet	Start	- - -		+ + +	- - -	+ + +	+ + +
	Continuation	+ +			+ + +		+ + +
Coronary and peripheral vascular diseases, anticoagulant	Start	- - -		+ + +		+ + +	+ + +
	Continuation			- - -	+		
Hypertension	Start		+ + +		-	+ +	-
	Continuation	+ + +		- - -	+ +		- - -
Hyperlipedemia	Start	- - -			- - -	- -	-
	Continuation	- - -	- - -	- - -	- - -	- - -	- - -
Anti-arrhythmic cardiac diseases	Start		+ + +	+ + +		+ + +	+ + +
	Continuation	+ + +		- -			
IHD/Angina	Start	- - -			- - -	+ + +	+ + +
	Continuation	+ + +			+ + +	+	
Congestive heart failure/hypertension	Start	- - -	+ + +	+ + +		+ + +	+ +
	Continuation	- - -	- - -	- - -	- - -	- - -	- - -
Other IHD/hypertension	Start	- - -	+ + +	+ + +	- - -	+ + +	+ +
	Continuation		- - -	- - -			- - -

[a]Discrete-time hazard models are estimated. The models also include age (in five-year groups), year (in one-year groups), and educational level (in five categories).

association between being never-married and purchasing medicine for hypertension (alone) or arrhythmic diseases. For both sexes, the sharpest negative effects were seen with respect to drugs for hyperlipidemia.

Among divorced men and women, the purchase of four types of medicine was lower than in the married reference group. These were medication for hypertension (alone), hyperlipidemia, heart failure (among men), and ischemic heart disease. On the other hand, three types of medicine were purchased to a larger extent by the divorced than the married, for one or both sexes: medicine for coronary and peripheral vascular diseases (antiplatelet as well as anticoagulant treatment), arrhythmic diseases and angina. However, with two exceptions (1.20 and 1.24), the positive estimates were not above 1.10.

The widowed were, on the whole, more likely than the married to purchase medicine for circulatory disorders. There was only one negative relationship: the use of medicine for hyperlipidemia. Relationships with respect to several other disorders were positive: hypertension, arrhythmic diseases, heart failure and ischemic heart disease for both sexes and coronary and peripheral vascular diseases and angina for women. Again, the positive relationships were not large; all effects were smaller than 1.12.

Associations between marital status and starting and continuing drug purchase
The lower chance of purchasing medicine among the never-married reflects a lower chance of making a first purchase (Table 3, Panel B). Once initiated, the chance of continuing to purchase the medication was significantly

higher than (at a 5% level) or as high among the never-married as the married for several disorders, exceptions being heart failure and, for men, hyperlipedemia.

For the divorced, who generally purchased about as much medicine for circulatory disorders as the married, there is an almost opposite pattern. Their chance of starting to purchase medicine was quite *high*. This was seen for several types of medicine for both men and women, and no effect runs in the other direction. On the other hand, they had a relatively *low* probability of *continuing* to purchase several types of the medicines considered, and there was only one example of the opposite.

The pattern for the widowed was similar to that for the divorced: there were several positive associations with the chance of starting to purchase medicine and one negative (as opposed to none for the divorced), and there was no positive association with the chance of continuing the purchases (as opposed to one for the divorced) and several negative ones. However, there were fewer of the latter associations (five in total, for three different conditions, as opposed to 10 in total for the divorced), so on the whole, the widowed appear to be less different from the married than are the divorced.

Discussion

These results show, consistent with other studies, large marital status variations in mortality from circulatory diseases with the highest risks, relative to married people, for the never-married followed by the divorced and then the widowed. Overall, in the age group considered here (50-79), the unmarried had rates of mortality from circulatory diseases 1.4-2.8 times higher than those of the married. However, never-married people in particular purchased less of the medicines that are typically used after such a circulatory disease has been diagnosed or risk factors for it identified. This was primarily because of a significantly lower chance of first purchase of most of these medicines The picture is more mixed for the divorced and widowed, who purchased less of some of these medicines but more of others, though the difference in the latter direction, which was seen especially among the widowed, was quite small (but statistically significant). In contrast to the never-married, the chances of starting to purchase these medicines were as least as high among the divorced and widowed as among married people, but adherence rates thereafter, indicated by continuing medication purchases, were lower (especially among the divorced).

We assume that purchases of medication are good measures of actual use of medication, and therefore refer to use in the remaining discussion. To the extent that there is a difference between purchase and use, it would seem likely, if anything, that the unmarried might be less inclined than the married to use the purchased medication, because of the lack of social support and control by

a spouse that is further discussed below. If so, marital status differences in actual use may be more pronounced than suggested by our analysis of purchases.

Interpretations of the observed patterns: underuse of medication?

To draw conclusions about underuse of medicine one should ideally compare actual use with need or recommended use. Unfortunately, we lack information on the actual prevalence and severity of the various circulatory disorders (and associated risk factors), which would be good indications of the need, and must instead compare differences in medication purchase, reflecting medication use, with those in mortality. As mentioned, one of our key findings is that the never-married use less medicine than the married for all disorders considered except a few. In theory, it is possible that they also *need* less of these medicines, despite their much higher mortality from all circulatory disease groups (and thus presumably also from the disorders under consideration). Let us assume that they to a larger extent than the married suffer from the *most severe* types of each of these disorders, but have a lower prevalence of the *less* severe types for which medication is nevertheless recommended. Then, even if they take medicine in accordance with recommendations or needs (i.e. no underuse), they could end up using less medicine than the married and have higher mortality. In other words, low usage coupled with high mortality does not *necessarily* mean underuse.

However, this situation seems improbable especially as there are common risk factors for many less and more serious conditions and evidence from numerous studies points to a higher, rather than lower, prevalence of circulatory diseases and associated risk factors among the unmarried than the married. More specifically, it has been shown that the unmarried have higher cholesterol levels than the married [42], higher prevalence of diabetes [43,44], and higher blood pressure [42,45-47], although other studies do not point so clearly in this direction [48-52]. A modest excess prevalence of stroke among the unmarried has also been reported [52,53], as well as an excess prevalence of heart failure [54]. Consistent with this, other studies have reported that lifestyle factors associated with higher circulatory disease risks are less common among married people. In particular, the unmarried are more likely than the married to be physically inactive [42,49,50] (but see [55] for an opposite result), to be obese [49,50,56], (but see [55] for an opposite result) to have a high intake of sodium [46], to eat more fast food [55] and to smoke [42,43,49].

Theoretically, the never-married could also have a lower prevalence of both the more and the less severe types of any disorder - thus taking less medicine even without any underuse - and still have a strong mortality disadvantage because of less adequate use of *other* types of treatment, such as angioplasty or bypass surgery. However, a study by Bearden et al. [57] that addressed the latter issue did not show any relationship between marital status and these kinds of surgical interventions. To conclude, we think the most plausible interpretation of our findings is that the unmarried, and especially the never-married, suffer from circulatory disorders to a larger extent than the married and therefore have a greater need for medication, but that they are on the whole less likely than the married to take the medication they need, which adds further to their mortality disadvantage.

If the unmarried are particularly inclined to use less medicine than recommended or needed for their circulatory disorders, the implications for mortality depend on whether this underuse is most pronounced with respect to the less severe or the more severe types of the disorder. The use of statins (for hyperlipidemia) may serve as a particularly relevant example. This drug is used both as primary prevention (i.e. in the absence of actual circulatory diseases and even at rather low cholesterol levels if other risk factors are identified) and secondary prevention (i.e. when a circulatory disease is diagnosed and presumably treated). The efficacy of this primary prevention has been highly disputed, though a recent Cochrane review pointed towards a mortality reduction [58], which would justify continuation of the practice. We have found that the married use more of this medicine than all groups of unmarried, despite the evidence summarised above that suggests higher cholesterol levels for the unmarried and thus more need for this medicine. Hypothetically, however, it could be that use of statins among the unmarried for the purposes of secondary prevention is consistent with their needs – and so higher than use among the married- whereas use for the purposes of primary prevention is much lower. Such a pattern would have fewer implications for mortality risks than a lower than recommended use for secondary prevention.

Finally, it should be noted that, if the unmarried to a larger extent than the married take too little medicine compared to their needs, they may of course still use somewhat more medicine per person. For example, we have found that some groups of unmarried use more medicine for arrhythmic diseases than the married, and no group less, which may reflect that there is a particularly large difference between the married and the unmarried in the actual prevalence of that disorder. The fact that mortality from "cardiovascular diseases other than ischemic heart diseases" varies particularly much according to marital status lends some support to this idea. Similarly, the unmarried use more diuretics for heart failure (a subgroup of medicines for that disease and not shown in the tables), alone or in combination with other medicine, and this may indicate a relatively high prevalence of right-sided heart failure, which may be linked to chronic obstructive pulmonary disease and thus smoking – the latter being more common among the unmarried according to some studies as already noted [42,43,49].

Factors underlying the differentials in use, and likely underuse, of medication

As mentioned above, studies of marital status differences in health and mortality consistently refer to economic benefits of marriage and the important role played by spouses in providing social support and exerting social control [5-7]. Such factors are thought to affect the disease or accident incidence - through lifestyle (including the use of explicit preventive strategies) - as well as the availability of care, use of medical treatment and other factors of importance for the further development of the diseases. The pathway of special relevance given our perspective is that a spouse's encouragement and monitoring – but perhaps not the more favourable economic position of the married - may affect the chance of seeking a consultation, receiving a diagnosis (or identifying risk factors) and prescription, cashing the initial prescription, and seeking and cashing further prescriptions. The reason for the probably modest importance of economic resources is that costs of prescriptions are typically not very high and for those with chronic diseases, there are subsidies as well as a cap on total annual expenses in Norway.

The evidence on such causal pathways is not large, but some studies of cardiovascular diseases suggest that spouses may encourage attendance at screening, prompt consultation after onset of symptoms or otherwise increase the chance of an early diagnosis [20,21]. Consistent with this, other studies have shown that the unmarried are often diagnosed later with cancer [22,23] and have lower participation rates in screening for various diseases [24]. Some, but not all, earlier investigations have also shown a poorer treatment adherence among the unmarried – within rather small patient samples and often based on self-reporting of drug use [26-28,31,32,59], see details in Introduction. One recent very large study found no differences between partnered and unpartnered women in reported use of common medications for IHD two years after first hospital admission for this condition [60], but it may be that differences in adherence are less marked for severe conditions which have resulted in acute admissions.

In the absence of a spouse, children may play a similar role in supporting consultation and treatment adherence, and as fewer of the never-married than the widowed or divorced have children, this might account for some of the differences we found between groups of the unmarried when it comes to the chance of using and starting to use the medicines for circulatory disorders. However there is little evidence from previous studies on this issue. Another possible reason for these differences between the never-married and formerly married is that the latter may persist with habits of health care seeking developed during their married life, though it is harder to understand why they are more inclined to *discontinue* the use of medicines.

Limitations and strengths of the analysis

The study has some limitations, the most important being the lack of information on actual disorders as discussed above. Furthermore, formal marital status does not tell us the full story about actual living arrangements. Some of the unmarried live in cohabiting unions (currently 29% in the age group 45-66 and 10% in the age group 67-79, according to Statistics Norway [61]), and if cohabitants use medicine to a larger extent than the unmarried who live alone and do not have a partner, the difference between the latter and the married will be even larger than the estimated difference between the unmarried and the married that we report. Some authors have shown that the lower prevalence of circulatory diseases or their risk factors among the married is restricted to those having a good marriage, whereas those in a poor marriage are in a worse position than the single [51,62,63]. With register data, it is of course impossible to consider the quality of the marriage. We also lacked data on other possibly relevant confounders, mediators or moderators such as lifestyle factors, values, prior health status or indicators of socio-economic status other than education.

Additionally, NorPD does not include drug purchases for individuals in health care institutions. Since the unmarried are more likely to be institutionalized, the actual use of medicine in this group may not be quite as modest compared to the married as indicated by our estimates. However, this bias must be small, as the analysis only includes persons younger than 80, and at age 75-79 only 5% live in institutions [64].

An important strength of the study is availability of data that covers the whole population in which the measure of drug use was based on recorded purchase, assumed to be a good indicator of use, rather than self-report of use.

Conclusion

Our results suggest that there is an underuse of medicine for circulatory disorders among the unmarried, and especially the never-married. The low usage of medication by the never-married particularly reflects low initial purchase of medication whereas for the divorced and widowed failure to continue with medication seemed more important. Inadequate use of these potentially very efficient medicines in such a large population group is, of course, a serious public health problem. Furthermore, underuse of medication for circulatory disorders among the unmarried in relatively recent years, combined with an increasing importance of such medicines, suggest a growing disadvantage for the unmarried when it comes to this type of medication (unless there was a much more pronounced underuse among these groups in earlier years, when the available medication was less efficient). This increasing disadvantage may have contributed to their falling behind with respect to mortality from circulatory diseases, and thus the widening marital status gap in all-cause mortality – which has been seen in a number of countries. In Norway, the excess mortality has increased particularly much for the group of unmarried also showing the clearest indications of underuse of medication for circulatory disorders, the never-married. Stated differently, the unmarried – and particularly the never-married- may not have benefited from recent life-saving improvements in medical treatment for circulatory disorders to the same extent as the married.

Further investigation of this issue is clearly warranted. A central element of such investigations should be to collect data that make it possible to better measure the potential underuse of medication. For that purpose, one would need information about the actual prevalence of the disorders as well as all types of treatment that are used. Obviously, it would also be an advantage if the data could shed light on the underlying mechanisms such as, for example, the role of spouses and children in prompting seeking of and adherence to treatment.

Competing interests
The authors declare that they have no competing interest.

Authors' contributions
Both authors have contributed to the planning of the analysis and the writing. ØK has done the estimation. The final manuscript is approved by both authors.

Acknowledgements
The project is partly funded by an ERC Advanced Grant to Emily Grundy. The advice from Håkon Kravdal is greatly appreciated.

Author details
[1]Norwegian Institute of Public Health, Oslo, Norway. [2]Department of Economics, University of Oslo, Oslo, Norway. [3]Department of Social Policy, London School of Economics and Political Science, London, UK. [4]Postal address: Department of Economics, P.O. Box 1095 Blindern, 0317 Oslo, Norway.

References
1. Ben-Shlomo Y, Smith GD, Shipley M, Marmot MG: **Magnitude and causes of mortality differences between married and unmarried men.** *J Epidemiol Community Health* 1993, **47**:200–205.
2. Joung IM, Glerum JJ, vanPoppel FW, Kardaun JW, Mackenbach JP, Glerum JJ, VanPoppel FW, Kardaun JW, Mackenbach JP: **The contribution of specific causes of death to mortality differences by marital status in the Netherlands.** *Eur J Pub Health* 1996, **6**:142–149.
3. Rendall MS, Weden MM, Favreault MM, Waldron H: **The protective effect of marriage for survival: a review and update.** *Demography* 2011, **48**:481–506.

4.　Brochmann H, Klein T: Love and death in Germany: the marital biography and its effect on mortality. *J Marriage Fam* 2004, 66:567–581.

5.　Wilmoth J, Koso G: Does marital history matter? Marital status and wealth outcomes among preretirement adults. *J Marriage Fam* 2002, 64:254–268.

6.　Umberson D, Montez JK: Social relationships and health: a flashpoint for health policy. *J Health Soc Behav* 2010, 51:S54–S66.

7.　Lewis MA, Butterfield RM: Social control in marital relationships: effect of one's partner on health behaviors. *J Appl Soc Psychol* 2007, 37:298–319.

8.　Fessler MT: Madmen: An Evolutionary Perspective on Anger and men's Violent Responses to Transgression. In *International Handbook of Anger: Constituent and Concomitant Biological, Psychological, and Social Processes.* Edited by Potegal M, Stemmler G, Speilberger C. New York: Springer; 2010:361–381.

9.　Love DA: The effects of marital status and children on savings and portfolio choice. *Rev Financ Stud* 2010, 23:385–432.

10.　Waite L, Gallagher M: *Why Married People are Happier, Healthier, and Better Off Financially.* New York: Broadway Books; 2002.

11.　Hoffmann R, Plug I, McKee M, Khoshaba B, Westerling R, Looman C, Mackenbach JP: Innovations in medical care and mortality trends from four circulatory diseases between 1970 and 2005. *Eur J Publ Health* 2013, 23:852–857.

12.　Lichtenberg FR: The impact of new drug launches on longevity: evidence from longitudinal, disease-level data from 52 countries, 1982-2001. *Int J Health Care Finance Econ* 2005, 5:47–73.

13.　O'Flaherty M, Buchan I, Capewell S: Contributions of treatment and lifestyle to declining CVD mortality: why have CVD mortality rates declined so much since the 1960s? *Heart* 2013, 99:159–162.

14.　Ford ES, Ajani UA, Croft JB, Critchley JA, Labarthe DR, Kottke TE, Giles WH, Capewll S: Explaining the decrease in U.S. deaths from coronary disease, 1980-2000. *New Engl J Med* 2007, 356:2388–2398.

15.　Laatikainen T, Critchley J, Vartiainen E, Solomaa V, Ketonen M, Capewell S: Explaining the decline in coronary heart disease mortality in Finland between 1982 and 1997. *Am J Epidemiol* 2005, 162:764–773.

16.　Capewell S, O'Flaherty M, Ford ES, Critchley JA: Potential reductions in United states coronary heart disease mortality by treating more patients. *Am J Cardiol* 2009, 103:1703–1709.

17.　Berntsen KN: Trends in total and cause-specific mortality by marital status among elderly Norwegian men and women. *BMC Public Health* 2011, 11:537.

18.　Murphy M, Grundy E, Kalogirou S: The increase in marital status differences in mortality up to the oldest age in seven European countries, 1990–99. *Popul Stud* 2007, 61:287–298.

19.　Roelfs DJ, Shor E, Kalish R, Yogev T: The rising relative risk of mortality for singles: meta-analysis and metaregression. *Am J Epidemiol* 2011, 174:379–389.

20.　Atzema CL, Austin PC, Huynh T, Hassan A, Chiu M, Wang JT, Tu JV: Effect of marriage on duration of chest pain associated with acute myocardial infarction before seeking care. *CMAJ* 2011, 183:1482–1491.

21.　Moser D, Kimble L, Alberts M, Alonzo A, Croft J, Dracup K, Evenson KR, Go AS, Hand MM, Kothari RU, Mensah GA, Morris DL, Pancioli AM, Riegel B, Zerwic JJ: Reducing delay in seeking treatment by patients with acute coronary syndrome and stroke: A scientific statement from the American Heart Association Council on cardiovasuclar Nursing and Stroke Council. *Circulation* 2006, 114:168–182.

22.　Abdollah F, Sun M, Thuret R, Abdo A, Morgan M, Jeldres C, Shariat SF, Perrotte P, Montorsi F, Karakiewicz PI: The effect of marital status on stage and survival of prostate cancer patients treated with radical prostatectomy: a population-based study. *Canc Causes Contr* 2011, 22:1085–1095.

23.　Ortiz CAR, Freeman JL, Kuo YF, Goodwin JS: The influence of marital status on stage at diagnosis and survival of older persons with melanoma. *J Gerontol: Medical Sciences* 2007, 62A:892–898.

24.　Stimpson JP, Wilson FA: Cholesterol screening by marital status and sex in the United States. *Preventing Chronic Disease* 2009, 6:1–9.

25.　Kulkarni SP, Alexander KP, Lytle B, Heiss G, Peterson ED: Long-term adherence with cardiovascular drug regimens. *Am Heart J* 2005, 151:185–191.

26.　Marcum ZA, Zheng Y, Perera S, Strotmeyer E, Newman AB, Simonsick EM, Shorr RI, Bauer DC, Donohue JM, Hanlon JT: Prevalence and correlates of self-reported medication non-adherence among older adults with coronary heart disease, diabetes mellitus, and/or hypertension. *Res Soc Admin Pharm* 2013, 9:817–827.

27.　Molloy GJ, Perkins-Porras L, Strike PC, Streptoe A: Social networks and partner stress as predictors of adherence to medication, rehabilitation attendance, and quality of life following acute coronary syndrome. *Health Psychol* 2008, 27:52–58.

28.　Wu JR, Lennie TA, Chung ML, Frazier SK, Dekker RL, Biddle MJ, Moser DK: Medication adherence mediates the relationship between marital status and cardiac event-free survival in patients with heart failure. *Heart & Lung* 2012, 41:107–114.

29.　Trivedi RB, Ayotte B, Edelman D, Bosworth HB: The association of emotional wellbeing and marital status with treatment adherence among patients with hypertension. *J Behav Med* 2008, 31:489–497.

30.　Simeonova E: Marriage, bereavement and mortality: the role of health care utilization. *J Health Econ* 2013, 32:33–50.

31.　Gallagher R, Warwick M, Chenoweth L, Stein-Parbury J, Milton-Wildey K: Medication knowledge, adherence and predictors among people with heart failure and chronic obstructive pulmonary disease. *J Nurs Healthc Chronic Illn* 2011, 3:30–40.

32.　Oksanen T, Kawachi I, Kouvonen A, Suzuki E, Takao S, Sjösten N, Virtanen M, Pentti J, Vahtera J, Kivimäki M: Workplace social contact and adherence to antihypertensive medication: a cohort study. *PLoS One* 2011, 6:e24732.

33.　Furu K, Wettermark B, Andersen M, Martikainen JE, Almarsdottir AB, Sørensen HAT: The Nordic countries as a cohort for pharmacoepidemiological research. *Basic Clin Pharmacol Toxicol* 2011, 106:86–94.

34.　Goldman N, Korenman S, Weinstein R: Marital status and health among the elderly. *Soc Sci Med* 1995, 40:717–730.

35.　Williams K, Umberson D: Marital status, marital transitions, and health:a gendered life course perspective. *J Health Soc Behav* 2004, 45:81–98.

36.　Lyngstad T, Jalovaara M: A review of the antecedents of union dissolution. *Demogr Res* 2010, 23:257–292.

37.　Sweeney MM: Two decades of family change: the shifting economic foundations of marriage. *Am Sociol Rev* 2002, 67:132–147.

38.　Elo IT: Social class differentials in health and mortality: patterns and explanations in comparative perspective. *Annu Rev Sociol* 2009, 35:553–572.

39.　Vikum E, Bjørngaard JH, Westin S, Krokstad S: Socio-economic inequalities in Norwegian health care utilization over 3 decades: the HUNT Study. *Eur J Pub Health* 2013, 23:1003–1010.

40.　Allison PD: Discrete-time methods for the analysis of event histories. *Sociol Methodol* 1982, 13:61–98.

41.　Kuo RN, Dong YH, Liu JP, Chang CH, Shau WY, Lai MS: Predicting healthcare utilization using a pharmacy-based metric with the WHO's anatomical therapeutic chemical algorithm. *Med Care* 2011, 49:1031–1039.

42.　Kamon Y, Okamura T, Tanaka T, Hozawa A, Yamagata Z, Takebayashi T, Kusaka Y, Urano S, Nakagawe H, Kadowaki T, Miyoshi Y, Yamato H, Okayama A, Ueshima H, the HIPOP.OHP Research Group: Marital status and cardiovascular risk factors among middle-aged Japanese male workers: The High-risk and Population Strategy for Occupational Health Promotion (HIPOP-OHP) Study. *J Occup Health* 2008, 50:348–356.

43.　Molloy GJ, Stamatakis E, Randall G, Hamer M: Marital status, gender and cardiovascular mortality: behavioural, psychological distress and metabolic explanations. *Soc Sci Med* 2009, 69:223–228.

44.　Choi BCK, Shi F: Risk factors for diabetes mellitus by age and sex: results of the national population health survey. *Diabetologica* 2001, 44:1221–1231.

45.　Keenan NL, Rosendorf KA: Prevalence of hypertension and controlled hypertension – United States, 2005-2008. *Morbidity and Mortality Weekly Report (Center for Disease Control)* 2011, 60:94–97.

46.　Lipowicz A, Lopuszanska M: Marital differences in blood pressure and the risk of hypertension among Polish men. *Eur J Epidemiol* 2005, 20:421–427.

47.　Kamiya Y, Whelan B, Timonen V, Kenny RA: The differential impact of subjective and objective aspects of social engagement on cardiovascular risk factors. *BMC Geriatr* 2010, 10:81.

48.　Ebrahim S, Wannamethee G, McCallum A, Walker M, Shaper AG: Marital status, change in marital status, and mortality in middle-aged British men. *Am J Epidemiol* 1995, 142:834–842.

49.　Cubbin C, Sundquist K, Ahlén H, Johansson SE, Winkleby MA, Sundquist J: Neighborhood deprivation and cardiovascular disease risk factors: protective and harmful effects. *Scand J Publ Health* 2006, 34:228–237.

50.　Gallo LC, Troxel WM, Matthews KA, Kuller LH: Marital status and quality in middle-aged women: associations with levels and trajectories of cardiovascular risk factors. *Health Psychol* 2003, 22:53–463.

51.　Gliksman MD, Lazarus R, Wilson A, Leeder SR: Social support, marital status and living arrangement correlates of cardiovascular disease risk factors in the elderly. *Soc Sci Med* 1995, 40:811–814.

52. Engström G, Khan FA, Zia E, Jerntorp I, Pessah-Rasmussen H, Norrving B, Janzon L: **Marital dissolution is followed by an increased incidence of stroke.** *Cerebrovasc Dis* 2004, **18**:318–324.

53. Maselko J, Bates LM, Avendano M, Glymour MM: **The intersection of sex, marital status, and cardiovascular risk factors in shaping stroke incidence: results from the heath and retirement study.** *J Am Geriatr Soc* 2009, **57**:2293–2299.

54. Ingelsson E, Lind L, Ärnlöv J, Sundström J: **Socioeconomic factors as predictors of incident heart failure.** *J Card Fail* 2006, **12**:540–545.

55. Yannakoulia M, Panagiotako D, Pitsavos C, Skoumas Y, Stafanadis C: **Eating patterns may mediate the association between matrital status, body mass index, and blood cholesterol levels in apparently healthy men and women from the ATTICA study.** *Soc Sci Med* 2008, **66**:2230–2239.

56. Hedblad B, Jonsson S, Nilsson P, Engström G, Berglund G, Janzon L: **Obesity and myocardial infarction – vulnerability related to occupational level and marital status. A 23-year follow-up of an urban male Swedish population.** *J Intern Med* 2002, **252**:542–550.

57. Bearden D, Allman R, McDonald R, Miller S, Pressel S, Petrovitch H: **Age, race, and gender variation in the utilization of coronary artery bypass surgery and angioplasty in SHEP. SHEP cooperative research group. Systolic Hypertension in the Elderly Program.** *J Am Geriatr Soc* 1994, **42**:1143–1149.

58. Taylor FC, Huffman M, Ebrahim S: **Statin therapy for primary prevention of cardiovascular disease.** *JAMA* 2013, **310**:2451–2452.

59. Ji R, Liu G, Shen H, Wang Y, Li H, Peterson E, Wang Y: **Persistence of secondary prevention medications after acute ischemic stroke or transient ischemic attack in Chinese population: data from China national stroke registry.** *Neurol Res* 2013, **35**:29–36.

60. Floud S, Balkwill A, Canoy D, Wright FL, Reeves GK, Green B, Beral V, Cairns BJ, the Million Women Study Collaborators: **Marital status and ischemic heart disease incidence and mortality in women: a large prospective study.** *BMC Med* 2014, **12**:42.

61. Statistics Norway: *Living Arrangements in Norway. 2012.* http://www.ssb.no/english/subjects/02/01/20/samboer_en/.

62. Gallo LC, Troxel WM, Kuller LH, Sutton-Tyrrell K, Edmundowicz D, Matthews KA: **Marital status, marital quality, and atherosclerotic burden in postmenopausal women.** *Psychosom Med* 2003, **65**:952–962.

63. Holt-Lunstad J, Birmingham W, Jones BQ: **Is there something unique about marriage? The relative impact of marital status, relationship quality, and network social support on ambulatory blood pressure and mental health.** *Ann Behav Med* 2008, **35**:239–244.

64. Ugreninov E: *Seniorer i Norge. Statistical Analyses 72.* Oslo-Kongsvinger: Statistics Norway; 2005.

10

Is the standard dose of amoxicillin-clavulanic acid sufficient?

Michiel Haeseker[1,3,5*], Thomas Havenith[2], Leo Stolk[2], Cees Neef[2], Cathrien Bruggeman[1,3] and Annelies Verbon[4]

Abstract

Background: The pharmacodynamic (PD) efficacy target of amoxicillin is 40% time above the minimal inhibition concentration (40%T > MIC). Recent studies of other antibiotics have shown that PD-efficacy targets are not always reached. The aim of this study was to evaluate the percentage of hospitalised patients, using amoxicillin/clavulanic acid intravenously (iv), that reach the pharmacodynamic efficacy target 40%T > MIC. Additionally, the association of demographic anthropomorphic and clinical parameters with the pharmacokinetics and pharmacodynamics of amoxicillin were determined.

Methods: In serum of 57 hospitalised patients amoxicillin concentrations were measured using high performance liquid chromatography. Patients were older than 18 years and most patients had an abdominal infection. The standard amoxicillin/clavulanic acid dose was 4 times a day 1000/200 mg iv. Pharmacokinetic parameters were calculated with maximum *a posteriori* Bayesian estimation (MW\Pharm 3.60). A one-compartment open model was used. Individual dosing simulations were performed with MW\Pharm.

Results: In our study population, the mean (±SD) age was 67 (±16) years and the mean clearance corrected for bodyweight was 0.17 (±0.07) L/h/kg. Only, 65% of the patients reached the proposed amoxicillin 40%T > MIC with amoxicillin/clavulanic acid for bacterial MICs of 8 mg/L. A computer simulated increase of the standard dose to 6 times daily, increased this percentage to 95%. In this small study group 40%T > MIC was not associated with clinical or microbiological cure.

Conclusion: A substantial proportion of the hospitalised patients did not reach the 40%T > MIC with the standard dose amoxicillin/clavulanic acid for a bacterial MIC of 8 mg/L. Therefore, we suggest increasing the standard dose of amoxicillin/clavulanic acid to 6 times a day in patients with severe Enterobacteriaceae infections.

Trial registration: Trial registration number: NTR1725 16th march 2009.

Keywords: Amoxicillin, Clavulanic acid, Pharmacokinetics, Age

Background

In vitro and animal studies have shown that β-lactam antibiotics for Gram-positive bacteria and Gram-negative bacteria are effective when the percentage time above the minimal inhibition concentration (%T > MIC) of the unbound serum concentration is more than 35-40%. Maximal effects are reached with %T > MIC above 60-70% [1-3]. Only sparse pharmacokinetic/pharmacodynamic (PK/PD) data are estimated in human clinical studies.

Pharmacokinetic analysis of amoxicillin/clavulanic acid has mostly been done in healthy individuals [4,5]. In human clinical studies amoxicillin/clavulanic acid has been found to cure *Streptococcus pneumoniae* and *Haemophilus influenza* infections clinically and microbiologically when %T > MIC was ≥40% [1]. To our knowledge, there are no human pharmacodynamic efficacy studies for Enterobacteriaceae.

Amoxicillin/clavulanic acid is a commonly used broad spectrum antibiotic. Clavulanic acid extends the spectrum of amoxicillin to β-lactamase producing strains, such as *E. coli*, *K. pneumoniae*, *H. influenzae* and *S. aureus*. Clavulanic acid has very little intrinsic antibacterial effect. Clavulanic acid irreversibly inhibits β-lactamase, protecting amoxicillin [6]. Therefore, amoxicillin is measured for

* Correspondence: m.haeseker@mumc.nl
[1]Department of Medical Microbiology, Maastricht University Medical Centre, Maastricht, the Netherlands
[3]Care and Public Health Research Institute (CAPHRI), Maastricht, the Netherlands
Full list of author information is available at the end of the article

determining the PD-efficacy target. Susceptibility patterns of Enterobacteriaceae have changed over time, and recent studies have shown that efficacy targets of other antibiotics, such as ciprofloxacin [7,8], ceftazidim [9] and gentamicin [10] are not reached in a significant percentage of patients. In the EUCAST rationale document the target attainment rates for different doses of amoxicillin for different MICs based on Monte Carlo simulations are reported [11]. Amoxicillin blood levels have not been measured in these simulations. The aim of this study was to measure the amoxicillin serum concentrations in hospitalised patients using amoxicillin/clavulanic acid intravenously (iv) and to determine if the efficacy target of $40\%T > MIC$ was reached. Additionally, we have investigated the association of demographic anthropomorphic and clinical parameters with pharmacokinetics and pharmacodynamics of amoxicillin.

Methods

Study design

Patients above 18 years of age treated with amoxicillin/clavulanic acid iv and hospitalised at the Maastricht University Medical Centre (MUMC), a 715 bed university hospital, were included from January 2010 until October 2010. Amoxicillin blood levels were measured in residual samples drawn for routine assays. Patients with at least two blood samples available were included and blood samples taken during or within 0.5 hours after infusion were excluded. Amoxicillin/clavulanic acid (Sandoz, Holzkirchen, Germany) was started at the discretion of the attending physician, either empirically or as therapy for bacteria susceptible to amoxicillin/clavulanic acid. The standard dose of amoxicillin/clavulanic acid was 1000/200 mg 4 times a day and 1000/200 mg 2 times a day was prescribed when the creatinine clearance (CLcr) was 10–50 ml/min. Amoxicillin/clavulanic acid 1000/200 mg/100 mL infusion was infused in 30 minutes. Demographic and clinical data, such as age, gender, weight, temperature, co-medication, length of hospital stay, time of administration of amoxicillin/clavulanic acid and laboratory parameters, such as, serum creatinine, C-reactive protein (CRP) were retrieved from the electronic patient file (iSoft, the Netherlands). Clinical outcome was defined by CRP normalisation, number of admission days, and discharge from the hospital, time to defeveresence and microbiological cure. CLcr was calculated with the Cockcroft-Gault formula using the lean body mass.

This study was registered at the Dutch Trial Register (NTR 1725) [12] and was approved by the Medical Ethical Committee of the Maastricht University Medical Centre (MEC 08-4-063). All data in this study were analysed anonymously and amoxicillin blood levels were measured in residual samples drawn for routine assays. Therefore, no consent was required from the patient.

This is in agreement with the Medical Research Involving Human Subjects Act, the code for proper use of human tissue as formulated by the Dutch Federation of Medical Scientific Societies and the policy of the Medical Ethics Committee of the Maastricht University Medical Centre.

HPLC analysis

A simple, fast and specific method for measuring amoxicillin serum levels has been validated for linearity, precision, accuracy and stability, following the guidelines for industry bioanalytical method validation recommended by the Food and Drug Administration (FDA) [13]. In short, serum samples were precipitated with perchloric acid 3%. A reverse phase high pressure liquid chromatography (RP-HPLC) method was used. The calibration range was 10 to 200 mg/L. Six quality controls (8, 20, 40, 60, 80 and 160 mg/L) were tested. The intra- and inter-assay variability was within 7.5%. The relationship between plasma concentration and sd was fitted with a polynomial of second order [14]. With this polynomial the lower limit of quantification with a precision of 20% has been calculated and was 0.8 mg/L [15]. All our measured concentrations were above 0.8 mg/L.

Pharmacokinetic analysis

Pharmacokinetic parameters of amoxicillin in individual patients were calculated with maximum *a posteriori* (MAP) Bayesian estimation program (computer program MW/Pharm 3.60, Mediware, the Netherlands). A one-compartment open pharmacokinetic model was used. With MAP Bayesian estimation [16,17] all patient characteristics and measured amoxicillin concentrations are fitted on an existing population model [4,5]. With two concentrations per patient individual pharmacokinetic parameters can be adequately calculated with MAP Bayesian estimation [17]. With these individual fitted pharmacokinetic parameters, dosing simulations were made to adjust the dose individually; this MAP Bayesian estimation is standard procedure in laboratories which provide therapeutic drug monitoring service. A population kinetic model from our population was not made. The free fraction of amoxicillin was fixed at 80%. The $\%T > MIC$ was determined with the formula of Turnidge; $\%T > MIC = \ln(Dose/Vd \times MIC) \times T\frac{1}{2}/\ln(2) \times 100/dosing\ interval$ [18]. Individual dosing simulations were performed with MW-Pharm (3 times 1000–2000 mg, 4 times 2000 mg, 5 times 1000–2000 mg, 6 times 1000–2000 mg).

Microbiological analysis

Identification of the causative bacterium (ID) and antibiotic susceptibility testing (AST) were performed with the Becton Dickinson Phoenix™ Automated Microbiology

System (Franklin Lakes, New Jersey, USA) using the ID/ AST Combo panels UNMIC/ID53 and NMIC/ID75 for Gram negative bacteria and the AST panel PMIC-58 for Gram positive bacteria. In urine cultures the lowest MIC detectable was 0.5 mg/L by the UNMIC/ID53 panel (standard clinical care). MIC values were not determined by the Becton Dickinson Phoenix™ for Streptococcal spp. and Anaerobes. Susceptibility testing for Streptococcal spp. and Anaerobes was done with the disc diffusion method.

Statistical analysis

Metric variables were tested for normality of distribution by the Shapiro-Wilk test and presented as mean (±SD). If not, median and ranges were also given. Categorical variables are presented as frequencies and percentages. Univariate analysis on the amoxicillin clearance corrected for bodyweight (CLam/W) with categorical variables was either done by Student t-test or by one-way ANOVA. Data analysis was done with SPSS-pc version 16.0. A P-value of <0.05 is considered to be statistically significant.

Results

Study group

A total of 57 patients with a mean (±SD) of 3 (±0.9) blood samples (median: 2, range 2–5 blood samples) were included. The mean age was 67 (±16) years (median: 69, range 23–93 years) and 70% were male (Table 1). About half of the patients had an abdominal infection, 18% a wound infection and 10% a pneumonia (Table 1).

Pharmacokinetic and pharmacodynamic analysis

The mean CLam/W was 0.17 (±0.07) L/h/kg (median: 0.16, range: 0.05-0.37 L/h/kg) and the mean volume of distribution corrected for bodyweight (V/W) was 0.31 (±0.07) L/kg (median: 0.30, range: 0.19-0.50 L/kg). The mean volume of distribution (V) was 24 (±5.6) L (median: 24, range: 14–36 L) and the mean elimination half-life (t½) was 1.5 (±0.6) h (median: 1.3, range: 0.6-3.29 h) which is in the same range as described in the EUCAST rationale document [11]. The mean serum creatinine was 90 (±36) μmol/L (median: 90, range: 49–210 μmol/L). Fifty-five (96%) patients received the standard dose of amoxicillin/ clavulanic acid 4 times a day 1000/200 mg iv, 1 patient 3 times 1000/200 mg iv and 1 patient 2 times a day 1000/ 200 mg iv, both because of renal insufficiency. Patients above 70 years had lower CLam/W (P = 0.02), Table 2. A significant correlation was found between CLam/W and age (P < 0.001).

The measured concentrations of amoxicillin were plotted against the sampling times in Figure 1. There was a good linear correlation (R^2 = 0.96) between the amoxicillin actual measured concentration and estimated concentration with MAP Bayesian fitting (MW/Pharm 3.60,

Table 1 Characteristics of 57 hospitalised patients

	Mean (±SD)	Median (range)
Age in years	67 (±16)	69 (23–93)
Weight in kg	78 (±20)	75 (43–153)
Number of blood levels	3 (±0.9)	2 (2–5)
Amoxicillin iv days	13 (±9)	10 (3–57)
Admission days	27 (±34)	19 (4–188)
Gender	Number (percentage)	
• Male	40 (70%)	
• Female	17 (30%)	
Infection	Number (percentage)	
• Abdominal infection	28 (49%)	
• Wound infection	10 (17.5%)	
• Pneumonia	6 (11%)	
• Urinary tract infection	3 (5%)	
• Other	10 (17.5%)	
Amoxicillin combination	Number (percentage)	
• Monotherapy	44 (78%)	
• Ciprofloxacin	4 (7%)	
• Erythromycin	3 (5%)	
• Gentamicin	3 (5%)	
• Other[a]	3 (5%)	
Co-medication	Number (percentage)	
• None	16 (28%)	
• Cardiovascular	27 (47%)	
• Diabetic mellitus	15 (26%)	
• Immunosuppressive	3 (5%)	
• Other[b]	8 (14%)	

[a]Other: rifampicin, cefuroxim and metronidazol.
[b]Other: haloperidol, levothyroxine, painkillers, anticoagulant.

Mediware, the Netherlands), Figure 2. The amoxicillin efficacy target (40%T > MIC) was reached in 100% of patients with a bacterial MIC ≤ 2 mg/L of Gram negative bacteria, in 93% of patients with a MIC = 4 mg/L and in 65% of patients with a MIC = 8 mg/L (Figure 3). When divided in age categories, arbitrarily set at 70 years; all patients older than 70 years reached the 40%T > MIC with a MIC of 4 mg/L and 87% of the patients younger than 70 years. For a MIC of 8 mg/L, the 40%T > MIC was reached in 81% of the patients older than 70 years and in 52% of the patients younger than 70 years (Figure 3).

Analysis of influence of co-variates on pharmacokinetic and pharmacodynamic parameters

To determine which co-variates have an effect on the pharmacokinetic parameters of amoxicillin, a univariate analysis was done using a predetermined set of predictors (Table 3). In the univariate analysis CLam/W was

Table 2 Mean (±SD) CLam/W[a], CLcr[b], V/W[c] and T½[d] for amoxicillin in patients using amoxicillin/clavulanic acid broken down per age group

Age group in years	N	CLam/W in L/h/kg	CLcr in mL/min	V/W in L/kg	T½ in h
<70	31	0.19 (±0.08)	82 (±25)	0.30 (±0.06)	1.26 (±0.44)
>70	26	0.14 (±0.06)	55 (±19)	0.32 (±0.08)	1.83 (±0.71)
P-value		0.02	<0.01	0.82	<0.01

[a]CLam/W: amoxicillin clearance corrected for bodyweight.
[b]CLcr: creatinine clearance.
[c]V/W: volume of distribution corrected for bodyweight.
[d]T½: amoxicillin half life.

related to age, creatinine, CLcr, V/W and 40%T > MIC. Linear correlations were found between CLam/W, creatinine and age (R^2 0.327), Vd (R^2 0.370) and age (R^2 0.227). In the univariate analysis age was not correlated to creatinine (R 0.10, $P = 0.467$) and no linear correlation (R^2 0.01) was found.

Dosing simulations

To determine whether increasing the dose of amoxicillin/clavulanic acid would lead to sufficiently high %T > MIC, the %T > MIC was calculated for all patients with increasing doses with the Turnidge formula [18]. When increasing the dosage frequency from 4 times to 6 times a day all patients with bacterial MIC ≤ 4 reach the efficacy target and 95% (54/57) of the patients with bacterial MIC ≤ 8 (Figure 4).

Microbiological analysis

Sixteen out of twenty one abdominal fluid cultures became positive, 8/10 wound cultures, 7/16 blood cultures, 4/5 urine cultures and 1/2 sputum cultures became positive. Of three patients no cultures were taken. In total thirty-six of the 57 patients (63%) had a positive culture. Of the positive cultures, 30 (83%) were Enterobacteriaceae; E. coli (n = 21), Klebsiella spp. (n = 6), Enterobacter spp. (n = 2) and Proteus spp. (n = 1). In three patients two bacteria were isolated. Of the Gram positive cultures, 6 were Enterococcus spp, 3 Staphylococcus aureus and 1 coagulase negative staphylococcus. Forty MIC values were available in 36 patients. Of the isolated Enterobactericeae 17/30 (57%) of had a MIC ≤ 4 mg/L, 4/30 (13%) had a MIC = 8 mg/L and 9/30 (30%) had a MIC ≥ 16 mg/L. Of the isolated Gram positive bacteria 8/10 (80%) of had a MIC ≤ 1 mg/L and 2/10 (20%) had a MIC ≥ 4 mg/L. Clinical cure was reached in 46 patients, 8 patients switched antibiotic therapy and in 3 patients cure was not reached (of which two died). No significant associations were found between 40%T > MIC and defevervescence, CRP decrease or increase, admission days and clinical outcome (data not shown).

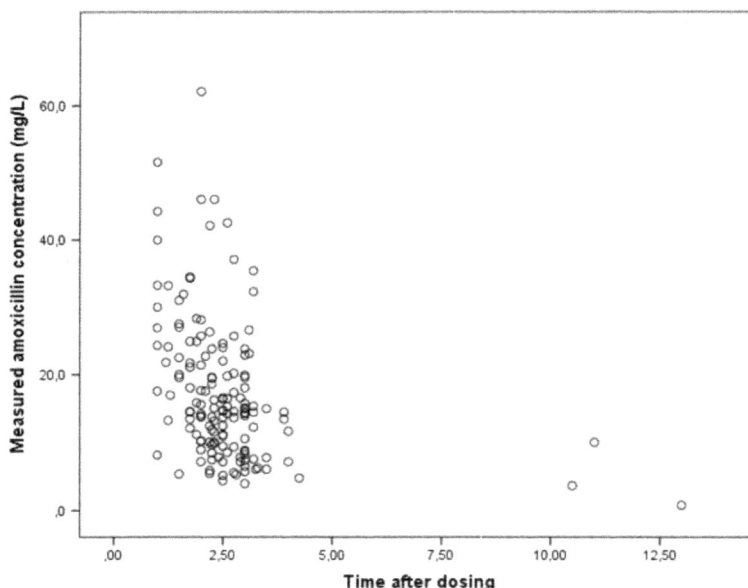

Figure 1 The measured concentrations of amoxicillin plotted against the time after amoxicillin administration.

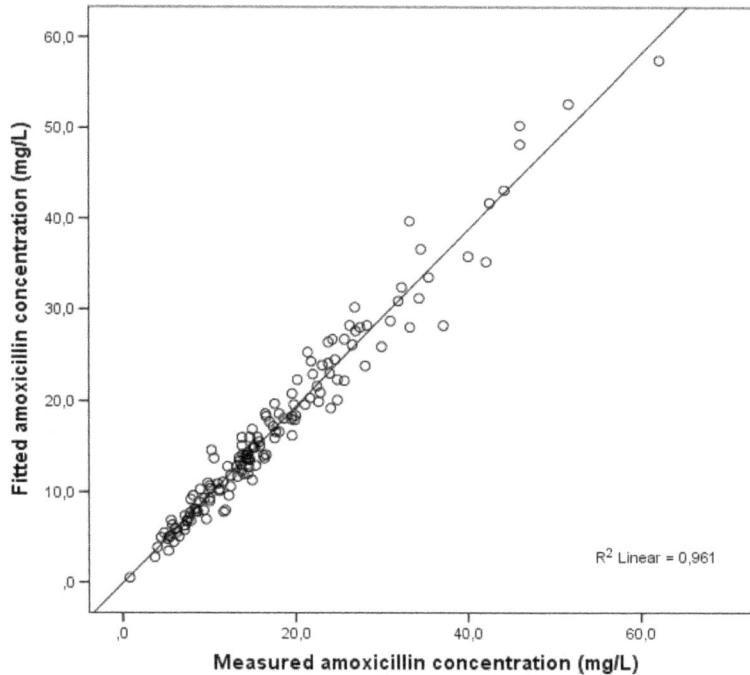

Figure 2 Correlation between amoxicillin actual measured concentration and estimated with maximum a posteriori Bayesian fitting (MW/Pharm 3.60, Mediware, the Netherlands).

Discussion

In this study, we demonstrate that the efficacy target of 40%T > MIC for amoxicillin/clavulanic acid was reached in 93% of the patients tested when the MIC was 4 mg/L and only in 65% of the patients tested when the MIC was 8 mg/L. In the EUCAST and CLSI criteria Enterobacteriaceae are considered to be susceptible for amoxicillin/clavulanic acid with bacterial MIC ≤ 8 mg/L [11]. High bacterial MICs for amoxicillin/clavulanic acid are an increasing problem in the Netherlands and in Europe [19,20]. To prevent treatment failure for individual patients and to prevent development of antibiotic resistance on population level, increasing the standard dose of amoxicillin/clavulanic acid seems warranted. Dosing simulation showed that increasing the standard dose of amoxicillin/clavulanic acid to 6 times a day 1000/200 mg increased the number of patients reaching 40%T > MIC to 100% for bacterial MIC ≤ 4 and to 95% with bacterial MIC ≤ 8. Continuous iv dosing is an alternative for frequent dosing of time dependent β-lactam antibiotics.

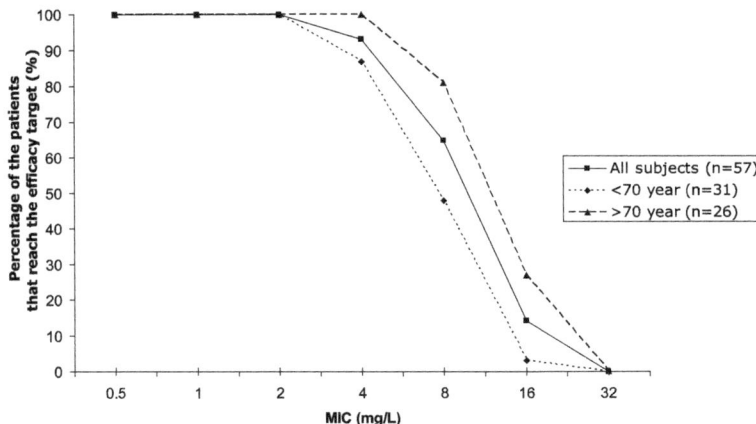

Figure 3 The percentage of patients that reach the 40%T > MIC for different age categories at different MICs.

Table 3 Univariate Pearson correlation coefficients between amoxicillin/clavulanic acid, CLam/W and predictors used in this study

	Univariate CLam/W	
	R	P-value
Creatinine	−0.584	<0.001
Age	−0.476	<0.001
Gender	−0.034	0.812
V/W	−0.608	<0.001
40%T > MIC	−0.424	0.025

CLam/W, amoxicillin/clavulanic acid clearance corrected for bodyweight.
V/W, amoxicillin/clavulanic acid volume of distribution corrected for bodyweight.

Unfortunately, amoxicillin is not very suitable for continuous iv dosing, because of the instability of amoxicillin at room temperature. Therefore, we suggest increasing the dose of amoxicillin/clavulanic acid to 6 times a day in patients with severe Enterobacteriacee sepsis or intra-abdominal infection.

In general amoxicillin/clavulanic acid is well tolerated. The most frequent adverse drug events are diarrhoea, nausea and vomiting. However, amoxicillin/clavulanic acid is also associated with liver injury, which is estimated to occur from 1 to 1.7 per 10.000 users [21,22]. Clavulanic acid seems to be responsible for the adverse drug reaction, since amoxicillin alone is rarely associated with liver injury and causes less gastrointestinal problems than the combination preparation [23-25]. In vitro pharmacodynamic studies demonstrate that low dose of clavulanic acid suffice and the β-lactamase inhibition of clavulanic acid lasts for 8–12 hours [26,27]. Therefore, increasing the standard dose of amoxicillin/clavulanic acid of 4 times a day 1000/200 mg iv with amoxicillin

twice daily 1000 mg iv may be a safe and effective alternative.

CLam/W is correlated with CLcr and the amoxicillin dose is adjusted with to the CLcr. However, other covariates also influence the CLam/W. CLam/W was significantly correlated with age. However, age and creatinine were not correlated to each other, meaning that elderly patients can have both a normal creatinine and a decreased CLam/W. Therefore, the correlation of age with CLam/W seems independent of the creatinine. Furthermore, the 4 patients that did not reach the efficacy target with bacterial MIC = 4 were all young patients with excellent clearance. Our measured attainment results are lower than those calculated attainment results in the EUCAST rationale document, in which Monte Carlo simulations were used to calculate the target attainment rates (40%T > MIC) of different dosing regimens (from 500 mg 3 times a day to 2 g 4 times a day) for different bacterial MICs (0.5-32 mg/L) [11]. The target attainment in the EUCAST rationale document for the standard dose (1000/200 mg 4 times a day) is 100% at bacterial MIC ≤ 4 and 75% with bacterial MIC ≤ 8 mg/L [11]. In our real life blood level determination study, these percentages were 93% and 65%, respectively. This difference may be explained by the larger interindividual variability of our population and in particular by a group of younger patients with normal renal clearance (CLcr > 60 mL/min). Remarkably, in the EUCAST rationale document, the interindividual variation is extremely small; t½ is 1.1 (±0.1) h, versus t½ is 1.5 (±0.6) h in our study. The higher t½ in our study may be due to the high mean age of our population.

No significant associations have been found between the target 40%T > MIC and clinical outcome. As expected, our study population was too small and too heterogeneous. A large number of patients are needed to draw

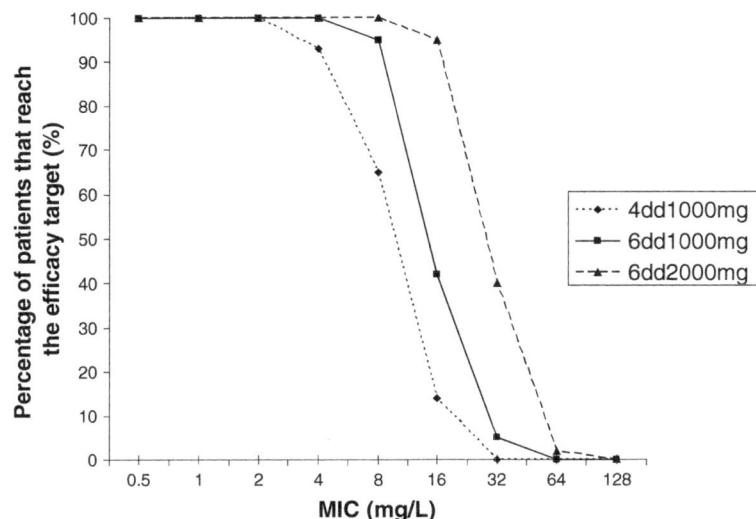

Figure 4 Calculated percentage of patients with 40%T > MIC at different MICs for increasing amoxicillin dosages.

conclusions for this endpoint. Moreover, in an in vitro study, ceftazidim has been shown to be maximally effective when 40%T > MIC was reached for concentrations four times the MIC or higher [28]. In our study, the target of 40%T > 4 × MIC was only reached in 100% for low MICs (≤1 mg/L), but never for bacterial MICs of 4 and 8 mg/L. Our study was not designed to isolate a large number of bacterial MICs and therefore only a limited number of clinical bacterial MICs were available in our study. Taken together a large clinical PK/PD study of amoxicillin/clavulanic acid is needed with microbiological and clinical cure endpoints to establish the association between clinical endpoints and the efficacy target 40%T > MIC.

Conclusions

The current standard dose of amoxicillin/clavulanic acid 4 times a day 1000/200 mg iv is too low to reach the 40%T > MIC for bacterial MIC of 8 mg/L in a high percentage of patients. To prevent treatment failure for individual patients and to prevent development of antibiotic resistance on population level, we suggest increasing the standard dose of amoxicillin/clavulanic acid to 6 times a day in patients with an Enterobacteriaceae sepsis or intra-abdominal infection.

Abbreviations

AST: Antibiotic susceptibility testing; CLam/W: Amoxicillin clearance corrected for bodyweight; CLcr: Creatinine clearance; CRP: C-reactive protein; ID: Identification of the causative bacterium; iv: Intravenous; MAP: Maximum a posteriori; MIC: Minimal inhibition concentration; MUMC: Maastricht University Medical Centre; PK: Pharmacokinetic; RP-HPLC: Reverse phase high pressure liquid chromatography; SD: Standard deviation; T: Time; V/W: Volume of distribution corrected for bodyweight.

Competing interests

The authors declare that they have no competing interests.

Authors' contributions

MH, TH and LS carried out the data analysis. CB, LS, CN an AV participated in design of the study. MH, TH, LS, CN, CB and AV drafted the manuscript. All authors have read and approved the final version manuscript.

Acknowledgements

We acknowledge the support provided by department of Clinical Chemistry and the Pharmacy laboratory. We also acknowledge the assistance of Dr. Bekers and the excellent technical assistance of Jeroen Welzen and Pauline Vinken. This work was supported by Care and Public Health Research Institute (CAPHRI), Maastricht, the Netherlands and the Medical University Centre Maastricht, the Netherlands.

Author details

[1]Department of Medical Microbiology, Maastricht University Medical Centre, Maastricht, the Netherlands. [2]Department of Clinical Pharmacy, Maastricht University Medical Centre, Maastricht, the Netherlands. [3]Care and Public Health Research Institute (CAPHRI), Maastricht, the Netherlands. [4]Department of Internal Medicine, Erasmus Medical Centre, Rotterdam, the Netherlands. [5]Present address: Maastricht University Medical Centre, P. Debyelaan 25, PO Box 58006202 AZ Maastricht, the Netherlands.

References

1. Craig WA: **Antimicrobial resistance issues of the future.** *Diagn Microbiol Infect Dis* 1996, **25**(4):213–217.
2. Vogelman B, Craig WA: **Kinetics of antimicrobial activity.** *J Pediatr* 1986, **108**(5 Pt 2):835–840.
3. Craig WA: **Interrelationship between pharmacokinetics and pharmacodynamics in determining dosage regimens for broad-spectrum cephalosporins.** *Diagn Microbiol Infect Dis* 1995, **22**(1–2):89–96.
4. Adam D, de Visser I, Koeppe P: **Pharmacokinetics of amoxicillin and clavulanic acid administered alone and in combination.** *Antimicrob Agents Chemother* 1982, **22**(3):353–357.
5. Sjovall J, Alvan G, Huitfeldt B: **Intra- and inter-individual variation in pharmacokinetics of intravenously infused amoxycillin and ampicillin to elderly volunteers.** *Br J Clin Pharmacol* 1986, **21**(2):171–181.
6. Matsuura M, Nakazawa H, Hashimoto T, Mitsuhashi S: **Combined antibacterial activity of amoxicillin with clavulanic acid against ampicillin-resistant strains.** *Antimicrob Agents Chemother* 1980, **17**(6):908–911.
7. van Zanten AR, Polderman KH, van Geijlswijk IM, van der Meer GY, Schouten MA, Girbes AR: **Ciprofloxacin pharmacokinetics in critically ill patients: a prospective cohort study.** *J Crit Care* 2008, **23**(3):422–430.
8. Haeseker M, Stolk L, Nieman F, Hoebe C, Neef C, Bruggeman C, Verbon A: **The ciprofloxacin target AUC : MIC ratio is not reached in hospitalized patients with the recommended dosing regimens.** *Br J Clin Pharmacol* 2013, **75**(1):180–185.
9. Aubert G, Carricajo A, Coudrot M, Guyomarc'h S, Auboyer C, Zeni F: **Prospective determination of serum ceftazidime concentrations in intensive care units.** *Ther Drug Monit* 2010, **32**(4):517–519.
10. Rea RS, Capitano B, Bies R, Bigos KL, Smith R, Lee H: **Suboptimal aminoglycoside dosing in critically ill patients.** *Ther Drug Monit* 2008, **30**(6):674–681.
11. EUCAST: **Amoxicillin Rationale for the EUCAST clinical breakpoints.** *www. eucast.org/documents/rd/*.
12. **Nederlands Trial Register. Antibiotic blood levels elderly.** http://www. trialregister.nl/trialreg/admin/rctview.asp?TC=1725.
13. FDA: *Guidance for Industry. Bioanalytical Method Validation, U.S. Department of Health and Food Science.* Rockville, MD, USA: Food and Drug Administration (FDA); 2001.
14. Martinez MN, Riviere JE: **Review of the 1993 veterinary drug bioequivalence workshop, held on march 29–31, 1993, in Rockville, Maryland.** *J Vet Pharmacol Ther* 1994, **17**(2):85–119.
15. Pullen J, Stolk LM, Neef C, Zimmermann LJ: **Microanalysis of amoxicillin, flucloxacillin, and rifampicin in neonatal plasma.** *Biomed Chromatogr* 2007, **21**(12):1259–1265.
16. Proost JH, Meijer DK: **MW/Pharm, an integrated software package for drug dosage regimen calculation and therapeutic drug monitoring.** *Comput Biol Med* 1992, **22**(3):155–163.
17. van der Meer AF, Marcus MA, Touw DJ, Proost JH, Neef C: **Optimal sampling strategy development methodology using maximum a posteriori Bayesian estimation.** *Ther Drug Monit* 2011, **33**(2):133–146.
18. Turnidge JD: **The pharmacodynamics of beta-lactams.** *Clin Infect Dis* 1998, **27**(1):10–22.
19. Blaettler L, Mertz D, Frei R, Elzi L, Widmer AF, Battegay M, Fluckiger U: **Secular trend and risk factors for antimicrobial resistance in Escherichia coli isolates in Switzerland 1997–2007.** *Infection* 2009, **37**(6):534–539.
20. SWAB: **Consumption of antimicrobial agents and antimicrobial resistance among medically important bacteria in the Netherlands.** http://www. swab.nl/swab/cms3.nsf/viewdoc/20BCD3983B5C390AC12575850031D33D.
21. de Abajo FJ, Montero D, Madurga M, Garcia Rodriguez LA: **Acute and clinically relevant drug-induced liver injury: a population based case–control study.** *Br J Clin Pharmacol* 2004, **58**(1):71–80.
22. Garcia Rodriguez LA, Stricker BH, Zimmerman HJ: **Risk of acute liver injury associated with the combination of amoxicillin and clavulanic acid.** *Arch Intern Med* 1996, **156**(12):1327–1332.
23. Salvo F, Polimeni G, Moretti U, Conforti A, Leone R, Leoni O, Motola D, Dusi G, Caputi AP: **Adverse drug reactions related to amoxicillin alone and in association with clavulanic acid: data from spontaneous reporting in Italy.** *J Antimicrob Chemother* 2007, **60**(1):121–126.
24. Bolzan H, Spatola J, Castelletto R, Curciarello J: **Intrahepatic cholestasis induced by amoxicillin alone.** *Gastroenterol Hepatol* 2000, **23**(5):237–239.
25. Schwarze C, Schmitz V, Fischer HP, Sauerbruch T, Spengler U: **Vanishing bile duct syndrome associated with elevated pancreatic enzymes after**

short-term administration of amoxicillin. *Eur J Gastroenterol Hepatol* 2002, **14**(11):1275–1277.

26. Aguilar L, Martin M, Balcabao IP, Gomez-Lus ML, Dal-Re R, Prieto J: **In vitro assessment of the effect of clavulanic acid at concentrations achieved in human serum on the bactericidal activity of amoxicillin at physiological concentrations against Staphylococcus aureus: implications for dosage regimens.** *Antimicrob Agents Chemother* 1997, **41**(6):1403–1405.

27. Cooper CE, Slocombe B, White AR: **Effect of low concentrations of clavulanic acid on the in-vitro activity of amoxycillin against beta-lactamase-producing Branhamella catarrhalis and Haemophilus influenzae.** *J Antimicrob Chemother* 1990, **26**(3):371–380.

28. Mouton JW, Punt N, Vinks AA: **Concentration-effect relationship of ceftazidime explains why the time above the MIC is 40 percent for a static effect in vivo.** *Antimicrob Agents Chemother* 2007, **51**(9):3449–3451.

11

Tobramycin exposure from active calcium sulfate bone graft substitute

Françoise Livio[1*], Peter Wahl[2], Chantal Csajka[1,3], Emanuel Gautier[2] and Thierry Buclin[1]

Abstract

Background: Bone graft substitute such as calcium sulfate are frequently used as carrier material for local antimicrobial therapy in orthopedic surgery. This study aimed to assess the systemic absorption and disposition of tobramycin in patients treated with a tobramycin-laden bone graft substitute (Osteoset® T).

Methods: Nine blood samples were taken from 12 patients over 10 days after Osteoset® T surgical implantation. Tobramycin concentration was measured by fluorescence polarization. Population pharmacokinetic analysis was performed using NONMEM to assess the average value and variability (CV) of pharmacokinetic parameters. Bioavailability (F) was assessed by equating clearance (CL) with creatinine clearance (Cockcroft CLCr). Based on the final model, simulations with various doses and renal function levels were performed. (ClinicalTrials.gov number, NCT01938417).

Results: The patients were 52 +/− 20 years old, their mean body weight was 73 +/− 17 kg and their mean CLCr was 119 +/− 55 mL/min. Either 10 g or 20 g Osteoset® T with 4% tobramycin sulfate was implanted in various sites. Concentration profiles remained low and consistent with absorption rate-limited first-order release, while showing important variability. With CL equated to CLCr, mean absorption rate constant (ka) was 0.06 h-1, F was 63% or 32% (CV 74%) for 10 and 20 g Osteoset® T respectively, and volume of distribution (V) was 16.6 L (CV 89%). Simulations predicted sustained high, potentially toxic concentrations with 10 g, 30 g and 50 g Osteoset® T for CLCr values below 10, 20 and 30 mL/min, respectively.

Conclusions: Osteoset® T does not raise toxicity concerns in subjects without significant renal failure. The risk/benefit ratio might turn unfavorable in case of severe renal failure, even after standard dose implantation.

Keywords: Tobramycin, Bone graft substitute, Pharmacokinetics, Renal failure

Background

Since the end of the sixties, bone cement such as polymethyl methacrylate (PMMA) and bone graft substitute such as calcium sulfate are frequently used as carrier material for local antimicrobial therapy in orthopedic surgery for osteomyelitis, infected arthroplasty, soft tissue infections or prophylaxis. Unlike PMMA, calcium sulfate is resorbable, thus obviating the need for surgical removal. Osteoset® T (Wright Medical Technology Inc, Arlington, TN, USA) is one of these products; it contains 4% tobramycin sulfate in calcium sulfate pellets. Most data on Osteoset® T come from animal studies, where high local and low systemic tobramycin concentrations have been observed [1]. No pharmacokinetic (PK) observations with patients treated with Osteoset® T have been published so far, despite well known concentration-related potential toxicity of aminoglycosides. Only concentrations have been described in patients implanted with a tobramycin-laden polymer carrier material (Simplex™ P Bone Cement with Tobramycin) showing high tobramycin levels at the operative site but low systemic absorption [2].

The aim of this study was to develop a population PK model for tobramycin in patients treated with an active calcium sulfate bone substitute and to predict tobramycin systemic exposure under various dose and renal function levels.

Method

Patients and sampling

The data were collected prospectively between October 2006 and March 2008 from all adult patients treated with

* Correspondence: francoise.livio@chuv.ch
[1]Division of Clinical Pharmacology, Biomedicine, Department of Laboratories, Centre Hospitalier Universitaire Vaudois, Lausanne 1011, Switzerland
Full list of author information is available at the end of the article

Osteoset® T in our orthopedic surgery department. Osteoset® T was implanted whenever estimated a useful adjunct to standard therapy for bone, soft tissues and prosthetic joint infections requiring surgical debridement. Either 10 g or 20 g of Osteoset® T with 4% tobramycin sulfate were implanted, representing 262 or 524 mg tobramycin repectively taking into account the salt factor (tobramycin/tobramycin sulfate = 0.655). Additional intravenous aminoglycosides were not used in these patients. No wound drains were used.

Blood samples were taken at 3 h, 6 h, 12 h, 24 h, 48 h and on days 3, 5, 7 and 10 after implantation. Whenever a tourniquet had been used during the operation, its release-time was taken into account instead of implantation time. Blood was sampled in BD Vacutainer® SST II Advance (Becton Dickinson AG, Allschwil, Switzerland) serum separator tubes.

The study protocol was approved by the Institutional Review Board of Fribourg Cantonal Hospital and all subjects gave their written informed consent. This study was registered in ClinicalTrials.gov under code number NCT01938417.

Drug assay

Tobramycin concentrations were measured on a COBAS INTEGRA 800 (Roche Diagnostics GmbH, Mannheim, Germany) fluorescence polarization detector, using a standard tobramycin measurement kit (ref. 20737925). The lower limit of quantification (LOQ) of the assay was 0.1 mg/L. Coefficient of variation (CV) within runs was 1.7% at 2.2 mg/L, while CV between runs were 6.2%, 2.6% and 2.5% at 0.9 mg/L, 2.8 mg/L and 4.5 mg/L, respectively. Accuracy was monthly checked by participating to the external quality control scheme provided by LGC Standards for antibiotics (LGC Standards Proficiency Testing, Bury, UK). Assays were processed within 6 hours after sampling.

Population pharmacokinetic analysis

The pharmacokinetic analysis was performed using nonlinear mixed-effects modeling with the NONMEM computer program (version VI) [3]. Models were fitted to the data with the first-order conditional estimation with interaction (FOCE INTER) method. One and two compartment models with first-order absorption were compared. The first tobramycin concentration below the LOQ was set to half of the LOQ value and subsequent points below the LOQ were dropped out. Average value and variability of clearance (CL), volume of distribution (V) and absorption rate constant (k_a) were assessed. As aminoglycosides are known to be completely and exclusively eliminated by glomerular filtration, tobramycin CL was equated to the creatinine clearance (CL_{cr}) value, thus enabling the estimation of absolute bioavailability (F) in

the absence of intravenous injection. CL_{cr} was estimated with the Cockcroft formula, based on patient's serum creatinine, body weight, and sex [4], with linear interpolation for days without creatinine measurement. The residual variability was adequately modeled using an additive plus proportional error model. The final model was then developed by testing in a stepwise fashion the potential influence of sex, age, body weight, Osteoset® T quantity and implantation site on the pharmacokinetic parameters.

Based on the final average parameters and variability, simulations using various tobramycin doses (262 mg; 786 mg; 1310 mg) at various CL_{cr} levels (120, 90, 60, 30, 20 and 10 mL/min) were performed, using 2000 virtual patients each to predict the doses associated with concentrations exceeding the 2 mg/L threshold over a prolonged period of time (5 days or more).

Results

Twelve patients (7 males, 5 females) were included in this observational study. Their mean age was 52 years (range 19–82, SD ± 20), body weight 73 kg (53–116, ± 17), and CL_{cr} 119 mL/min (34–288, ± 55).

Osteoset® T implantation sites were tibia/fibula (6 patients), hip (2), calcaneum (2), femur (1) and lumbar spine (1), either for established infections (9) or prophylaxis (3). Eight patients were implanted 10 g Osteoset® T containing 262 mg tobramycin, while 4 were implanted 20 g Osteoset® T containing 524 mg tobramycin.

Osteoset® T was well tolerated; further clinical details have been presented elsewhere [5]. Systemic tobramycin concentrations measured remained low (<2 mg/L at 24 h) in all patients. Concentration profiles were consistent with a one compartement model with absorption rate-limited first-order release, while showing important variability. A two compartment model was also tested but did not improve the fit. With CL equated to CL_{Cr}, mean estimated k_a was 0.0603 h^{-1}, volume of distribution 16.6 L (CV 89%) and F was 63% and 32% (CV 74%) in the 8 patients having received 10 g Osteoset® T and in the 4 patients having received 20 g, respectively. Sex, age, body weight or implantation site did not seem to affect tobramycin absorption or disposition when introduced as covariates. Population pharmacokinetic parameter estimates and variability are summarized in Table 1. The concentration values observed are represented on Figure 1, along with mean population prediction and 90% prediction intervals for CL_{Cr} 120 mL/min.

The simulations of concentration profiles (using an average F estimate of 47%) showed that more than 5% patients would maintain concentrations over 2 mg/L during at least five days post implantation with tobramycin 262, 786 and 1310 mg when CL_{cr} was respectively set at 10, 20 and 30 mL/min.

Table 1 Tobramycin population pharmacokinetic parameter estimates

Population mean		
Parameter	Estimate	s.e%[b]
CL (L h^{-1})	7.14[d]	–
V (L)	16.6	35
K$_a$ (h$^{-1)}$)	0.0603	19
F (if cast 10 g)	0.63	19
F (if cast 20 g)	0.32	19
Interpatient variability		
Parameter	CV%[a]	s.e%[c]
CL	–	–
V	89	74
k$_a$	–	–
F	74	72
Residual variability		
Error type		s.e%
σ$_{prop}$ (CV%)[e]	29	50[c]
σ$_{add}$ (SD in mg/L)[f]	0.062	22[b]

CL, mean apparent clearance; V, mean apparent volume of distribution; k$_a$, mean absorption rate constant; F, mean bioavailability.
[a]estimates of variability expressed as coefficient of variation (CV%).
[b]s.e = standard error of the estimates (S.E), defined as S.E/estimate and expressed as percentage.
[c]s.e = standard error of the coefficient of variations, taken as $\sqrt{s.e_{estimate}/estimate}$, expressed as a percentage.
[d]equated to creatinine clearance (CL$_{cr}$).
[e]residual variability in the plasma concentrations associated with the proportional error term, expressed as a coefficient of variation (CV%).
[f]residual variability in the plasma concentrations associated with the additive error term, expressed as a standard deviation (SD).

Discussion and conclusions

This is the first tobramycin pharmacokinetic study after Osteoset® T implantation in a clinical setting. Tobramycin systemic concentration values were measured well below the traditional toxicity threshold of 2 mg/L from 24 h and later on, which was not unexpected considering the low tobramycin dose implanted and the good renal function of the study subjects. Whether continuous systemic exposure to low concentrations below minimal inhibitory concentration may favor antimicrobial resistance remains an issue [6].

Prominent inter-individual variability was observed, probably due to heterogeneity of patients, indications, surgical techniques and implantation sites. There have probably been too few patients included for reliably testing the influence of all covariates. Loss through wound oozing has been neglected (not measured) but could represent another source of variability. Imprecision on low tobramycin levels measurement, very close to the LOQ, could also have increased residual variability.

The significant difference in bioavailability between 10 g and 20 g Osteoset® T (63% versus 32% respectively) could indicate that higher amounts of bone graft substitute either limit tobramycin release to some extent, or slow it down sufficiently for the resulting concentrations to fall below the LOQ. Unbalanced loss through wound oozing could also partly account for this difference. Implantation site and tissue perfusion could also play a role, although this could not be demonstrated in our analysis, due to limited data.

Our model gained in credibility when tobramycin CL was equated to CL$_{cr}$; indeed there is no argument to think of a different elimination route for the drug absorbed from Osteoset® T compared to intravenous delivery [7]. The Cockcroft equation that we used has yet its limitations, in particular in obese or bedridden patients. Our model found a distribution volume of 0.22 L/kg body weight, consistent with previously published values [7]. The large inter-patient variability found in both V and F is likely to incorporate some amount of variability in CL and k$_a$.

High sustained potentially toxic concentrations were predicted by simulations with standard doses Osteoset®

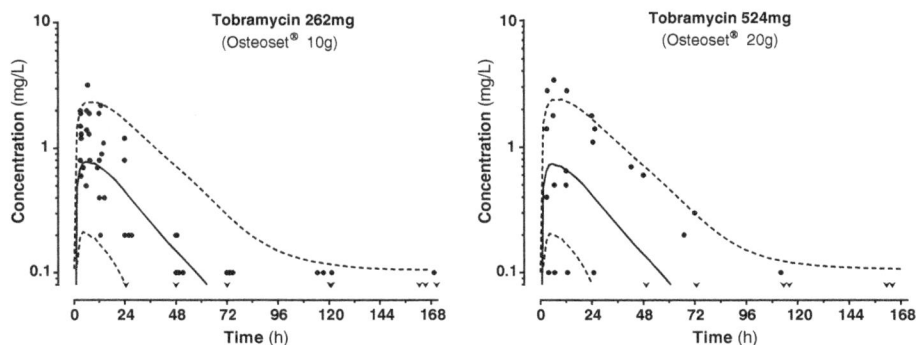

Figure 1 Concentrations versus time plot of tobramycin with mean population prediction (solid line) and 90% prediction interval (dashed lines) after Osteoset® 10 g (left) or 20 g (right) in patients with normal renal function. Dose difference is almost fully compensated by different bioavailability, giving similar predictions. Superimposed points show the concentrations observed in 8 patients after 10 g and 4 patients after 20 g. v : first concentration below the limit of detection.

T at renal failure stages 4 and 5. Considering the limited study power, this simulation should be taken as a rough estimate of the potential for toxicity of this product. Our model is probably too imprecise to deduce precise dose adjustment guidelines. However, it indicates that caution is warranted when Osteoset® T implant is considered for patients with severe renal failure, as its benefit/risk ratio could turn out unfavourable [8].

Competing interests
The authors declare that they have no competing interests.

Authors' contributions
FL performed the pharmacokinetic analysis and was involved in drafting the manuscript. PW designed the study and was involved in the acquisition of data. CC revised the pharmacokinetic analysis. EG was involved in the study design and coordination. TB gave final approval of the version to be published. All authors read and approved the final manuscript.

Acknowledgements
We thank Ali Maghraoui for technical assistance.

Author details
[1]Division of Clinical Pharmacology, Biomedicine, Department of Laboratories, Centre Hospitalier Universitaire Vaudois, Lausanne 1011, Switzerland.
[2]Department of Orthopedic Surgery, Cantonal Hospital, Fribourg, Switzerland.
[3]Department of Pharmaceutical Sciences, Clinical Pharmacy Unit, University of Geneva, Rue du Général- Dufour 24, Genève 4 1211, Switzerland.

References
1. Nelson CL, McLaren SG, Skinner RA, Smeltzer MS, Thomas JR, Olsen KM: **The treatment of experimental osteomyelitis by surgical debridement and the implantation of calcium sulfate tobramycin pellets.** *J Orthop Res* 2002, **20:**643–647.
2. Sterling GJ, Crawford S, Potter JH, Koerbin G, Crawford R: **The Pharmacokinetics of Simplex-tobramycin bone cement.** *J Bone Joint Surg* 2003, **85-B:**646–649.
3. Beal SL, Sheiner LB, Boeckmann AJ: *NONMEM Users Guides 1989–2006.* Ellicott City, Maryland, USA: Eds Icon Development Solutions.
4. Cockcroft DW, Gault MH: **Prediction of creatinine clearance from serum creatinine.** *Nephron* 1976, **16:**31–41.
5. Wahl P, Livio F, Jacobi M, Gautier E, Buclin T: **Systemic exposure to tobramycin after local antibiotic treatment with calcium sulfate as carrier material.** *Arch Orthop Trauma Surg* 2011, **131:**657–662.
6. Freeman CD, Nicolau DP, Belliveau PP, Nightingale CH: **Once-daily dosing of aminoglycosides: review and recommendations for clinical practice.** *J Antimicrob Chemother* 1997, **39:**677–686.
7. Burton ME, Shaw LM, Schentag JJ, Evans WE: **Aminoglycosides.** In *Applied Pharmacokinetics and Pharmacodynamics – Principles of Therapeutic Drug Monitoring.* 4th edition. Edited by Troy D, Hauber M, Remsberg C. Philadelphia: Lippincott Williams and Wilkins; 2006:285–327.
8. Wu IM, Marin EP, Kashgarian M, Brewster UC: **A case of an acute kidney injury secondary to an implanted aminoglycoside.** *Kidney Int* 2009, **75:**1109–1112.

12

Cost analysis of voriconazole versus liposomal amphotericin B for primary therapy of invasive aspergillosis among patients with haematological disorders in Germany and Spain

Helmut Ostermann[1], Carlos Solano[2], Isidro Jarque[3], Carolina Garcia-Vidal[4], Xin Gao[5], Jon Andoni Barrueta[6], Marina De Salas-Cansado[7], Jennifer Stephens[5*], Mei Xue[5], Bertram Weber[8] and Claudie Charbonneau[9]

Abstract

Background: The current healthcare climate demands pharmacoeconomic evaluations for different treatment strategies incorporating drug acquisition costs, costs incurred for hospitalisation, drug administration and preparation, diagnostic and laboratory testing and drug-related adverse events (AEs). Here we evaluate the pharmacoeconomics of voriconazole versus liposomal amphotericin B as first-line therapies for invasive aspergillosis (IA) in patients with haematological malignancy and prolonged neutropenia or who were undergoing haematopoietic stem-cell transplantation in Germany or Spain.

Methods: A decision analytic model based on a decision tree was constructed to estimate the potential treatment costs of voriconazole versus liposomal amphotericin B. Each model pathway was defined by the probability of an event occurring and the costs of clinical outcomes. Outcome probabilities and cost inputs were derived from the published literature, clinical trials, expert panels and local database costs. In the base case, patients who failed to respond to first-line therapy were assumed to experience a single switch between comparator drugs or the other drug was added as second-line treatment. Base-case evaluation included only drug-management costs and additional hospitalisation costs due to severe AEs associated with first- and second-line therapies. Sensitivity analyses were conducted to assess the robustness of the results. Cost estimates were inflated to 2011 euros (€).

Results: Based on clinical trial success rates of 52.8% (voriconazole) and 50.0% (liposomal amphotericin B), voriconazole had lower total treatment costs compared with liposomal amphotericin B in both Germany (€12,256 versus €18,133; length of therapy [LOT] = 10-day intravenous [IV] + 5-day oral voriconazole and 15-day IV liposomal amphotericin B) and Spain (€8,032 versus €10,516; LOT = 7-day IV + 8-day oral voriconazole and 15-day IV liposomal amphotericin B). Assuming the same efficacy (50.0%) in first-line therapy, voriconazole maintained a lower total treatment cost compared with liposomal amphotericin B. Cost savings were primarily due to the lower drug acquisition costs and shorter IV LOT associated with voriconazole. Sensitivity analyses showed that the results were sensitive to drug price, particularly the cost of liposomal amphotericin B.

Conclusions: Voriconazole is likely to be cost-saving compared with liposomal amphotericin B when used as a first-line treatment for IA in Germany and Spain.

Keywords: Aspergillosis, Cost-effectiveness, Decision-analytic model, Invasive fungal disease, Pharmacoeconomics

* Correspondence: jstephens@pharmerit.com
[5]Pharmerit International, Bethesda, MD, USA
Full list of author information is available at the end of the article

Background

Invasive fungal diseases (IFDs) are a significant cause of morbidity and mortality in immunocompromised patients, and are associated with increased healthcare costs [1]. The frequency of IFDs has increased substantially over recent years, largely due to the increasing size of the population at risk, which includes transplant recipients, patients with haematological malignancies, and patients with HIV [2].

Invasive aspergillosis (IA) is the most significant IFD in immunocompromised patients, with an incidence rate of approximately 10% in allogeneic bone marrow transplant recipients [3], and an overall case-fatality rate of 58% (range 43–87% depending on underlying disease) [4]. As a result, patients with IA have a significantly increased length of stay (LOS) in hospital and increased healthcare costs compared with patients without IA [5-8]. The direct costs associated with IA are substantial and include inpatient and outpatient costs, such as increased LOS in hospital, costs of antifungal therapy, and costs related to the treatment of drug-related adverse events (AEs) [9].

Effective treatment of IFD is an ongoing challenge to the clinical community from both a clinical and cost perspective. Across Europe, treatment recommendations are managed at a national level and are based on a range of factors including: clinical outcomes (e.g. infection resolution and mortality), economic outcomes (e.g. treatment costs and hospital LOS) and quality of life information. In Germany, the Infectious Diseases Working Party of the German Society of Haematology and Oncology provides guidelines for the diagnosis [10] and treatment [11] of IFD in patients with haemato-oncological disorders. In Spain, the Third European Conference on Infections and Leukaemia [12] and the Spanish Society of Infectious Diseases and Clinical Microbiology [13] provide specific therapies and disease-management strategies.

Voriconazole (Vfend®, Pfizer Inc) and liposomal amphotericin B (Ambisome®, Gilead Sciences) are licensed for the treatment of IFD, including IA. In a prospective, randomised trial of voriconazole versus amphotericin B deoxycholate for the primary treatment of IA, voriconazole demonstrated superior efficacy and improved survival, and resulted in fewer side effects, compared with amphotericin B [14].

Health economic-based models are designed to address questions of economic relevance, and integrate efficacy and safety data from clinical trials with medical resource use and quality of life information from the published literature, expert opinion and database analysis. Here, we evaluate the pharmacoeconomics of voriconazole versus liposomal amphotericin B as first-line therapies for IA in patients with haematological malignancy and prolonged neutropenia, or those undergoing haematopoietic stem cell transplantation (HSCT), from German and Spanish hospital perspectives.

Methods

Study design

This analysis was conducted from German and Spanish hospital perspectives. The study population comprised patients with haematological malignancy and prolonged neutropenia or those undergoing HSCT. Eligible patients met the criteria for proven or probable IA defined in the key randomised clinical trials of voriconazole [14] and liposomal amphotericin B [15]. Briefly, the key voriconazole trial enrolled immunocompromised patients aged ≥12 years with definite or probable IA. Patients were excluded if they had chronic aspergillosis, aspergilloma or allergic bronchopulmonary aspergillosis [14]. The key liposomal amphotericin B trial enrolled patients who met the criteria for proven or probable invasive mould infections as established by the European Organisation for Research and Treatment of Cancer/Mycosis Study Group; in addition, a protocol-defined modification allowed a diagnosis of probable IA in patients with a halo or air crescent sign on chest computed tomography scan who had undergone allogeneic stem cell transplantation or who had neutropenia within 14 days of study entry [15].

To estimate the potential therapy costs of voriconazole versus liposomal amphotericin B, a decision analytic model based on a decision tree was developed (Figure 1). Each pathway in the model was defined by the probability of an event occurring and the costs associated with each clinical outcome defined as: (1) treatment success or (2) treatment failure, which included add-on treatment due to lack of response, switching to second-line therapy due to serious AEs or for other reasons, and mortality.

The model inputs were treatment options, length of therapy (LOT), additional LOS in hospital, other efficacy and safety inputs, and drug costs. Outcome measures were the total hospital costs (e.g. drug and hospitalisation costs) associated with each therapy in 2011 euros (€). Outcome probabilities and cost inputs were derived from the published literature, clinical trials, expert panel discussions and local database costs.

Key model assumptions

The model time horizon was the 30-day inpatient follow-up period based on the mean LOS for HSCT patients with IA and haematological malignancy in a United States claims database analysis [16].

In the base-case scenario, patients who failed to respond to first-line therapy were assumed to undergo a single switch between comparator drugs or the other drug was added as a second-line therapy. Drug dosages were based on patients having an average weight of 70 kg, as defined in the key randomised clinical trials of voriconazole [14] and liposomal amphotericin B [15]. Voriconazole was administered intravenously at doses of 6 mg/kg twice daily (BID; Day 1) and 4 mg/kg BID (Day 2+), and orally at a

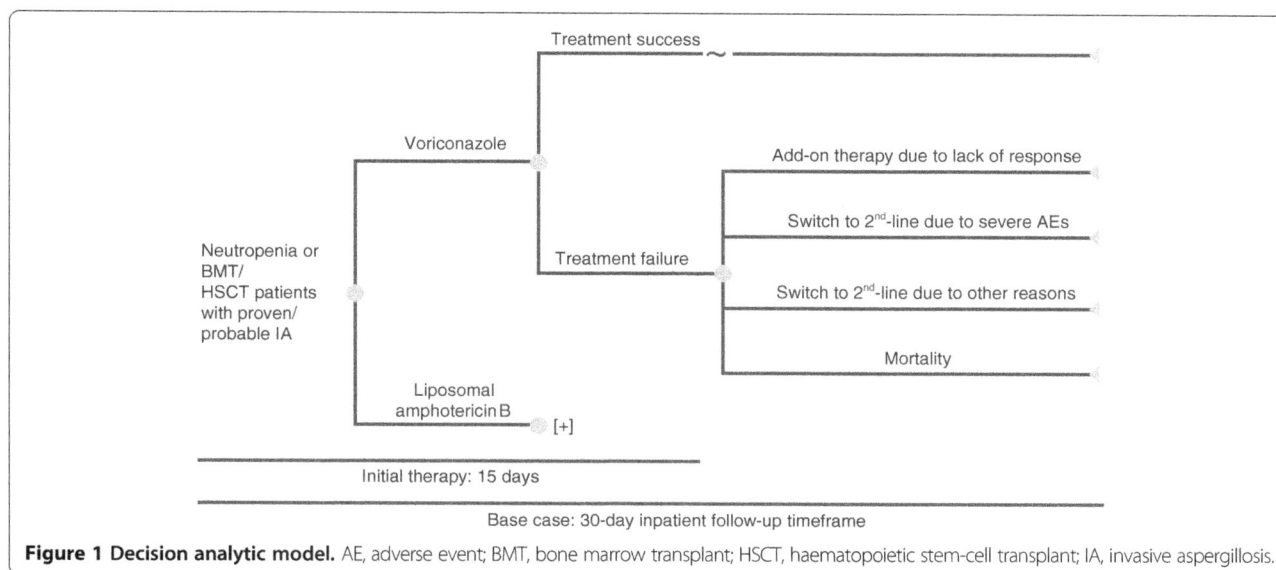

Figure 1 Decision analytic model. AE, adverse event; BMT, bone marrow transplant; HSCT, haematopoietic stem-cell transplant; IA, invasive aspergillosis.

dose of 200 mg BID. Intravenous (IV) liposomal amphotericin B was administered at a dose of 3 mg/kg once daily. It was assumed that there was no vial wastage during use.

The first-line drugs, voriconazole and liposomal amphotericin B, were only used in an inpatient setting (mean LOS = 30 days). Second-line therapies could be used in both inpatient and outpatient settings. IV LOT was determined by clinical experts from each country. In the German base-case scenario, first-line LOT was 10 days of IV voriconazole followed by 5 days of oral voriconazole and 15 days of IV liposomal amphotericin B. Second-line LOT was 15 days of IV voriconazole, liposomal amphotericin B or caspofungin. In the Spanish base-case scenario, first-line LOT was 7 days of IV voriconazole followed by 8 days of oral voriconazole and 15 days of IV liposomal amphotericin B. Second-line LOT was 7 days of IV voriconazole followed by 8 days of oral voriconazole and 15 days of IV liposomal amphotericin B or caspofungin.

After the initial success of IV voriconazole, conversion to oral voriconazole could be used as a first-line therapy, and it could also be used as a second-line add-on or switch-to therapy. If the comparator drug was added as second-line combination therapy due to lack of response with the first-line monotherapy, the first-line drug (voriconazole or liposomal amphotericin B) was continued as IV therapy (liposomal amphotericin B) or as a combination of IV and oral therapy (voriconazole) for the same duration as the add-on drug.

Cost calculation assumptions

The base-case evaluation included only drug-management costs and additional hospitalisation costs due to severe AEs associated with first- and second-line therapies.

Based on the results of the key randomised clinical trials, severe AEs with first- and second-line therapies included nephrotoxicity and hypokalaemia [14,15]. Although the effects of infusion-related reactions (e.g. visual disturbances, chest pain and back pain) were reported to be significantly different between the two treatment arms, it was assumed that the impact of moderate/severe infusion-related reactions would be captured by the pathway of treatment failure/switch due to AEs, and that additional costs incurred due to mild infusion-related reactions were minimal.

Hospital LOS was not included in the cost calculation as it was assumed to be similar across the different therapies. Based on a previously published study that assessed additional resource utilisation associated with AEs, an additional 2.2 days of hospital stay was applied to both treatment arms in the base-case scenario to reflect the impact of severe AEs [17].

Clinical input

Clinical efficacy, safety and mortality data in this model were based on the default drug dosages and were obtained from the key randomised clinical trials of voriconazole [14] and liposomal amphotericin B [15] (Table 1). The probability of adding another antifungal drug to the regimen due to lack of response was calculated as 1 minus the switch rate to second-line therapy.

Costs of medical resource and drug acquisition

Hospitalisation costs and outpatient IV administration costs were based on economic research on the treatment of IA in Germany [1,18,19] and Spain [20] (Table 2). Drug acquisition costs in Germany were derived from the LAUER-Taxe, Pharmindex for Germany drug costs

Table 1 Efficacy and safety input data

Treatment	Treatment success rate (%)	Add-on rate (%)	Severe AEs/switch due to severe AEs (%)	Switch (due to other reason) (%)	AE rate (%)	Mortality rate (%)
Voriconazole	52.8	19.2	13.4	9.0	13.4	5.6
Liposomal amphotericin B	50.0	8.7	20.0	16.0	20.0	5.3

Data sources: [14,15].
AE, adverse event.

(Table 3) [21]. Drug acquisition costs in Spain were derived from the Bot Plus database (Table 3) [22].

Sensitivity analysis

The effects of individual parameters (e.g. drug price and hospital costs) were examined by varying estimates by ±30%. Sensitivity results for each input were ranked from the most sensitive to the least sensitive via a tornado diagram.

Results

German hospital perspective

Based on clinical trial success rates of 52.8% for voriconazole and 50.0% for liposomal amphotericin B and a LOT of 10 days for IV voriconazole followed by 5 days for oral voriconazole and 15 days for IV liposomal amphotericin B, voriconazole had a lower total treatment cost compared with liposomal amphotericin B (€12,256 versus €18,133) (Figure 2A). If the same LOT of 10 days was assumed for both arms (IV only), voriconazole maintained a lower total treatment cost of €9,472 compared with the total treatment cost of €12,250 for liposomal amphotericin B. If the same efficacy (50.0%) was assumed for both first-line therapies, voriconazole maintained a lower total treatment cost compared with liposomal amphotericin B (€12,836 versus €18,133, respectively, over 15 days of treatment, and €9,862 versus €12,250, respectively, over 10 days of treatment) (Figure 3A).

When total treatment costs were broken down by line of therapy, first-line therapy costs were substantially lower for voriconazole versus liposomal amphotericin B, whereas second-line therapy costs were lower for liposomal amphotericin B versus voriconazole. These observations remained consistent regardless of whether LOT was 10 or 15 days and whether efficacy assumptions were based on clinical trial success rates or equivalency. AEs accounted for 3.9% (€199 of €5,094) and 2.1% (€297 of €13,816) of the

total costs of first-line treatment with voriconazole and liposomal amphotericin B, respectively.

The cost savings associated with voriconazole were primarily due to lower drug acquisition costs and a shorter IV LOT combined with the use of a cheaper oral formulation. AE savings accounted for 1.0% of the total cost saving associated with first-line voriconazole versus liposomal amphotericin B.

Spanish hospital perspective

Based on clinical trial success rates of 52.8% for voriconazole and 50.0% for liposomal amphotericin B and a LOT of 7 days for IV voriconazole followed by 8 days of oral voriconazole and 15 days for IV liposomal amphotericin B, voriconazole had a lower total treatment cost compared with liposomal amphotericin B (€8,032 versus €10,516) (Figure 2B). When the same efficacy of 50.0% was assumed for both first-line therapies, voriconazole maintained a lower total treatment cost compared with liposomal amphotericin B (€8,425 versus €10,516, respectively) (Figure 3B).

Similar to the German hospital perspective, when total treatment costs were broken down by therapy line, first-line therapy costs were substantially lower for voriconazole versus liposomal amphotericin B, whereas second-line therapy costs were lower for liposomal amphotericin B versus voriconazole. AEs accounted for 4.9% (€167 of €3,443) and 3.0% (€249 of €8,225) of the total costs of first-line treatment with voriconazole and liposomal amphotericin B, respectively.

Cost savings with voriconazole were primarily due to lower drug acquisition costs and a shorter IV LOT combined with the use of a cheaper oral formulation.

Table 3 Drug acquisition costs (2011 €)

Treatment	Dosage	Unit price (per vial or tablet) (€)	
		Germany	Spain
Voriconazole	200 mg IV	156.00	133.32
	Oral tablet 200 mg	45.00	35.68
Liposomal amphotericin B	50 mg IV	220.47	130.06
Caspofungin	70 mg IV	793.24	570.81
	50 mg IV	625.70	448.76

Data sources: [21,22].
IV, intravenous.

Table 2 Inpatient and outpatient costs (2011 €)

Setting	Description	Price (€)	
		Germany	Spain
Inpatient	Hospitalisation cost per day	674.10	566.52
Outpatient	Intravenous administration cost per unit	34.90	34.90

Data sources: [1,18-20].

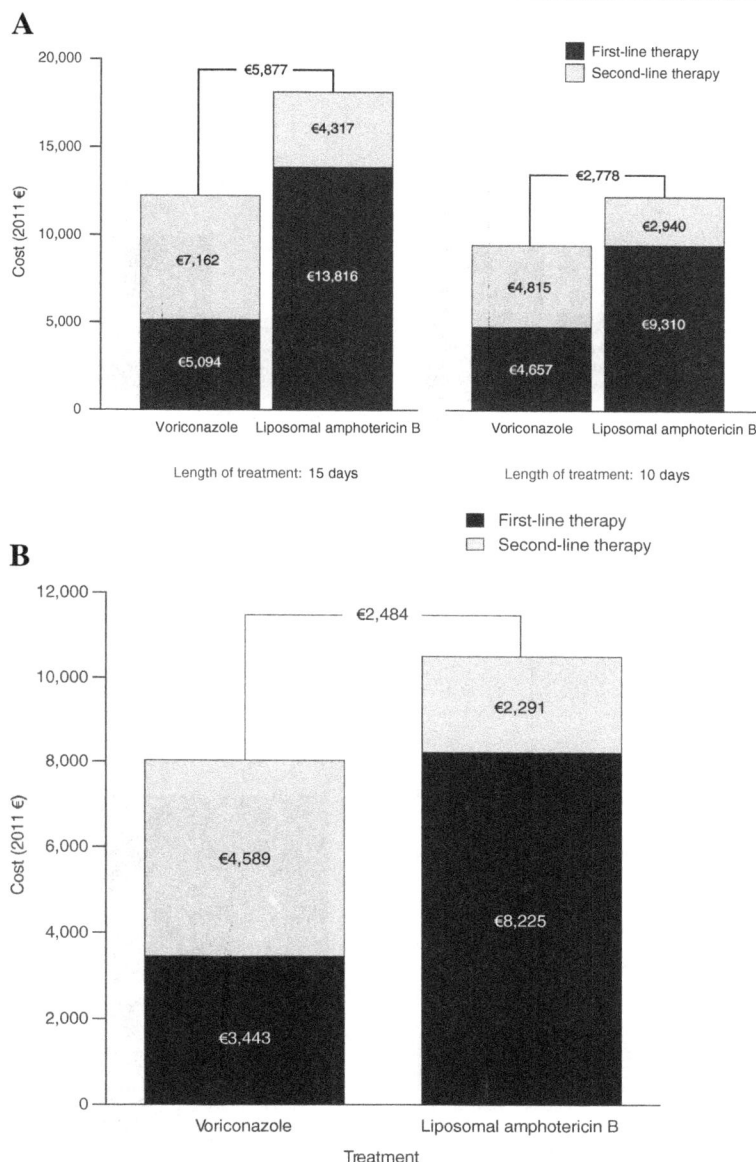

Figure 2 Cost comparison for base-case scenario in (A) Germany and (B) Spain.

AE savings accounted for 2.0% of the total cost saving associated with first-line voriconazole versus liposomal amphotericin B.

Sensitivity analyses
Sensitivity analyses showed that the results of the model were sensitive to drug price, particularly the cost of liposomal amphotericin B. In the German hospital scenario (LOT = 15 days) a variation in drug price of ±30% resulted in upper and lower bounds for the €5,878 total cost saving of €8,561 and €3,194 for liposomal amphotericin B, €5,070 and €6,685 for the IV formulation of voriconazole, and €5,746 and €6,009 for the oral formulation

of voriconazole. Similarly, in the Spanish hospital scenario (LOT = 15 days), a variation in drug price of ±30% resulted in upper and lower bounds for the €2,483 total cost saving of €4,066 and €900 for liposomal amphotericin B, €1,719 and €3,247 for the IV formulation of voriconazole, and €2,393 and €2,573 for the oral formulation of voriconazole.

Discussion
Pharmacoeconomic analyses are increasingly important in the clinical arena where decision-makers face growing pressure to optimise value and quality of care. In addition, pharmacoeconomic analyses can also provide information to support clinical decision-making to promote the

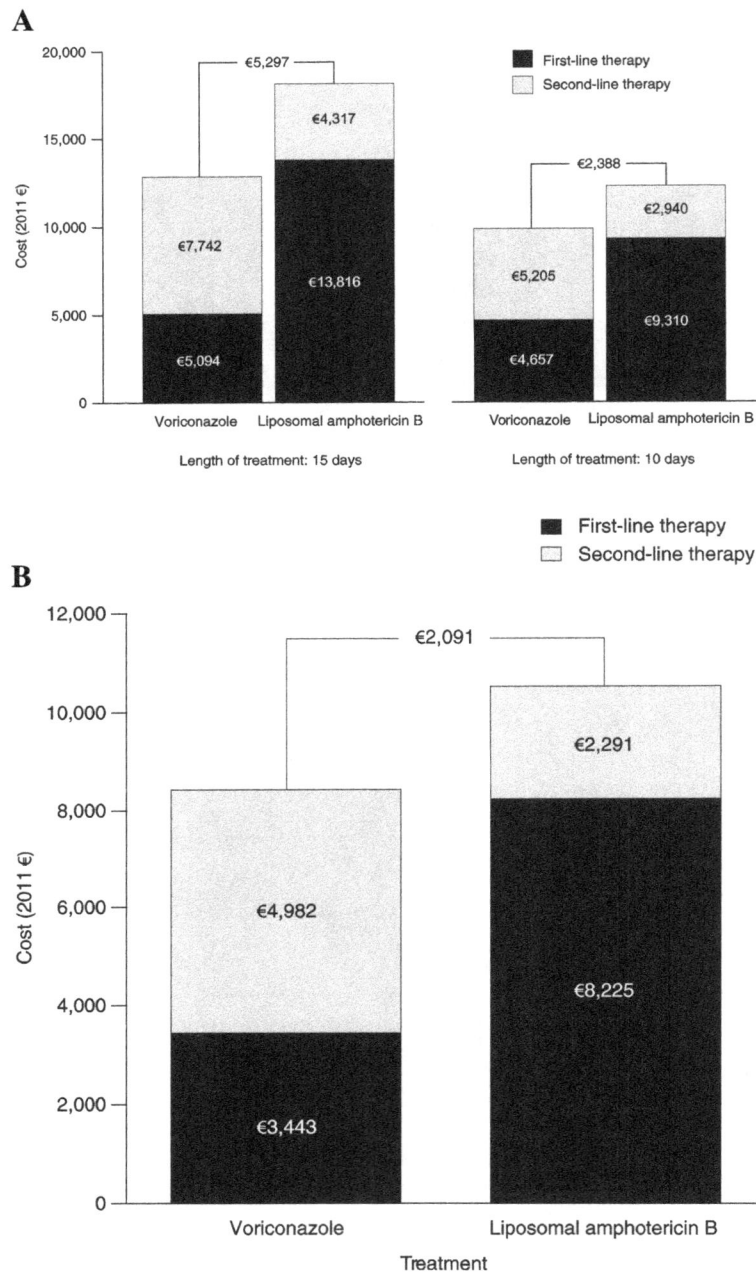

Figure 3 Cost comparison assuming equal efficacy in (A) Germany and (B) Spain.

most effective and appropriate treatment for patients. Improvements in efficacy and reductions in hospital LOS and costs associated with AEs are clearly also desirable outcomes for patients and clinicians.

The pharmacoeconomic evaluation described in this article applies to the treatment of IA infections in patients with haematological disorders in Germany and Spain. The findings from our model, together with the previously reported results from a randomised clinical trial [14], suggest that voriconazole is likely to be

cost-saving as first-line therapy compared with liposomal amphotericin B, and is a better treatment option from a clinical, safety and economic perspective. This observation was consistent across all scenarios tested in this analysis.

To the best of our knowledge, this is the first analysis to directly compare the pharmacoeconomic costs of voriconazole and liposomal amphotericin B for the treatment of IA. Wingard and colleagues compared the resource use and cost of treatment for voriconazole with conventional amphotericin B for IA and found that using voriconazole as a first-line therapy resulted in significantly fewer deaths and similar treatment costs [23]. Surviving patients who were treated with voriconazole spent fewer days in intensive care and more days out of hospital than those who received amphotericin B [23]. In addition, decision-tree modelling has suggested that voriconazole is cost-saving overall compared with conventional amphotericin B in clinical trial populations in the United States, Canada, Germany and the Netherlands [18,24-26].

Cost savings associated with voriconazole were thought to be attributable to its lower drug acquisition costs and shorter IV LOT due to the availability of an oral formulation of voriconazole. In the German model, a reduction in the IV LOT from 15 to 10 days had a great impact on the total treatment cost for liposomal amphotericin B, reducing the total cost by approximately one-third. In clinical practice, the IV LOT for voriconazole is often shorter than 10 days, which could lead to even greater cost savings. In addition to cost savings, the availability of an oral formulation of voriconazole offers several other advantages, including ease of delivery, reduced infection risk in an already immunocompromised patient population, and improved patient compliance.

The limitations of this study included the use of clinical trial data that may not be representative of the general population, the absence of head-to-head data comparing voriconazole with liposomal amphotericin B, and the assumption of 100% efficacy with second-line therapy. However, this assumption was required to prevent extrapolation of the time horizon beyond 30 days and was considered acceptable by clinical experts as no large trials evaluating efficacy data for second-line therapies have been conducted in this patient population.

Several factors, including drug-drug interactions and AEs, contribute to the long-term costs of IA. As voriconazole is an inhibitor of CYP3A4 liver enzymes, its concurrent use with other agents that are metabolized by the same system may result in substantial drug-drug interactions (e.g., concomitant use with immunosuppressive transplant medications) [27-29]. Voriconazole has also been associated with an increased risk of hepatotoxicity, with studies reporting significant transaminase abnormalities in 12.4% of patients [30]; however, most instances of drug-induced hepatotoxicity are unpredictable and vary considerably depending on the population, indication, formulation, and dosage [31,32]. Although liposomal amphotericin B has been shown to be substantially less toxic than conventional amphotericin B, particularly with respect to infusion-related reactions and nephrotoxicity, its use is still limited by these AEs [33]. Furthermore, concurrent use of liposomal amphotericin B with other nephrotoxic agents (e.g., cyclosporine, aminoglycosides, polymixins, tacrolimus and pentamidine) has been shown to increase the potential for drug-induced nephrotoxicity in some patients [34].

Conclusions

This study showed that voriconazole is likely to be cost-saving compared with liposomal amphotericin B for the first-line treatment of IA infections in patients with haematological disorders in Germany and Spain. These conclusions are valid for countries with a comparable healthcare system and comparable drug costs; however, studies using observational real-world data are required to confirm these findings.

Abbreviations
AE: Adverse event; BID: Twice daily; HSCT: Haematopoietic stem cell transplantation; IA: Invasive aspergillosis; IFD: Invasive fungal disease; IV: Intravenous; LOS: Length of stay; LOT: Length of therapy.

Competing interests
Helmut Ostermann has received research grants from Gilead Sciences and MSD; has received compensation for attending advisory boards for Astellas Pharma, Gilead Sciences, and MSD; and has served on the speaker's bureau for Astellas Pharma, Gilead Sciences, MSD, and Pfizer Inc. Carlos Solano has served as a consultant for Astellas Pharma, Gilead Sciences, MSD, and Pfizer Inc; has received research grants from Astellas Pharma, Gilead Sciences, Pfizer Inc and the Instituto de Salud Carlos III (Spanish Ministry of Economy and Competitiveness); and has received honoraria for talks from Astellas Pharma, Gilead Sciences, MSD, and Pfizer Inc. Isidro Jarque has served as a consultant for Astellas Pharma, Gilead Sciences, MSD, and Pfizer Inc. Carolina Garcia-Vidal has no competing interests. Jon Andoni Barrueta, Marina De Salas-Cansado, Bertram Weber, and Claudie Charbonneau are employees of Pfizer Inc. Xin Gao, Jennifer Stephens, and Mei Xue are employees of Pharmerit International, and have served as consultants for Pfizer Inc.

Authors' contributions
XG and JS contributed to model conceptualisation, design, and assumptions. XG and MX conducted the model programming and analyses. All authors contributed to the review and interpretation of the results, and the development and critical review of the manuscript. All authors read and approved the final manuscript.

Acknowledgements
The authors would like to thank Maria Echave (Pfizer Spain, Madrid, Spain), Joscha Gussmann (Pfizer Germany, Berlin, Germany) and Michal Kantecki (Pfizer International Operations, Paris, France) for their valuable contributions.

Funding source
This study was sponsored by Pfizer Inc. Editorial support was provided by Karen Irving of Complete Medical Communications and was funded by Pfizer Inc.

Author details
[1]Medical Clinic III, Department of Haematology and Oncology, University Hospital Munich – Grosshadern, Munich, Germany. [2]Haematology and Oncology Department, Hospital Clínico Universitario INCLIVA, University of Valencia, Valencia, Spain. [3]Haematology Service, Hospital Universitari i Politècnic La Fe, Valencia, Spain. [4]Hospital Universitari de Bellvitge, Universitat de Barcelona, Barcelona, Spain. [5]Pharmerit International, Bethesda, MD, USA. [6]Medical Unit, Pfizer Spain, Madrid, Spain. [7]Health Economics and Outcomes Research Department, Pfizer Spain, Madrid, Spain. [8]Health Technology Assessment and Outcomes Research Department, Pfizer Germany, Berlin, Germany. [9]Health Economics and Outcomes Research Department, Pfizer International Operations, Paris, France.

References
1. Rieger CT, Cornely OA, Hoppe-Tichy T, Kiehl M, Knoth H, Thalheimer M, Schuler U, Ullmann AJ, Ehlken B, Ostermann H: **Treatment cost of invasive fungal disease (Ifd) in patients with acute myelogenous leukaemia (Aml) or myelodysplastic syndrome (Mds) in German hospitals.** *Mycoses* 2012, 55:514–520.

2. Warnock DW: Trends in the epidemiology of invasive fungal infections. *Nippon Ishinkin Gakkai Zasshi* 2007, 48:1–12.

3. Marr KA, Carter RA, Boeckh M, Martin P, Corey L: Invasive aspergillosis in allogeneic stem cell transplant recipients: changes in epidemiology and risk factors. *Blood* 2002, 100:4358–4366.

4. Lin SJ, Schranz J, Teutsch SM: Aspergillosis case-fatality rate: systematic review of the literature. *Clin Infect Dis* 2001, 32:358–366.

5. Wilson LS, Reyes CM, Stolpman M, Speckman J, Allen K, Beney J: The direct cost and incidence of systemic fungal infections. *Value Health* 2002, 5:26–34.

6. Morgan J, Meltzer MI, Plikaytis BD, Sofair AN, Huie-White S, Wilcox S, Harrison LH, Seaberg EC, Hajjeh RA, Teutsch SM: Excess mortality, hospital stay, and cost due to candidemia: a case-control study using data from population-based candidemia surveillance. *Infect Control Hosp Epidemiol* 2005, 26:540–547.

7. Zaoutis TE, Argon J, Chu J, Berlin JA, Walsh TJ, Feudtner C: The epidemiology and attributable outcomes of candidemia in adults and children hospitalized in the United States: a propensity analysis. *Clin Infect Dis* 2005, 41:1232–1239.

8. Menzin J, Meyers JL, Friedman M, Perfect JR, Langston AA, Danna RP, Papadopoulos G: Mortality, length of hospitalization, and costs associated with invasive fungal infections in high-risk patients. *Am J Health Syst Pharm* 2009, 66:1711–1717.

9. Rubio-Terrés C, Grau S: Pharmacoeconomics of voriconazole. *Expert Opin Pharmacother* 2010, 11:877–887.

10. Ruhnke M, Böhme A, Buchheidt D, Cornely O, Donhuijsen K, Einsele H, Enzensberger R, Hebart H, Heussel CP, Horger M, Hof H, Karthaus M, Krüger W, Maschmeyer G, Penack O, Ritter J, Schwartz S: Diagnosis of invasive fungal infections in hematology and oncology–guidelines from the Infectious Diseases Working Party in Haematology and Oncology of the German Society for Haematology and Oncology (AGIHO). *Ann Oncol* 2012, 23:823–833.

11. Mousset S, Buchheidt D, Heinz W, Ruhnke M, Cornely OA, Egerer G, Krüger W, Link H, Neumann S, Ostermann H, Panse J, Penack O, Rieger C, Schmidt-Hieber M, Silling G, Sudhoff T, Ullmann AJ, Wolf HH, Maschmeyer G, Böhme A: Treatment of invasive fungal infections in cancer patients-updated recommendations of the Infectious Diseases Working Party (AGIHO) of the German Society of Hematology and Oncology (DGHO). *Ann Hematol* 2014, 93:13–32.

12. Maertens J, Marchetti O, Herbrecht R, Cornely OA, Flückiger U, Frère P, Gachot B, Heinz WJ, Lass-Flörl C, Ribaud P, Thiebaut A, Cordonnier C: European guidelines for antifungal management in leukemia and hematopoietic stem cell transplant recipients: summary of the ECIL 3–2009 update. *Bone Marrow Transplant* 2011, 46:709–718.

13. Fortún J, Carratalá J, Gavaldá J, Lizasoain M, Salavert M, de la Cámara R, Borges M, Cervera C, Garnacho J, Lassaleta Á, Lumbreras C, Sanz MÁ, Ramos JT, Torre-Cisneros J, Aguado JM, Cuenca-Estrella M: Guidelines for the treatment of invasive fungal disease by Aspergillus spp. and other fungi issued by the Spanish Society of Infectious Diseases and Clinical Microbiology (SEIMC). 2011 Update. *Enferm Infecc Microbiol Clin* 2011, 29:435–454.

14. Herbrecht R, Denning DW, Patterson TF, Bennett JE, Greene RE, Oestmann JW, Kern WV, Marr KA, Ribaud P, Lortholary O, Sylvester R, Rubin RH, Wingard JR, Stark P, Durand C, Caillot D, Thiel E, Chandrasekar PH, Hodges MR, Schlamm HT, Troke PF, de Pauw B: Voriconazole versus amphotericin B for primary therapy of invasive aspergillosis. *N Engl J Med* 2002, 347:408–415.

15. Cornely OA, Maertens J, Bresnik M, Ebrahimi R, Ullmann AJ, Bouza E, Heussel CP, Lortholary O, Rieger C, Boehme A, Aoun M, Horst HA, Thiebaut A, Ruhnke M, Reichert D, Vianelli N, Krause SW, Olavarria E, Herbrecht R: Liposomal amphotericin B as initial therapy for invasive mold infection: a randomized trial comparing a high-loading dose regimen with standard dosing (AmBiLoad trial). *Clin Infect Dis* 2007, 44:1289–1297.

16. Stephens JM, Gao X, Ji X, Baddley J, Schlamm H, Tarallo M: Hospital database analysis of haematologic malignancy and bone marrow transplant/stem cell transplant (BMT/SCT) patients with invasive aspergillosis (IA). Vancouver, BC, Canada: Poster presented at the 48th IDSA Annual Meeting; 2010.

17. Bates DW, Spell N, Cullen DJ, Burdick E, Laird N, Petersen LA, Small SD, Sweitzer BJ, Leape LL: The costs of adverse drug events in hospitalized patients. Adverse Drug Events Prevention Study Group. *JAMA* 1997, 277:307–311.

18. Jansen JP, Kern WV, Cornely OA, Karthaus M, Ruhnke M, Ullmann AJ, Resch A: Economic evaluation of voriconazole versus conventional amphotericin B in the treatment of invasive aspergillosis in Germany. *Value Health* 2006, 9:12–23.

19. Schürmann D, Sorensen SV, De Cock E, Duttagupta S, Resch A: Cost-effectiveness of linezolid versus vancomycin for hospitalised patients with complicated skin and soft-tissue infections in Germany. *Eur J Health Econ* 2009, 10:65–79.

20. Oblikue Consulting: E-Salud. Spanish Cost Database. Available at: http://www.oblikue.com/bddcostes/.

21. Lauer Taxe: Pharmindex for Germany drug cost. Available at: http://www.lauer-fischer.de/lf/Seiten/WEBAPO-Lauer-Taxe/WEBAPO-Lauer-Taxe-demo.aspx.

22. General Council of Official Colleges of Pharmacists: Bot Plus database. Available at: https://botplusweb.portalfarma.com.

23. Wingard JR, Herbrecht R, Mauskopf J, Schlamm HT, Marciniak A, Roberts CS: Resource use and cost of treatment with voriconazole or conventional amphotericin B for invasive aspergillosis. *Transpl Infect Dis* 2007, 9:182–188.

24. Wenzel R, Del Favero A, Kibbler C, Rogers T, Rotstein C, Mauskopf J, Morris S, Schlamm H, Troke P, Marciniak A: Economic evaluation of voriconazole compared with conventional amphotericin B for the primary treatment of aspergillosis in immunocompromised patients. *J Antimicrob Chemother* 2005, 55:352–361.

25. Jantunen E, Salonen J, Juvonen E, Koivunen E, Siitonen T, Lehtinen T, Kuittinen O, Leppä S, Anttila VJ, Itälä M, Wiklund T, Remes K, Nousiainen T: Invasive fungal infections in autologous stem cell transplant recipients: a nation-wide study of 1188 transplanted patients. *Eur J Haematol* 2004, 73:174–178.

26. Rotstein C, Laverdière M, Marciniak A, Ali F: An economic evaluation of voriconazole versus amphotericin B for the treatment of invasive aspergillosis in Canada. *Can J Infect Dis Med Microbiol* 2004, 15:277–284.

27. Capone D, Tarantino G, Gentile A, Sabbatini M, Polichetti G, Santangelo M, Nappi R, Ciotola A, D'Alessandro V, Renda A, Basile V, Federico S: Effects of voriconazole on tacrolimus metabolism in a kidney transplant recipient. *J Clin Pharm Ther* 2010, 35:121–124.

28. Dodds-Ashley E: Management of drug and food interactions with azole antifungal agents in transplant recipients. *Pharmacotherapy* 2010, 30:842–854.

29. Pieri M, Miraglia N, Polichetti G, Tarantino G, Acampora A, Capone D: Analytical and pharmacological aspects of therapeutic drug monitoring of mTOR inhibitors. *Curr Drug Metab* 2011, 12:253–267.

30. Pfizer Inc: Vfend full prescribing information. Available at: http://www.accessdata.fda.gov/drugsatfda_docs/label/2010/021266s032lbl.pdf.

31. Potoski BA, Brown J: The safety of voriconazole. *Clin Infect Dis* 2002, 35:1273–1275.

32. Tarantino G, Di Minno MN, Capone D: Drug-induced liver injury: is it somehow foreseeable? *World J Gastroenterol* 2009, 15:2817–2833.

33. Moen MD, Lyseng-Williamson KA, Scott LJ: Liposomal amphotericin B: a review of its use as empirical therapy in febrile neutropenia and in the treatment of invasive fungal infections. *Drugs* 2009, 69:361–392.

34. Gilead Sciences Ltd: Summary of Product Characteristics: Ambisome. Available at: http://www.medicines.org.uk/emc/medicine/1236/SPC/ambisome/.

13

Hydrocarbon molar water solubility predicts NMDA vs. GABA$_A$ receptor modulation

Robert J Brosnan[*] and Trung L Pham

Abstract

Background: Many anesthetics modulate 3-transmembrane (such as NMDA) and 4-transmembrane (such as GABA$_A$) receptors. Clinical and experimental anesthetics exhibiting receptor family specificity often have low water solubility. We hypothesized that the molar water solubility of a hydrocarbon could be used to predict receptor modulation in vitro.

Methods: GABA$_A$ ($\alpha_1\beta_2\gamma_{2s}$) or NMDA (NR1/NR2A) receptors were expressed in oocytes and studied using standard two-electrode voltage clamp techniques. Hydrocarbons from 14 different organic functional groups were studied at saturated concentrations, and compounds within each group differed only by the carbon number at the ω-position or within a saturated ring. An effect on GABA$_A$ or NMDA receptors was defined as a 10% or greater reversible current change from baseline that was statistically different from zero.

Results: Hydrocarbon moieties potentiated GABA$_A$ and inhibited NMDA receptor currents with at least some members from each functional group modulating both receptor types. A water solubility cut-off for NMDA receptors occurred at 1.1 mM with a 95% CI = 0.45 to 2.8 mM. NMDA receptor cut-off effects were not well correlated with hydrocarbon chain length or molecular volume. No cut-off was observed for GABA$_A$ receptors within the solubility range of hydrocarbons studied.

Conclusions: Hydrocarbon modulation of NMDA receptor function exhibits a molar water solubility cut-off. Differences between unrelated receptor cut-off values suggest that the number, affinity, or efficacy of protein-hydrocarbon interactions at these sites likely differ.

Background

Inhaled anesthetics interact with putative cell receptor targets in a manner uncharacteristic of most other pharmacologic agents. They exhibit immobilization efficacy in all animals, both vertebrates and invertebrates, and even in protozoa and plants. The inhaled agents range in diversity from single elements to diatomic molecules to complex hydrocarbons and share no conserved size, shape, or functional groups. Most agents also modulate multiple phylogenetically unrelated cell targets and generally inhibit excitatory channels or receptors and potentiate inhibitory ones, complicating the identification of a drug-receptor structural motif predictive of anesthetic molecular action [1].

Attempts to determine how disparate drugs act on so many unrelated receptors—and to define those targets

essential to inhaled anesthetic actions—have thus far proved illusory. Consequently, in the present study, we posed the opposite question: Why are some anesthetics unable to modulate certain anesthetic-sensitive ion channels or receptors, even at supra-pharmacologic concentrations? To answer this question, we restricted consideration to two unrelated ion channels in particular: the N-methyl-d-aspartate (NMDA) receptor, a member of the 3-transmembrane (TM3) ion channel family, and the γ-aminobutyric acid type A (GABA$_A$) receptor, a member of the 4-transmembrane (TM4) ion channel family. Strong evidence supports the role of both receptors in mediating various endpoints of general anesthesia, including immobility and amnesia [2-6]. Within the NMDA and GABA$_A$ channel proteins, hydrophilic or amphipathic cavities or pockets have been postulated near the solvent interface and within transmembrane segments of several subunits [7,8]. Presumably, such cavities might conceivably contain solvent molecules or nothing at all, though it should be

* Correspondence: rjbrosnan@ucdavis.edu
Department of Surgical and Radiological Sciences, School of Veterinary Medicine, University of California, Davis, CA 95616, USA

thermodynamically less favorable to maintain a vacuum within a pocket that is sufficiently large and polar enough to accommodate water.

The binding affinity of water within each pocket on an ion channel can be expressed as a standard dissociation constant, and the ability of a drug to displace water and either completely or partially fill the pocket can be expressed as a standard equilibrium constant. Since structures of phylogenetically unrelated channels are different, the hydrophilicity of their respective pockets should not be conserved. Therefore, dissociation constants are expected to be different for water bound within pockets of different channels. Consequently, the minimum concentration of drug necessary to displace water within a pocket capable of inducing a functional conformational change should be different between unrelated channels. If the drug cannot reach a concentration within the aqueous phase sufficient to displace water within the protein modulatory pocket, then that drug should exert no pharmacologic effect on the channel, even when delivered at a saturated aqueous phase concentration. The physical property that defines this maximum (saturated) concentration of a drug in the aqueous phase is the molar water solubility.

The effects of a number of conventional (modern and historic) and experimental anesthetics on NMDA and GABA$_A$ receptors have been studied previously. When plotted in order of their calculated molar water solubilities (Figure 1), there is an abrupt change in the ability of compounds to modulate NMDA receptors. Drugs with water solubility greater than about 1 mM all modulate NMDA and GABA$_A$ currents when administered in sufficiently large concentrations. However, drugs with lower molar water solubility modulate only GABA$_A$ or neither receptor type. These data suggest that molar water solubility may predict an NMDA receptor cut-off effect at values less than 1 mM and are consistent with non-specific interactions in which water displaced from modulatory pockets on the NMDA receptor contribute, at least in part, to molecular mechanisms of action. Compounds unable to reach approximately 1 mM aqueous concentration may thus be unable to competitively displace water within any of the NMDA critical modulatory sites.

We hypothesized that hydrocarbon molar water solubility below this critical cut-off value is associated with loss of NMDA receptor modulation, but not GABA$_A$ receptor modulation. As tests agents, we considered 14 different series of normal hydrocarbon chains or rings, where molecules within each series differed only by the length of the Ω chain or substitutent alkyl groups (Table 1). Because different functional groups differ in hydrophilicity, the length and volume of the hydrocarbon chain needed to achieve a given molar water solubility will likewise differ. Thus, if the hypothesis is correct, then observed cut-off responses should correlate with hydrocarbon molar water solubility rather than hydrocarbon size.

Although generally advocated to study anesthetic effects at clinically-relevant concentrations, we proposed to test this hypothesis at saturated aqueous drug concentrations for 3 reasons. First, because an aqueous binding site is postulated, it is important to study drug effects at an interfacial concentration that can be directly related to a bulk aqueous concentration. However, anesthetics do not distribute equally through the lipid bilayer. Halothane shows a preference for the phospholipid headgroup interface [27]. Xenon atoms prefer regions at the lipid-water interface and the central region of the bilayer [28]. The anesthetics cyclopropane, nitrous oxide, desflurane, isoflurane, and 1,1,2-trifluoroethane all preferentially

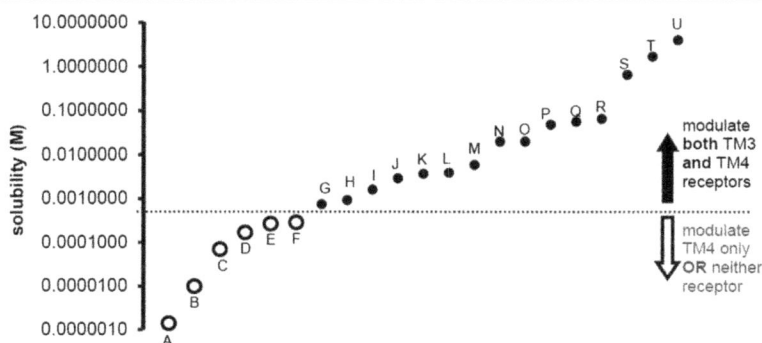

Figure 1 Summary of ion channel modulation as a function of calculated anesthetic molar solubility in unbuffered water at 25°C (values from SciFinder Scholar). Drugs that modulate 4-transmembrane receptors (TM4) or neither receptor type are shown as open circles (o, A-F) below the dotted horizontal solubility line. Drugs that modulate both 3-transmembrane (TM3) and TM4 receptors are shown as small black circles (●, G-U) above the dotted horizontal solubility line. A = nonane (unpublished data), B = midazolam [9], C = diazepam [10], D = undecanol [11], E = etomidate [12], F = 1,2-dichlorohexafluorocyclobutane [13], G = sevoflurane [14-17], H = propofol [18,19], I = ketamine [12,16,20], J = isoflurane [14-16,21,22], K = enflurane [15,23], L = dizocilpine [20,24], M = desflurane [16,17], N = halothane [14,22,23], O = cyclopropane [22,25], P = chloroform [22], Q = 2,6-dimethylphenol [26], R = methoxyflurane [14,15,23], S = diethyl ether [15,23], T = nitrous oxide [21,22], U = ethanol [21].

Table 1 Source, purity and physical properties of study compounds

Compound	CAS#	MW (amu)	P_{vap} (mmHg)	Solubility (M)	Carbon (#)	Volume (Å^3)	Source	Purity (%)
Alcohols								
1-decanol	112-30-1	158.28	1.48×10^{-2}	6.5×10^{-4}	10	317	Aldrich	>99
1-undecanol	112-42-5		5.10×10^{-3}	1.7×10^{-4}	11	344	Acros	98
1-dodecanol	112-53-8	172.31 186.33	2.09×10^{-3}	4.1×10^{-5}	12	372	TCI	99
Alkanes								
butane	106-97-8	58.12	1.92×10^{3}	1.4×10^{-3}	4	156	Matheson	99.99
pentane	109-66-0	72.15	5.27×10^{2}	4.3×10^{-4}	5	184		>99
hexane	110-54-3	86.18	1.51×10^{2}	1.2×10^{-4}	6	211	Aldrich Acros	>99
Aldehydes								
octanal	124-13-0	128.21	2.07×10^{0}	5.4×10^{-3}	8	262	Aldrich	99
nonanal	124-19-6	142.24	$5.32 \times 10^{-}$	2.3×10^{-3}	9	289	Aldrich	95
decanal	112-31-2	156.27	^{1}	9.8×10^{-4}	10	316	Aldrich	98
undecanal	112-44-7	170.29	2.07×10^{-1} 8.32×10^{-2}	4.2×10^{-4}	11	344	Aldrich	97
Alkenes								
1-pentene	109-67-1	70.13	6.37×10^{2}	1.4×10^{-3}	5	176	Aldrich	99
1-hexene	592-41-6	84.16	1.88×10^{2}	4.2×10^{-4}	6	203	Aldrich	>99
Alkynes								
1-hexyne	693-02-7	82.14	1.35×10^{2}	2.9×10^{-3}	6	184	Aldrich	97
1-heptyne	628-71-7	96.17	4.35×10^{1}	6.6×10^{-4}	7	212	Acros	99
1-octyne	629-05-0	110.2	1.44×10^{1}	1.9×10^{-4}	8	239	Acros	99
Amines								
1-octadecanamine	124-30-1	269.51	4.88×10^{-5}	1.3×10^{-3}	18	546	TCI	97
1-eicosanamine	10525-37-8	297.56	8.96×10^{-6}	2.7×10^{-4}	20	601	Rambus	95
Benzenes								
1,3-dimethylbenzene	108-38-3	106.17	7.61×10^{0}	1.2×10^{-3}	8	202	Aldrich	>99
1,3-diethylbenzene	141-93-5	134.22	1.15×10^{0}	6.6×10^{-5}	10	257	Fluka	>99
Cycloalkanes								
cyclopentane	287-92-3	70.13	3.14×10^{2}	3.3×10^{-3}	5	147	Aldrich	>99
cyclohexane	110-82-7	84.16	9.37×10^{1}	1.0×10^{-3}	6	176	Aldrich	>99.7
Ethers								
dibutylether	142-96-1	130.23	7.10×10^{0}	1.6×10^{-2}	8	277	Aldrich	99.3
dipentylether	693-65-2		1.00×10^{0}	3.0×10^{-3}	10	331	Fluka	>98.5
dihexylether	112-58-3	158.28 186.33	1.48×10^{-1}	5.8×10^{-4}	12	386	Aldrich	97
Esters								
ethyl heptanoate	106-30-9	158.24	6.02×10^{-1}	5.4×10^{-3}	9	299	MP Bio	99
ethyl octanoate	106-32-1		2.24×10^{-1}	2.1×10^{-3}	10	327	Aldrich	>99
ethyl decanoate	110-38-3	172.26 200.32	3.39×10^{-2}	4.4×10^{-4}	12	381	TCI	98
Haloalkanes								
1-fluoropentane	592-50-7	90.14	1.84×10^{2}	3.9×10^{-3}	5	193	Aldrich	98
1-fluorohexane	373-14-8	104.17	6.06×10^{1}	1.2×10^{-3}	6	220	Acros	>99
1-fluoroctane	463-11-6	132.22	7.09×10^{0}	1.3×10^{-4}	8	275	Aldrich	98

Table 1 Source, purity and physical properties of study compounds (Continued)

	CAS#	MW	P_{vap}	molar solubility		molecular volume	source	purity
Ketones								
2-decanone	693-54-9	156.27	2.48×10^{-1}	3.2×10^{-3}	10	316	TCI	>99
2-undecanone	112-12-9		9.78×10^{-2}	1.4×10^{-3}	11	343	Acros	98
2-dodecanone	6175-49-1	170.29 184.32	3.96×10^{-2}	5.8×10^{-4}	12	371	TCI	95
Sulfides								
1-(ethylthio)-hexane	7309-44-6	146.29	8.16×10^{-1}	2.8×10^{-3}	8	289	Pfaltz	97
1-(ethylthio)-octane	3698-94-0	174.35	1.08×10^{-1}	5.0×10^{-4}	10	344	Pfaltz	97
Thiols								
1-pentanethiol	110-66-7	104.21	1.42×10^{1}	1.5×10^{-3}	5	207	Aldrich	98
1-hexanethiol	111-31-9	118.24	4.50×10^{0}	5.1×10^{-4}	6	235	TCI	96

Chemical Abstracts Service number (CAS#), molecular weight (MW), vapor pressure at 25°C (P_{vap}), molar solubility in pure water at pH = 7, and molecular volume are calculated estimates (rather than measured values) referenced by SciFinder Scholar.

concentrate at the interface between water and hexane, [29] but the nonimmobilizer perfluoroethane does not exhibit a hydrophilic-hydrophobic interfacial maxima [29]. Nonetheless, even without knowing the membrane distribution profile of an anesthetic, the interfacial concentration can be assumed maximal at a saturating aqueous phase concentration at equilibrium; thus drug responses are compared at their respective relative maximum interfacial concentrations.

Second, different anesthetic endpoints are achieved at different drug concentrations. Thus, a drug could exhibit relative receptor specificity; that is to say, a drug may act preferentially at one receptor to achieve one endpoint—such as amnesia—but act on additional receptors when administered at higher concentrations to achieve other endpoints—such as immobility. Failure to modulate a receptor when a drug is delivered at a saturated concentration implies a null receptor response at lower drug concentrations and for any therapeutic endpoint.

Third, the drug concentrations that produce different anesthetic endpoints—amnesia, unconsciousness and immobility—are unknown for many experimental compounds. Some anesthetic endpoints may not even be achievable with some compounds, such as the nonimmobilizers. Absolute receptor specificity means that there is also relative specificity for any drug effect produced. Accordingly, comparisons of receptor effects using saturated concentrations *in vitro* are not prepositioned upon knowledge of *in vivo* drug anesthetic effects.

Hence, this study aimed to test whether NMDA versus $GABA_A$ receptor modulation was correlated with calculated molar water solubility "cut-off" values for diverse series of hydrocarbon functional groups.

Methods

Oocyte collection and receptor expression
An ovary from tricaine-anesthetized *Xenopus laevis* frogs was surgically removed using a protocol approved by the Institutional Animal Care and Use Committee at the University of California, Davis (Protocol #12030). Following manual disruption of the ovarian lobule septae, the ovary was incubated in 0.2% Type I collagenase (Worthington Biochemical, Lakewood, NJ) to defolliculate oocytes which were washed and stored in fresh and filtered modified Barth's solution composed of 88 mM NaCl, 1 mM KCl, 2.4 mM $NaHCO_3$, 20 mM HEPES, 0.82 mM $MgSO_4$, 0.33 mM $Ca(NO_3)_2$, 0.41 mM $CaCl_2$, 5 mM sodium pyruvate, gentamycin, penicillin, streptomycin, and corrected to pH = 7.4. All salts and antibiotics were A.C.S. grade (Fisher Scientific, Pittsburgh, PA).

Clones used were provided as a gift from Dr. R.A. Harris (University of Texas, Austin) and were sequenced and compared to references in the National Center for Biotechnology Information database to confirm the identity of each gene. $GABA_A$ receptors were expressed using clones for the human $GABA_A$ $\alpha 1$ and the rat $GABA_A$ $\beta 2$ and $\gamma 2s$ subunits in pCIS-II vectors. Approximately 0.25-1 ng total plasmid mixture containing either α_1, β_2, or γ_2 genes in a respective ratio of 1:1:10 was injected intranuclearly through the oocyte animal pole and studied 2–4 days later. These plasmid ratios ensured incorporation of the γ subunit into expressed receptors, as confirmed via receptor potentiation to 10 μM chlordiazepoxide or insensitivity to 10 μM zinc chloride during co-application with GABA. In separate oocytes, glutamate receptors were expressed using rat NMDA NR1 clones in a pCDNA3 vector and rat NMDA NR2A clones in a Bluescript vector. RNA encoding each subunit, prepared using a commercial transcription kit (T7 mMessage mMachine, Ambion, Austin, TX), was mixed in a 1:1 ratio, and 1–10 ng of total RNA was injected into oocytes and studied 1–2 days later. Oocytes injected with similar volumes of water served as controls.

$GABA_A$ receptor electrophysiology studies
Oocytes were studied in a 250 μL linear-flow perfusion chamber with solutions administered by syringe pump at

1.5 ml/min with gastight glass syringes and Teflon tubing. Oocyte GABA$_A$ currents were studied using standard two-electrode voltage clamping techniques at a holding potential of -80 mV using a 250 μL channel linear-flow perfusion chamber with solutions administered by syringe pump at 1.5 mL/min.

Frog Ringer's (FR) solution composed of 115 mM NaCl, 2.5 mM KCl, 1.8 mM CaCl$_2$, and 10 mM HEPES prepared in 18.2 MΩ H$_2$O and filtered and adjusted to pH = 7.4 was used to perfuse oocytes. Agonist solutions also contained 20-to-40 μM, equal to an EC$_{10-20}$, of 4-aminobutanoic acid (FR-GABA) [30-32]. After FR perfusion for 5 min, oocytes were exposed to 30 sec FR-GABA followed by another 5 min FR washout; this was repeated until stable GABA$_A$-elicited peaks were obtained. Next, FR containing a saturated solution of the study drug (Table 1)—or for gaseous study compounds a vapor pressure equal to 90% of barometric pressure with balance oxygen—was used to perfuse the oocyte chamber for 2 min followed by perfusion with a FR-GABA solution containing the identical drug concentration for 30 sec. FR was next perfused for 5 min to allow drug washout, and oocytes were finally perfused with FR-GABA for 30 sec to confirm return of currents to within 10% of the initial baseline response.

NMDA receptor electrophysiology studies

Methods for measurement of whole-cell NMDA receptor currents have been described [33,34]. Briefly, baseline perfusion solutions were the same as for GABA$_A$ with the substitution of equimolar BaCl$_2$ for calcium salts and the addition of 0.1 mM EGTA; this constituted barium frog Ringer's solution (BaFR). Agonist solutions for NMDA studies also contained 0.1 mM glutamate (E) and 0.01 mM glycine (G) to constitute a BaFREG solution that produced a NMDA receptor current ≥ EC$_{99}$.

The syringe pump and perfusion chamber apparatus as well as the clamp holding potential and baseline-agonist exposure protocols were identical to that described for the GABA$_A$ studies. The same test compounds, concentrations, and preparative methods were used in NMDA voltage clamp studies as in the GABA$_A$ voltage clamp studies (Table 1).

Response calculations and data analysis

Modulating drug responses were calculated as the percent of the control (baseline) peak as follows: $100 \cdot \frac{I_D}{I_B}$, where I_D and I_B were the peak currents measured during agonist + drug and agonist baseline perfusions, respectively. When present, direct receptor activation by a drug was similarly calculated as a percent of the agonist response. Average current responses for each drug and channel were described by mean ± SD. A lack of receptor

response (cut-off) was defined as a <10% change from baseline current that was statistically indistinguishable from zero using a two-tailed Student t-test. Hence, drug responses ≥110% of the baseline peak showed potentiation of receptor function, and drug responses ≤90% of the baseline peak showed inhibition of receptor function.

The log$_{10}$ of the calculated solubility (log$_{10}$S) for compounds immediately below and above the cut-off for each hydrocarbon functional group were used to determine the receptor cut-off. For each hydrocarbon, there was a "grey area" of indeterminate solubility effect (Figure 2) between sequentially increasing hydrocarbon chain lengths. Mean solubility cut-offs were calculated as the average log$_{10}$S for the least soluble compound that modulated receptor function and the most soluble neighboring compound for which no effect was observed. From this result, a 95% confidence interval for log$_{10}$S was calculated for receptor solubility cut-offs.

Results

Hydrocarbon effects on NMDA and GABA$_A$ receptors are summarized in Table 2, and sample recordings are presented in Figure 2. All of the compounds tested positively modulated GABA$_A$ receptor function, and a few of the 5-to-6 carbon compounds caused mild direct GABA$_A$ receptor activation, particularly the 1-fluoroalkanes and thiols. Mild direct receptor activation also occurred with dibutylether. With the exception of the aldehydes, alkynes, and cycloalkanes, GABA$_A$ receptor inhibition tended to decrease with increasing hydrocarbon chain length. No water solubility cut-off effect was observed for GABA$_A$ receptors for the compounds tested.

In contrast, NMDA receptors currents were decreased by the shorter hydrocarbons within each functional group (Table 1), but lengthening the hydrocarbon chain eventually produced a null response—a cut-off effect. No direct hydrocarbon effects on NMDA receptor function were detected in the absence of glutamate and glycine agonist.

The cut-off effect for NMDA receptor current modulation was associated with a hydrocarbon water solubility of 1.1 mM with a 95% confidence interval between 0.45 mM and 2.8 mM (Figure 3). More soluble hydrocarbons consistently inhibited NMDA receptor currents when applied at saturated aqueous concentrations, and hydrocarbons below this range had no appreciable effect on NMDA receptor function. Moreover, during the course of the study, water solubility was sufficiently predictive of an NMDA receptor cut-off so as to require identify and testing of only single pair of compounds bracketing this critical solubility value, as occurred with the alkenes, amines, cyclic hydrocarbons, and sulfur-containing compounds.

Increasing hydrocarbon chain length decreases water solubility, but also increases molecular size. However,

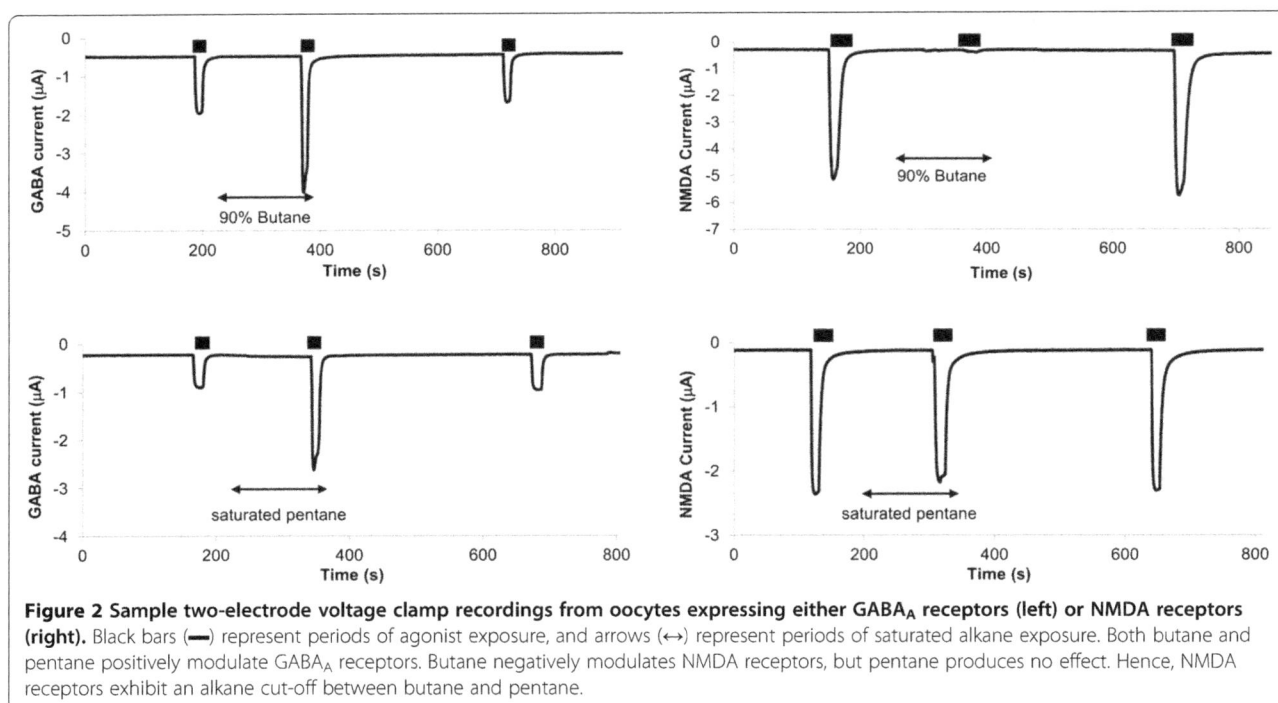

Figure 2 Sample two-electrode voltage clamp recordings from oocytes expressing either GABA$_A$ receptors (left) or NMDA receptors (right). Black bars (━) represent periods of agonist exposure, and arrows (↔) represent periods of saturated alkane exposure. Both butane and pentane positively modulate GABA$_A$ receptors. Butane negatively modulates NMDA receptors, but pentane produces no effect. Hence, NMDA receptors exhibit an alkane cut-off between butane and pentane.

when graphed as a function of either carbon number (Figure 4) or molecular volume (Figure 5), the observed NMDA receptor cut-off effects show no consistent pattern. For example, the n-alkanes, 1-alkenes, and 1-alkynes show progressive lengthening of the hydrocarbon chain cut-off, presumably as a result of the increasing aqueous solubility conferred by the double and triple carbon bonds, respectively. There was also tremendous variation in molecular size of compounds exhibiting NMDA receptor cut-off. Alkanes exhibited NMDA receptor cut-off between butane and pentane, respectively 4 and 5 carbons in length, whereas the primary amines exhibited cut-off between 1-octadecanamine and 1-eicosanamine, respectively 18 and 20 carbons in length. As expected, the molecular volume of these compounds associated with NMDA receptor cut-off is also quite different, with the primary amine being over 3 times larger than the alkane.

Discussion

NMDA receptor modulation is associated with an approximate 1.1 mM water solubility cut-off (Figure 3). In contrast, GABA$_A$ receptors potentiated all study compounds; this may be because a GABA$_A$ cut-off occurs at a lower water solubility value. Sequentially increasing hydrocarbon length to find a receptor cut-off effect potentially introduces confounding factors of carbon number and molecular volume that could in turn be responsible for the cut-off effect [35-38]. However, an aggregate comparison of cut-off values for all hydrocarbon groups as a function of carbon number (Figure 4) or molecular

volume (Figure 5) shows no discernible pattern, suggesting that these physical properties are unlikely the primary limiting factors for drug-receptor modulation.

The correlation between molar water solubility and the NMDA receptor cut-off suggests hydrocarbons compete with water for amphipathic binding pockets within anesthetic-sensitive ion channels. Most inhaled anesthetics exhibit low-affinity binding on receptors as evidenced by generally large median effective concentrations for anesthesia—in the 230–290 μM range for isoflurane and halothane [39]—as compared to agents that exert narcotic effects via a singular or primary molecular targets. These specific interactions—exemplified by ketamine antagonism of NMDA receptors [12], etomidate agonism of GABA$_A$ receptors [40], dexmedetomidine agonism of α$_2$-adrenoreceptors [41], and morphine agonism of μ-opioid receptors [42]—typically require only a few μM or less of drug and are consistent with high affinity interactions to resulting in induced fit binding. Instead, volatile anesthetics likely bind to pre-existing pockets and surfaces on or within the protein [43]. Amphipathic pockets likely contain water molecules; when these are displaced by amphipathic drugs, fewer strong hydrophilic interactions and more hydrophobic interactions are possible with amino acid side chains in the cavity. We propose such nonspecific binding causes a change in pocket shape and, in consequence, the larger three-dimensional protein structure that affects channel gating or conductance.

Hydrocarbons act as hydrogen bond donors—or in the case of electrophiles, as hydrogen bond acceptors—with

Table 2 Mean responses (±SEM) produced by 14 different functional groups on NMDA and GABA$_A$ receptor modulation, expressed as a percent of the control agonist peak, using standard two-electrode voltage clamp techniques with 5–6 oocytes each

Compound	NMDA			GABA$_A$		
	% Direct effect	% Agonist effect	Drug response	% Direct effect	% Agonist effect	Drug response
Alcohols						
1-decanol	None	70 ± 3	-	None	386 ± 20	+
1-undecanol	None	101 ± 2	0	None	181 ± 13	+
1-dodecanol	None	98 ± 1	0	None	177 ± 4	+
Alkanes						
butane	None	7 ± 2	-	None	623 ± 68	+
pentane	None	94 ± 3	0	None	321 ± 10	+
hexane	None	100 ± 1	0	None	129 ± 5	+
Aldehydes						
octanal	None	71 ± 3	-	6 ± 3	357 ± 20	+
nonanal	None	104 ± 2	0	None	219 ± 29	+
decanal	None	97 ± 3	0	None	159 ± 5	+
undecanal	None	97 ± 8	0	None	299 ± 29	+
Alkenes						
1-pentene	None	69 ± 1	-	2 ± 3	453 ± 38	+
1-hexene	None	97 ± 0	0	None	132 ± 2	+
Alkynes						
1-hexyne	None	41 ± 6	-	5 ± 2	418 ± 21	+
1-heptyne	None	68 ± 10	-	None	172 ± 8	+
1-octyne	None	96 ± 2	0	None	259 ± 11	+
Amines						
1-octadecanamine	None	73 ± 4	-	None	146 ± 5	+
1-eicosanamine	None	108 ± 1	0	None	166 ± 7	+
Benzenes						
1,3-dimethylbenzene	None	58 ± 3	-	None	366 ± 21	+
1,3-diethylbenzene	None	101 ± 2	0	None	305 ± 24	+
Cycloalkanes						
cyclopentane	None	83 ± 2	-	3 ± 2	196 ± 11	+
cyclohexane	None	101 ± 2	0	None	421 ± 17	+
Ethers						
dibutylether	None	59 ± 4	-	14 ± 13	347 ± 33	+
dipentylether	None	97 ± 2	0	None	211 ± 9	+
dihexylether	None	112 ± 4	0	None	113 ± 1	+
Esters						
ethyl heptanoate	None	78 ± 3	-	None	370 ± 34	+
ethyl octanoate	None	90 ± 1	-	None	285 ± 18	+
ethyl decanoate	None	98 ± 1	0	None	137 ± 2	+
Haloalkanes						
1-fluoropentane	None	76 ± 2	-	None	539 ± 35	+
1-fluorohexane	None	101 ± 1	0	11 ± 4	207 ± 13	+
1-fluoroctane	None	98 ± 1	0	None	182 ± 18	+

Table 2 Mean responses (±SEM) produced by 14 different functional groups on NMDA and GABA$_A$ receptor modulation, expressed as a percent of the control agonist peak, using standard two-electrode voltage clamp techniques with 5–6 oocytes each *(Continued)*

Ketones						
2-decaNone	None	81 ± 1	-	None	476 ± 52	+
2-undecaNone	None	98 ± 2	0	None	230 ± 16	+
2-dodecaNone	None	97 ± 3	0	None	325 ± 30	+
Sulfides						
1-(ethylthio)-hexane	None	87 ± 1	-	None	350 ± 57	+
1-(ethylthio)-octane	None	101 ± 1	0	None	120 ± 3	+
Thiols						
1-pentanethiol	None	85 ± 4	-	22 ± 8	466 ± 57	+
1-hexanethiol	None	102 ± 3	0	8 ± 2	290 ± 41	+

The % Direct Effect is the drug response without co-administration of the receptor agonist. The % Agonist Effect is the drug response with co-administration of agonist (glutamate and glycine for NMDA receptors; γ-aminobutyric acid for GABA$_A$ receptors). The Drug Response denotes inhibition (−) for drug + agonist responses less than the control agonist peak, potentiation (+) for drug + agonist responses greater than the control agonist peak, and no response (0) for drug + agonist responses that differ by <10% from the control agonist peak.

amino acid residues on anesthetic-sensitive receptors, resulting in displacement of water molecules from these binding pockets and alteration of protein function [44-46]. These low energy anesthetic-protein interactions are postulated to be enthalpically favorable since the displaced water molecules should be better able to hydrogen bond with like molecules in the bulk solvent rather than with amino acids [44,46]. Halothane and isoflurane both have been shown to bind in water accessible pockets formed between α-helices in δ-subunits of the nicotinic acetylcholine receptor [47], a member of the 4-transmembrane receptor superfamily that includes the GABA$_A$ receptor. Models of nicotinic acetylcholine receptors and GABA$_A$ receptors further suggest that endogenous agonist or anesthetic binding might increase water accumulation in hydrophilic pockets and increase the number and accessibility of hydrophilic sites that are important for channel gating [48,49]. However, molecules

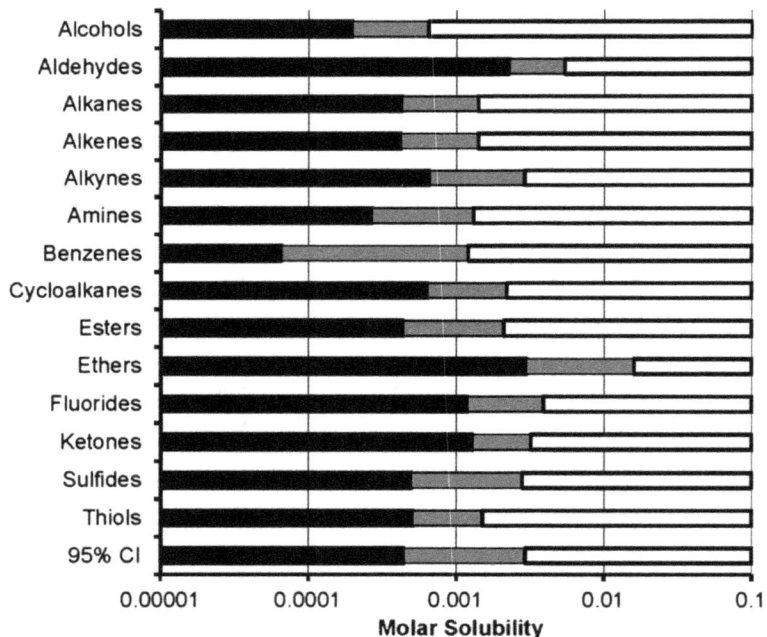

Figure 3 Summary of receptor cut-off effects as a function of molar water solubility for compounds tested in Tables 1 and 2. For each hydrocarbon functional group, white bars represent compounds that modulate both GABA$_A$ and NMDA receptors, and black bars represent compounds that modulate GABA$_A$ receptors but have no effect on NMDA receptors at a saturating concentration. Intervening grey bars represent solubility values for which no data exist.

Hydrocarbon molar water solubility predicts NMDA vs. GABAA receptor modulation

107

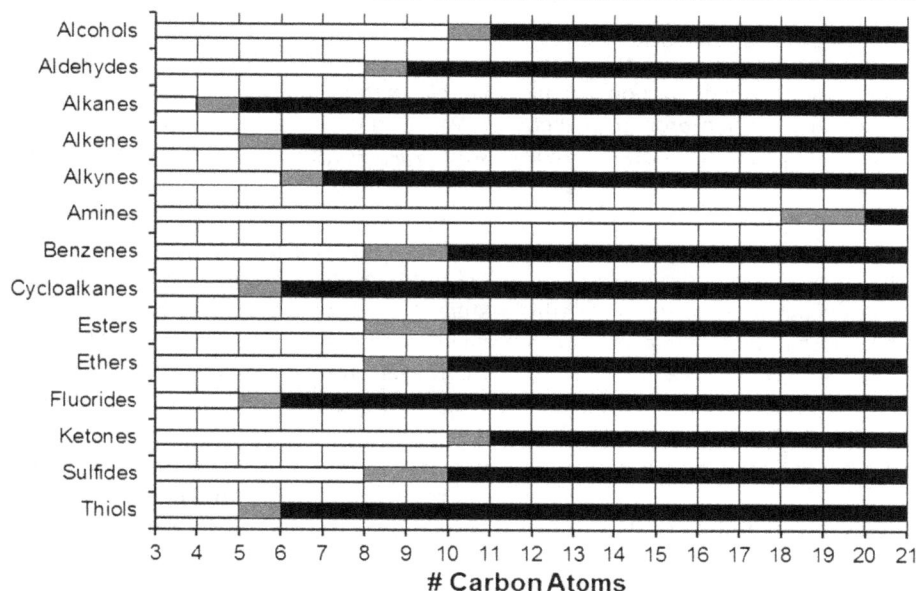

Figure 4 Summary of receptor cut-off effects as a function of the number of drug carbon atoms for compounds tested in Tables 1 and 2. For each hydrocarbon functional group, white bars represent compounds that modulate both GABA$_A$ and NMDA receptors, and black bars represent compounds that modulate GABA$_A$ receptors but have no effect on NMDA receptors at a saturating concentration. Intervening grey bars represent solubility values for which no data exist. No receptor cut-off pattern is evident as a function of the number of drug carbon atoms.

that are insufficiently water soluble may not be able to displace enough water molecules at enough critical sites in order to modulate channel function.

NMDA receptor modulation by inhaled anesthetics such as isoflurane, xenon, and carbon dioxide occurs—

at least in part—at hydrophilic agonist binding sites [33,50]. However, data from the present study show that less hydrophilic drugs—those with lower molar water solubilities—are still able to modulate GABA$_A$ receptor currents even when NMDA receptor efficacy is lost. Since

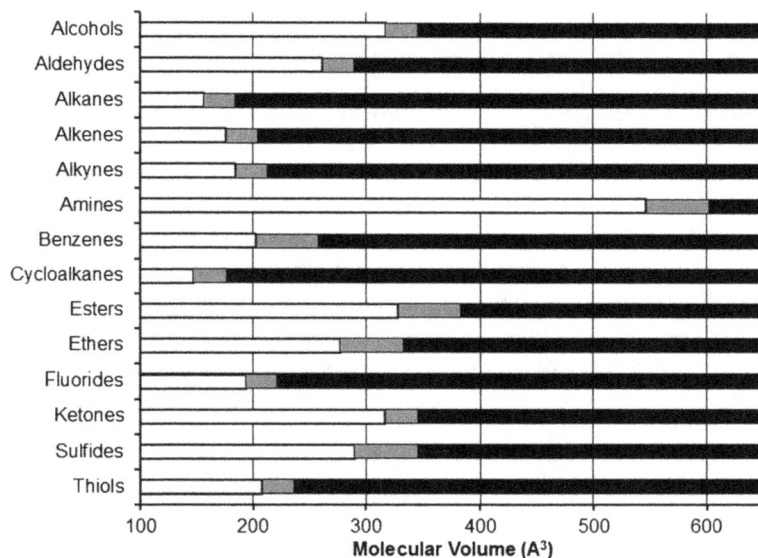

Figure 5 Summary of receptor cut-off effects as a function of the calculated molecular volume of each drug for compounds tested in Tables 1 and 2. For each hydrocarbon functional group, white bars represent compounds that modulate both GABA$_A$ and NMDA receptors, and black bars represent compounds that modulate GABA$_A$ receptors but have no effect on NMDA receptors at a saturating concentration. Intervening grey bars represent solubility values for which no data exist. No receptor cut-off pattern is evident as a function of molecular volume.

these receptors belong to different and phylogenetically distinct superfamilies, it seems likely that either the number of displaced water molecules required to effect modulation, the relative affinities of the hydrocarbon versus water molecule for a critical hydrophilic protein pocket, and/or the number of hydrophilic sites necessary for allosteric modulation should also be different between proteins. Simply stated, there is no reason to suppose that unrelated channels are likely to have conserved affinity constants for water within protein cavities capable of inducing an effect on ion conductance. As evidence, GABA receptors currents, but not those of NMDA receptors, can be modulated by compounds with molar aqueous solubilities much less than 1.1 mM. Presumably, the water dissociation constant in the NMDA receptor binding site is lower than that in the analogous $GABA_A$ receptor binding site.

The locations within NMDA receptor subunits responsible for anesthetic-mediated modulation of protein function remain unresolved. However, it is likely that volatile anesthetics bind at multiple extracellular and transmembrane interfacial sites and cavities, as has been observed with nicotinic acetylcholine receptors [47,51], Gloeobacter ligand-gated ion channels [52], and voltage-gated sodium channels [53]. Whether an anesthetic positively or negatively modulates an ion channel may be a function of competing drug interactions at different sites within the protein [54]. The protein cavities must to some extent be hydrophilic so that they are occupied by water in the native state. However, if these sites are too hydrophilic, then the energy necessary for a low-affinity drug to displace the water molecules becomes too great, requiring either very high drug concentrations that alter cell effects due to changes in serum osmolality or highly polar or charged drugs which, by virtue of these properties, are impermeable to the cell membrane and therefore cannot access critical transmembrane modulatory sites.

Although the present study assessed the association between water solubility and drug efficacy on anesthetic-sensitive ion channels, a relationship between solubility and potency may exist as well. For example, site-directed mutagenesis of the Ala825 residue on the M4 domain of the NR2A subunit, a region at which alcohols bind and can negatively modulate NMDA receptor currents [55,56], affects potency of the slightly water-soluble hypnotic agent tribromoethanol. In fact, the hydrophobicity of the substituted amino acid negatively correlates with tribromoethanol potency as an NMDA receptor inhibitor [57]. Interestingly, except when replaced by the extremely hydrophobic tryptophan residue, which may change binding or access of water itself to the cavity, mutagenesis at this same site had no effect on the infinitely water-soluble anesthetic ethanol. Perhaps the small and highly polar ethanol molecule mimics many of the

intramolecular forces, such as hydrogen bonding, of the water molecules it displaces within the binding site, thus extreme changes within the pocket are required to affect potency.

Water and lipid solubility also affect drug potency for wild-type receptors. Increasing chain length of straight-chain alcohols or diols increases hydrophobicity and is initially associated with increased inhibitory potency of NMDA receptors [58,59]. Similarly, the magnitude of $GABA_A$ receptor positive modulation in the present study tended to increase as hydrocarbon chains lengthened within any functional group. This is consistent with the Meyer-Overton prediction of increased anesthetic potency as a function of increasing hydrophobicity [60,61]. The probability of a hydrocarbon passively entering a lipid cell membrane is parabolically related to hydrocarbon hydrophobicity; more hydrophobic molecules—up to a point—may be able to more easily access transmembrane modulatory sites [62]. However, drug solubility in the lipid membrane should not affect drug concentration in the amphipathic protein pocket, since the net energy involved in moving into and out of the lipid membrane are equal and opposite. The change in state—in this case, drug diffusion in a reversible path from perfusate to lipid membrane to protein pocket—is thermodynamically defined only by the initial state (free energy in perfusate) and final state (free energy of receptor binding), and the change in free energy is independent of the membrane path between these two states [63]. However, increasingly hydrophobic molecules should differ more in their intermolecular interactions with surrounding amino acid side chains compared to the water molecules they displaced. Therefore, if they can successfully access this amphipathic pocket, increasingly hydrophobic molecules may be capable of producing larger conformational changes in the protein and greater modulation of protein function. However, as molecules become even more hydrophobic and water solubility falls below the cutoff value, there are simply insufficient molecules in the aqueous phase to successfully compete with water at hydrophilic modulation or transduction sites on a receptor to alter its function. There is progressive loss of modulatory efficacy at sites with higher cut-offs that reduces the maximum drug-effect magnitude. Finally, when the drug water solubility becomes such that it is insufficient in concentration to out-compete the water in the lowest-cut-off site, the drug effect is reduced to zero.

Likewise, in the whole animal, this plausibly explains why transitional compounds and nonimmobilizers predicted by the Meyer-Overton correlation to produce anesthesia either have lower than expected potency or lack anesthetic efficacy altogether. As with the NMDA cut-off hydrocarbons presented in the present study, transitional compounds and nonimmobilizers all share a common property of low aqueous solubility [64]. Nonimmobilizers such as 1,2-dichlorohexafluorocyclobutane fail to depress GABA$_A$-dependent pyramidal cells [65] or NMDA-dependent CA1 neurons [66] in the hippocampus, and likely lack these effects elsewhere in the central nervous system. With decreasing water solubility, there is differential loss of receptor effects—such as occurred with NMDA receptors versus GABA$_A$ receptors in the present study. The anesthetic cut-off effect in whole animal models correlates with agent water solubility, and might be explained by the loss of one or more anesthetic-receptor contributions to central nervous system depression. Conversely, receptor molar water solubility cut-off values may be used to define those ion channels that are not essential for volatile anesthetic potency. Inhaled agents likely act via low affinity interactions with multiple cell receptors and ion channels to decrease neuronal excitability in the brain and spinal cord, but a loss or inadequate contribution from certain targets—perhaps GABA$_A$ or glycine receptors—as water solubility decreases may render a drug a nonimmobilizer. Additionally, agents having a water solubility below the cut-off value for some anesthetic-sensitive receptors may also produce undesirable pharmacologic properties, such as seizures following the loss of GABA$_A$ receptor modulation [67]. In contrast, NMDA receptors can contribute to immobilizing actions of conventional volatile anesthetics [3], but they are not as a general principle essential for inhaled anesthetic action since an agent like pentane does not modulate NMDA receptors—even at a saturated aqueous concentration (Table 2)—yet has a measurable minimum alveolar concentration [68,69].

As shown in Figure 3, the different hydrocarbon series exhibit small variability about the 1.1 mM cut-off. Some variability is due simply to the lack of compounds of intermediate solubility within a functional group series. For example, pentanethiol inhibited NMDA receptors, whereas the 1-carbon longer hexanethiol did not (Table 2). This pre-cut-off thiol is nearly 3-times more soluble in water than its post-cut-off cognate; yet it is not possible to obtain a more narrowly defined cut-off delineation for 1-thiols. Even larger variability was observed with the dialkylbenzene series, to which 1 additional carbon was added to each 1- and 3-alkyl group. The solubility ratio between the NMDA antagonist 1,3-dimethylbenzene and its cut-off cognate 1,3-diethylbenzene is more than 18 (Table 2).

Variability about the molar water solubility NMDA receptor cut-off may also have arisen from the use of calculated, rather than measured, values for hydrocarbon molar water solubility. Aqueous solubility is difficult to measure accurately, particularly for poorly soluble substances. Calculated solubilities are more accurate for small uncharged compounds, but still can have an absolute error within 1 log unit [70]. However, even predicted

values for nonpolar n-alkanes may show large deviations from experimental data as the hydrocarbon chain length increases [71].

Furthermore, the molar solubility values used in the present study were calculated for pure water at 25°C and at pH = 7.0. These were not the conditions under which drug-receptor effects were studied. Ringer's oocyte perfusates contained buffers and physiologic concentrations of sodium, potassium, and chloride resulting in a 250 mOsm solution. The solubility of haloether and haloalkane anesthetic vapors vary inversely with osmolarity [72], as do the water-to-saline solubility ratio of benzenes, amines, and ketones [73]. The presence of salts could have caused overestimation of aqueous solubility for some compounds when using values calculated for pure water. Likewise, solubility is also temperature-dependent. Studies were conducted at 22°C; solubility of gases in water should be greater than values calculated at 25°C. In contrast, most solutes used in the present study have negative enthalpy for dissolution [74], so solubility should be decreased at the lower ambient temperature. The reverse should occur for exothermic solutions, as predicted by the Le Chatelier principle. As for hydronium ion concentration, the solubility of most study compounds is trivially affected at pH values between 7-to-8. However, hydrocarbons containing an amine group have pK$_a$ values that are closer to physiologic pH, and the calculated aqueous solubility of 1-eicosanamine and 1-octadecanamine (Table 1) decreases by about 66% as pH increases from 7 to 8. Calculated molar water solubilities for the amines in this study were probably modestly overestimated at a physiologic pH equal to 7.4.

Only water solubility reliably predicted the NMDA receptor cut-off. Yet, molecular size and shape still likely influence this effect to some lesser degree. Most of the hydrocarbons examined in the present study had functional groups located on the 1- or 2-carbon position. However, the ethers were all 1,1'-oxybisalkanes; each member of the ether consisted of symmetrical 1-carbon additions to alkyl groups on either side of the oxygen atom (Table 1). Consequently, this electron-rich oxygen atom allowing hydrogen bonding with water molecules or amino acid residues with strong partial positive charges lies buried in the middle of the ether. For hydrocarbons with equivalent molar water solubilities, it may be more difficult for dialkyl ether to form hydrogen bonds in hydrophilic receptor pockets compared to a long primary amine (Table 1) that might more easily insert its nucleophilic terminus into the anesthetic-binding pocket while the long hydrophobic carbon chain remains in the lipid membrane. This may explain why ethers in this study appear to exhibit an NMDA cut-off that is slightly greater than hydrocarbons with other functional groups. Perhaps if a methyl-alkyl ether series were used instead of a dialkyl ether series, the apparent molar water solubility cut-off for this group would have been lower. Nonetheless, the cut-off variability is sufficiently small to allow *a priori* predictions of low-affinity hydrocarbon modulation of NMDA receptors. It remains to be shown whether other anesthetic-sensitive ion channels exhibit distinct cut-off effects that may also be predicted by a single physical property: molar water solubility.

Conclusion

Cut-off responses for NMDA receptor inhibition by diverse hydrocarbons occurs when drug molar water solubility is less than approximately 1.1 mM. However, hydrocarbons having lower molar water solubilities are still able to potentiate GABA$_A$ receptors. This finding supports a hypothesis that volatile compounds, such as inhaled anesthetics, access one or more amphipathic "pockets" within a protein, such as the NMDA receptor, to displace resident water molecules and induce a conformational change. Volatile anesthetics and other compounds with insufficient molar water solubility can never achieve sufficient concentration at the amphipathic pocket site to displace water and modulate protein function—even when such compounds are administered at a saturated aqueous phase concentration.

Competing interests
The authors declare that they have no competing interests.

Authors' contributions
RB: Developed hypothesis, designed experiments, assisted with experiments, analyzed data, and wrote the manuscript. TP: Conducted experiments and reviewed the manuscript. Both authors read and approved the final manuscript.

Acknowledgements
This entirety of this work was funded by the National Institutes of Health National Institutes of General Medical Sciences (Grant GM092821-02).

References
1. Brosnan RJ: Inhaled anesthetics in horses. *Vet Clin North Am Equine Pract* 2013, **29**(1):69–87.
2. Chau PL: New insights into the molecular mechanisms of general anaesthetics. *Br J Pharmacol* 2010, **161**(2):288–307.
3. Stabernack C, Sonner JM, Laster MJ, Zhang Y, Xing Y, Sharma M, Eger EI 2nd: Spinal N-methyl-d-aspartate receptors may contribute to the immobilizing action of isoflurane. *Anesth Analg* 2003, **96**(1):102–107.
4. Rau V, Oh I, Liao M, Bodarky C, Fanselow MS, Homanics GE, Sonner JM, Eger EI 2nd: Gamma-aminobutyric acid type A receptor beta3 subunit forebrain-specific knockout mice are resistant to the amnestic effect of isoflurane. *Anesth Analg* 2011, **113**(3):500–504.
5. Rau V, Iyer SV, Oh I, Chandra D, Harrison N, Eger EI 2nd, Fanselow MS, Homanics GE, Sonner JM: Gamma-aminobutyric acid type A receptor alpha 4 subunit knockout mice are resistant to the amnestic effect of isoflurane. *Anesth Analg* 2009, **109**(6):1816–1822.
6. Dutton RC, Laster MJ, Xing Y, Sonner JM, Raines DE, Solt K, Eger EI 2nd: Do N-methyl-D-aspartate receptors mediate the capacity of inhaled anesthetics to suppress the temporal summation that contributes to minimum alveolar concentration? *Anesth Analg* 2006, **102**(5):1412–1418.
7. Mayer ML: Glutamate receptors at atomic resolution. *Nature* 2006, **440**(7083):456–462.
8. Ernst M, Bruckner S, Boresch S, Sieghart W: Comparative models of GABAA receptor extracellular and transmembrane domains: important insights in pharmacology and function. *Mol Pharmacol* 2005, **68**(5):1291–1300.
9. Nistri A, Berti C: Potentiating action of midazolam on GABA-mediated responses and its antagonism by Ro 14–7437 in the frog spinal cord. *Neurosci Lett* 1983, **39**(2):199–204.
10. Macdonald R, Barker JL: Benzodiazepines specifically modulate GABA-mediated postsynaptic inhibition in cultured mammalian neurones. *Nature* 1978, **271**(5645):563–564.
11. Dildy-Mayfield JE, Mihic SJ, Liu Y, Deitrich RA, Harris RA: Actions of long chain alcohols on GABAA and glutamate receptors: relation to in vivo effects. *Br J Pharmacol* 1996, **118**(2):378–384.
12. Flood P, Krasowski MD: Intravenous anesthetics differentially modulate ligand-gated ion channels. *Anesthesiology* 2000, **92**(5):1418–1425.
13. Kendig JJ, Kodde A, Gibbs LM, Ionescu P, Eger EI 2nd: Correlates of anesthetic properties in isolated spinal cord: cyclobutanes. *Eur J Pharmacol* 1994, **264**(3):427–436.
14. Jenkins A, Franks NP, Lieb WR: Effects of temperature and volatile anesthetics on GABA(A) receptors. *Anesthesiology* 1999, **90**(2):484–491.
15. Krasowski MD, Harrison NL: The actions of ether, alcohol and alkane general anaesthetics on GABAA and glycine receptors and the effects of TM2 and TM3 mutations. *Br J Pharmacol* 2000, **129**(4):731–743.
16. Hollmann MW, Liu HT, Hoenemann CW, Liu WH, Durieux ME: Modulation of NMDA receptor function by ketamine and magnesium. Part II: interactions with volatile anesthetics. *Anesth Analg* 2001, **92**(5):1182–1191.
17. Nishikawa K, Harrison NL: The actions of sevoflurane and desflurane on the gamma-aminobutyric acid receptor type A: effects of TM2 mutations in the alpha and beta subunits. *Anesthesiology* 2003, **99**(3):678–684.
18. Yamakura T, Sakimura K, Shimoji K, Mishina M: Effects of propofol on various AMPA-, kainate- and NMDA-selective glutamate receptor channels expressed in Xenopus oocytes. *Neurosci Lett* 1995, **188**(3):187–190.
19. Hales TG, Lambert JJ: The actions of propofol on inhibitory amino acid receptors of bovine adrenomedullary chromaffin cells and rodent central neurones. *Br J Pharmacol* 1991, **104**(3):619–628.
20. Yamakura T, Chavez-Noriega LE, Harris RA: Subunit-dependent inhibition of human neuronal nicotinic acetylcholine receptors and other ligand-gated ion channels by dissociative anesthetics ketamine and dizocilpine. *Anesthesiology* 2000, **92**(4):1144–1153.
21. Yamakura T, Harris RA: Effects of gaseous anesthetics nitrous oxide and xenon on ligand-gated ion channels. Comparison with isoflurane and ethanol. *Anesthesiology* 2000, **93**(4):1095–1101.
22. Ogata J, Shiraishi M, Namba T, Smothers CT, Woodward JJ, Harris RA: Effects of anesthetics on mutant N-methyl-D-aspartate receptors expressed in Xenopus oocytes. *J Pharmacol Exp Ther* 2006, **318**(1):434–443.
23. Martin DC, Plagenhoef M, Abraham J, Dennison RL, Aronstam RS: Volatile anesthetics and glutamate activation of N-methyl-D-aspartate receptors. *Biochem Pharmacol* 1995, **49**(6):809–817.
24. Wong EH, Kemp JA, Priestley T, Knight AR, Woodruff GN, Iversen LL: The anticonvulsant MK-801 is a potent N-methyl-D-aspartate antagonist. *Proc Natl Acad Sci U S A* 1986, **83**(18):7104–7108.
25. Hara K, Eger EI 2nd, Laster MJ, Harris RA: Nonhalogenated alkanes cyclopropane and butane affect neurotransmitter-gated ion channel and G-protein-coupled receptors: differential actions on GABAA and glycine receptors. *Anesthesiology* 2002, **97**(6):1512–1520.
26. Krasowski MD, Jenkins A, Flood P, Kung AY, Hopfinger AJ, Harrison NL: General anesthetic potencies of a series of propofol analogs correlate with potency for potentiation of gamma-aminobutyric acid (GABA) current at the GABA(A) receptor but not with lipid solubility. *J Pharmacol Exp Ther* 2001, **297**(1):338–351.
27. Vemparala S, Saiz L, Eckenhoff RG, Klein ML: Partitioning of anesthetics into a lipid bilayer and their interaction with membrane-bound peptide bundles. *Biophys J* 2006, **91**(8):2815–2825.
28. Stimson LM, Vattulainen I, Rog T, Karttunen M: Exploring the effect of xenon on biomembranes. *Cell Mol Biol Lett* 2005, **10**(4):563–569.
29. Pohorille A, Wilson MA, New MH, Chipot C: Concentrations of anesthetics across the water-membrane interface; the Meyer-Overton hypothesis revisited. *Toxicol Lett* 1998, **100**–101:421–430.
30. Brosnan R, Gong D, Cotten J, Keshavaprasad B, Yost CS, Eger EI 2nd, Sonner JM: Chirality in anesthesia II: stereoselective modulation of ion

Hydrocarbon molar water solubility predicts NMDA vs. GABAA receptor modulation

111

channel function by secondary alcohol enantiomers. *Anesth Analg* 2006, 103(1):86–91.

31. Yang L, Milutinovic PS, Brosnan RJ, Eger EI 2nd, Sonner JM: The plasticizer di(2-ethylhexyl) phthalate modulates gamma-aminobutyric acid type A and glycine receptor function. *Anesth Analg* 2007, 105(2):393–396.

32. Yang L, Zhao J, Milutinovic PS, Brosnan RJ, Eger EI 2nd, Sonner JM: Anesthetic properties of the ketone bodies beta-hydroxybutyric acid and acetone. *Anesth Analg* 2007, 105(3):673–679.

33. Brosnan RJ, Pham TL: Does anesthetic additivity imply a similar molecular mechanism of anesthetic action at N-methyl-D-aspartate receptors? *Anesth Analg* 2011, 112(3):568–573.

34. Brosnan RJ, Pham TL: Carbon dioxide negatively modulates N-methyl-D-aspartate receptors. *Br J Anaesth* 2008, 101(5):673–679.

35. Eger EI 2nd, Halsey MJ, Harris RA, Koblin DD, Pohorille A, Sewell JC, Sonner JM, Trudell JR: Hypothesis: volatile anesthetics produce immobility by acting on two sites approximately five carbon atoms apart. *Anesth Analg* 1999, 88(6):1395–1400.

36. Jenkins A, Greenblatt EP, Faulkner HJ, Bertaccini E, Light A, Lin A, Andreasen A, Viner A, Trudell JR, Harrison NL: Evidence for a common binding cavity for three general anesthetics within the GABAA receptor. *J Neurosci* 2001, 21(6):RC136.

37. Wick MJ, Mihic SJ, Ueno S, Mascia MP, Trudell JR, Brozowski SJ, Ye Q, Harrison NL, Harris RA: Mutations of gamma-aminobutyric acid and glycine receptors change alcohol cutoff: evidence for an alcohol receptor? *Proc Natl Acad Sci U S A* 1998, 95(11):6504–6509.

38. Eger EI 2nd, Laster MJ: The effect of rigidity, shape, unsaturation, and length on the anesthetic potency of hydrocarbons. *Anesth Analg* 2001, 92(6):1477–1482.

39. Franks NP, Lieb WR: Selective actions of volatile general anaesthetics at molecular and cellular levels. *Br J Anaesth* 1993, 71(1):65–76.

40. Tomlin SL, Jenkins A, Lieb WR, Franks NP: Stereoselective effects of etomidate optical isomers on gamma-aminobutyric acid type A receptors and animals. *Anesthesiology* 1998, 88(3):708–717.

41. Tonner PH, Scholz J, Koch C, Schulte am Esch J: The anesthetic effect of dexmedetomidine does not adhere to the Meyer-Overton rule but is reversed by hydrostatic pressure. *Anesth Analg* 1997, 84(3):618–622.

42. Pert CB, Snyder SH: Properties of opiate-receptor binding in rat brain. *Proc Natl Acad Sci U S A* 1973, 70(8):2243–2247.

43. Trudell JR, Bertaccini E: Molecular modelling of specific and non-specific anaesthetic interactions. *Br J Anaesth* 2002, 89(1):32–40.

44. Bertaccini EJ, Trudell JR, Franks NP: The common chemical motifs within anesthetic binding sites. *Anesth Analg* 2007, 104(2):318–324.

45. Abraham MH, Lieb WR, Franks NP: Role of hydrogen bonding in general anesthesia. *J Pharm Sci* 1991, 80(8):719–724.

46. Streiff JH, Jones KA: Volatile anesthetic binding to proteins is influenced by solvent and aliphatic residues. *J Chem Inf Model* 2008, 48(10):2066–2073.

47. Chiara DC, Dangott LJ, Eckenhoff RG, Cohen JB: Identification of nicotinic acetylcholine receptor amino acids photolabeled by the volatile anesthetic halothane. *Biochemistry* 2003, 42(46):13457–13467.

48. Williams DB, Akabas MH: Gamma-aminobutyric acid increases the water accessibility of M3 membrane-spanning segment residues in gamma-aminobutyric acid type A receptors. *Biophys J* 1999, 77(5):2563–2574.

49. Willenbring D, Xu Y, Tang P: The role of structured water in mediating general anesthetic action on alpha4beta2 nAChR. *Phys Chem Chem Phys* 2010, 12(35):10263–10269.

50. Dickinson R, Peterson BK, Banks P, Simillis C, Martin JC, Valenzuela CA, Maze M, Franks NP: Competitive inhibition at the glycine site of the N-methyl-D-aspartate receptor by the anesthetics xenon and isoflurane: evidence from molecular modeling and electrophysiology. *Anesthesiology* 2007, 107(5):756–767.

51. Brannigan G, LeBard DN, Henin J, Eckenhoff RG, Klein ML: Multiple binding sites for the general anesthetic isoflurane identified in the nicotinic acetylcholine receptor transmembrane domain. *Proc Natl Acad Sci U S A* 2010, 107(32):14122–14127.

52. Chen Q, Cheng MH, Xu Y, Tang P: Anesthetic binding in a pentameric ligand-gated ion channel: GLIC. *Biophys J* 2010, 99(6):1801–1809.

53. Raju SG, Barber AF, LeBard DN, Klein ML, Carnevale V: Exploring volatile general anesthetic binding to a closed membrane-bound bacterial voltage-gated sodium channel via computation. *PLoS Comput Biol* 2013, 9(6):e1003090.

54. Bromstrup T, Howard RJ, Trudell JR, Harris RA, Lindahl E: Inhibition versus potentiation of ligand-gated ion channels can be altered by a single mutation that moves ligands between intra- and intersubunit sites. *Structure* 2013, 21(8):1307–1316.

55. Xu M, Smothers CT, Trudell J, Woodward JJ: Ethanol inhibition of constitutively open N-methyl-D-aspartate receptors. *J Pharmacol Exp Ther* 2012, 340(1):218–226.

56. Ren H, Zhao Y, Dwyer DS, Peoples RW: Interactions among positions in the third and fourth membrane-associated domains at the intersubunit interface of the N-methyl-D-aspartate receptor forming sites of alcohol action. *J Biol Chem* 2012, 287(33):27302–27312.

57. Salous AK, Ren H, Lamb KA, Hu XQ, Lipsky RH, Peoples RW: Differential actions of ethanol and trichloroethanol at sites in the M3 and M4 domains of the NMDA receptor GluN2A (NR2A) subunit. *Br J Pharmacol* 2009, 158(5):1395–1404.

58. Peoples RW, Ren H: Inhibition of N-methyl-D-aspartate receptors by straight-chain diols: implications for the mechanism of the alcohol cutoff effect. *Mol Pharmacol* 2002, 61(1):169–176.

59. Peoples RW, Weight FF: Cutoff in potency implicates alcohol inhibition of N-methyl-D-aspartate receptors in alcohol intoxication. *Proc Natl Acad Sci U S A* 1995, 92(7):2825–2829.

60. Mihic SJ, McQuilkin SJ, Eger EI 2nd, Ionescu P, Harris RA: Potentiation of gamma-aminobutyric acid type A receptor-mediated chloride currents by novel halogenated compounds correlates with their abilities to induce general anesthesia. *Mol Pharmacol* 1994, 46(5):851–857.

61. Horishita T, Eger EI 2nd, Harris RA: The effects of volatile aromatic anesthetics on voltage-gated Na + channels expressed in Xenopus oocytes. *Anesth Analg* 2008, 107(5):1579–1586.

62. Hansch C, Fujita T: p-σ-π Analysis. A Method for the Correlation of Biological Activity and Chemical Structure. *J Am Chem Soc* 1964, 86(8):1616–1626.

63. Fermi E: *Thermodynamics*. New York, NY: Prentice-Hall; 1937.

64. Eger EI 2nd: Mechanisms of Inhaled Anesthetic Action. In *The Pharmacology of Inhaled Anesthetics. Volume 1*. Edited by Eger EI 2nd. IL, USA: Baxter Healthcare Corporation; 2002:33–42.

65. Perouansky M, Banks MI, Pearce RA: The differential effects of the nonimmobilizer 1,2-dichlorohexafluorocyclobutane (F6, 2 N) and isoflurane on extrasynaptic gamma-aminobutyric acid A receptors. *Anesth Analg* 2005, 100(6):1667–1673.

66. Taylor DM, Eger EI 2nd, Bickler PE: Halothane, but not the nonimmobilizers perfluoropentane and 1,2-dichlorohexafluorocyclobutane, depresses synaptic transmission in hippocampal CA1 neurons in rats. *Anesth Analg* 1999, 89(4):1040–1045.

67. Raines DE: Anesthetic and nonanesthetic halogenated volatile compounds have dissimilar activities on nicotinic acetylcholine receptor desensitization kinetics. *Anesthesiology* 1996, 84(3):663–671.

68. Liu J, Laster MJ, Taheri S, Eger EI 2nd, Koblin DD, Halsey MJ: Is there a cutoff in anesthetic potency for the normal alkanes? *Anesth Analg* 1993, 77(1):12–18.

69. Taheri S, Laster MJ, Liu J, Eger EI 2nd, Halsey MJ, Koblin DD: Anesthesia by n-alkanes not consistent with the Meyer-Overton hypothesis: determinations of the solubilities of alkanes in saline and various lipids. *Anesth Analg* 1993, 77(1):7–11.

70. Delaney JS: Predicting aqueous solubility from structure. *Drug Discov Today* 2005, 10(4):289–295.

71. Ferguson AL, Debenedetti PG, Panagiotopoulos AZ: Solubility and molecular conformations of n-alkane chains in water. *J Phys Chem* 2009, 113(18):6405–6414.

72. Lerman J, Willis MM, Gregory GA, Eger EI 2nd: Osmolarity determines the solubility of anesthetics in aqueous solutions at 37 degrees C. *Anesthesiology* 1983, 59(6):554–558.

73. Long FA, McDevit WF: Activity coefficients of nonelectrolyte solutes in aqueous salt solutions. *Chem Rev* 1952, 51(1):119–169.

74. Abraham MH: Free energies, enthalpies, and entropies of solution of gaseous nonpolar nonelectrolytes in water and nonaqueous solvents The hydrophobic effect. *J Am Chem Soc* 1982, 104(8):2085–2094.

14

The effectiveness and cost-effectiveness of treatments for idiopathic pulmonary fibrosis: systematic review, network meta-analysis and health economic evaluation

Emma Loveman[1]*, Vicky R Copley[1], Jill L Colquitt[1], David A Scott[2], Andy J Clegg[1], Jeremy Jones[1], Katherine MA O'Reilly[3], Sally Singh[4], Claudia Bausewein[5] and Athol Wells[6]

Abstract

Background: Idiopathic pulmonary fibrosis (IPF) is a life-limiting lung disease with considerable impact on patients and carers as the disease progresses. Currently few treatments are available. We aimed to evaluate the clinical and cost-effectiveness of available treatments for IPF.

Methods: Systematic reviews of clinical effectiveness, quality of life and cost effectiveness were undertaken. Eleven bibliographic databases were searched from inception to July 2013 and studies were assessed for eligibility against a set of pre-defined criteria. Two reviewers screened references, extracted data from included studies and appraised their quality. An advisory group was consulted about the choice of interventions. A narrative review was undertaken and where feasible fixed effect and random effects meta-analysis were undertaken including a network meta-analysis (NMA).

A decision-analytic Markov model was developed to estimate cost-effectiveness of pharmacological treatments for IPF. Following best practice recommendations, the model perspective was of the national health service and personal social services, a discount rate of 3.5% for costs and health benefits was applied and outcomes were expressed as cost per quality adjusted life-year gained. Parameter values were obtained from the NMA and systematic reviews. Sensitivity analyses were undertaken.

Results: Fourteen studies were included in the review of clinical effectiveness, of which one evaluated azathioprine, three N-acetylcysteine [NAC] (alone or in combination), four pirfenidone, one nintedanib, one sildenafil, one thalidomide, two pulmonary rehabilitation, and one a disease management programme. Study quality was generally good. Evidence suggests that some effective treatments are available. In NMA only nintedanib and pirfenidone show statistically significant improvements. The model results show increased survival for five pharmacological treatments (NAC triple therapy, inhaled NAC, nintedanib, pirfenidone, and sildenafil) compared with best supportive care, at increased cost. Only inhaled NAC was cost-effective at current willingness to pay thresholds but it may not be clinically effective.

Conclusions: Few interventions have any statistically significant effect and the cost-effectiveness of treatments is uncertain. A lack of studies on palliative care approaches was identified and there is a need for further research into pulmonary rehabilitation and thalidomide in particular. A well conducted RCT on inhaled NAC therapy should also be considered.

Keywords: Idiopathic pulmonary fibrosis, Systematic review, Meta-analysis, Cost-effectiveness

* Correspondence: emma.loveman@soton.ac.uk
[1]Southampton Health Technology Assessments Centre (SHTAC), University of Southampton, Southampton, UK
Full list of author information is available at the end of the article

Background

Idiopathic pulmonary fibrosis (IPF) is a debilitating respiratory condition for which there is no cure. IPF is characterised by aberrant wound healing in which excessive (and perhaps abnormal) extracellular matrix is deposited in the lung thereby distorting the architecture and disrupting function. This lung injury and scarring eventually leads to a decline in lung function which culminates in respiratory failure [1]. Shortness of breath on exercise and a chronic dry cough are the prominent symptoms [2]. IPF is known to affect males more than females and in particular affects people over 60 years of age. The prevalence of IPF is increasing, although the cause of this increase is uncertain, [3,4] and with a poor prognosis (estimated mean survival of between 2–5 years) IPF has become an area of focus with recent UK national guidelines on the diagnosis and management of IPF published, [5] and international consensus guidelines [6] due to be updated in 2014.

IPF is a difficult condition to manage, particularly in the latter stages. Early and accurate diagnosis is important to maximise the potential for a better outcome but there is an unmet need with few recommended treatments [5]. In the UK all patients should be given best supportive care (BSC) from the point of diagnosis, which includes information and support, symptom relief, management of co-morbidities, withdrawal of ineffective therapies and end-of-life care. In addition individuals should be assessed for pulmonary rehabilitation if appropriate and have a clinical nurse specialist available to them [5]. For those without contraindications lung transplantation should be considered as this is the only treatment shown to improve survival [7]. However, with donor organs being in short supply there is a need for alternative treatments that aim to modify the disease and prolong survival. Few treatments are available to the clinician and patient currently, and the evidence for the effectiveness of such treatments is unclear. We aimed to evaluate the current state of the clinical and cost-effectiveness of treatments for people with IPF through three systematic reviews, a network meta-analysis (NMA) and economic modelling.

Methods

The *a priori* methods for this evidence synthesis are described in the research protocol which is registered with PROSPERO (reference: 42012002116). Search strategies were developed and applied to 11 electronic bibliographic databases (including the Cochrane library, MEDLINE and EMBASE) from inception to July 2013 with no language restrictions. Bibliographies of retrieved papers were screened and experts contacted to identify additional studies. Systematic reviews were undertaken of clinical effectiveness (including only randomised controlled trials [RCTs] and controlled clinical trials [CCTs]), economic evaluations and health related quality of life (HRQoL) studies. Eligible participants were those with a diagnosis of IPF and includable interventions were as deemed relevant by a clinical and patient advisory group. Best supportive care, placebo or any of the interventions were eligible as comparators and outcomes of relevance included measures of survival, measures of symptoms (breathlessness, cough), HRQoL, lung function, exercise performance, adverse events and measures of costs and cost-effectiveness. Studies reporting HRQoL in people with IPF were eligible for inclusion if they used either generic preference-based measures or the St Georges Respiratory Questionnaire (SGRQ) which is a disease specific instrument used in IPF. Other disease specific instruments were not eligible for inclusion as there are currently no methods to map results of these to utility measures required for economic evaluation.

Titles and abstracts were screened for potential eligibility by two reviewers using a pre-defined inclusion criteria, retrieved articles were assessed for eligibility, data were extracted and methodological quality assessed by one reviewer and checked by a second. Study quality was assessed using recognised methods [8-10]. For the review of clinical effectiveness we developed a check-list to assess the methodological quality of the studies based on the criteria recommended by the Centre for Reviews and Dissemination, [8] (Quality assessment/risk of bias section) and summarised the risk of bias (as per Cochrane collaboration recommendations [11]) within each study according to the risk of selection bias. We developed a check-list to assess the methodological quality of the cost effectiveness studies based on the check-list of Drummond and colleagues [9] and recommendations by Phillips and colleagues [10]. Data items extracted included study details (design, follow-up, funding), participant details (numbers, eligibility, characteristics), intervention details (including dose and duration of treatment), outcomes reported and results. Narrative syntheses were undertaken and in the review of clinical effectiveness meta-analysis was performed where appropriate with heterogeneity assessed. FVC was measured on two continuous scales and these were meta-analysed using the standardised mean difference (SMD). A NMA focusing on pharmacological treatments for IPF and assessing forced vital capacity (FVC) endpoints was undertaken [12].The NMA focused on FVC as it is correlated with disease progression [6] and was therefore relevant to the economic model. For FVC endpoints the NMA used the SMD in a Bayesian framework using code adapted from published sources [13]. Vague normal priors were used for the treatment effects and a vague uniform prior for the random effect standard deviation. Model code is provided in the Additional file 1. Fixed and random effects models were applied with best model fit determined using the deviance information criterion (DIC). The SMDs output from the NMA were then converted to log odds ratios using standard methods for ease of interpretation within the context of an NMA [14].

Quality assessment/risk of bias

1. Was the method used to generate random allocations adequate?
2. Was the allocation adequately concealed?
3. Were the groups similar at the outset of the study in terms of prognostic factors
4. Was the care provider blinded?
5. Was the patient blinded?
6. Were outcome assessors blinded to the treatment allocation?
7. i) Were there any unexpected imbalances in drop-outs between groups? ii) If so, were they explained or adjusted for?
8. Is there any evidence to suggest that the authors measured more outcomes than they reported?
9. i) Did the analysis include an intention to treat analysis? ii) If so, was this defined?
10. i) Did the analysis account for missing data? ii) If so, were the methods appropriate?

A decision-analytic model was developed to compare the cost-effectiveness of pharmacological interventions in patients with initially unprogressed IPF. The model perspective is that of the UK National Health Service and Personal Social Services. The model structure was informed by the available literature and expert opinion on the clinical progression of the disease. It uses four distinct health states: unprogressed IPF; progressed IPF; lung-transplant; and dead. Health states except death are associated with a HRQoL utility and a cost estimate. Progression is defined by an absolute decline in FVC per cent predicted of ≥10% from a baseline (recently-diagnosed) value, based on the included RCTs. Published sources were used to inform the probability of a lung transplant; survival after lung transplant; and all-cause mortality by age. Acute exacerbations are not modelled as separate health states but are associated with a cost and utility decrement. Model cycle length is one month and a lifetime horizon of 30 years was adopted to capture all clinically and economically important events. A half-cycle correction is applied. Key assumptions are that all patients are in in the unprogressed state initially; those experiencing a ≥10% absolute decline in FVC% predicted are considered to be in the progressed health state; and treatment has a constant effect on relative rate of FVC% decline, FVC% predicted was used as a proxy for disease severity when assigning utilities to the health states. In addition, where treatment costs for any individual treatment were not available an assumed cost was used and tested in threshold analysis.

Treatment effects were obtained from the NMA. Utility values from the systematic review of HRQoL are applied to the modelled health states to estimate the benefits measured as quality adjusted life years (QALYs). Costs are included for treatments, treatment monitoring, acute exacerbations, lung transplant and adverse events, based on the UK health system. Future costs and benefits are discounted at 3.5% per annum. The outcome is reported as cost per QALY gained against the next best alternative treatment using incremental cost effectiveness ratios (ICERs). The model examines uncertainty in deterministic and probabilistic sensitivity analyses. Model validation was undertaken by checking structure, calculations and data inputs. In addition the advisory group reviewed the structure and internal consistency was examined by varying input values. Model results were compared with trial outputs and other publications [15-17].

Results
Clinical effectiveness
Searches identified 905 unique references and 64 of these were retrieved after screening of titles and abstracts. Fourteen studies (13 RCTs and 1 CCT) were included (Figure 1). Four RCTs evaluated the use of pirfenidone, [15,18,19] three the use of n-acetylcysteine (alone or in combination), [20-22] one azathioprine, [23] one nintedanib, [16] one sildenafil, [24] one thalidomide, [25] one a pulmonary rehabilitation programme, [26] and one a disease management programme [27]. In addition one CCT of pulmonary rehabilitation was included [28]. This study was published in Polish and translation of key methods and results only were undertaken due to resource and time constraints. Therefore caution is recommended in interpreting our assessment of this study. No studies of palliative care interventions were identified that met the inclusion criteria. Study quality was generally good with a low risk of bias. Ten studies were undertaken in populations that would likely be classed as mild to moderate IPF [29]. The majority of these studies had reasonable sample sizes and duration of follow was between nine months and 16 months. Four studies were undertaken in populations that would be classed as moderate to severe IPF. Three of these were the non-pharmacological intervention studies, and one the drug sildenafil. Sample sizes were generally smaller in the non-pharmacological studies, and there was no long-term follow up. Across all studies the mean ages of participants ranged from approximately 54–69 years, the gender ratio of males to females was generally 3:1, and the duration of diagnosis tended to be between 1 and 3 years. In the ten studies in mild-to-moderate IPF the baseline FVC ranged between 65-90% and in the four studies in moderate-to-severe IPF this ranged from 55-70%. The populations were deemed to be reasonably similar to those seen in clinical

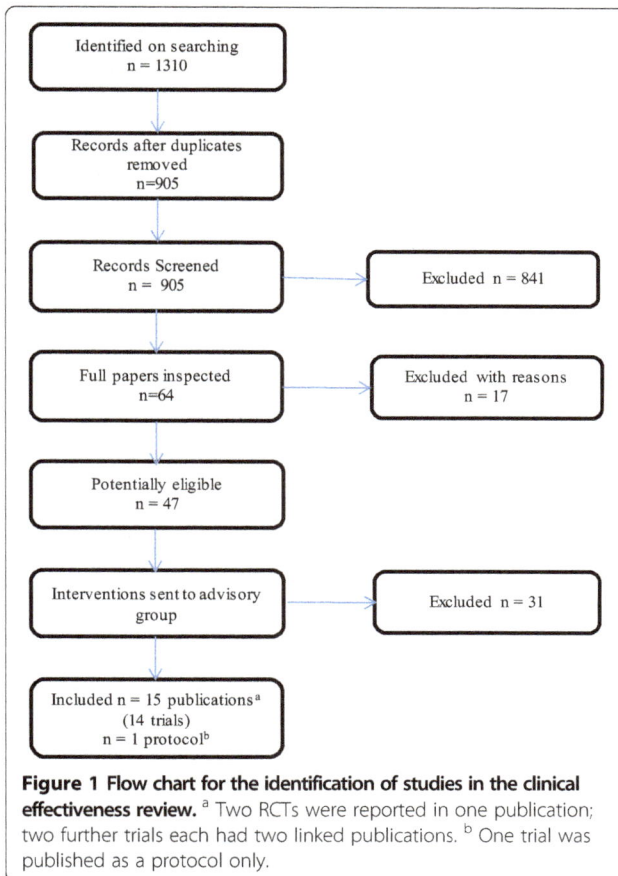

Figure 1 Flow chart for the identification of studies in the clinical effectiveness review. [a] Two RCTs were reported in one publication; two further trials each had two linked publications. [b] One trial was published as a protocol only.

practice by our advisory group. For further summary details see Table 1.

Results for the clinical effectiveness of the five pharmacological interventions in patients with mild to moderate IPF were mixed. In clinical practice azathioprine is only used in restricted circumstances, in one RCT [23] azathioprine and prednisolone led to an improvement in survival compared with placebo and prednisolone when an age adjusted analysis was used. There was no effect on lung function. This trial had an unclear risk of bias, a small sample size, and it is uncertain whether all patients had a diagnosis of IPF based on current recommendations. Consequently, caution is recommended when interpreting results. Nintedanib 300 mg/day was more favourable than placebo on some FVC measures, acute exacerbations and mortality, however, the primary outcome of annual rate of decline in FVC was not statistically significant [16]. Treatment with NAC was evaluated in three studies, [20-22] in combination with azathioprine and prednisolone in two (triple therapy) and in an inhaled format in one. Study results were mixed and establishing the stand-alone effect of NAC is difficult due to the differences between the three studies. There was no benefit from triple therapy on FVC compared to placebo in one trial, however, there was a

benefit on vital capacity (VC) when compared to azathioprine and prednisolone in another. The treatment effect of inhaled NAC was not statistically different from that of a control group (p = 0.05). The study using inhaled NAC had an unclear risk of bias which should be considered when interpreting results. Four RCTs [15,18,19] evaluated the use of pirfenidone and meta-analysis shows that pirfenidone appears to demonstrate a significant effect on FVC when compared to placebo (SMD 0.24, 95% CI 0.06, 0.41, p = 0.008). This should be cautiously interpreted as the outcomes pooled were different, the timing of assessment varied (from 48 weeks to 72 weeks) and there was moderate statistical heterogeneity (I^2 = 45%). The effect of pirfenidone on secondary outcomes was more uncertain. Thalidomide was assessed in those with cough in a small crossover RCT [25]. HRQoL outcomes related to cough were improved with thalidomide compared to placebo. There is no evidence relating to any subgroups in any of the published studies.

One study [24] assessed sildenafil for those with moderate to severe IPF. No statistically significant benefit of sildenafil was seen on the primary outcome, a 20% improvement on the six minute walk test. Results on secondary outcomes were mixed with some favourable to sildenafil but others being not statistically significant.

Adverse events were generally mild to moderate and reasonably well balanced between the treatments and controls with the exception of thalidomide which led to a greater proportion of people experiencing at least one adverse event (77%) than the placebo treated participants (22%) [25]. Severe adverse events appeared to be more common in one study in those treated with triple therapy [21].

Ten studies of pharmacological interventions were included in NMA; the resulting evidence network is shown in Figure 2. Thalidomide was excluded as the focus of treatment is not on lung function. Inhaled NAC was considered separately from triple therapy owing to its different method of administration. Both direct and indirect evidence was used to assess the treatment effect compared to placebo. Only the fixed effect results for nintedanib and pirfenidone were statistically significant, odds ratios for reducing the rate of decline in FVC compared to placebo are shown in (Table 2). The random effects model did not demonstrate a better fit than the fixed effect model and there was no evidence of inconsistency within the evidence network. A head-to-head comparison of nintedanib versus pirfenidone suggested a trend favouring nintedanib, but this was not statistically significant and should be cautiously interpreted in the light of the various differences between the studies (Table 2). Further trial evidence could be used to test this further.

Three non-pharmacological intervention studies compared a pulmonary rehabilitation programme or disease management programme to control interventions in moderate-to-severe IPF. Results from the two pulmonary

Table 1 Study characteristics of included interventions

Study and intervention details	Baseline characteristics	Outcomes	Risk of bias (selection bias)
Pharmacological agents			
Azathioprine			
Raghu et al. 1991 [21] *Country:* USA *Design:* RCT *Number of centres:* 2 *Funding:* Grant from Virginia Mason ResearchCentre, Seattle, USA *Interventions:* *1.* Prednisone and placebo, n = 13 *2.* Prednisone and azathioprine, n = 14 *Duration of treatment:* 12 months	Mean Age: 56 years M/F%: 55/45 Time since diagnosis: 2 years FVC: 67%	*Primary outcomes:* not stated as primary or secondary: measurable change in lung function (FVC, DLCO, P[A-a]O2) at 12 months; survival *Length of follow-up:* 12 months	Unclear risk
BIBF-1120			
Richeldi et al. 2011 [22] *Country:* 25 countries including Italy, Mexico, Germany, USA, Korea, UK, France. *Design:* RCT (dose finding phase II study) *Number of centres:* 92 *Funding:* supported by Boehringer Ingelheim *Interventions:* *1.* BIBF 1120 50 mg/day, n = 86 *2.* BIBF 1120 50 mg twice per day (100 mg/day), n = 86 *3.* BIBF 1120 100 mg twice per day (200 mg/day), n = 86 *4.* BIBF 1120 150 mg twice per day (300 mg/day), n = 85 *5.* Placebo, n = 85 *Duration of treatment:* 52 weeks	Mean Age: 65 years M/F%: 75/25 Time since diagnosis: 1.2 years FVC: 80%	*Primary outcomes:* annual rate of decline in FVC *Secondary outcomes:* % predicted FVC; DLCO; SpO2; TLC; 6MWT, SGRQ, decrease in FVC of more than 10% or more than 200 ml; SpO2 decrease of more than 4%; acute exacerbations; survival; death from a respiratory cause; adverse events *Length of follow-up:* 54 weeks	Low risk
N-Acetylcysteine (alone or in combination)			
Demedts et al. 2005 [18] *Country:* Belgium, France, Germany, Italy, Spain, the Netherlands *Design:* RCT *Number of centres:* 36 *Funding:* sponsored by the Zambon group *Interventions:* *1.* N-acetylcysteine, prednisolone, azathioprine, n = 92 (80 analysed) *2.* Placebo, prednisolone, azathioprine, n = 90 (75 analysed) *Duration of treatment:* not stated, assume 12 months.	Mean Age: 63 years M/F%: 72/28 Time since diagnosis: 1.6 years FVC: 66%	*Primary outcomes:* absolute changes in VC and DLCO at 12 months *Secondary outcomes:* % predicted VC, % predicted DLCO, alveolar volume change and % predicted, CRP score, dyspnoea score, maximum exercise indexes, HRCT outcomes, SGRQ, adverse events, withdrawals, and mortality *Length of follow-up:* 12 months	Low risk
Raghu et al., (IPFCRN) 2012 [19]	Mean Age: 68 years	*Primary outcomes:* change in FVC at 60 weeks	Low risk

Table 1 Study characteristics of included interventions *(Continued)*

Country: USA	M/F%: 75/25	*Secondary outcomes:* rate of death, time until death, frequency of acute exacerbation, frequency of maintained FVC response, time to disease progression, clinical and physiological measures including: DLCO, 6MWT, CPI, UCSD SBQ, SGRQ, SF-36, EQ-5D. Adverse events.	
Design: RCT (PANTHER study)	Time since diagnosis: 1 year		
Number of centres: 25	FVC: 71%		
Funding: grants from the NHLBI; the Cowlin Family fund. NAC and placebo donated by Zambon			
Interventions:			
1. N-acetylcysteine and placebo (data not presented in article as 'ongoing' data collection), n = 81			
2. N-acetylcysteine/prednisolone/azathioprine, n = 77		*Length of follow-up:* 60 weeks in the planned analysis. The study was stopped early. The mean follow-up was 32 weeks.	
3. Placebo, n = 78			
Duration of treatment: up to 60 weeks			
Homma et al. 2012 [20]	Mean Age: 68 years	*Primary outcomes:* absolute change in FVC at 48 weeks	Unclear risk
Country: Japan	M/F%: 76/24		
Design: RCT	Time since diagnosis: 3 years		
Number of centres: 27	FVC: 89%	*Secondary outcomes:* changes in lowest aterial O2 saturation, 6MWT distance, PFT parameters (VC, % predicted VC, TLC, % predicted TLC, DLCO, predicted DLCO), serum markers of pneumocyte injury; disease progression as determined by HRCT; subjective changes in symptoms such as dyspnoea, adverse events.	
Funding: grant from Ministry of Health, Labour and Welfare			
Interventions:			
1. N-acetylcysteine inhaled, n = 51 (38 analysed)			
2. Control, n = 49 (38 analysed) *Duration of treatment:* 48 weeks			
		Length of follow-up: 48 weeks	

Pirfenidone

Noble et al., 2011 [15]	Mean Age: 67 years	*Primary outcomes:* change in per cent predicted FVC	Low risk
Capacity study 006	M/F%: 72/28		
Country: Australia, Belgium, Canada, France, Germany, Ireland, Italy, Mexico, Poland, Spain, Switzerland, UK, USA	Time since diagnosis: ≤1 year: 59%	*Secondary outcomes:* categorical FVC (5-point scale), progression-free survival, worsening IPF, dyspnoea, 6MWT distance, worst peripheral oxygen saturation (SpO2) during the 6MWT, per cent predicted DLco, fibrosis, mortality.	
	FVC: 74%		
Design: RCT			
Number of centres: 110 centres			
Funding: InterMune			
Interventions:			
1. Pirfenidone 2403 mg/day, n = 171		*Length of follow-up:* 72 weeks from the date the last patient was enrolled.	
2. Placebo, n = 173			
Duration of treatment: 72 weeks			
Noble et al., 2011 [15]	Mean Age: 66 years	*Primary outcomes:* change in per cent predicted FVC	Low risk
Capacity study 004	M/F%: 71/29		
Country: Australia, Belgium, Canada, France, Germany, Ireland, Italy, Mexico, Poland, Spain, Switzerland, UK, USA	Time since diagnosis: ≤1 year: 48%	*Secondary outcomes:* categorical FVC (5-point scale), progression-free survival, worsening IPF, dyspnoea, 6MWT distance, worst peripheral oxygen saturation (SpO2) during the 6MWT, per cent predicted DLco, mortality.	
	FVC: 75%		
Design: RCT			
Number of centres: 110 centres			
Funding: InterMune			
Interventions:			
1. Pirfenidone 2403 mg/day, n = 174		*Length of follow-up:* 72 weeks from the date thelast patient was enrolled	
2. Pirfenidone 1197 mg/day, n = 87			

Table 1 Study characteristics of included interventions *(Continued)*

3. Placebo, n = 174

Duration of treatment: 72 weeks

Taniguchi et al., 2010 [16]	Mean Age: 65 years	*Primary outcomes:* change in vital capacity to week 52	Unclear risk
Country: Japan	M/F%: 78/22		
Design: RCT	Time since diagnosis: <1		
Number of centres: 73	year: 37%	*Secondary outcomes:* Progression-free survival time, change in lowest SpO2 during the 6MET. Pa,O2, PA-a,O2, TLC and DLCO, acute exacerbation, markers of interstitial pneumonias, symptoms.	
Funding: public sector grants. Drug and placebo from Shionogi & Co, Ltd.	FVC: 78%		
1. Pirfenidone 1800 mg/day, n = 108			
2. Pirfenidone 1200 mg/day, n = 55			
3. Placebo, n = 104		*Length of follow-up:* 52 weeks	
Duration of treatment: 52 weeks			
Azuma et al., 2005 [17]	Mean Age: 64 years	*Primary outcomes:* change in the lowest SpO2 during the 6MET	Unclear risk
Country: Japan	M/F%: 90/10		
Design: RCT	Time since diagnosis: <1		
Number of centres: 25	year: 22%	*Secondary outcomes:* resting PFTs while breathing air (VC, TLC, DLCO PaO2), disease progression by HRCT patterns, acute exacerbation, serum markers of pneumocyte damage, QoL	
Funding: Shionogi & co, Ltd	FVC: 80%		
Interventions:			
1.Pirfenidone 1800 mg/day, n = 73			
2. Placebo, n = 36			
Duration of treatment: 9 months			
		Length of follow-up: minimum of 9 months	

Thalidomide

Horton *et al.,* 2012 [24]	Mean Age: 68 years	*Primary outcomes:* cough-specific quality of life (CQLQ)	Low risk
Country: USA	M/F%: 78/22		
Design: randomised cross-over trial	Time since diagnosis: 1.7		
Number of centres: one	years	*Secondary outcomes:* cough, respiratory quality of life.	
Funding: Celgene Corporation	FVC: 70%		
Interventions:			
1. Thalidomide, n = 23		*Method of assessing outcome:* Cough-specific quality of life measured by CQLQ. Cough measured by 10 cm VAS. Respiratory quality of life measured by SGRQ.	
2. Placebo, n = 23			
Duration of treatment: 12 weeks each treatment with a 2 week washout period between treatments.			
		Length of follow-up: 12 weeks.	

Sildenafil (severe IPF)

Zisman and colleagues IPFCRN, 2010 [23]	Mean Age: 69 years	*Primary outcomes:* presence or absence of an improvement of at least 20% in the 6MWT distance at 12 weeks.	Unclear risk
Country: USA	M/F%: 84/16		
Design: RCT	Time since diagnosis: 1.9		
Number of centres: 14	years		
Funding: NHLBI; the Cowlin Fund (Chicago Community trust); Pfizer; Masimo.	FVC: 57%	*Secondary outcomes:* changes in the 6MWT distance, degree of dyspnoea, quality of life, FVC, DLCO, arterial partial pressure of oxygen and arterial oxygen saturation, and the alveolar-arterial oxygen gradient while breathing ambient air, adverse events, hospitalisations, death.	
1. Sildenafil, n = 89			
2. Placebo, n = 91			
Duration of treatment: 12 weeks.			
		Length of follow-up: 12 weeks	

Table 1 Study characteristics of included interventions *(Continued)*

Non-pharmacological interventions

Disease management programme/Pulmonary Rehabilitation

Lindell et al. 2010 [26]	Mean Age: 66 years	*Primary outcomes:* Not specified as primary or secondary outcomes. Dyspnoea (UCSDSBQ); Anxiety (BAI); Depression (BDI-II); Stress (PSS); QoL (SF-36)	Unclear risk
Country: USA	M/F%: 76/24		
Design: RCT	Time since diagnosis: NR		
Number of centres: one	FVC: >55: 70%		
Funding: Fairbanks-Horix Foundation			
Interventions:		Length of follow-up: Unclear	
1. Program to Reduce IPF Symptoms and Improve Management (PRISIM), n = 10 pairs			
2. Usual care, n = 11 pairs			
Duration of treatment: 6 weeks			
Jastrzebski et al. 2008 [27]	Mean Age: 56 years	*Primary outcomes:* not specified as primary or secondary. Dyspnoea (oxygen cost diagram, baseline dyspnoea index). QoL (SF-36), 6MWT (distance, dyspnoea in Borg's scale), maximal inspiratory pressure, lung function tests (IC, TLC, VC, FEV1, DLCOSB, DLCO/VA).	High risk
Country: Poland	M/F%: 64/36		
Design: CCT	Time since diagnosis: >2		
Number of centres: one	years		
Funding: not translated	FVC: 68%		
Interventions:			
1. Inspiratory muscle training, n = 16			
2. Control, n = 14		Length of follow-up: 12 weeks	
Duration of treatment: 12 weeks (two six week cycles)			
Nishiyama et al. 2008 [25]	Mean Age: 66 years	*Primary outcomes:* not specified as primary or secondary. Pulmonary function tests (FVC, FEV1, TLC, PaO2,PaCO2,) DLCO, 6MWT; BDI; SGRQ	Unclear risk
Country: Japan	M/F%: 76/24		
Design: RCT	Time since diagnosis: NR		
Number of centres: one	FVC: 67%		
Funding: Japanese ministry of health, labor and welfare		Length of follow-up: 10 weeks after the start of the programme.	
Interventions:			
1. Pulmonary rehabilitation programme (PRP), n = 15 (13 analysed)			
2. Control, n = 15			
Duration of treatment: 10 week programme.			

rehabilitation studies were inconclusive; some outcomes were favourable to pulmonary rehabilitation but not others. The risk of bias was uncertain and endpoints were only assessed immediately after the interventions finished. Limited evidence of the effectiveness of a disease management programme was demonstrated. This study had an uncertain risk of bias and follow-up was immediate.

Cost effectiveness and HRQoL systematic reviews

One economic evaluation was identified, which examined a testing strategy prior to treatment with triple therapy but did not examine the cost-effectiveness of treatment. The systematic review of HRQoL included 23 studies that examined HRQoL using either a generic preference-based tool (EuroQol five dimensions [EQ-5D], Short Form-36 [SF-36]) or a disease specific instrument (SGRQ) that

could be mapped to utility for the economic model. Results varied between the studies, given the different populations under study and the different measures and time points of measurement, however, results generally showed that IPF has an adverse effect on HRQoL which increases with severity.

Cost-effectiveness of pharmacological treatments for IPF

The baseline risk of disease progression in the unprogressed state was taken from two of the pirfenidone trials included in the systematic review of clinical effectiveness [15] as the population most closely met the model definition of unprogressed IPF and the RCTs had large sample sizes. The probabilities of progression free survival were obtained from the Kaplan Meier survival curve published for the pooled placebo population of two RCTs [15].

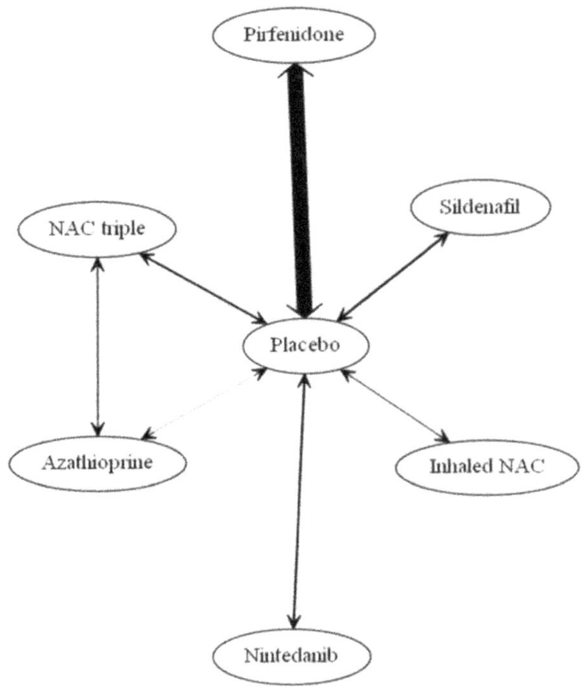

Figure 2 Evidence network for FVC endpoint. Legend: The width of the lines connecting treatment pairs is proportional to the number of participants within each trial comparison.

This study was an observational study but followed a larger sample than other published studies that differentiate survival by FVC decline and was deemed the most appropriate for the evaluation. Five parametric survival curves were fitted using the distributions noted above. The exponential distribution was selected (using AIC and face validity) to extrapolate beyond the five years of observed data. Probabilities of acute exacerbations in both unprogressed and progressed health states, and probabilities of lung transplant and survival from lung transplant, were taken from published sources.

HRQoL utility values were applied to each of the alive health states. These were not differentiated by treatment; the impact of treatment on utility was assumed to occur because of delay to disease progression which the model accounts for. The HRQoL values used for the unprogressed and progressed IPF health states were taken from EQ-5D values reported in two trials included in the systematic reviews of clinical effectiveness and HRQoL [21,24]. These trials were conducted by the same clinical network and it is likely that the estimates of EQ-5D are consistent and can therefore be contrasted in our economic model. The utility values applied in the model can be seen in Table 3. Utility associated with lung transplant is taken from a UK-based study [31] which assessed HRQoL using the EQ-5D. We weighted the utility to account for a greater proportion of single lung transplants in the IPF population than the proportion seen in the study, based on clinical opinion. Utility data for acute exacerbations were not identified in the literature and therefore a utility decrement was applied that was in line with decrements seen in those with asthma and chronic obstructive pulmonary disease (Table 3). Sensitivity analyses were used to test these utility decrements.

Five types of cost are considered in the economic model. The costs associated with each treatment were made up of the costs of the drug and the monitoring costs associated with the treatment. Dose information and unit costs were taken from published sources where available [32,33]. Unit

Parametric survival curves were fitted to this curve in Stata using maximum likelihood estimation in order to extrapolate beyond the 72 weeks follow-up. Exponential, Weibull, loglogistic, lognormal and Gompertz parametric models were examined. Goodness of fit was assessed using the Akaike Information Criterion (AIC). The Weibull model was selected because of the balance of good fit (AIC) and face validity (comparison of predicted survival with known survival in IPF). In the progressed state the monthly probability of death was taken from the overall survival curve in a recent study reporting survival for those experiencing a 10% or greater decline in FVC [30].

Table 2 NMA Fixed effects results, SMDs converted to log odds ratios for slowing the decline in FVC

Comparator (vs. placebo)	N studies	Total N participants	Log odds ratios			Odds ratios		
			Mean	95% CrI		Mean	95% CrI	
Azathioprine	1	19	0.44	−0.30	1.19	1.56	0.74	3.29
Nintedanib	1	170	−0.97	−1.52	−0.41	0.38	0.22	0.66
NAC triple therapy	2	294	−0.06	−0.60	0.48	0.94	0.55	1.62
Inhaled NAC	1	76	−0.42	−1.24	0.40	0.66	0.29	1.49
Pirfenidone	4	1006	−0.39	−0.62	−0.16	0.68	0.54	0.85
Sildenafil	1	180	−0.12	−0.65	0.41	0.89	0.52	1.51
Head-to-head comparison								
Nintedanib vs. Pirfenidone	−0.58			−1.18	0.03	0.56	0.31	1.03

Table 3 EQ-5D utility values by model health state

Model health state	EQ-5D (SD)
Unprogressed IPF (corresponds with an FVC ~72%)	0.80 (0.20)
Progressed IPF (corresponds with an FVC ~59%)	0.74 (0.19)
Lung transplant	
0-6 months after transplant	0.71 (0.38)
7-18 months after transplant	0.72 (0.31)
19-36 months after transplant	0.70 (0.33)
>36 months after transplant	0.68 (0.38)
Acute exacerbation decrement	0.20 (not available)

costs and data sources were unavailable for nintedanib and an assumed cost was used which was also subject to full sensitivity analysis. Hospital admission costs arising from acute exacerbations were estimated from NHS reference costs for all treatments as no treatment-specific acute exacerbation costs were available (£1361.04) [34]. Ongoing non-pharmacological treatment costs for management of the condition were included and covered annual home oxygen costs (£824.30) and the costs of long-term oxygen monitoring (£173.94) for the progressed IPF state. The costs associated with lung transplant were calculated using NHS reference costs [34] excluding outpatient procedures (£35,468.61). Costs of adverse events were attributed to the pharmacological interventions. Based on the incidence of serious adverse events seen in the trials included in the systematic review of clinical effectiveness, costs were applied for each event per patient in the first cycle of the model [34].

The model base-case results show increased survival for five of the treatments compared with BSC, at increased cost (see Table 4). The combination of azathioprine and prednisolone is dominated by BSC (treatment is more costly and less effective than BSC). Triple therapy is associated with an ICER of £41,811 per QALY gained when compared to BSC. Inhaled NAC is associated with an ICER of £5,037 per QALY gained when compared to BSC. Sildenafil, pirfenidone and nintedanib are not cost-effective at a willingness to pay (WTP) threshold of £30,000/QALY when compared to BSC. Therefore only one treatment, inhaled NAC, is cost-effective at a £30,000 WTP threshold, but its treatment effect is not statistically significant in the RCT, a small study with undetermined risk of bias.

Deterministic and probabilistic sensitivity analyses tested uncertainty in model parameter values, including costs and probabilities of acute exacerbation and lung transplant. Treatment effects and utilities were also varied in sensitivity analyses. The parameters were varied between the 2.5th and 97.5th percentiles of the mean value and analyses found that results were generally robust but were particularly sensitive to changes in the value of the treatment effect parameters.

The monthly cost of nintedanib was assumed (£3,274). Results demonstrate that, given a WTP of £30,000 per QALY, nintedanib must cost less than £736 per month to be considered as the cost-effective treatment option compared to BSC and pirfenidone.

Discussion

We systematically reviewed evidence for the clinical effectiveness of six pharmacological interventions and two non-pharmacological interventions for IPF. Participants in most of these studies would likely be classed as having mild-to-moderate IPF and generally were similar to those seen in clinical practice. There was a range of treatments under investigation in these trials with only one treatment, pirfenidone, providing evidence from more than one trial that was suitable for a formal meta-analysis to be undertaken. The outcomes reported in these studies differed however, and therefore caution is required when considering the results of the meta-analysis and the narrative synthesis of each of the included studies. In a network meta-analysis of the pharmacological treatments only pirfenidone and nintedanib had a statistically significant treatment effect, reducing the rate of decline in FVC compared to placebo. One pharmacological treatment was excluded from the network meta-analysis as the focus of treatment was not on lung function but on the symptom cough. In this study thalidomide appeared to improve cough, and quality of life compared with a placebo treatment. Results of three studies investigating two non-pharmacological treatments show mixed results and it is therefore unclear how effective these interventions are. There are differences between the studies in terms of the interventions, the participants, and the outcomes reported together with study design issues (e.g. short follow-up) and uncertain risk of bias that may account for some of the results seen.

Evidence from systematic reviews of cost effectiveness and HRQoL identified one economic evaluation of limited relevance and 23 HRQoL studies. These latter studies varied in their populations and study methods but generally

Table 4 Summary of base case results

Treatment	Total costs (£)	Total QALYs	ICER vs. BSC (£/QALY)	ICER vs. next best option (£/QALY)
BSC	3,084	2.98	-	-
Azathioprine & prednisolone	4,313	2.66	Dominated	Dominated
NAC triple therapy	5,021	3.03	41,811	Extended Dominance
Inhaled NAC	5,029	3.37	5,037	5,037
Sildenafil	12,008	3.11	68,116	Dominated
Pirfenidone	70,118	3.34	190,146	Dominated
Nintedanib	139,613	4.01	132,658	209,246

NB: Nintedanib uses an assumed cost.

showed that IPF has an adverse effect on HRQoL compared to population norms, and that HRQoL diminishes as IPF progresses. A new decision analytic health economic model was developed to assess the cost-effectiveness of six pharmacological treatments for IPF. Results show increased survival for five of the treatments compared with best supportive care, at increased cost. Only one treatment, inhaled NAC, is cost-effective at a WTP threshold of £30,000 but no statistically significant treatment effect was seen in the RCT or our NMA. Probabilistic sensitivity analysis showed that inhaled NAC has a 65% probability of being cost-effective if a decision threshold of £20,000 per QALY gained is used. Although pirfenidone and nintedanib achieve a statistically significant treatment effect in NMA they each have a probability of 0% of being cost-effective at a threshold of £30,000 per QALY. This is based on an assumed cost for nintedanib. A sensitivity analysis indicated that nintedanib must cost less than £736 per month to be considered cost-effective.

The past few years have seen an increasing interest in the management of IPF, with pharmacological companies evaluating a range of potential interventions, and a number of influential bodies producing guidelines. However, this systematic review demonstrates that at present there are few treatments which have any effect on surrogate outcomes which can be linked through evidence to patient related outcomes such as mortality. The findings of our research also suggest that under current willingness to pay thresholds only one treatment is likely to be cost effective, although, general recommendations cannot be made due to limitations in the evidence base. In terms of a cure it is considered that lung transplantation is the only intervention available which has curative intent. However, no evidence on lung transplant was eligible for inclusion in this evidence synthesis and so this could not be evaluated formally. There is also a scarcity of studies on interventions for symptom management and palliative care in IPF despite this being a recommended approach in recent clinical guidance [5].

No previous systematic reviews have included all potentially relevant treatments for IPF, and there has only been limited economic evaluation previously. Our results are useful to clinicians and patients, and complement recent national guidance by NICE in the UK [5]. In addition to standard synthesis we undertook a network meta-analysis to compare the pharmacological therapies to a common comparator. Our results show that only two treatments (nintedanib and pirfenidone) significantly slow the decline in FVC compared to placebo under a fixed effect model. However, with few studies it was not possible to fully explore heterogeneity within these data and the results should be cautiously interpreted. We also undertook an illustrative analysis comparing nintedanib with pirfenidone through an indirect comparison. While this showed a

trend favouring nintedanib, it was not statistically significant and should be interpreted with caution until such time that a more complete analysis can be undertaken on more robust data. We identified a number of ongoing trials of potential relevance. Our evidence synthesis has highlighted the current evidence base in which these new trials can be contextualised once they report.

There were numerous differences between the studies included in this review. However we applied a rigorous approach to the inclusion, quality assessment and data synthesis of the studies (laid out in a research protocol), to ensure that our work was as unbiased as possible. Our research was guided by an advisory group from its initiation, in particular to ensure that the interventions included were appropriate to current or future management in the NHS. We ensured that only the highest quality studies were included to limit uncertainty in the results.

Our study has several limitations. The meta-analysis and NMA used the standardised mean difference to express findings from studies on a common scale. In this case we combined mean change in FVC% predicted with absolute change in FVC, albeit the former is adjusted for certain baseline characteristics, and this should be considered when interpreting the results. Many of the included studies compared treatments to placebo. Few direct comparisons were identified and results of an indirect comparison via the NMA approach are presented. However there are known limitations to the use of indirect comparisons which should also be considered in interpreting our findings [35]. The economic model assumes that treatments have a constant effect on the relative rate of FVC% decline compared to BSC, but treatment may in fact become less effective with time or as the condition progresses. (This would make the treatments less cost-effective than shown in our results.) Finally, because of limitations in the data the absolute decline in FVC% predicted was used as the measure of disease progression in the model. It is possible that use of this measure may introduce bias because the starting FVCs of patients (which might vary widely) is not taken into account.

Conclusions

This evidence synthesis reports on the effectiveness of a range of interventions for IPF and complements recent UK guidance [5]. The current evidence suggests that there are currently few treatments which are clinically and cost-effective. Pirfenidone and nintedanib offer the potential for hope to sufferers and their clinicians, however, their cost-effectiveness is likely to be prohibitive. This research has thoroughly examined the current evidence and can be seen as a platform from which the clinical importance of newer treatments can be assessed when ongoing trials report. The systematic review has highlighted the need for further research into interventions to help alleviate or control symptoms of this debilitating condition, in particular pulmonary rehabilitation programmes and thalidomide. Given the results of our study and the weaknesses of the inhaled NAC trial, a well-designed RCT of inhaled NAC should also be considered; our search of ongoing RCTs failed to identify any such studies currently underway.

Additional file

Additional file 1: NMA model code. Random effects model code for the NMA.

Abbreviations

BSC: Best supportive care; CCT: Controlled clinical trial; EQ-5D: EuroQol five dimensions; FVC: Forced vital capacity; HRQoL: Health related quality of life; ICER: Incremental cost-effectiveness ratio; IPF: Idiopathic pulmonary fibrosis; UK: United Kingdom; NAC: N-acetylcysteine; NHS: National health service; NICE: National institute for health and care excellence; NMA: Network meta-analysis; QALY: Quality adjusted life Year; RCT: Randomised controlled trial; SD: Standard deviation; SF-36: Short Form-36; SMD: Standardised mean difference; VC: Vital capacity; WTP: Willingness to pay.

Competing interests

KOR and AW have previously been members of the Intermune advisory board for pirfenidone and received payment for research travel expenses only. All authors have completed the unified competing interest form at www.icmje.org/coi_disclosure.pdf (available on request from the corresponding author) and declare 1) no financial support for the submitted work from anyone other than their employer; 2) no financial relationships with commercial entities that might have an interest in the submitted work; 3) no spouses, partners, or children with relationships with commercial entities that might have an interest in the submitted work; and 4) no non-financial interests that may be relevant to the submitted work.

Authors' contributions

EL (Senior Research Fellow) developed the original research application, developed the research protocol, contributed to the background section, assisted in the development of the search strategy, assessed studies for inclusion, extracted data from and quality assessed included studies, synthesised evidence, drafted and edited the final report, project managed the study and is the guarantor of the study; VRC (Senior Research Fellow, Health Economics) assessed studies for inclusion, extracted data from and quality assessed included studies, synthesised evidence, developed the economic evaluation, drafted the report; JLC (Senior Research Fellow) developed the original research application, contributed to the development of the research protocol, contributed to the background section, assessed studies for inclusion, extracted data from and quality assessed included studies, synthesised evidence and drafted the report; DAS (Senior Director, Health Economics, Icon PLC) contributed to the development of the research protocol, synthesised evidence, assisted in developing the economic evaluation, drafted the report; AJC (Professor/Director of SHTAC) developed the original research application, contributed to developing the research protocol, extracted data from and quality assessed included studies, synthesised evidence, drafted the report, provided quality assurance for the project; JJ (Principal Research Fellow, Health Economics) developed the original research application, developed the research protocol, assisted in developing the economic evaluation, drafted the report; KMAO (Consultant Physician) drafted the background section, assisted with the interpretation of the clinical effectiveness evidence, provided clinical advice to the project, drafted the report; SS (Professor of Pulmonary and Cardiac Rehabilitation) drafted the background section, assisted with the interpretation of the clinical effectiveness evidence, provided expert advice to the project, drafted the report; CB (Professor of Palliative Medicine) drafted the background section, assisted with the interpretation of the clinical effectiveness evidence, provided expert advice to the project, drafted the report; AW (Professor/Consultant Physician) assisted with the interpretation of the clinical effectiveness evidence, provided expert advice to the project, drafted the report. All authors read and approved the final manuscript.

Acknowledgements

We would like to thank members of our advisory group who provided expert advice and comments on the protocol and the interpretation of the findings of this research. We are also grateful to Karen Welch, Information Specialist, SHTAC, University of Southampton, for generating and running the literature searches, Stuart Mealing, Health Economics, Oxford Outcomes for technical assistance with the economic model, Fiona Boyle, Finance Manager, University Hospitals Southampton Foundation Trust, for sourcing information on relevant costs for the economic evaluation, Helen Thomas, NHS Blood and Transplant for assistance with data related to lung transplantation, and Jonathan Shepherd, Principal Research Fellow, SHTAC, University of Southampton, for reviewing a draft of the full report that this paper is taken from.

This project was funded by the National Institute for Health Research Health Technology Assessment (NIHR HTA) programme. It will be published in full in the Health Technology Assessment journal series (www.nets.nihr.ac.uk/programmes/hta) in late 2014. The views and opinions expressed therein are those of the authors and do not necessarily reflect those of the HTA programme, NIHR, NHS or the Department of Health.

Author details

[1]Southampton Health Technology Assessments Centre (SHTAC), University of Southampton, Southampton, UK. [2]Icon PLC, Oxford, UK. [3]Mater Misericordiae University Hospital, Dublin, Ireland. [4]University Hospitals of Leicester NHS Trust, Leicester, UK. [5]Department of Palliative Medicine, University Hospital of Munich, Munich, Germany. [6]Green Lane Hospital, London, UK.

References

1. Swigris JJ, Stewart AL, Gould MK, Wilson SR: Patients' perspectives on how idiopathic pulmonary fibrosis affects the quality of their lives. *Health Qual Life Outcomes* 2005, 3:61.
2. Meltzer EB, Noble PW: Idiopathic pulmonary fibrosis. *Orphanet J Rare Dis* 2008, 3:8. www.ojrd.com/content/3/1/8.
3. Navaratnam V, Fleming KM, West J, Smith CJ, Jenkins RG, Fogarty A, Hubbard RB: The rising incidence of idiopathic pulmonary fibrosis in the U.K. *Thorax* 2011, 66:462–467.
4. Raghu G, Weycker D, Edelsberg J, Bradford WZ, Oster G: Incidence and prevalence of idiopathic pulmonary fibrosis. *Am J Respir Crit Care Med* 2006, 174:810–816.
5. NICE: *Diagnosis and management of suspected idiopathic pulmonary fibrosis. CG 163.* London: NICE; 2013.
6. Raghu G, Collard HR, Egan JJ, Martinez FJ, Behr J, Brown KK, Colby TV, Cordier JF, Flaherty KR, Lasky JA, Lynch DA, Ryu JH, Swigris JJ, Wells AU, Ancochea J, Bouros D, Carvalho C, Costabel U, Ebina M, Hansell DM, Johkoh T, Kim DS, King TE Jr, Kondoh Y, Myers J, Muller NL, Nicholson AG, Richeldi L, Selman M, Dudden RF, et al: An official ATS/ERS/JRS/ALAT statement: idiopathic pulmonary fibrosis: evidence-based guidelines for diagnosis and management. *Am J Respir Crit Care Med* 2011, 183:788–824.
7. Christie JD, Edwards LB, Kucheryavaya AY, Benden C, Dipchand AI, Dobbels F, Kirk R, Rahmel AO, Stehlik J, Hertz MI: The registry of the international society for heart and lung transplantation: 29th adult lung and heart-lung transplant report-2012. *J Heart Lung Transplant* 2013, 31:1073.
8. Centre for Reviews and Dissemination: *Systematic reviews: CRD's guidance for undertaking reviews in health care.* Third edition. York: York Publishing Services Ltd., CRD; 2009.
9. Drummond MF, Jefferson TO: Guidelines for authors and peer reviewers of economic submissions to the BMJ. The BMJ economic evaluation working party. *BMJ* 1996, 313:275–283.
10. Philips Z, Ginnelly L, Sculpher M, Claxton K, Golder S, Riemsma R, Woolacoot N, Glanville J: Review of guidelines for good practice in decision-analytic modelling in health technology assessment. *Health Technol Assess* 2004, 8:1–158.
11. Higgins JP, Green S: Cochrane handbook for systematic reviews of interventions version 5.1.0 [updated march 2011]. *Cochrane Collaboration* 2011, Available from www.cochrane-handbook.org.
12. Caldwell D, Ades AE, Higgins JPT: Simultaneous comparison of multiple treatments: combining direct and indirect evidence. *BMJ* 2005, 331:897–900.

13. Dias S, Welton NJ, Sutton AJ, Ades AE: *NICE DSU technical support document 2: a generalised linear modelling framework for pairwise and network meta-analysis of randomised controlled trials*. 2011. http://www.nicedsu.org.uk .14-6-0013.

14. Chinn S: **A simple method for converting an odds ratio to effect size for use in meta-analysis.** *Stat Med* 2000, **19**:3127–3131.

15. Noble PW, Albera C, Bradford WZ, Costabel U, Glassberg MK, Kardatzke D, King TE Jr, Lancaster L, Sahn SA, Szwarcberg J, Valeyre D, du Bois RM: **Pirfenidone in patients with idiopathic pulmonary fibrosis (CAPACITY): two randomised trials.** *Lancet* 2011, **377**:1760–1769.

16. Richeldi L, Costabel U, Selman M, Kim DS, Hansell DM, Nicholson AG, Brown KK, Flaherty KR, Noble PW, Raghu G, Brun M, Gupta A, Juhel N, Kluglich M, du Bois RM: **Efficacy of a tyrosine kinase inhibitor in idiopathic pulmonary fibrosis.** *N Engl J Med* 2011, **365**:1079–1087.

17. Hagaman JT, Kinder BW, Eckman MH: **Thiopurine S-methyltransferase testing in idiopathic pulmonary fibrosis: a pharmacogenetic cost-effectiveness analysis.** *Lung* 2010, **188**:125–132.

18. Taniguchi H, Ebina M, Kondoh Y, Ogura T, Azuma A, Suga M, Taguchi Y, Takahashi H, Nakata K, Sato A, Takeuchi M, Raghu G, Kudoh S, Nukiwa T: **Pirfenidone in idiopathic pulmonary fibrosis.** *Eur Respir J* 2010, **35**:821–829.

19. Azuma A, Nukiwa T, Tsuboi E, Suga M, Abe S, Nakata K, Taguchi Y, Nagai S, Itoh H, Ohi M, Sato A, Kudoh S: **Double-blind, placebo-controlled trial of pirfenidone in patients with idiopathic pulmonary fibrosis.** *Am J Respir Crit Care Med* 2005, **171**:1040–1047.

20. Demedts M, Behr J, Buhl R, Costabel U, Dekhuijzen R, Jansen HM, MacNee W, Thomeer M, Wallaert B, Laurent F, Nicholson AG, Verbeken EK, Verschakelen J, Flower CD, Capron F, Petruzzelli S, De Vuyst P, van den Bosch JM, Rodriguez-Becerra E, Corvasce G, Lankhorst I, Sardina M, Montanari M: **High-dose acetylcysteine in idiopathic pulmonary fibrosis.** *N Engl J Med* 2005, **353**:2229–2242.

21. Raghu G, Anstrom KJ, King J, Lasky JA, Martinez FJ: **Prednisone, azathioprine, and N-acetylcysteine for pulmonary fibrosis.** *N Engl J Med* 2012, **366**:1968–1977.

22. Homma S, Azuma A, Taniguchi H, Ogura T, Mochiduki Y, Sugiyama Y, Nakata K, Yoshimura K, Takeuchi M, Kudoh S: **Efficacy of inhaled N-acetylcysteine monotherapy in patients with early stage idiopathic pulmonary fibrosis.** *Respirology* 2012, **17**:467–477.

23. Raghu G, Depaso WJ, Cain K, Hammar SP, Wetzel CE, Dreis DF, Hutchinson J, Pardee NE, Winterbauer RH: **Azathioprine combined with prednisone in the treatment of idiopathic pulmonary fibrosis: a prospective double-blind, randomized, placebo-controlled clinical trial.** *Am Rev Respir Dis* 1991, **144**:291–296.

24. Zisman DA, Schwarz M, Anstrom KJ, Collard HR, Flaherty KR, Hunninghake GW: **A controlled trial of sildenafil in advanced idiopathic pulmonary fibrosis.** *N Engl J Med* 2010, **363**:620–628.

25. Horton MR, Santopietro V, Matthew L, Horton KM, Polito AJ, Liu MC, Danoff SK, Lechtzin N: **Thalidomide for the treatment of cough in idiopathic pulmonary fibrosis.** *Ann Intern Med* 2012, **157**:398–406.

26. Nishiyama O, Kondoh Y, Kimura T, Kato K, Kataoka K, Ogawa T, Watanabe F, Arizono S, Nishimura K, Taniguchi H: **Effects of pulmonary rehabilitation in patients with idiopathic pulmonary fibrosis.** *Respirology* 2008, **13**:394–399.

27. Lindell KO, Olshansky E, Song MK, Zullo TG, Gibson KF, Kaminski N, Hoffman LA: **Impact of a disease-management program on symptom burden and health-related quality of life in patients with idiopathic pulmonary fibrosis and their care partners.** *Heart Lung* 2010, **39**:304–313.

28. Jastrzebski D, Kozielski J, Zebrowska A: **[Pulmonary rehabilitation in patients with idiopathic pulmonary fibrosis with inspiratory muscle training]. [Polish].** *Pneumonol Alergol Pol* 2008, **76**:131–141.

29. Nathan SD, Shlobin OA, Weir N, Ahmad S, Kaldjob JM, Battle E, Sheridan MJ, du Bois RM: **Long-term course and prognosis of idiopathic pulmonary fibrosis in the New millennium.** *Chest* 2011, **140**:221–229.

30. Richeldi L, Ryerson CJ, Lee JS, Wolters PJ, Koth LL, Ley B, Elicker BM, Jones KD, King TE Jr, Ryu JH, Collard HR: **Relative versus absolute change in forced vital capacity in idiopathic pulmonary fibrosis.** *Thorax* 2012, **67**:407–411.

31. Anyanwu AC, McGuire A, Rogers CA, Murday AJ: **Assessment of quality of life in lung transplantation using a simple generic tool.** *Thorax* 2001, **56**:218–222.

32. Department of Health: *National health service England and wales electronic drug tariff May 2013.* ; 2013. 14-6-2013. www.ppa.org.uk/edt/May_2013/mindex.htm.

33. Joint Formulary Committee: *British national formulary (BNF) 65. No. 65.* London: British Medical Association and Royal Pharmaceutical Society of Great Britain; 2013.

34. Department of Health: *NHS reference costs 2011–2012.* https://www.gov.uk/government/publications/nhs-reference-costs-financial-year-2011-to-2012. 8-11-2012.

35. Mills EJ, Thorlund K, Ionnidis JPA: **Demystifying trial networks and network meta-analysis.** *BMJ* 2013, **346**:f2914.

15

Anti-TNF inhibits the Airways neutrophilic inflammation induced by inhaled endotoxin in human

Olivier Michel[1*], Phong Huy Duc Dinh[3], Virginie Doyen[1] and Francis Corazza[2]

Abstract

Background: Inhaled endotoxin induces airways'neutrophilia, in human. TNF-a being a key cytokine in the response to endotoxin, the effect of anti-TNF on the endotoxin-induced neutrophilic response was evaluated among healthy volunteers.

Methods: Among a population of 30 healthy subjects, an induced-sputum was collected 2 weeks before, and 24 hours after an inhalation of 20 mcg endotoxin (E coli 026:B6). Then, the subjects were randomized into 3 parallel groups treated with control, oral methylprednisolone 20 mg/day during 7 days or anti-TNF (adalimumab, Humira®, Abbott) 40 mg SC. One week later, an induced-sputum was sampled, 24 hours after an inhalation of endotoxin.

Results: After endotoxin inhalation, the number of total cells, neutrophils and macrophages was significantly increased (p <0.001). Compared to the response to endotoxin among the control group, anti-TNF inhibited the endotoxin-induced neutrophil influx, both in relative (51.3 (±6.4)% versus 26.2 (±5.3)%, p <0.002) and in absolute values (1321 (443–3935) cells/mcL versus 247 (68–906) cells/mcL, p <0.02). The endotoxin-induced neutrophilic response was not significantly modified among the control group and oral corticosteroid group.

Conclusions: While oral corticosteroid had no effect, anti-TNF inhibited the neutrophil influx in sputum, induced by inhalation of endotoxin, in human subject. The endotoxin model could be an early predictor of clinical efficacy of novel therapeutics.

Trial registration: ClinicalTrials.gov NCT02252809 (EudraCT2008-005526-37)

Keywords: Endotoxin inhalation, Neutrophilic inflammation, Corticosteroids, Anti-TNF

Background

Over one bilion people through the World suffer from chronic respiratory diseases (CRD), mainly chronic obstructive pulmonary diseases (COPD) and asthma [1]. Currently there is no satisfactory treatment for COPD and severe asthma. Airways' neutrophilic inflammation is a risk factor of severity of several CRD. The number of neutrophils in sputum correlates with the severity [2] and accelerated decrease of FEV1 [3] in COPD and with severe exacerbations in asthma [4]. Neither oral corticosteroids (CS), nor a high dose inhaled CS has an effect on the airways' neutrophilic inflammation in COPD [5,6], and neutrophilic exacerbations of asthma are refractory to increasing the dose of inhaled corticosteroids [7]. Through the activation of NF-kB, TNF-a induces the IL-8 chemokine that is a chemoattractant for the neutrophils. Consistently, some studies reported that the concentrations of TNF-a and its soluble receptor are raised in the sputum of COPD patients [8]. The lack of anti-inflammatory effects of CS in COPD could be related to the reduction in recruitment of histone desacetylase-2 by CS, resulting in the absence of control of NFkB transcription, leading to expression of cytokines such as TNF-a and IL-8 [9]. Thus, TNF-a appears to participate to the mechanism of airways neutrophilic inflammation in COPD and severe asthma.

The endotoxin-induced airways' inflammation mimicks several aspects of acute exacerbation of COPD [10]. This

* Correspondence: omichel@ulb.ac.be
[1]Clinic of Allergology and Immunology, CHU Brugmann (Université Libre de Bruxelles - ULB), 4 pl Van Gehuchten, B –1020, Brussels, Belgium
Full list of author information is available at the end of the article

neutrophilic inflammation is not modified by oral prednisolone [11]. In an ex-vivo model, using endotoxin exposure of lung tissue from COPD, TNF was the initial cytokine and was predicitive for the following release of IL-6, CXCL8 and IL-10. It was inhibited by the neutralisation of the TNFα [12]. The concentration of TNF in the broncho-alveolar lavage was significantly increased during the early phase [2 hours] after bronchial endotoxin instillation in human [13]. Recently the involvement of NF-kB activation in the neutrophilic response to inhaled endotoxin has been reported among smokers [14].

Since TNF-a seems to be a key cytokine in endotoxin-induced neutrophilic inflammation, the current study evaluated the inhibiting effect of anti-TNF on the neutrophilic response among healthy volunters exposed to inhaled endotoxin.

Methods
Subjects
A population of 49 healthy, male and female, non-smoker volunteers (age 18 to 50 years) was screened, after a written informed consent was obtained from each subject. They were excluded if they used drugs within 2 weeks or over-the counter medication.

Study design
During the screening phase, an induced-sputum was collected 2 weeks before, and 24 hours after an inhalation of 20 mcg endotoxin. On day 1, among the 49 healthy volunteers, 40 were selected after having produced a valid sputum (defined as a 80% or more viability, with less than 50% squamous cells, and less than 70% neutrophils). A significant inflammatory response to inhaled endotoxin was defined as an increase of 10% or more of the absolute count of neutrophils in the sputum. By doing so, 30 subjects were included (mean age: 31.0 (28 – 34) years; females/males: 16/14) (Figure 1).

After a wash-out period of 7 days, they were randomised into 3 open parallel groups: control or treated with 20 mg oral prednisolone (Medrol®, Pfizer-Upjohn) once daily for

7 days (PDN) or a single sub-cutaneous anti-TNF antibody, 40 mg adalimumab (Humira®, Abbott) on day 1. On day 14, a challenge test with inhaled endotoxin was performed in each subject and an induced-sputum was obtained 24 hours later. A clinical follow-up visit was performed after 5 weeks.

Induced sputum
Hypertonic sterile saline (5%) was nebulized for 30 minutes with an ultrasonic nebulizer (Fisoneb; Karapharm, Marseille, France); subjects rinsed their mouth with water every 10 minutes and tried to cough sputum directly into a sterile plastic box. After selection of all portions of sputum as free as possible of saliva, the plugs were weighed, mixed with 4 volumes of dithiotreitol 0.1% (Sputolysin; Behring Diagnostics, Somerville, NJ), homogenised and rocked for 15 min. before adding 4 volumes of Dulbecco's PBS. After filtration and centrifugation (15 minutes at 800 g) the supernatant was frozen at -80°C while the pelleted cells were resuspended in PBS. The number of total cells was measured with a Thoma's hemocytometer. The cell viability was assessed by the Trypan blue method. A slide was prepared by centrifugation (Cytospin, Shandon Inc, Pittsburgh, PA) and stained with May-Grünwald-Giemsa. The differential cells were counted on 400 cells.

Endotoxin challenge tests
The procedure of endotoxin challenge has been previously reported [15]: briefly 20 μg of a suspension of lipopolysaccharide (LPS Escherichia coli 026:B6 from Sigma Chemical, St Louis, MO -ref L-2654), the active derivative of endotoxin, was administered by a dosimeter Mefar MB3 (Mefar, Brescia, Italy). The dose of inhaled endotoxin corresponded to 17 inhalations of a calibrated aerosol of 6 mcL/inhalation containing a solution of 0.2 mg/mL endotoxin. Outputs was checked by weighing the nebulizer containing 2 ml of sterile normal saline before and after 10 actuations [16]. The endotoxin dose was selected according to data published on the dose–response relationship to inhaled endotoxin [17]. The objective was to cause only minimal systemic responses,

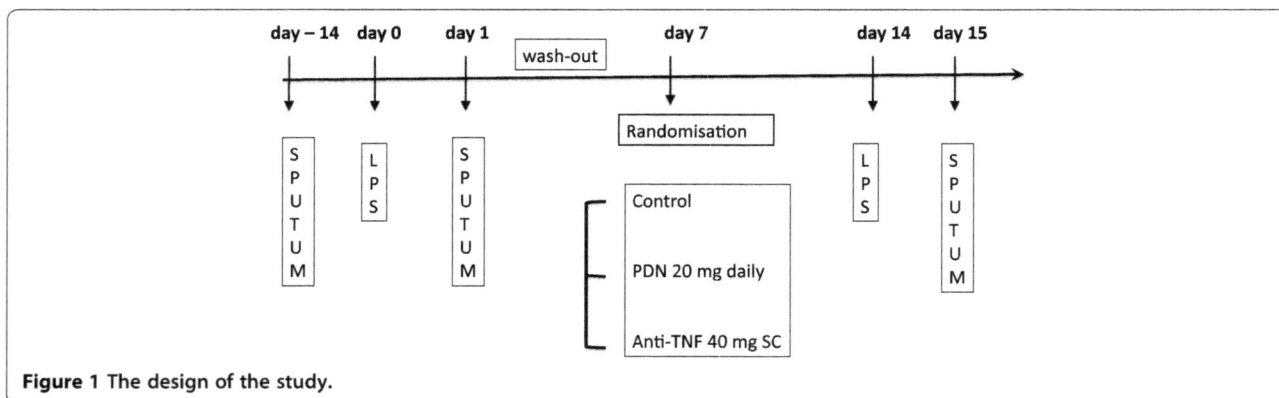

Figure 1 The design of the study.

though with a significant but sub-maximal inflammatory responses in the lung, to allow prednisolone and/or adalimumab to significantly reduce these responses. At the end of the procedure, the volunteers were instructed to rinse their mouth to eliminate residual endotoxin trapped on the oral mucosa. Symptoms, oral temperature, forced vital capacity (FVC), forced expiratory volume in 1 second (FEV1) and the FEV1/FVC were recorded before and hourly after endotoxin.

Good clinical practice

This study was conducted according to with Good Clinical Practice Guidelines of the International Conference on Harmonisation. The study was registered in the non-public database of all drugs trials in the European Community (EudraCT: 2008-005526-37), as an exploratory phase study, in 2008, and then in the public database form the Clinical-Trials.gov NCT02252809. It was approved by the Ethics Committee of the CHU Brugmann (decision number CE2008/49) and the competent authorities in Belgium. Written informed consent was obtained in each subject. The Clinical Research Unit of the Institution was responsible for study coordination.

Statistics

The results were expressed as mean or geometric mean ±95% confidence interval. The absolute values of the cells were Log transformed. Repeatability of the response to LPS was assessed, among the control group, by plotting the differences between repeated measurements against the mean of the repeated measures, and testing whether the mean differences was significantly different from 0 (method of Bland and Altman) [18]. ANOVA was used to compare change from baseline among the three groups (control, PDN, anti-TNF), followed by paired t-tests between each active treatments and the control group. P values smaller than 0.05 were considered statistically significant.

Results

The demographics of the population is shown in Table 1. There was no significant difference among the 3 randomised groups for age, sex ratio, sputum characterictics at the basal state.

Except a slight headache among 5 subjects, there was no significant symptom or change in lung function. The temperature increased slighly from 36.3 (36.0-36.6) immediately before LPS to 36.3 (36.0-36.5) (p = NS), 36.3 (36.2-36.7) (p = NS), 36.4 (36.1-36.6) (p = NS) , 36.5 (26.2-36.8) (p <0.05), at 2, 4, 8 and 24 hours after inhaled LPS, respectively. There was no significant drug effect on the symptoms and/or the temperature.

Among the 30 subjects, during the screening phase, the endotoxin inhalation induced a significant rise of the geometric means of total viable cells (p <0.0001), neutrophils (p <0.0001), macrophages (p <0.001), and lymphocytes (p <0.0001) (Figure 2A). The arithmetic means of the percentage of neutrophils increased from 35.0 (26.9 – 43.1)% to 52.4 (44.6 – 60.3)%, (p <0.0001), while there was a decrease of macrophages from 60.7 (52.2 – 62.2)% to 43.8 (35.9 – 51.8)%, (p <0.0001) (Figure 2A). Among the subjects of the control group, the neutrophilic (%) response correlated significantly between the 2 endotoxin challenges (i.e. the endotoxin challenge before and after randomisation, r = 0.78; p <0.02), suggesting that the response was reproducible. The intra-subject repeatability of the method was evaluated in the control group, by comparing the neutrophilic response on day 1 and day 14 (Figure 2B). The Bland and Altman analysis showed that the measurements of percentage and absolute values of neutrophils were not statistically different between day 1 and day 14 (t-test = –0.179 and –0.585, respectively).

Anti-TNF inhibited the neutrophil influx both in relative (51.3 (36.8 - 65.8)% versus 26.2 (14.1 – 38.2)% , p <0.002), and in absolute value (1321 (443–3935) cells/mcL versus 247 (68–906) cells/mcL, p <0.02) (Figure 3). While anti-TNF increased the percentage of macrophages (44.7(29.8 – 59.6)% versus 71.3 (58.4 – 84.1)% ; p <0.002), it had no significant effect on the absolute count of macrophages (1180 (661–2089) cells/mcL versus 873 (457–1660) cells/mcL;

Table 1 Demography and sputum characteristics at the basal state in the whole population and among each randomized group

	Whole population	Control	PDN	Anti-TNF
Subjects (n)	30	10	10	10
Sex (F/M)	16/14*	4/6	5/5	7/3
Age (years, 95% CI)[†]	31 (28–34)	29 (23–34)	33 (27–40)	31 (25–37)
Weight of sputum plugs (mg, 95% CI)[‡]	469 (389–553)	564 (378–750)	422 (309–535)	433 (260–606)
Cells viability (%, 95% CI)[†]	80.4 (76.0-84.7)	80.7 (73.7-87.6)	85.6 (78.3-92.8)	74.8 (65.5-84.2)
Total cells (cells/µL, 95% CI)[‡]	2280 (1496–3467)	4083 (1749–9506)	2138 (933–4909)	1356 (764–2404)

[†]arithmetic means; [‡]geometric means.
*age, sputum characteristics were not significantly different among female (F) compared to male (M).

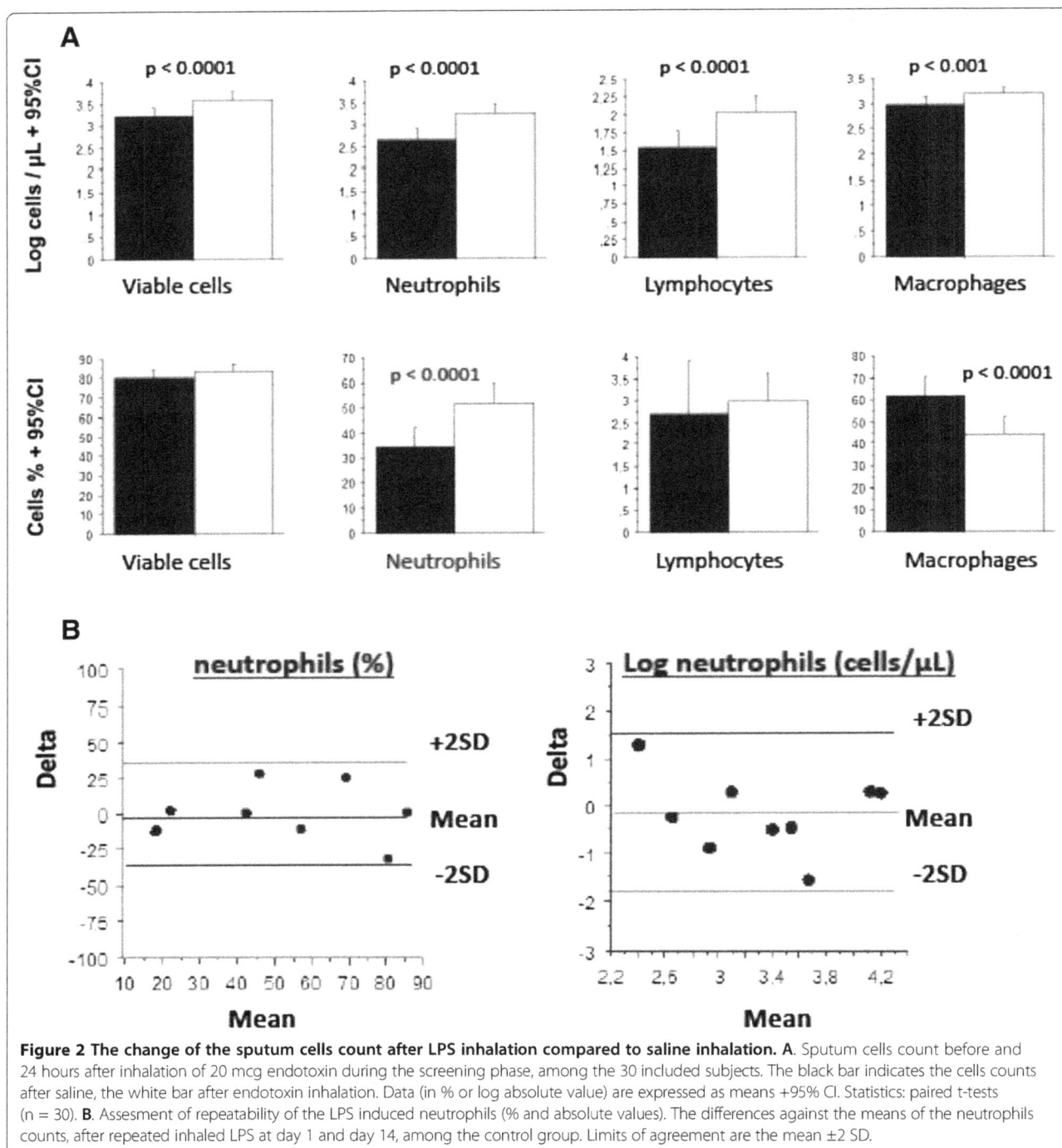

Figure 2 The change of the sputum cells count after LPS inhalation compared to saline inhalation. A. Sputum cells count before and 24 hours after inhalation of 20 mcg endotoxin during the screening phase, among the 30 included subjects. The black bar indicates the cells counts after saline, the white bar after endotoxin inhalation. Data (in % or log absolute value) are expressed as means +95% CI. Statistics: paired t-tests (n = 30). **B.** Assesment of repeatability of the LPS induced neutrophils (% and absolute values). The differences against the means of the neutrophils counts, after repeated inhaled LPS at day 1 and day 14, among the control group. Limits of agreement are the mean ±2 SD.

p = NS) (Figure 3). Oral corticosteroid had no significant effect on the neutrophils and macrophages response to endotoxin, while it inhibited significantly the percentage but not the absolute count of lymphocytes (Figure 3). The data of the endotoxin-induced cells count response in sputum before and after a treatment are shown in Table 2.

The endotoxin-induced changes of the cell counts of the control group were compared to the changes after

treatment with corticosteroids or anti-TNF (Figure 4, ANOVA for repeated measurements). The F-tests were significant for PMN % (F^2_{26} = 8.07, p <0.01), macrophages % (F^2_{27} = 8.27, p <0.01), viability % (F^2_{26} = 5.69, p <0.01), and Log PMN (F^2_{26} = 4.33 , p <0.03), but not for Log macrophages, Log lymphocytes and lymphocytes %.

The amplitude of the neutrophil response to endotoxin, expressed in absolute values was variable among

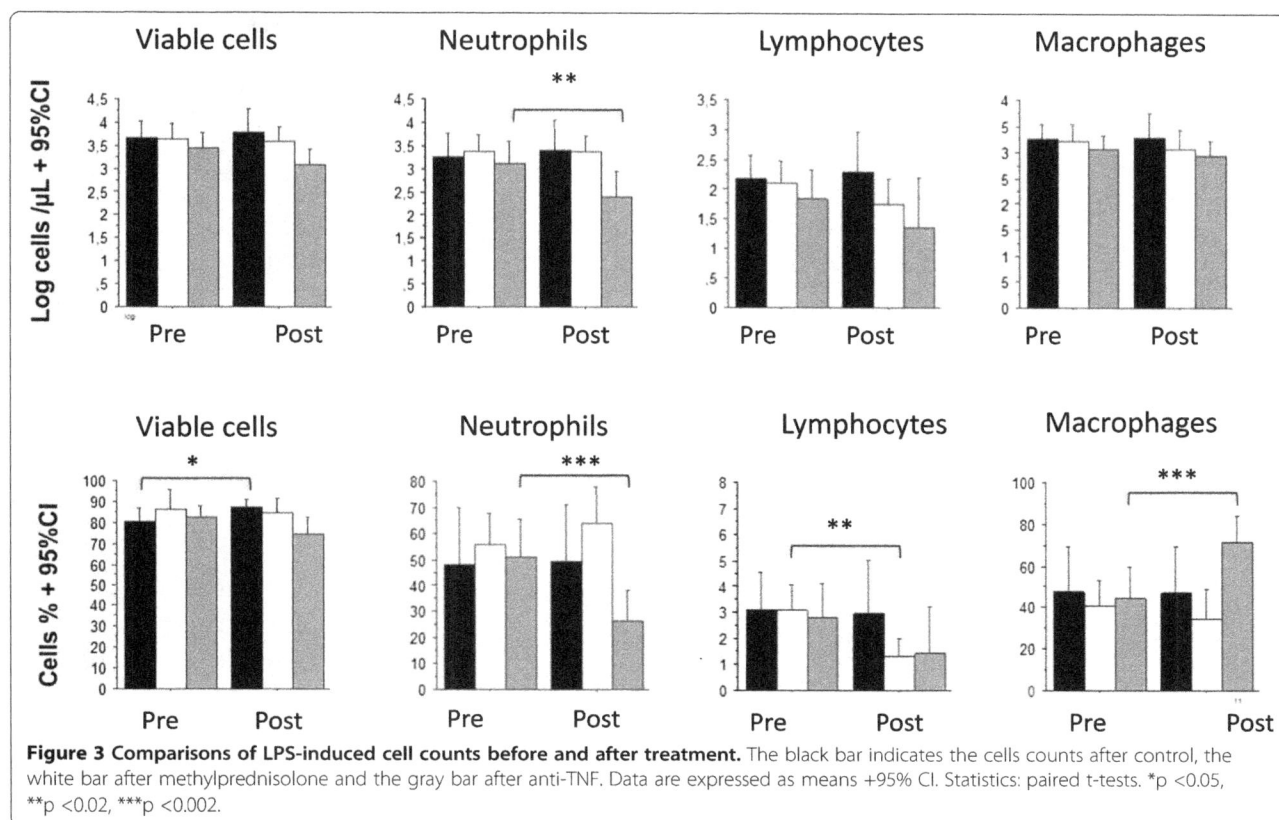

Figure 3 Comparisons of LPS-induced cell counts before and after treatment. The black bar indicates the cells counts after control, the white bar after methylprednisolone and the gray bar after anti-TNF. Data are expressed as means +95% CI. Statistics: paired t-tests. *p <0.05, **p <0.02, ***p <0.002.

the subjects and not related with the neutrophil count at the basal state (Figure 5A). Anti-TNF totally inhibited the endotoxin-induced rise of neutrophils, in each subject (exept one). The rise of the neutrophilic count after endotoxin (Figure 5B) was significantly related to the amplitude of the anti-TNF blocking effect, suggesting that anti-TNF was mainly active on the endotoxin-induced change in neutrophils but not, on the airways neutrophils count at the basal state. There was no significant change of the amplitude of the neutrophil response to endotoxin in both the control groups and the oral steroids treated subjects (Figure 5C and D).

Discussion

The study shown that a pretreatment with anti-TNF inhibited the endotoxin-induced neutrophil influx in induced sputum, among healthy subjects. Conversely, oral corticosteroid had no effect on the endotoxin induced inflammation.

In human, a bronchial instillation of endotoxin induced an early phase reaction, occuring after 2 hours and characterized by a local increase in neutrophils and cytokines, such as TNF-a, IL1-b, IL-6 and IL-8 [13]; TNF-a increased more than 300 fold, compared to the control [13]. It was followed by a later phase (24–48 hours) characterized by

the presence of neutrophils, macrophages, macrophages and lymphocytes [13,19], recovering within 7 days [19]. In ex vivo lung tissue, stimulated with endotoxin (100 ng/ml), TNF-a was the initial cytokine, expressed by the macrophages and mastocytes as early as 1 hour, rising at 2 and 4 hours and peaking at 6 hours and it was also predictive for the following release of cytokines, after endotoxin exposure [12]. Since TNF-a is a key cytokine in endotoxin-induced airway' inflammation, we hypothesised that anti-TNF could attenuate the endotoxin induced airways' neutrophilia.

The current data confirmed the airways' neutrophilic response in absolute and relative value, 24 hours after an inhalation of 20 mcg endotoxin. Firstly, we evaluated the repeatability of the PMN response. It is well known that the amplitude of the neutrophilic response to inhaled endotoxin is highly variable between subjects [20], as also confirmed by the present results. Nevertheless,in the current study, among the 10 subjects submitted to repeated endotoxin challenges, at 14 days interval, the intra-subject repeatability of the sputum neutrophilia was significant, consistently with recent data [14,21,22].

Secondly, we investigated the effect of oral corticosteroids on the endotoxin-induced airways' neutrophilia. A 7 days pretreatment with methylprednisolone 20 mg daily

Table 2 The endotoxin-induced cells count response in sputum before and after a treatment with control, oralsteroids and anti-TNF

Parameters	Total	Control .(1)	PDN .(2)	p value[‡] (1) vs (2)	Anti-TNF .(3)	p value[‡] (1) vs (3)
n	30	9	10		10	
Total viable cells (cells/μL)						
Before LPS	1811 (1191–2748)	2716 (1132–6741)	1820 (805–4111)		1000 (607–1648)	
After LPS	4188 2754–6368)	4570 (2004–10399)	4447 (2060–9571)		2884 (1352–6152)	
After LPS + treatment		6039 1883–19408)	3963 (2004–7834)	NS	1261 (591–2691)	0.052
p value[†]	< 0.0001					
Neutrophils (cells/μL)						
Before	520 (299)906)	789 (229–2710)	561 (207–1517)		244 (120–498)	
After LPS	1954 (1135–3357)	1795 (560–5768)	2387 (1019–5598)		1321 (443–3935)	
After LPS + treatment		2594 (614–10990)	2313 (1084–5284)	NS	247 (68–906)	< 0.02
p value[†]	p <0.0001					
Macrophages (cells/μL)						
Before	993 (681–1449)	1438 (692–2985)	914 (395–2113)		656 (396–1089)	
After LPS	1618 (1138–2296)	1786 (939–3396)	1644 (807–3350)		1180 (661–2089)	
After LPS + treatment		1892 (647–5508)	1185 (528–2654)	NS	873 (457–1660)	NS
p value[†]	p <0.001					
Lymphocytes (cells/μL)						
Before	39 (23–65)	65 (29–147)	33 (12–91)		21 (8–54)	
After LPS	119 (71–201)	155 (64–378)	125 (54–299)		67 (20–219)	
After LPS + treatment		198 (42–929)	54(18–156)	NS	22 (3–159)	NS
p value[†]	p <0.0001					
Neutrophils (%)						
Before	35 .0 (26.9-43.1)	36.8 (18.3-55.3)	37.3 19.0-55.3)		28.2 (18.2-38.1)	
After LPS	52.4 (44.6-60.3)	48.4 (27.1-69.8)	55.9 (44.0-67.8)		51.3 (36.8-65.8)	
After LPS + treatment		49.6 (28.2-70.9)	63.8 (49.8-77.8)	NS	26.2 (14.1-38.2)	< 0.002
p value[†]	p <0.0001					
Macrophages (%)						
Before	60.7 (52.2-62.2)	58.6 (39.8-77.5)	59.5 (39.5-79.5)		67.1 (57.2-77.0)	
After LPS	43.8 (35.9-51.8)	47.8 (26.2-69.3)	40.8 (28.7-52.8)		44.7 (29.8-59.6)	
After LPS + treatment		46.9 (24.5-69.3)	34.6 23.4-48.8)	< 0.002	71.3 (58.4-84.1)	NS
p value[†]	p <0.0001					
Lymphocytes (%)						
Before	2.7 (1.5-3.9)	2.1 (0.8-3.4)	2.7 (0.6-4.8)		3.3 (0.1-6.3)	
After LPS	3.0 (2.3-3.6)	3.1 (1.6-4.6)	3.1 (2.4-4.1)		2.8 (1.4-4.1)	
After LPS + treatment		2.9 (0.9-5.0)	1.3 (0.6-2.0)	NS	1.5 (0.3-3.2)	0.052
p value[†]	NS					

The % and absolute values are expressed as arithmetic or geometric means, respectively (95% Confidence Interval). PDN, methylprednisolone.
[‡]Unpaired t-tests were used to compare the changes among control (1) with the changes after prednisolone (2) or anti-TNF (3).
[†]Paired t-test to compare the cell counts before and after LPS, among the whole population.

had no significant effect. In a previous study the same drug regiment did not have an effect on the response to 50 mcg LPS, a dose that has been associated with clinical symptoms [11]. It was thought that exposure to a subclinical (and consequently sub-maximal) dose of LPS could be blocked by oral steroids but it was not confirmed by the current data. We can not excluded that for a lower level of LPS exposure (such as 5 μg), an effect of oral

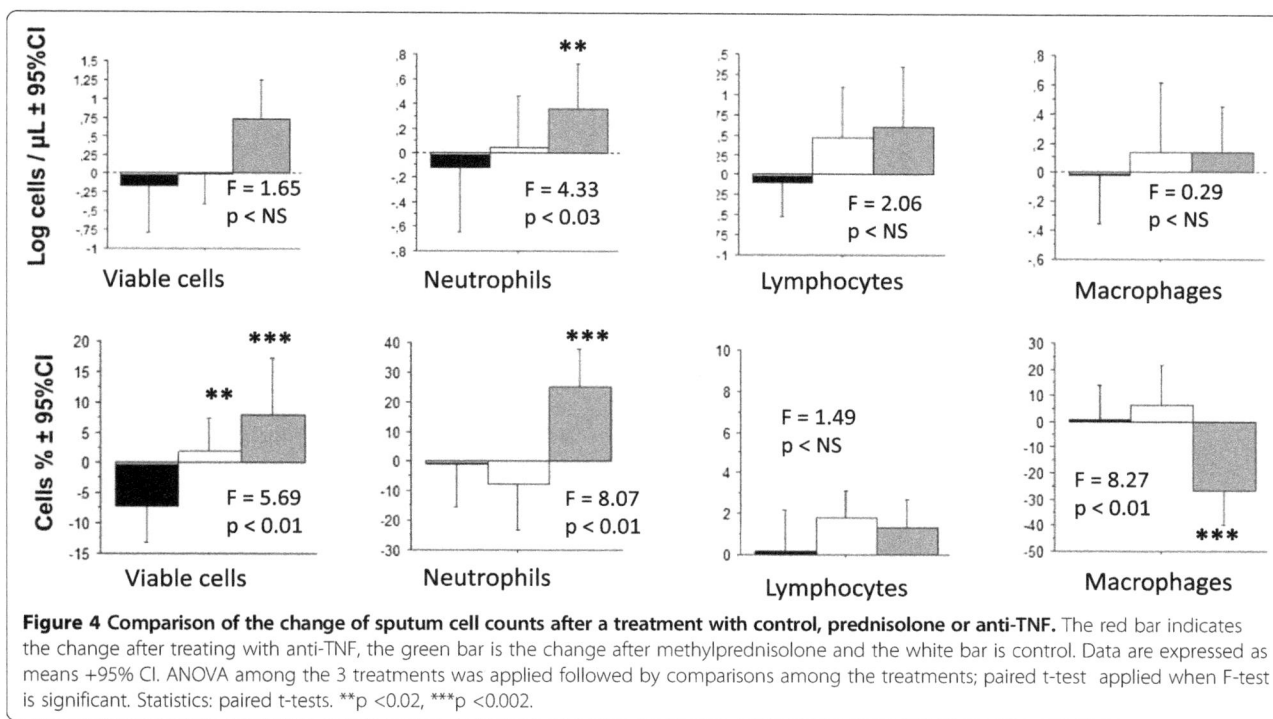

Figure 4 Comparison of the change of sputum cell counts after a treatment with control, prednisolone or anti-TNF. The red bar indicates the change after treating with anti-TNF, the green bar is the change after methylprednisolone and the white bar is control. Data are expressed as means +95% CI. ANOVA among the 3 treatments was applied followed by comparisons among the treatments; paired t-test applied when F-test is significant. Statistics: paired t-tests. **p <0.02, ***p <0.002.

corticosteroids on biomarkers of inflammation could be significant; though at this level of exposure, the response is inconsistent between subjects [14,17].

Thirdly, we have shown that, in contrast to corticosteroids, a pretreatment with anti-TNF blocked the neutrophilic response, both in relative and absolute values. In mirror with the decrease of the neutrophils, the percentage of macrophages increased, though the absolute number of macrophages remained unchanged after anti-TNF treatment. Interestingly the current data shown that anti-TNF had a blocking effect mainly on the rise of the neutrophils rather than the basal sputum neutrophilia. This suggests that anti-TNF could be active rather on neutrophilic exacerbations, than on the basal state.

Patients with refractory asthma have evidence of upregulation of the TNF-α axis since they had increased expression of membrane-bound TNF-α, TNF-α receptor 1, and TNF-α−converting enzyme by peripheral-blood monocytes and a 10 weeks of treatment with the soluble TNF receptor, etanercept, was associated with a significant improve in non specific bronchial hyperresponsiveness, post bronchodilator FEV1 and asthma-related quality of life [23]. In moderate asthma, the anti-TNF infliximab had no effect on morning peak expiratory flow, though it reduced of more than 50% the number of moderate exacerbations [24]. A recent case series suggesting that anti-TNF may improve the condition of severe steroid-dependent refractory asthma, with frequent exacerbations and daily symptoms despite close repeated medical evaluation and maximal treatment including oral steroids

[25]. In animal model of allergen sensitization, on the contrary to corticosteroids, anti-TNF does not modify the allergen ovalbumin-induced airways reaction. Though, when ovalbumin is mixed with endotoxin, anti-TNF significantly blocked the inflammatory reaction, suggesting that TNF may play a more prominent pathogenic role in patients with an environmental exposure to endotoxin [26].

The importance of TNF in severe corticoresistant asthma was also suggested by increased protein and gene expression in the airways [27]. The gene expression profiling in induced sputum, shown that upregulation of TNF was associated with neutrophilic asthma [28]. TNF-a is also believed to play a central role in the pathophysiology of COPD [29]. Since, on one side severe asthma and COPD are heterogeneous diseases with different phenotypes and endotypes and, on the other side the TNF inhibitor have blocking effect on endotoxin-induced airways' neutrophilic inflammation, future studies could investigate what kind of patient can benefit from anti-TNF, in regard to their inflammatory sensitivity to endotoxin [30].

Other anti-inflammatory drugs have been evaluated on endotoxin induced airways' inflammation in human. Salmeterol was shown to have a significant anti-inflammatory effect, even when a 100 µg dose of inhaled endotoxin was used [31]. It has been reported that neutrophilic inflammation induced by intra-nasal instillation was reduced by inhibition of CXCR2 (a chemokine receptor antagonist) [32]. Recently an oral CXCR2 antagonist inhibited the induced sputum inflammation, induced by inhaled endotoxin, among healthy

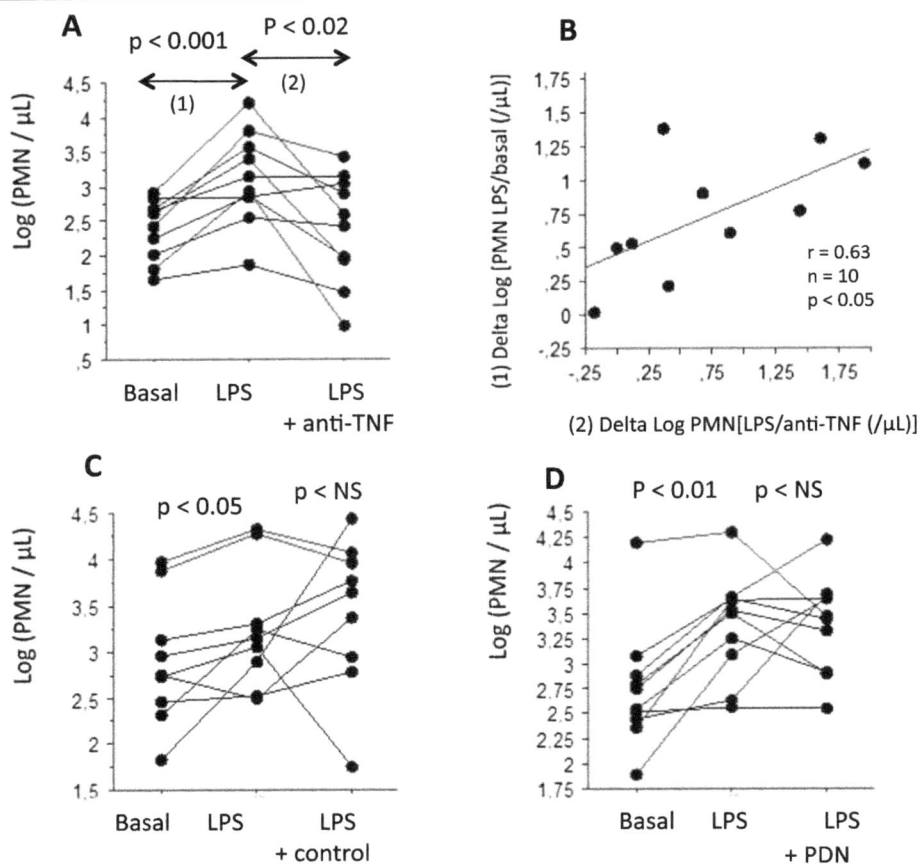

Figure 5 The individual values of the PMN response after endotoxin. A. The individual values of Log count of neutrophils in sputum at the basal state, after endotoxin inhalation(LPS) and after LPS with a previous treatment with anti-TNF (LPS + anti-TNF). **B**. The relationship between the rise of the Log count of neutrophils in sputum after endotoxin (LPS) (vertical axis) with the inhibiting effect of anti-TNF on the LPS response (horizontal axis). **C**. The individual values of Log count of neutrophils in sputum at the basal state, after endotoxin inhalation(LPS) and after LPS among the control group. **D**. The individual values of Log count of neutrophils in sputum at the basal state, after endotoxin inhalation(LPS) and after LPS with a previous treatment with oral steroids (PDN).

volunteers [33]. Simvastatin inhibits inflammatory responses in vitro and in murine models of lung inflammation in vivo; a pretreatment with simvastatinreduced the lung neutrophilic response induced by LPS inhalation in human volunteers [34]. The PDE-4 inhibitors have been also evaluated on the LPS model. Roflumilast reduced the neutrophilic into the airways after segmental bronchial challenge with endotoxin [35] – however not confirmed in a recent study using GMP-grade LPS [21] -, while cilomilast had no effet on the endotoxin-induced sputum neutrophila [11]. Interestingly, the phase III development of cilomilast have been stopped due to a lack of efficacy, while roflumilast has received post-phase III market autorisation. Recently it has been reported that in human volunteers, a pretreatment with vitamin E decreased the neutrophilic airways' response induced by endotoxin [36].

The data obtained with the endotoxin model among healthy subjects have been extrapolated to the COPD patients. Based on their own data, R Kitz et al. concluded

that the endotoxin inflammation is a model to investigate the inflammatory response in human and to improve our understanding of the mechanism of chronic respiratory diseases [37]. Because inhalation of endotoxin induced inflammation mimicking several characteristics of COPD, Korsgen et al. considered that the endotoxin model in human could be used for initial human studies of novel COPD-drugs [38]. According to Aul et al., the endotoxin response could be a suitable model of bacterial exacerbations of COPD since the response is safe, reproducible and associated to translocation of the NF-kB subunit p65 in sputum cells [14]. In a brief review comparing the endotoxin model with ozone and rhinovirus challenges, the endotoxin is the model of choice for new drugs involving the TLR4 receptor, and NF-kB pathway [39]. Since the current data show that endotoxin inflammation is inhibited by adalimumab, a TNF inhibitor, this last could be used as a positive control, in future studies evaluating novel agents.

Conclusions

While oral corticosteroid was not effective, the TNF inhibitor adalimumab blocks the endotoxin-induced neutrophilic airways' inflammation.

Firstly, this endotoxin model could be used to understand the biological effects of compounds that inhibit the LPS induced NF-kB pathway and/or be a model of acute exacerbation of COPD and it could be an early predictor of clinical efficacy of novel therapeutics. Secondly, an anti-TNF treatment could be indicated in chronic respiratory diseases with acute neutrophilic airways' exacerbations, in particular related to endotoxin sensitivity and/or environmental exposure.

Abbreviations

COPD: Chronic obstructive pulmonary disease; CRD: Chronic respiratory diseases; CS: Corticosteroids; FEV1: Forced expiratory volume in one second; FVC: Forced vital capacity; LPS: Lipopolysaccharide; PDN: Prednisolone; PMN: Polymorphonuclear neutrophils; TNF: Tumor necrosis factor.

Competing interests

OM has received research funding from Funxional Therapeutics Ltd. PHDD, VD, FC have declared that they have no competing interests.

Authors' contributions

OM conceived of the study, participated in its design and redaction of the manuscript. PHDD carried out the technical aspects of the sputum induction and LPS challenges. VD participated to the redaction of the manuscript. FC carried out the processing and cellular analysis of the induced sputum. All authors read and approved the final manuscript.

Acknowledgements

Phong Huy Duc Dinh was supported by the Belgium CUD (Commission Universitaire au Développement). The study was partially supported by a grant from Funxional Therapeutics Ltd, Cambridge, United Kingdom.

Author details

[1]Clinic of Allergology and Immunology, CHU Brugmann (Université Libre de Bruxelles - ULB), 4 pl Van Gehuchten, B –1020, Brussels, Belgium. [2]Laboratory of Immunology, CHU Brugmann (Université Libre de Bruxelles - ULB), Brussels, Belgium. [3]Department of Immunology, Pham Ngoc Thach University of Medicine (PNTU), Ho Chi Minh, Vietnam.

References

1. Bousquet J, Kiley J, Bateman ED, Viegi G, Cruz AA, Khaltaev N, Aït Khaled N, Baena-Cagnani CE, Barreto ML, Billo N, Canonica GW, Carlsen KH, Chavannes N, Chuchalin NA, Drazen J, Fabbri LM, Gerbase MW, Humbert M, Joos G, Masjedi MR, Makino S, Rabe K, To T, Zhi L: Prioritised research agenda for prevention and control of chronic respiratory diseases. Eur Respir J 2010, 36:995–1001.
2. Keatings VM, Collins PD, Scott DM, Barnes PJ: Differences in interleukin-8 and tumor necrosis factor-in induced sputum from patients with chronic obstructive pulmonary disease or asthma. Am J Respir Crit Care Med 1996, 153:530–534.
3. Stanescu D, Sanna A, Veriter C, Kostianev S, Calcagni PG, Fabbri LM, Maestrelli P: Airways obstruction, chronic expectoration, and rapid decline of FEV1 in smokers are associated with increased levels of sputum neutrophils. Thorax 1996, 51:267–271.
4. Fraenkel DJ, Bardin PG, Sanderson G, Lampe F, Johnston SL, Holgate ST: Lower airways inflammation during rhinovirus colds in normal and in asthmatic subjects. Am J Respir Crit Care Med 1995, 151:879–886.
5. Keatings VM, Jatakanon A, Worsdell YM, Barnes PJ: Effects of inhaled and oral glucocorticoids on inflammatory indices in asthma and COPD. Am J Respir Crit Care Med 1997, 155:542–8.
6. Culpitt SV, Maziak W, Loukidis S, Nightingale JA, Matthews JL, Barnes PJ: Effect of high dose inhaled steroid on cells, cytokines, and proteases in induced sputum in chronic obstructive pulmonary disease. Am J Respir Crit Care Med 1999, 160:1635–1639.
7. Doull IJ, Lampe FC, Smith S, Schreiber J, Freezer NJ, Holgate ST: Effect of inhaled corticosteroids on episodes of wheezing associated with viral infection in school age children: randomised double blind placebo controlled trial. BMJ 1997, 315:858–862.
8. Vernooy JH, Kucukaycan M, Jacobs JA, Chavannes NH, Buurman WA, Dentener MA, Wouters EF: Local and systemic inflammation in patients with chronic obstructive pulmonary disease: soluble tumor necrosis factor receptors are increased in sputum. Am J Respir Crit Care Med 2002, 166:1218–1224.
9. Barnes PJ, Ito K, Adcock IM: Corticosteroid resistance in chronic obstructive pulmonary disease: inactivation of histone deacetylase. Lancet 2004, 363:731–33.
10. Groneberg DA, Chung KF: Models of chronic obstructive pulmonary disease. Respir Res 2004, 5:18.
11. Michel O, Dentener M, Cataldo D, Cantinieaux B, Vertongen F, Delvaux C, Kelly J: Effects of oral Prednisolone and Cilomilast on LPS-induced inflammation in human. Pulm Pharm Ther 2007, 20:676–83.
12. Hackett TL, Holloway R, Holgate ST, Warner JA: Dynamics of pro-inflammatory and anti-inflammatory cytokine release during acute inflammation in chronic obstructive pulmonary disease: an ex vivo study. Respir Res 2008, 9:47–61.
13. O'Grady NP, Preas HL, Pugin J, Fiuza C, Tropea M, Reda D, Banks SM, Suffredini AF: Local inflammatory responses following bronchial endotoxin instillation in humans. Am J Respir Crit Care Med Vol 2001, 163:1591–8.
14. Aul R, Armstrong J, Duvoix A, Lomas D, Hayes B, Miller BE, Jagger C, Singh D: Inhaled LPS challenges in smokers: a study of pulmonary and systemic effects. Br J Clin Pharmacol 2012, 74:1023–32.
15. Michel O, Duchateau J, Sergysels R: Effect of inhaled endotoxins on bronchial reactivity in asthmatic and normal subjects. J Appl Physiol 1989, 66:1059–1064.
16. Crapo RO, Casaburi R, Coates AL, Enright PL, Hankinson JL, Irvin CG, MacIntyre NR, McKay RT, Wanger JS, Anderson SD, Cockcroft DW, Fish JE, Sterk PJ: Guidelines for methacholine and exercise challenge testing-1999. This official statement of the American Thoracic Society was adopted by the ATS Board of Directors, July 1999. Am J Respir Crit Care Med 2000, 161:309–29.
17. Michel O, Nagy AM, Schroeven M, Duchateau J, Neve J, Fondu P, Sergysels R: Dose–response relationship to inhaled endotoxin in normal subjects. Am J Respir Crit Care Med 1997, 156:1157–1164.
18. Bland JM, Altman DG: Statistical methods to assessing agreement beween two methods of clinical measurement. Lancet 1986, 1(8476):307–10.
19. Doyen V, Kassengera Z, Dinh DHP, Michel O: Time course of endotoxin-induced airways' inflammation in healthy subjects. Inflammation 2012, 35:33–8.
20. Arbour NC, Lorenz E, Schutte BC, Zabner J, Kline JN, Jones M, Frees K, Watt JL, Schwartz DA: TLR4 mutations are associated with endotoxin hyporesponsiveness in humans. Nat Genet 2000, 25:187–91.
21. Janssen O, Schaumann F, Holz O, Lavae-Mokhtari B, Welker L, Winkler C, Winkler C, Biller H, Krug N, Hohlfeld JM: Low-dose endotoxin inhalation in healthy volunteers - a challenge model for early clinical drug development. BMC Pulmonary Medicine 2013, 13:19.
22. Michel O, Doyen V, Leroy B, Bopp B, Dinh DHP, Corazza F, Wattiez R: Expression of calgranulin A/B heterodimer after acute inhalation of endotoxin: proteomic approach and validation. BMC Pulm Med 2013, 13:65.
23. Berry MA, Hargadon B, Shelley M, Parker D, Shaw DE, Green RH, Bradding P, Brightling CE, Wardlaw AJ, Pavord ID: Evidence of a role of tumor necrosis factor alpha in refractory asthma. N Engl J Med 2006, 354:697–708.
24. Erin EM, Leaker BR, Nicholson GC, Tan AJ, Green LM, Neighbour H, Zacharasiewicz AS, Turner J, Barnathan ES, Kon OM, Barnes PJ, Hansel TT: The effects of a monoclonal antibody directed against tumor necrosis factor-alpha in asthma. Am J Respir Crit Care Med 2006, 174:753–62.
25. Taillé C, Poulet C, Marchand-Adam S, Borie R, Dombret MC, Crestani B, Aubier M: Monoclonal anti-TNF-α antibodies for severe steroid-dependent asthma: a case series. Open Respir Med J 2013, 7:21–5.
26. Long AJ, McCarthy R, Rundell L, Goess C, Cuff CA: The efficacy of TNF blockade in asthma models depends on endotoxin levels in the allergic challenge. Proc Am Thorac Soc 2009, 6:331–332.

27. Holgate ST, Polosa R: **The mechanisms, diagnosis, and management of severe asthma in adults.** *Lancet* 2006, **368**(9537):780–93.

28. Baines KJ, Simpson JL, Wood LG, Scott RJ, Gibson PG: **Transcriptional phenotypes of asthma defined by gene expression profiling of induced sputum samples.** *J Allergy Clin Immunol* 2011, **127**:153–160.

29. Murugan V, Peck MJ: **Signal transduction pathways linking the activation of alveolar macrophages with the recruitment of neutrophils to lungs in chronic obstructive pulmonary disease.** *Exp Lung Res* 2009, **35**:439–85.

30. Matera MG, Calzetta L, Cazzola M: **TNF-a inhibitors in asthma and COPD: we must not throw the baby out with the bath water.** *Pulm Pharm Ther* 2010, **23**:121–128.

31. Maris NA, de Vos AF, Dessing MC, Spek CA, Lutter R, Jansen HM, van der Zee JS, Bresser P, van der Poll T: **Anti-inflammatory effects of salmeterol after inhalation of lipopolysaccharide by healthy volunteers.** *Am J Respir Crit Care Med* 2005, **172**:878–84.

32. Virtala R, Ekman AK, Jansson L, Westin U, Cardell LO: **Airway inflammation evaluated in a human nasal lipopolysaccharide challenge model by investigating the effect of a CXCR2 inhibitor.** *Clin Exp Allergy* 2012, **42**:590–6.

33. Leaker BR, Barnes PJ, O'Connor B: **Inhibition of LPS-induced neutrophilic inflammation in healthy volunteers with an oral CXCR2 antagonist.** *Respir Res* 2013, **14**:137.

34. Shyamsundar M, McKeown ST, O'Kane CM, Craig TR, Brown V, Thickett DR, Matthay MA, Taggart CC, Backman JT, Elborn JS, McAuley DF: **Simvastatin decreases lipopolysaccharide-induced pulmonary inflammation in healthy volunteers.** *Am J Respir Crit Care Med* 2009, **179**:1107–14.

35. Hohlfeld JM, Schoenfeld K, Lavae-Mokhtari M, Schaumann F, Mueller M, Bredenbroeker D, Krug N, Hermann R: **Roflumilast attenuates pulmonary inflammation upon segmental endotoxin challenge in healthy subjects: a randomized placebo-controlled trial.** *Pulm Pharmacol Ther* 2008, **21**:616–23.

36. Hernandez ML, Wagner JG, Kala A, Mills K, Wells HB, Alexis NE, Lay JC, Jiang Q, Zhang H, Zhou H, Peden DB: **Vitamin E, γ-tocopherol, reduces airway neutrophil recruitment after inhaled endotoxin challenge in rats and in healthy volunteers.** *Free Radic Biol Med* 2013, **60**:56–62.

37. Kitz R, Rose MA, Placzek K, Schulze J, Zielen S, Schubert R: **LPS inhalation challenge: a new tool to characterize the infammatory response in humans.** *Med Microbiol Immunol* 2008, **197**:13–19.

38. Korsgren M, Linden M, Entwistle N, Cook J, Wollmer P, Andersson M, Larsson B, Greiff L: **Inhalation of LPS induces inflammatory airway responses mimicking characteristics of chronic obstructive pulmonary disease.** *Clin Physiol Funct Imaging* 2012, **32**:71–9.

39. van der Merwe R, Molfino NA: **Challenge models to assess new therapies in chronic obstructive pulmonary disease.** *Int J Chron Obstruct Pulmon Dis* 2012, **7**:597–605.

16

Microbiological contamination in counterfeit and unapproved drugs

Dieter Pullirsch[1*], Julie Bellemare[2], Andreas Hackl[1], Yvon-Louis Trottier[2], Andreas Mayrhofer[1], Heidemarie Schindl[1], Christine Taillon[2], Christian Gartner[1], Brigitte Hottowy[1], Gerhard Beck[1] and Jacques Gagnon[2*]

Abstract

Background: Counterfeit and unapproved medicines are inherently dangerous and can cause patient injury due to ineffectiveness, chemical or biological contamination, or wrong dosage. Growth of the counterfeit medical market in developed countries is mainly attributable to life-style drugs, which are used in the treatment of non-life-threatening and non-painful conditions, such as slimming pills, cosmetic-related pharmaceuticals, and drugs for sexual enhancement. One of the main tasks of health authorities is to identify the exact active pharmaceutical ingredients (APIs) in confiscated drugs, because wrong API compounds, wrong concentrations, and/or the presence of chemical contaminants are the main risks associated with counterfeit medicines. Serious danger may also arise from microbiological contamination. We therefore performed a market surveillance study focused on the microbial burden in counterfeit and unapproved medicines.

Methods: Counterfeit and unapproved medicines confiscated in Canada and Austria and controls from the legal market were examined for microbial contaminations according to the US and European pharmacopoeia guidelines. The microbiological load of illegal and legitimate samples was statistically compared with the Wilcoxon rank-sum test.

Results: Microbial cultivable contaminations in counterfeit and unapproved phosphodiesterase type 5 inhibitors were significantly higher than in products from the legal medicines market ($p < 0.0001$). Contamination levels exceeding the USP and EP limits were seen in 23% of the tested illegal samples in Canada. Additionally, microbiological contaminations above the pharmacopoeial limits were detected in an anabolic steroid and an herbal medicinal product in Austria (6% of illegal products tested).

Conclusions: Our results show that counterfeit and unapproved pharmaceuticals are not manufactured under the same hygienic conditions as legitimate products. The microbiological contamination of illegal medicinal products often exceeds USP and EP limits, representing a potential threat to consumer health.

Background

The counterfeiting of pharmaceuticals has been a known problem for decades. In recent years, the challenge has escalated and the numbers of counterfeit drugs have increased continuously, not only in developing but also in developed countries [1]. Available estimates on the value of the global market for counterfeit drugs are in the range of US$ 75 to US$ 200 billion, indicating the significance of the problem [1,2]. In West Africa alone, the illegal anti-malarial drug market may exceed US$ 400 million [3,4]. In developed countries, life-style drugs, such as phosphodiesterase type 5 (PDE5) inhibitors used for the treatment

of erectile dysfunction, seem to be the main targets for counterfeiting [5]. In the face of rising drug costs, counterfeit versions of cancer drugs and other life-saving medicines are also on the rise worldwide [6]. Overall, any medication that is in high demand is an attractive target for counterfeiters [5].

According to the definition by the World Health Organization (WHO), a counterfeit medicine is "one which is deliberately and fraudulently mislabelled with respect to identity and/or source. Counterfeiting can apply to both branded and generic products and counterfeit products may include products with the correct ingredients or with the wrong ingredients, without active ingredients, with insufficient active ingredients or with fake packaging" [7]. However, "a counterfeit drug is defined differently in different countries" [7].

---

* Correspondence: Dieter.Pullirsch@ages.at; Jacques.Gagnon@hc-sc.gc.ca
[1]AGES - Austrian Agency for Health & Food Safety, Austrian Medicines and Medical Devices Agency, Traisengasse 5, Vienna AT-1200, Austria
[2]Health Canada, 1001 St-Laurent West, Longueuil, Qc J4K 1C7, Canada

Unapproved medicines are drugs sold or imported without having been granted a marketing authorisation by health authorities [8]. Unapproved drugs are often marketed as being similar to, or a foreign version of, an approved drug. Such medicines may indeed comply with the quality standards in their country of origin, but because they are not imported or sold through the legal supply chain, their origin often remains unclear and their compliance with the quality standards of the target country cannot be verified [9,10].

Consumers are generally unaware of the dangers associated with the use of counterfeit and unapproved life-style drugs. Next to treatments for erectile dysfunction, appearance-enhancing medications such as slimming pills or anabolic steroids are in high demand. While non-treatment with these drugs does not lead to detrimental health effects, their use can result in dangerous adverse effects caused by overdosed content or contaminations [6]. Additionally, consumers of life-style drugs often bypass the healthcare system, so that underlying diseases, such as coronary artery disease, obesity, or anorexia, cannot be detected and pharmacodynamic or pharmacokinetic interactions with other drugs or substances cannot be identified and prevented [5].

Security and encryption experts are continuously working to devise new methods to protect originator drugs from being counterfeited. Thus, secret colour compositions and packaging materials as well as holograms interpretable only with laser readers have been developed to prevent counterfeits from entering the legal supply chain [11]. Yet, counterfeit drugs in developed countries are mainly detected on the illegal pharmaceutical market. Consumers buy medications via the internet to save money or time or because they are too embarrassed about their health problems to seek professional help [5]. The WHO estimates that 50% of medicines bought from online pharmacies that do not list their physical address are counterfeits [12].

The pharmacological content of counterfeit medicines has been examined by both authorities and manufacturers of original products [5]. For example, with PDE5 inhibitors being a main target for counterfeiting, they have been extensively studied [13,14]. A serious incident with counterfeit PDE5 inhibitors occurred in Singapore in 2008, when 4 people died due to hypoglycaemia caused by counterfeits contaminated with glyburide [15].

Microbial contamination and infection are known to be serious risks associated with illegal drug use, the legal use of pharmaceuticals distributed under poor hygienic conditions, and counterfeit medicines for parenteral administration [16-18]. For example, according to a recently published report from Shanghai, China, intravitreal injection of counterfeit bevacizumab contaminated with endotoxin caused acute intraocular inflammation in a series of 80 patients, 21 of whom had to undergo vitrectomy as a result [19]. Whereas parenteral pharmaceuticals must be sterile, non-sterile products may be administered to regions of the human body that are rich in microbial flora and have physical or immunological barriers to infection [20]. However, the US and European pharmacopoeiae state that even in non-sterile preparations, the presence of certain microorganisms "may have the potential to reduce or even inactivate the therapeutic activity of the product and has a potential to adversely affect the health of the patient. Manufacturers therefore have to ensure a low bioburden of finished dosage forms by implementing current guidelines on Good Manufacturing Practice during the manufacture, storage and distribution of pharmaceutical preparations" [21,22]. Microbiological contamination levels above pharmacopoeial limits may lead to alterations and spoilage of active ingredients and cause adverse effects by infections or toxins.

We here present the results from marketing surveillance studies performed by the Canadian and Austrian official control laboratories between 2008 and 2011 on microbiological contaminations in illegal medicines. Because microbial contamination is a well-known and already widely documented threat for sterile parenteral medicines and because counterfeit and unapproved drugs are frequently sold as solid dosage forms, the main focus of our studies was on solid life-style drugs.

Methods

All experiments were performed by Health Canada and by the AGES Austrian Medicines and Medical Devices Agency. Both organizations are responsible for market surveillance in their respective countries.

Canadian study design

Health Canada defines a counterfeit health product as one that is represented as, and likely to be mistaken for, an authentic product [23]. Analyses focused on randomly selected counterfeit and unapproved drugs for the treatment of erectile dysfunction from the illegal market. Twenty-one counterfeit and 31 unapproved PDE5 inhibitors were analysed for microbial contamination. As controls, samples of all available PDE5 inhibitors were obtained from the legal market (Viagra® 25, 50, 100 mg; Cialis® 2.5, 5, 10, 20 mg; Levitra® 5, 10, 20 mg) and analysed. All counterfeit and unapproved samples had been seized by the Royal Canadian Mounted Police or Border Integrity Officers between 2008 and 2010.

The drugs were tested for compliance with the US Pharmacopoeia. A total of five microbiological analyses were performed on the samples: total aerobic microbial count (TAMC), total yeast and mould count (TYMC), pathogens (Escherichia coli, Pseudomonas aeroginosa, Salmonella, and Staphylococcus aureus), and enumeration of enterobacteriae and anaerobic bacteria. All analyses, including handling procedures, dilutions, and culture media, were conducted in accordance with the US Pharmacopoeia (USP), Chapters 61 and 62 [24,25], which are harmonized with the European Pharmacopoeia (EP). The assay for sildenafil citrate content was performed according to the corresponding USP monograph.

Austrian study design

According to the European Medicines Agency, counterfeit medicines are medicines that fail to comply with intellectual-property rights or infringe trademark law [26].

Seven counterfeit PDE5 inhibitors and 26 unapproved medicines (25 solid dosage forms and 1 herbal tea) from the illegal market were randomly selected and analysed for microbial contamination. Unapproved medicines consisted of suspected performance-enhancing drugs or slimming agents (Table 1). As a reference, PDE5 inhibitor products (Viagra® 50 mg; Cialis® 10 mg; Levitra® 10 mg) were obtained from the legal market and examined for microbial contaminations. The drugs had been seized by the Austrian police and the Austrian customs agency between 2008 and 2011. All samples were tested for EP compliance. As in the Canadian study, analyses for TAMC, TYMC, pathogens (*Escherichia coli, Pseudomonas aeroginosa, Salmonella* and *Staphylococcus aureus*), enterobacteriae, and anaerobic bacteria were performed as applicable. All analyses, including handling procedures, dilutions and culture media, were conducted in accordance with the EP, Chapters 2.6.12, 2.6.13, and 2.6.31 [27-29], which are harmonized with the USP. The assay for sildenafil citrate content was performed according to the corresponding EP monograph.

Acceptance criteria in the USP and EP

According to the USP and EP, the acceptance criteria for non-aqueous preparations for oral use are 10^3 colony-forming units (CFU)/g in the TAMC test and 10^2 CFU/g in the TYMC test. The acceptance criterion for herbal products with cold extraction is 10^5 CFU/g in the TAMC test, 10^4 in the TYMC test, and 10^4 for bile-tolerant gram-negative bacteria.

According to the USP and EP, the acceptance criteria of 10^3 CFU/g were interpreted as a maximum acceptable count of 2000 CFU/g. The acceptance criterion of 10^5 CFU/g for herbal products with cold extraction was interpreted as a maximum acceptable count of 500 000 CFU/g.

Statistical analysis

Due to the skewed distribution of microbiological burden, the non-parametric Wilcoxon rank-sum test, applying the normal approximation, was used to test for differences between medicines in the degree of microbiological contamination. In addition, Fisher's exact test was used to compare contamination after dichotomization, both with respect to no/any microbiological burden as well as

Table 1 Microbiological contamination in counterfeit and unapproved drugs in the Austrian study

Product	Microbial load		
	TAMC (CFU/g)	TYMC (CFU/g)	Pathogens
Approved PDE5 inhibitors			
Sildenafil 50 mg	< 5	< 5	nd
Tadalafil 10 mg	< 5	< 5	nd
Vardenafil 10 mg	< 5	< 5	nd
Counterfeit PDE5 inhibitors			
Sildenafil 100 mg #1	< 5	< 5	nd
Sildenafil 100 mg #2	< 5	10	negative
Sildenafil 100 mg #3	< 5	< 5	nd
Sildenafil 100 mg #4	< 5	< 5	nd
Sildenafil 100 mg #5	< 5	< 5	nd
Sildenafil 100 mg #6	170	< 5	negative
Tadalafil 80 mg #7	< 5	< 5	nd
Other unapproved products			
Zinc gluconate #8	< 5	< 5	nd
Nicotic acid #9	< 5	< 5	nd
Methandienone #10	80	< 5	negative
Methandienone #11	11 000	< 5	negative
Mephedrone HCl #12	n/a	n/a	n/a
Butylone HCl #13	n/a	n/a	n/a
Methandienone #14	80	60	negative
Stanozolol #15	100	< 5	negative
Stanozolol #16	110	< 5	negative
Clenbuterole 0.02 mg #17	< 5	< 5	nd
Sibutramine, phenolphtalein #18	20	40	negative
Sildenafil 100 mg #19	< 5	< 5	nd
4-Methylethcathinone #20	< 5	< 5	nd
4-Methylcathinone/Coffein #21	< 5	< 5	n/a
4-Methylcathinone/Coffein #22	< 5	< 5	n/a
4-Methylcathinone/Coffein #23	< 5	< 5	nd
3-Fluoromethcathinone/ Lidocaine/Coffein #24	< 5	< 5	nd
Coffein/Acetylsalicylic acid #25	< 5	< 5	nd
Slimming herb #26 (herbal product)	720 000	4 000	>10^4 bile-tolerant gram-negative bacteria

TAMC: Total aerobic microbial count; TYMC: Total yeast and mould count; nd: Not determined; n/a: Not applicable (interfering substance prevented successful completion of the test).
Illegal medicines confiscated in Austria were analysed for microbiological contaminations by microbial enumeration tests and tests for specific pathogens.

with respect to the acceptance limit of < = 2000 CFU/g versus >2000 CFU/g as defined according to the USP and EP. All statistical tests are presented with two-sided significance levels. The Wilcoxon rank-sum test comparing microbiological contamination of legal versus illegal (counterfeit and unapproved) medicines was considered the primary analysis.

Results

Only counterfeit and unapproved PDE inhibitors showed increased contamination

Not a single CFU was detected in the approved PDE5 inhibitor products obtained through the legal pharmaceutical supply chain—neither in the Canadian nor in the Austrian study. Thus, although the USP and EP allow an upper limit of 10^3 CFU/g, no cultivable microbial contaminations were detected for these pharmaceuticals produced under controlled GMP conditions (Figure 1).

In the Canadian study, 12 of the 31 unapproved PDE5 inhibitor samples (39%) were contaminated with more than 10^3 CFU/g (Figure 1). Taking counterfeit and unapproved drugs together, 12 of the 52 samples (23%) were contaminated with more than 10^3 CFU/g, 36 samples (69%) showed increased levels of microbial contamination that were within the acceptable limits, and only 4 of the 52 illegal products (8%) showed excellent results with no cultivable contamination.

In the Austrian study, none of the 7 counterfeit PDE5 inhibitor samples tested showed a microbial contamination above the EP limit. Contamination with colony-forming microorganisms within EP limits was found in 2 of the 7 samples (29%, Table 1).

Statistical analysis of increased microbiological burden in counterfeit and unapproved PDE5 inhibitors in Canada

Wilcoxon rank-sum and Fisher's exact tests were performed to test for statistical significance of observed differences between legal and illegal (counterfeit and unapproved) PDE5 inhibitors in Canada. In the Wilcoxon rank-sum test, the degree of microbiological contamination (CFU/g) in illegal medicines was significantly higher than in the legal products ($p < 0.0001$, two-sided). The Fisher's exact test demonstrated that the number of contaminated illegal samples (>0 CFU/g; as opposed to no contamination at all) was statistically significantly higher than in legal samples ($p < 0.0001$, two-sided). Overall, therefore, both the number of cultivable contaminations (Wilcoxon rank-sum test) and the number of contaminated samples (>0 CFU/g; Fisher's exact test) were significantly higher among illegal PDE5 inhibitors.

Comparison for non-compliance with the pharmacopoeia limits (>2000 CFU/g) did not show a statistically significant difference between illegal and legal medicines, but a clear trend was observed ($p = 0.1864$, two-sided Fisher's exact test). Unapproved medicines showed a clear statistically significant increase of non-compliance when compared to the counterfeit products ($p < 0.0001$, two-sided Fisher's exact test).

Due to the limited number of PDE5 inhibitors from Austria, statistical analysis was only performed for the Canadian market.

Bacillus contaminations were frequent in counterfeit and unapproved PDE5 inhibitors

The identified species are summarized in Table 2. None of the pathogens specifically defined in the pharmacopeiae were detected. Amongst others, mainly contaminations with *Bacillus* ssp. were observed. Identified *Bacillus* species included *B. firmus, B. lentus, B. megaterium, B. pumilus, B. polymyxa, B. subtillis/amyloliquefaciens/atrophaeus, B. licheniformis, B. cereus/thuringensis/mycoides, B. pumilus, B. coagulans, B. fusiformis, B. circulans,* and *B. glucanolyticus.*

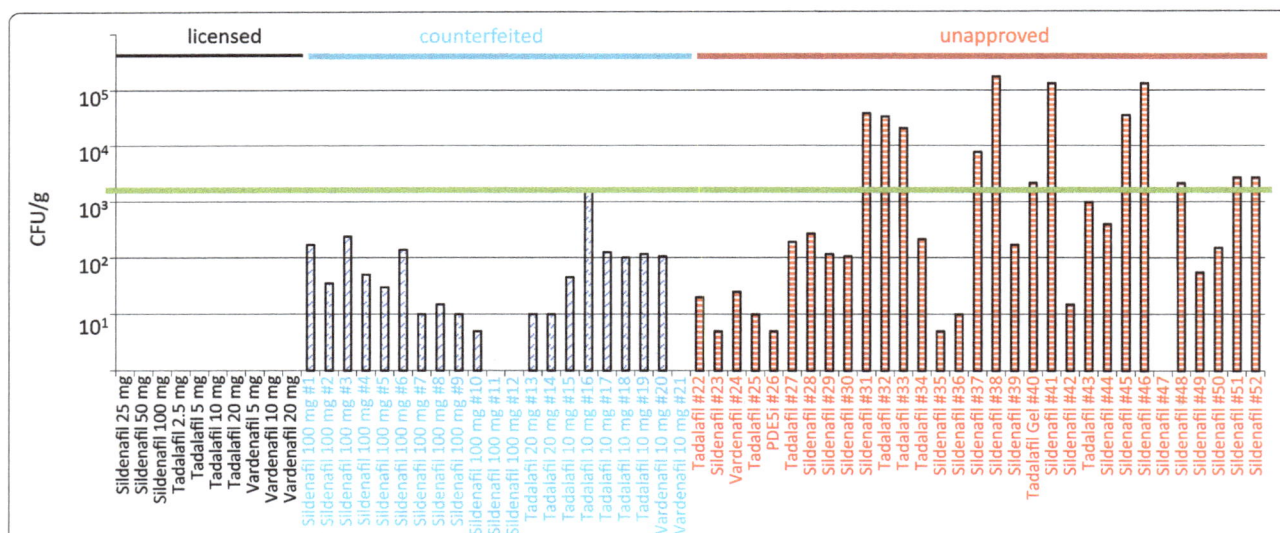

Figure 1 Microbiological load in PDE5 inhibitors in Canada. Products from the legal market (black), counterfeit (blue), and unapproved (red) drugs were tested for microbiological contamination. The pharmacopoeial limits of 10^3 CFU (2000 counts)/g are indicated by the green line.

Table 2 Identified bacterial species in counterfeit and illegal PDE inhibitors in the Canadian study

Product	Identified bacteria
Approved PDE5 inhibitors	
Sildenafil 25 mg	n/a
Sildenafil 50 mg	n/a
Sildenafil 100 mg	n/a
Tadalafil 2.5 mg	n/a
Tadalafil 5 mg	n/a
Tadalafil 10 mg	n/a
Tadalafil 20 mg	n/a
Vardenafil 5 mg	n/a
Vardenafil 10 mg	n/a
Vardenafil 20 mg	n/a
Counterfeit PDE5 inhibitors	
Sildenafil 100 mg #1	Bacillus spp.
Sildenafil 100 mg #2	Serratia spp., Paenibacillus polymyxa, Paenibacillus amylolyticus, Bacillus ssp., Paenibacillus gluconolyticus, Corynebacterium spp., Brevibacillus borstelensis
Sildenafil 100 mg #3	Brevibacillus choshinensys, Bacillus spp.
Sildenafil 100 mg #4	Bacillus ssp.
Sildenafil 100 mg #5	Bacillus spp.
Sildenafil 100 mg #6	Bacillus ssp., Brevibacillus choshinensys, Virgibacillus pantothenticus, Alicyclobacillus acidoterrestris, Sphingomonas paucimobilis, Paenibacillus polymyxa, Propionibacterium acnes, Brevibacillus borstelensis, Bacillus spp.
Sildenafil 100 mg #7	Micrococcus luteus
Sildenafil 100 mg #8	Bacillus ssp., Propionibacterium acnes
Sildenafil 100 mg #9	Paenibacillus amylolyticus
Sildenafil 100 mg #10	Brevibacillus choshinensys
Sildenafil 100 mg #11	n/a
Sildenafil 100 mg #12	n/a
Tadalafil 20 mg #13	Bacillus ssp.
Tadalafil 20 mg #14	Kocuria rosea, Bacillus pumilus
Tadalafil 10 mg #15	Bacillus spp
Tadalafil 10 mg #16	Bacillus spp
Tadalafil 10 mg #17	Granulicatella adiacens, Streptococcus salivarus, Bacillus spp
Tadalafil 10 mg #18	Bacillus spp
Tadalafil 10 mg #19	Bacillus spp
Vardenafil 20 mg #20	Bacillus spp
Vardenafil 20 mg #21	n/a
Unapproved PDE5 inhibitors	
Tadalafil #22	Paenibacillus lautus, Paenibacillus durus, Paenibacillus glucanolyticus, Bacillus spp.
Sildenafil #23	Bacillus ssp., Paenibacillus spp.
Vardenafil #24	Bacillus ssp.
Tadalafil #25	Staphylococcus epidermidis, Bacillus spp.

Table 2 Identified bacterial species in counterfeit and illegal PDE inhibitors in the Canadian study *(Continued)*

PDE5 inhibitor #26	Bacillus spp.,
Tadalafil #27	Bacillus spp.
Sildenafil #28	Bacillus spp.
Sildenafil #29	Bacillus spp.
Sildenafil #30	Bacillus spp., Sphingomonas paucimobilis, aerobic Actinomycetes
Sildenafil #31	Bacillus spp.
Tadalafil #32	Bacillus spp.
Tadalafil #33	Bacillus spp.
Tadalafil #34	Granulicatella adiacens, Streptococcus salivarus, Bacillus spp.
Sildenafil #35	Bacillus spp.
Sildenafil #36	Bacillus spp., Micrococcus spp.
Sildenafil #37	Bacillus spp.
Sildenafil #38	Bacillus spp.
Sildenafil #39	Bacillus spp.
Tadafenil #40	Bacillus spp.
Sildenafil #41	Bacillus spp.
Sildenafil #42	Bacillus spp.
Tadafenil #43	Bacillus spp., Staphylococcus hominis
Sildenafil #44	Bacillus spp.
Sildenafil #45	Bacillus spp.
Sildenafil #46	Bacillus spp.
Sildenafil #47	Bacillus spp.
Sildenafil #48	Bacillus spp.
Sildenafil #49	Bacillus spp.
Sildenafil #50	Bacillus spp.
Sildenafil #51	Bacillus spp.
Sildenafil #52	Bacillus spp.

n/a: Not applicable.
Bacterial species identified in the contaminated samples of Figure 1.

Inconsistent doses of active pharmaceutical ingredients in counterfeit PDE5 inhibitors

Although this was not the main focus of our study, we also examined the content of active ingredients in the counterfeit samples (Additional file 1). Of all 26 counterfeits tested, 24 (92%) did not contain the labelled amount of PDE5 inhibitor (acceptance criterion ± 10% of the labelled amount). In 21 samples (81%), a reduced content of the active ingredient was detected, whereas 3 samples (12%) were about 2-fold over-dosed. Interestingly, 14 of the 26 samples (54%) also contained trace amounts of a second PDE5 inhibitor.

Microbiological contamination in other product classes tested

When examining the 25 non-PDE5-inhibitor unapproved medicines with solid dosage forms from the Austrian market, one product containing methandienone was contaminated with 1.1×10^4 CFU/g in the TAMC test, thus exceeding the EP limit of 10^3 CFU/g. Of the 25 unapproved medicines, one (4%) did not comply with EP standards and an additional 7 (28%) showed a microbial load higher than that seen in the legal products manufactured under defined GMP conditions.

Increased microbiological burden in an unapproved herbal product

One unapproved herbal medicinal product was tested in Austria. The product contained brown-coloured dried plant tissue and was contaminated with 720 000 CFU/g in the TAMC test (Table 1), exceeding the acceptance criterion of 10^5 CFU/g (maximum of 500 000 counts). Besides, the sample also exceeded the EP limit of 10^4 CFU/g of bile-tolerant gram-negative bacteria. *Klebsiella pneumonia* was identified as the prevalent bile-tolerant species.

Discussion

The microbiological content in non-sterile products has to be controlled to a level consistent with patient safety [20]. Microbial enumeration tests are required to demonstrate production under acceptable hygienic conditions. Whenever pharmacopoeial limits are exceeded, the microbiological quality of manufacturing was not sufficiently controlled and adverse effects on product and patient safety cannot be excluded. Additionally, according to the US and European pharmacopoeiae, the significance of recovered microorganisms must be evaluated and the absence of specific pathogens demonstrated depending on the route of administration [21,22]. Microbiological contaminations may be introduced by the raw material, through the manufacturing process, or during packaging and transport, and risk-based control points should be incorporated into the manufacturing process [20].

Our data, derived from independent studies performed in two different pharmaceutical markets, confirm that counterfeit and unapproved medicines are not manufactured under the same hygienic condition as genuine products. The Canadian and Austrian studies presented both showed that none of the PDE5 inhibitors from the legitimate supply chain produced under GMP conditions contained any microbial burden detectable by routine pharmacopoeial testing, whereas 92% of Canadian and 29% of Austrian PDE5 inhibitor samples seized from the illegal market contained cultivable contaminations. Also, 23% of counterfeit and unapproved PDE5 inhibitors seized in Canada and 6% of all tested samples from the Austria illegal market failed to comply with the pharmacopoeial limits in microbial enumeration tests.

In the Canadian study, the microbiological contaminations in unapproved products were higher than in counterfeit products. It may be hypothesized that individuals producing counterfeit products may be more intent on using reasonably safe production conditions than those trading in unapproved products. However, the difference between counterfeit and unapproved products seen in our study may not be generalizable. Thus, we found that both product groups contained higher amounts of microbiological contaminations than products from the legal market, indicating that both groups may be expected to be prepared under less hygienic production conditions than genuine medicinal products. In the Austrian study, a higher rate of contaminations above EP limits was also observed for unapproved than in counterfeit products, but due to the different nature of the products tested in Austria, direct statistical comparison was not performed.

Most identified contaminating bacteria in PDE5 inhibitors belong to the *Bacillus* genus. *Bacillus ssp.* can form resistant endospores and are part of the normal environmental flora [30]. This may be indicative of contamination by human manipulators. Although no major pathogens were isolated, some of the identified *Bacillus species* are capable of causing human infection [30]. Besides, *Serratia* species, *Propionibacterium acnes*, *Granulicatella adiacens*, *Streptococcus salivarus*, *Staphylococcus epidermidis*, *Staphylococcus hominis*, *Enterococcus gallinarum*, and *Sphingomonas paucimobilis* were identified and have the potential to cause clinical symptoms of infection [31,32]. In view of the oral route of administration of PDE5 inhibitors, the bacterial species detected may not pose an increased risk to consumers, provided that the total counts do not exceed pharmacopoeial limits.

Klebsiella pneumoniae was identified in an unapproved herbal medicinal tea, with the included package leaflet recommending extraction with cold water. This method of extraction may not be expected to reduce viable contaminations. *K. pneumoniae* is a gram-negative bacterium that can cause bacterial pneumonia and hospital-acquired urinary tract and wound infections [33]. *K. pneumoniae* mainly attacks immunocompromised patients and individuals with underlying diseases, such as diabetes mellitus [33]. The examined infusion failed to comply with the EP limits for bile-tolerant gram-negative bacteria and for total bacterial counts (TAMC). Although the concentrations of *K. pneumoniae* detected in this product are unlikely to lead to clinical infection in healthy humans [34], a potential threat cannot be excluded, especially when storage conditions are not monitored and further bacterial growth might occur.

Two potential threats arise from microbiological contaminations in pharmaceutical products. First, certain microorganisms may alter the quality of the active ingredients and even lead to spoilage of the product. Second, microbiological contaminations may directly cause adverse effects by producing toxins or causing infections. Product alterations are less likely in solid PDE5 inhibitors but may occur in herbal products. In general, the threats from microbiological contaminations are higher for herbal products and products with a moisture content that supports bacterial survival and growth than for solid dosage forms. Accordingly, a recent study found high levels of bacterial contaminations in counterfeit toothpaste [35], and an outbreak of *Salmonella montevideo* has been associated with a dietary herbal food supplement [36]. Herbal products show higher levels and limits of contamination because of the raw materials they contain and the mild production methods used. In contrast, PDE5 inhibitors are less likely to be contaminated with bacteria due to the synthetisation process of the active substances, the chemicals used, and the low moisture content. Even in synthesised medicines, however, contaminations by excipients or cutting agents and human manipulation during manufacture and transport pose a risk when hygienic production conditions are not guaranteed. In recent years, several cases of injectional anthrax most likely caused by contaminated heroin have been described in Europe [37]. Suggested routes of contaminations included animal-derived sources, such as bone meal or animal hides [38]. Although this is clearly a worst-case scenario associated with injectional administration of an illicit drug, it illustrates that the lack of controls during manufacturing and/or transport of pharmaceutical active substances can lead to contamination with severe pathogens. Interestingly, despite good evidence for the cause of infection, neither *B. anthracis* nor its genome was detected in any of the heroin samples tested [37]. The production of illegal drugs and illegal pharmaceuticals might differ, but for both, in the absence of strictly quality-controlled hygienic production conditions, even testing for specific pathogens may not be sufficient to detect serious contaminations.

Conclusions

Based on our studies, it may be assumed that various groups of illegal medications contain increased levels of microbial contaminations. Our results demonstrate that illegal pharmaceuticals are produced under less hygienic conditions than legitimate products manufactured under controlled and defined GMP conditions.

To gain broader insights into the microbiological burden in counterfeit drugs, we recommend the risk-based inclusion of microbiological quality studies in the surveillance of the illegal pharmaceutical market.

Additional file

Additional file 1: PDE5 inhibitor content in counterfeit drugs from Canada and Austria. Inconsistent doses of active pharmaceutical ingredients were detected in counterfeit PD5 inhibitors.

Competing interests
The authors declare that they have no competing interests.

Authors' contributions
All authors read and approved the final manuscript. DP collected and analysed the data and drafted the article. YLT and CT analysed the results, drafted the study report by Health Canada, and critically revised the article. JB and JG planned and designed the Canadian study part, analysed the Canadian results, and critically revised the article. AH, HS, GB, and AM planned and designed the Austrian part of the study and analysed the data. BG performed the experiments and analysed the results. CG performed the statistical analyses of the results and critically revised the article.

Acknowledgements
The authors wish to thank Geneviève Dufour, Catherine Deschênes, Karine Lebel, and Isabelle Disnard for technical analysis and Daniel Plante, France Gaudreault, Petra Schlick, and Samantha Hewavitharana for critical reading of the article.

Disclaimer
This publication does not necessarily reflect the opinion of the AGES, Health Canada, or other authorities.

References

1. World Health Organization: Growing threat from counterfeit medicines. *Bull World Health Organ* 2010, **88**(4):247–248.
2. Mackey TK, Liang BA: Improving global health governance to combat counterfeit medicines: a proposal for a UNODC-WHO-Interpol trilateral mechanism. *BMC Med* 2013, **11**:233.
3. Gostin LO, Buckley GJ, Kelley PW: Stemming the global trade in falsified and substandard medicines. *JAMA* 2013, **309**(16):1693–1694.
4. United Nations Office on Drugs and Crime: Transnational trafficking and the rule of law in West Africa: a threat assessment. 2009, https://www.unodc.org/documents/data-and-analysis/Studies/West_Africa_Report_2009.pdf (accessed on 2013-02-12).
5. Jackson G, Patel S, Khan S: Assessing the problem of counterfeit medications in the United Kingdom. *Int J Clin Pract* 2012, **66**(3):241–250.
6. Jackson G: Faking it: the dangers of counterfeit medicine on the internet. *Int J Clin Pract* 2009, **63**(2):181.
7. World Health Organization: General information on counterfeit medicines. http://www.who.int/medicines/services/counterfeit/overview/en/ (accessed 2013-02-04).
8. Jung C: Evaluating FDA Communications to Reduce Counterfeit and Unapproved Drugs in the Clinical Setting. In *Risk Communication Advisory Committee Meeting*; 2013. http://www.fda.gov/downloads/AdvisoryCommittees/CommitteesMeetingMaterials/RiskCommunicationAdvisoryCommittee/UCM370232.pdf (accessed 2013-11-29).
9. U.S. Food and Drug Administration: Letters to doctors about risks of purchasing unapproved versions of botox and other medications from foreign or unlicensed suppliers. http://www.fda.gov/Drugs/DrugSafety/DrugIntegrityandSupplyChainSecurity/ucm330610.htm, (accessed 02-12-2013).
10. U.S. Food and Drug Administration: Fraudulent versions of botox found in the United States. http://www.fda.gov/drugs/drugsafety/ucm349503.htm , accessed 02-12-2013.
11. Schubert C: New countermeasures considered as drug counterfeiting grows. *Nat Med* 2008, **14**(7):700.
12. Mackey TK, Liang BA: The global counterfeit drug trade: patient safety and public health risks. *J Pharm Sci* 2011, **100**(11):4571–4579.
13. Jackson G, Arver S, Banks I, Stecher VJ: Counterfeit phosphodiesterase type 5 inhibitors pose significant safety risks. *Int J Clin Pract* 2010, **64**(4):497–504.
14. Low MY, Zeng Y, Li L, Ge XW, Lee R, Bloodworth BC, Koh HL: Safety and quality assessment of 175 illegal sexual enhancement products seized in red-light districts in Singapore. *Drug Saf* 2009, **32**(12):1141–1146.
15. Kao SL, Chan CL, Tan B, Lim CC, Dalan R, Gardner D, Pratt E, Lee M, Lee KO: An unusual outbreak of hypoglycemia. *N Engl J Med* 2009, **360**(7):734–736.
16. Liang BA: Fade to black: importation and counterfeit drugs. *Am J Law Med* 2006, **32**(2–3):279–323.
17. Kaushik KS, Kapila K, Praharaj AK: Shooting up: the interface of microbial infections and drug abuse. *J Med Microbiol* 2011, **60**(Pt 4):408–422.

18. Mugoyela V, Mwambete KD: **Microbial contamination of nonsterile pharmaceuticals in public hospital settings.** *Ther Clin Risk Manag* 2010, 6:443–448.

19. Wang F, Yu S, Liu K, Chen FE, Song Z, Zhang X, Xu X, Sun X: **Acute intraocular inflammation caused by endotoxin after intravitreal injection of counterfeit bevacizumab in Shanghai China.** *Ophthalmology* 2013, 120(2):355–361.

20. U.S. Pharmacopoeial Convention: **Bioburden Control of Non-sterile Drug Substances and Products - Draft.** In *United States Pharmacopoeia*. Rockville: USP 39 (4) In-Process Revision, U.S. Pharmacopoeial Convention; 2013.

21. U.S. Pharmacopoeial Convention: **Microbiological Examination of non-sterile Products: Acceptance Criteria for pharmaceutical Preparations and Substances for pharmaceutical use.** In *United States Pharmacopoeia*. Rockville: General Chapter 1111((USP 35): 1733), U.S. Pharmacopoeial Convention; 2012.

22. European Directorate for the Quality of Medicines & HealthCare: **Microbiological Quality of non-sterile Pharmaceutical Preparations and Substances for Pharmaceutical use.** In *European Pharmacopoeia 70*. Strasbourg: Chapter 5.1.4, EDQM; 2011.

23. Health Canada: *Policy on Counterfeit Health Products POL-0048*. Ottawa, Ontario: Policy and Strategic Planning Division, Health Products and Food Branch Inspectorate; 2010.

24. U.S. Pharmacopoeial Convention: **Microbiological examination of nonsterile products: microbiological enumeration tests.** In *United States Pharmacopeia*. Rockville: General Chapter 61(USP 35), U.S. Pharmacopoeial Convention; 2012:56–60.

25. U.S. Pharmacopoeial Convention: **Microbiological examination of nonsterile products: tests for specified microorganisms.** In *United States Pharmacopeia*. Rockville: General Chapter 62 (USP 35), U.S. Pharmacopoeial Convention; 2012:60–61.

26. European Medicines Agency: **Falsified medicines.** EMA Homepage, http://www.emea.europa.eu/ema/index.jsp?curl=pages/special_topics/general/general_content_000186.jsp&mid=WC0b01ac058002d4e8. (accessed 2013-04-26).

27. European Directorate for the Quality of Medicines & HealthCare: **Microbiological examination of non-sterile products: microbial enumeration tests.** In *European Pharmacopoeia 70*. Strasbourg: Chapter 2.6.12, EDQM; 2011:163–167.

28. European Directorate for the Quality of Medicines & HealthCare: **Microbiological examination of non-sterile products: test for specified micro-organisms.** In *European Pharmacopoeia 70*. Strasbourg: Chapter 2.6.13, EDQM; 2011:167–171.

29. European Directorate for the Quality of Medicines & HealthCare: **Microbiological examination of herbal medicinal products for oral use.** In *European Pharmacopoeia 70*. Strasbourg: Chapte 2.6.31, EDQM; 2011:197–198.

30. Ozkocaman V, Ozcelik T, Ali R, Ozkalemkas F, Ozkan A, Ozakin C, Akalin H, Ursavas A, Coskun F, Ener B, Tunali A: **Bacillus spp. among hospitalized patients with haematological malignancies: clinical features, epidemics and outcomes.** *J Hosp Infect* 2006, 64(2):169–176.

31. American Society For Microbiology: *Manual of Clinical Microbiology*. 10th edition. Washington DC: ASM Press Editor in Chief: James Versalovic; 2011.

32. Mandell GL, Bennett JE, Dolin R: *Principles and Practice of Infections and Diseases*. 7th edition. Churchill Livingstone, Elsevier, Philadelphia: Imprint; 2010.

33. Podschun R, Ullmann U: **Klebsiella spp. as nosocomial pathogens: epidemiology, taxonomy, typing methods, and pathogenicity factors.** *Clin Microbiol Rev* 1998, 11(4):589–603.

34. Public Health Agency of Canada: **Klebsiella ssp. pathogen safety datasheet - infectious substances.** http://www.phac-aspc.gc.ca/lab-bio/res/psds-ftss/klebsiella-eng.php (accessed 2014-04-16).

35. Brzezinski JL, Craft DL: **Characterization of microorganisms isolated from counterfeit toothpaste.** *J Forensic Sci* 2012, 57(5):1365–1367.

36. Stocker P, Rosner B, Werber D, Kirchner M, Reinecke A, Wichmann-Schauer H, Prager R, Rabsch W, Frank C: **Outbreak of Salmonella Montevideo associated with a dietary food supplement flagged in the Rapid Alert System for Food and Feed (RASFF) in Germany, 2010.** *Euro Surveill* 2011, 16(50):20040.

37. Hanczaruk M, Reischl U, Holzmann T, Frangoulidis D, Wagner DM, Keim PS, Antwerpen MH, Meyer H, Grass G: **Injectional anthrax in heroin users, europe, 2000–2012.** *Emerg Infect Dis* 2014, 20(2):322–323.

38. Price EP, Seymour ML, Sarovich DS, Latham J, Wolken SR, Mason J, Vincent G, Drees KP, Beckstrom-Sternberg SM, Phillippy AM, Koren S, Okinaka RT, Chung WK, Schupp JM, Wagner DM, Vipond R, Foster JT, Bergman NH, Burans J, Pearson T, Brooks T, Keim P: **Molecular epidemiologic investigation of an anthrax outbreak among heroin users, Europe.** *Emerg Infect Dis* 2012, 18(8):1307–1313.

17

Cohort study of consistency between the compliance with guidelines for chemotherapy-induced nausea and vomiting and patient outcome

Masahiro Inoue[1,2], Manabu Shoji[2,3], Naomi Shindo[2], Kazunori Otsuka[1,2], Masatomo Miura[3] and Hiroyuki Shibata[1,2]*

Abstract

Background: Chemotherapy-induced nausea and vomiting is one of the most influential factors that affect patient quality of life; thus, preventing this adverse event could lead to better patient outcome. Standard preventive guidelines for antiemetic treatment have already been established based on the emetogenicity of chemotherapeutic agents. It is important that compliance with in-house guidelines and their effect on patient outcome is monitored.

Methods: In 3 years since the Akita university hospital antiemetic guidelines were outlined, we assessed the incidence of chemotherapy-induced nausea and vomiting using the antiemesis tool of the Multinational Association of Supportive Care in Cancer. Compliance of the guidelines was extracted from the hospital clinical record, and the chemotherapy-induced nausea and vomiting was examined by the patient reported outcome.

Results: Seventy-three patients answered the questionnaire. The overall compliance rate with the guidelines for early nausea and vomiting was 98.6% and with the delayed nausea and vomiting was 87.7%. The complete response rate for the early and delayed chemotherapy-induced nausea and vomiting was 77.8% and 73.8%, respectively. The overall relative risk of early nausea and vomiting was 0.22 (P < 0.05), whereas the relative risk for delayed nausea and vomiting was 2.09 (P < 0.05). Breakthrough vomiting was observed in 3 cases in the low-risk group only. These data suggest that delayed nausea and vomiting is difficult to prevent, particularly in the low-risk group. Further, it seems that the individual sensitivity for emetogenicity might differ among patients.

Conclusions: In addition to standard prevention guidelines based on emetogenicity, individual care based on patient reports should be considered for the complete prevention of chemotherapy-induced nausea and vomiting.

Keywords: Chemotherapy-induced nausea and vomiting, Guidelines, Emetogenicity

Background

One of the most devastating effects on the quality of life (QOL) of cancer patients is chemotherapy-induced nausea and vomiting (CINV). CINV is believed to affect 70%–80% of patients that receive cancer chemotherapy [1]. In addition, even effective chemotherapy may be stopped because of severe CINV, and the clinical losses may be significant in these cases [2].

The underlying mechanisms that cause CINV have been determined gradually, and many neurotransmitters such as 5-hydroxytryptamine (5-HT$_3$, serotonin) and substance P are involved in CINV [3]. 5-HT3 receptor antagonists (5-HT3RA) such as granisetron, ondansetron, and palonosetron have been approved for the treatment of CINV [4]. In addition, aprepitant was approved as a substance P blocker and a neurokinin 1 (NK1) receptor antagonist (NK1RA) for the prevention of acute and delayed CINV [4]. These agents have greatly improved patient outcome regarding CINV. For example, it was reported that a complete response of CINV occurred in 53.6%–53.7% of patients that received moderately

* Correspondence: hiroyuki@med.akita-u.ac.jp
[1]Department of Clinical Oncology, Graduate School of Medicine, Akita University, Akita, Japan
[2]Division of Chemotherapy for Outpatient, Akita University, Akita, Japan
Full list of author information is available at the end of the article

emetogenic chemotherapy using palonosetron plus dexamethasone (DEX) [5]. It was also reported that, among patients receiving cisplatin-based chemotherapy, the advantage achieved by the use of aprepitant was 20 percentage points [6].

Since the Multinational Association of Supportive Care in Cancer (MASCC) released their antiemetic guidelines in 1998, the American Society of Clinical Oncology (ASCO) and the National Comprehensive Cancer Network (NCCN) also released guidelines for the prevention and treatment of CINV [7]. Antiemetic strategies primarily using 5-HT3RA, NK1RA, and DEX have been established and recommended based on four emetogenicities (high, moderate, low, and minimal risk) for each chemotherapeutic agent [7]. In individual institutions, in-house guidelines for the prevention and treatment of CINV according to the MASCC, ASCO, and NCCN guidelines have been created and implemented, including in our hospital. Added to these guidelines, it is very important to monitor both patient outcome and their compliance with the guidelines [8]. However, because awareness of the occurrence of CINV depends only on patient declarations, it is difficult to know the severity of the CINV without patient-reported outcomes. In the current study, we assessed the consistency between the CINV compliance guidelines set in 2010 in Akita University Hospital and the outcome of patients visiting the Division of Chemotherapy for Outpatients. In this observational study, we revealed that the individual monitoring of CINV, even in low-risk emetogenicity patients, is very important to improve patient QOL during chemotherapy.

Methods

Patients who visited the Division of Chemotherapy for Outpatients, Akita University Hospital, between November 2013 and March 2014 were asked about their early and delayed CINV using the Japanese version of the MASCC Antiemesis Tool (MAT) [9], which was administered at a usual medical examination using a questionnaire. The grade of nausea was rated from 1 to 10 (1, minimum; 10, maximum), and the number of times of vomiting was recorded by the patients themselves. Questions were asked at any time during treatment, but only once for each patient. Conducted chemotherapeutic and anti-emetic agents were extracted from electronic clinical record of hospital, and the compliance of guideline was examined. Further, comparison was made between the patient reported outcome and the compliance of guideline (Figure 1). Stat Mate III (ATMS, Tokyo, Japan) was used to calculate the relative risk. The level of statistical significance was set as $P < 0.05$. This retrospective study was approved by the Ethics Committee of the School of Medicine of Akita University. Written informed consent for participation in the study was obtained from participants.

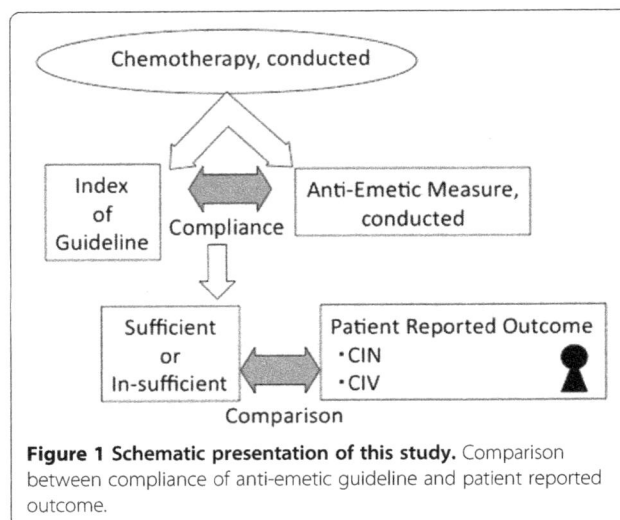

Figure 1 Schematic presentation of this study. Comparison between compliance of anti-emetic guideline and patient reported outcome.

Results and discussion

Patients

The patients included 36 males and 37 females aged 28–79 years, with a median age of 62 years (Table 1). The patients were diagnosed with the malignancies listed in Table 1. Colorectal cancer was most frequent (16/73), followed by breast (13/73), lung (9/73), and gastric cancers (9/73). All participants were diagnosed as suitable for chemotherapy as outpatients, without any clinical signs of brain metastasis or intestinal obstructions. The performance status of all participants was below 2, according to the Eastern Cooperative Oncology Group. The detailed clinical information such as clinical stages,

Table 1 Patients' characteristics

Number of participant	73
Age (median)	28-79 (62)
Male: Female	36: 37
Chemotherapy naïve patients	3
Primary leasion	
Esophageal cancer	2
Gastric cancer	9
Colorectal cancer	16
Bile duct carcinoma	1
Pancreatic cancer	7
Breast cancer	13
Lung cancer	9
Malignant lymphoma	3
Acute lymphoblastic leukemia	1
Malignant myeloma	2
Prostate cancer	5
Renal cell carcinoma	1
Cancer of unknown primary	4

previous treatment is listed in Additional file 1: Table S1. Chemotherapy naïve, and the other patients experienced ≥2 cycles of chemotherapy.

Regimens

The regimens used to treat the patients and their emetic risks are listed in Table 2. The most frequent regimen was docetaxel alone (9/73), followed by gemcitabine (8/73). The regimens were divided into four emetic risk groups: high, moderate, low, and minimal risks. The number of patients receiving high-, moderate-, low-, and minimal-risk regimens was 11, 17, 38, and 7, respectively.

Compliance with the antiemetic guideline

The compliance of the antiemetic guideline was examined. Our anti-emetic guideline is indicated in Table 3. Sufficient antiemetic treatments were performed for the minimal-risk regimens in all patients. In the low-risk group, all except 1 case received sufficient treatments; one under treatment was performed in the early phase, and no under treatments were performed in the delayed phase. For the moderate-risk group, sufficient treatments were performed in 14 of cases (82.4%); no under treatments occurred in the early phase, whereas three under treatments were performed in the delayed phase. For the high-risk group, sufficient treatments were performed in 6 cases (54.5%); no under treatments occurred in the early phase, whereas five under treatments were performed in the delayed phase. The overall compliance rate was 87.7%; the compliance rate was 98.6% with early phase CINV. The compliance rate for delayed phase CINV was 87.7%; specifically, 97.4% in the low-risk group, 82.4% in the moderate group, and 54.5% in the high-risk group.

Comparison between patient outcome and compliance with the guidelines

We next compared the patient-reported CINV and the compliance of guideline. As shown in Figure 2, early CINV was not prevented in 22.2% of cases, although the sufficient antiemetic treatment against was conducted. However, early CINV was not prevented at all in the under treatment case. The overall relative risk for compliance with the guidelines was calculated to be 0.22 ($P <$ 0.05). Specifically, in the minimal-risk group, CIN was not prevented in one of 7 cases (14.3%), in spite of sufficient treatment (the grade of nausea was 2 (G2)). In the low-risk group, CIN was not prevented in 8 of 37 cases (21.6%) (G1 to G5; median = G2.5). Among these, one patient vomited once (2.7%). In the moderate-risk group, CIN was not prevented in 2 of 7 cases (11.8%) (G2 to G4; median = G3), but no CIV was observed. In the high-risk group, CIN was not prevented in 5 of 11 cases (45.5%) (G1 to G6; median = G3), but no CIV was observed.

Table 2 Treatment regimens and emetogenisity

Emetogenisity	Index of anti-emetic guideline	Regimen	Number
Minimal (n = 7)	Early; (−), Delayed; (−)	Tmab + VNR	2
		Tmab	2
		VNR	1
		MTX + VCR + PSL	1
		temsirolimus	1
Low (n = 38)	Early; DEX, Delayed; (−)	GEM	8
		S-1 + GEM	1
		nab-PTX + GEM	1
		nab-PTX	3
		Tmab + PTX	2
		PTX	1
		DTX + S-1	2
		DTX + EMP	1
		DTX + PSL	4
		DTX	9
		eribulin	1
		Bmab + sLV5FU2	1
		sLV5FU2	3
		VTD	1
Moderate (n = 17)	Early; NK1RA + 5-HT$_3$RA + DEX, or 5-HT$_3$RA + DEX, Delayed; NK1RA + 5-HT$_3$RA + DEX, or 5-HT$_3$RA + DEX	Bmab + CBDCA + PTX	3
		Pmab + FOLFOX6	2
		Bmab + CapeOX	1
		CapeOX	3
		SOX	1
		Bmab + FOLFIRI	1
		Bmab + IRIS	1
		IRIS	2
		CPT-11	2
		VCD	1
High (n = 11)	Early; NK1RA + 5-HT$_3$RA + DEX, Delayed; NK1RA + 5-HT$_3$RA + DEX	CDDP + CPT-11	4
		FEC	2
		EC	2
		R-CHOP	3

Tmab; Trastuzumab, VNR; vinorelbine, MTX; Methotrexate, VCR; Vincristine, PSL; Prednisolone, GEM; Gemcitabine, nab-PTX; nab-Paclitaxel, DTX; Docetaxel, EMP; estramustine, Bmab; Bevacizumab, sLV5FU2; simplified biweekly 5-FU & leucovorin, VTD; bortezomib, thalidomide, dexamethasone, CBDCA; Carboplatin, FOLFOX6; combination of Oxaliplatin and 5FU, CapeOX; capecitabine plus intermittent oxaliplatin, SOX; S-1 plus intermittent oxaliplatin, FOLFIRI; combination of Irinotecan and 5FU IRIS; CPT-11; Irinotecan, VCD; bortezomib, Cyclophosphamide, dexamethasone, CDDP; Cisplatin, FEC; 5FU, Epirubicin, Cyclophosphamide, EC; Epirubicin, Cyclophosphamide, R-CHOP; Rituximab, Cyclophosphamide, Doxorubicin, Vincristine, Prednisolone.

Delayed CINV was not prevented in 17 of the 65 cases (26.2%), even though sufficient antiemetic treatments were conducted (Figure 3). In the under treatment cases, CINV (G1) was not prevented in 1 of 8 cases (12.5%).

Table 3 Compliance of antiemetic treatment

Emetogenisity	Actual measure (Early)	Actual measure (Delayed)	n	Compliance
Minimal	5-HT$_3$RA + DEX	no	2	Sufficient
	5-HT$_3$RA	no	1	Sufficient
	DEX	no	1	Sufficient
	no	no	3	Sufficient
Low	5-HT$_3$RA + DEX	no	29	Sufficient
	5-HT$_3$RA + DEX	DEX	3	Sufficient
	5-HT$_3$RA + DEX	D2RA	1	Sufficient
	DEX	DEX	1	Sufficient
	DEX	no	3	Sufficient
	no	no	1	**Insufficient**
Moderate	5-HT$_3$RA + DEX	DEX	6	Sufficient
	5-HT$_3$RA + DEX	NK1RA + DEX	3	Sufficient
	NK1RA + 5-HT$_3$RA + DEX	NK1RA	2	Sufficient
	NK1RA + 5-HT$_3$RA + steroid (MM)	NK1RA	1	Sufficient
	NK1RA + 5-HT$_3$RA + DEX	5-HT$_3$RA + DEX + NK1RA	1	Sufficient
	5-HT$_3$RA + DEX	no	3	**Insufficient**
	5-HT$_3$RA + DEX	DEX + D2RA	1	Sufficient
High	NK1RA + 5-HT$_3$RA + DEX	NK1RA	2	**Insufficient**
	NK1RA + 5-HT$_3$RA + steroid (ML)	NK1RA	2	Sufficient
	NK1RA + 5-HT$_3$RA + steroid (ML)	NK1RA + D2RA	1	Sufficient
	5-HT$_3$RA + DEX	DEX	2	**Insufficient**
	5-HT$_3$RA + DEX	no	1	**Insufficient**

5-HT$_3$RA; 5-HT$_3$ receptor antagonist, DEX; Dexamethasone, D2RA; Dopamine receptor D2 receptor antagonist, NK1RA; Neurokinin 1 receptor antagonist, MM; multiple myeloma, ML; malignant lymphoma.

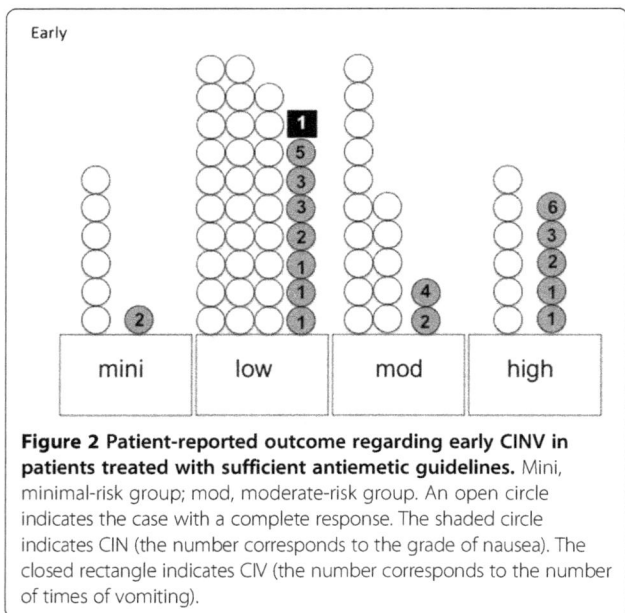

Figure 2 Patient-reported outcome regarding early CINV in patients treated with sufficient antiemetic guidelines. Mini, minimal-risk group; mod, moderate-risk group. An open circle indicates the case with a complete response. The shaded circle indicates CIN (the number corresponds to the grade of nausea). The closed rectangle indicates CIV (the number corresponds to the number of times of vomiting).

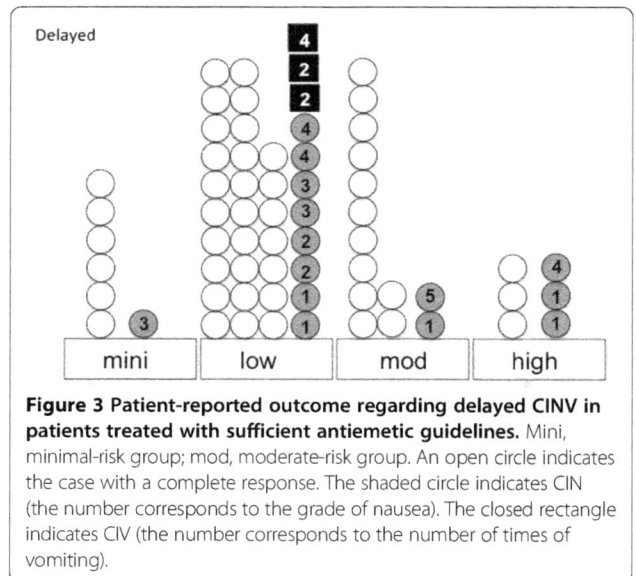

Figure 3 Patient-reported outcome regarding delayed CINV in patients treated with sufficient antiemetic guidelines. Mini, minimal-risk group; mod, moderate-risk group. An open circle indicates the case with a complete response. The shaded circle indicates CIN (the number corresponds to the grade of nausea). The closed rectangle indicates CIV (the number corresponds to the number of times of vomiting).

The overall relative risk for delayed CINV was 2.22 ($P <$ 0.05). Specifically, in the minimal-risk group, CIN was not prevented in 1 of 7 cases (14.3%) (G3). In the low-risk group, CIN was not prevented in 11 of 38 cases (29.0%) (G1 to G4; median = G3). Among these, three patients vomited (two patients twice and one patient once). In the moderate-risk group, CIN was not prevented in 2 of 14 cases (14.3%) (G1 to G5; median = G3), but there were no instances of vomiting. In the high-risk group, CIN was not prevented in 3 of 6 cases (50%) (G1 to G4; median = G4), but there was no vomiting.

In this observational study, CIV occurred only in the patients that received low emetogenic chemotherapeutic agents. One male patient (71 years old) that reported early CIV was treated for the second time with nab-pactlitaxel for his carcinoma of unknown origin, mediastinal lymph node metastasis, and pleural dissemination. The remaining three patients claimed breakthrough CIV. Of these, one female patient (42 years old) was treated for the fourth time with eribulin for breast cancer with bone and liver metastases. Another female patient (61 years old) was treated with docetaxel for the second time for lung cancer with asymptomatic and multiple micrometastases in the brain. Finally, one male patient (55 years old) was treated for the twelfth time with docetaxel for lung cancer and cancerous pleuritis. The compliance rate of our hospital was better than that reported previously [10]. Preventive treatment against early CINV was almost completely effective; however, the prevention of delayed CINV was not sufficient in the high-risk group according to the current guidelines. It is necessary to prevent delayed CINV. According to the patient-reported outcome, delayed CINV occurred in only 12.5% of the patients that were treated with anti-emetic agents insufficiently. However, early and delayed CIN occurred in 22.2% and 26.2% of patients, respectively, in spite of conduction of sufficient anti-emetic treatment, particularly, in the high-risk group, early and delayed CIN occurred in 45.5% and 50.0% of patients, respectively. However, the grade of CIN was not so severe (The median grade of early CIN = G3. and delayed CIN = G4). Moreover, no CIV (breakthrough CIV) was reported. The guidelines for the prevention of CINV in the high-risk group appeared to be effective to comparable extent. In the low-risk group, early and delayed CINV occurred in 21.6% and 28.9% of patients, respectively, in spite of sufficient anti-emetic treatment (The median grade of the early and the delayed CIN = G2.5 and G3, respectively). Moreover, 3 cases of breakthrough CIV were reported. Among these, all three vomited several times. These data suggest that compliance with the guideline alone could not prevent emetogenicity. Consistent with this, a previous study also reported that sufficient measures could not prevent breakthrough CIV completely, even in low-risk patients [11]. In addition, some reports have discussed the difficulty of prevention using antiemetic guidelines for delayed CINV [12,13]. In particular, prevention in low-risk patients remains controversial.

Current guidelines are based primarily on the emetogenicity of chemotherapeutic agents. Data suggested that individual differences in the sensitivity to antiemetic treatments may occur. There are also too many individual parameters, including exposure to chemotherapy, alcohol use, age, and gender [14,15]. As such, data should be gathered and analyzed regarding CINV cases. Such factors may include individual sensitivities to the preventive agents, tumor status, and the physical condition of patient. Refining the antiemetic measures is also necessary; accordingly, some methods have been proposed [13,16]. However, the establishment of the personalized precautions as well as the standard one is likely to be necessary for the complete prevention of CINV.

Conclusions

The generation of antiemetic guidelines might contribute toward patient compliance with antiemetic measures. However, complete prevention remains challenging because individual factors should be considered.

Additional file

Additional file 1: Table S1. Detailed characteristics of participants.

Abbreviations

QOL: Quality of life; CINV: Chemotherapy-induced nausea and vomiting; 5-HT3: 5-hydroxytryptamine; 5-HT3RA: 5-HT3 receptor antagonists; NK1: Neurokinin 1; NK1RA: NK1 receptor antagonist; MASCC: Multinational association of supportive care in cancer; ASCO: the American society of clinical oncology; NCCN: National comprehensive cancer network; DEX: Dexamethasone; MAT: MASCC antiemesis tool.

Competing interests

The authors declare that they have no competing interests.

Authors' contributions

MI, MS, and NS gathered the patient data. MS, NS, KO, MM, and HS set the in-house guidelines. HS planned the study and wrote the manuscript. All authors read and approved the final manuscript.

Authors' information

MI is an assistant professor, KO is a lecturer, and HS is a professor in the Department of Clinical Oncology. MM is a professor in the Department of Pharmacy. HS is a Japanese Society of Medical Oncology certified specialist in Medical Oncology. MS was Board-Certified as a Pharmacist in Oncology Pharmacy by the Japanese Society of Hospital Pharmacist. NS is a Japanese Nursing Association-certified nurse for cancer chemotherapy.

Acknowledgments

The authors would like to thank Enago (http://www.enago.jp) for English language review.

Author details
[1]Department of Clinical Oncology, Graduate School of Medicine, Akita University, Akita, Japan. [2]Division of Chemotherapy for Outpatient, Akita University, Akita, Japan. [3]Department of Pharmacy, Akita University, Akita, Japan.

References
1. Morran C, Smith DC, Anderson DA, McArdle CS. Incidence of nausea and vomiting with cytotoxic chemotherapy: a prospective randomised trial of antiemetics. Br Med J. 1979;1:1323–4.
2. Richardson JL, Marks G, Levine A. The influence of symptoms of disease and side effects of treatment on compliance with cancer therapy. J Clin Oncol. 1988;6:1746–52.
3. Baker PD, Morzorati SL, Ellett ML. The pathophysiology of chemotherapy-induced nausea and vomiting. Gastroenterol Nurs. 2005;28:469–80.
4. Basch E, Prestrud AA, Hesketh PJ, Kris MG, Feyer PC, Somerfield MR, et al. American Society of Clinical Oncology guideline for antiemetics in oncology: update 2006. J Clin Oncol. 2006;24:2932–47.
5. Aapro M, Fabi A, Nolè F, Medici M, Steger G, Bachmann C, et al. Double-blind, randomised, controlled study of the efficacy and tolerability of palonosetron plus dexamethasone for 1 day with or without dexamethasone on days 2 and 3 in the prevention of nausea and vomiting induced by moderately emetogenic chemotherapy. Ann Oncol. 2010;21:1083–8.
6. Gralla RJ, De Wit R, Herrstedt J, Carides AD, Ianus J, Guoguang-Ma J, et al. Antiemetic efficacy of the neurokinin-1 antagonist, aprepitant, plus a 5-HT3 antagonist and a corticosteroid in patients receiving anthracy-clines or cyclophosphamide in addition to high-dose cisplatin: analysis of combined data from two phase III randomized clinical trials. Cancer. 2005;104:864–8.
7. Jordan K, Sippel C, Schmoll HJ. Guidelines for antiemetic treatment of chemotherapy-induced nausea and vomiting: past, present, and future recommendations. Oncologist. 2007;12:1143–50.
8. Liau CT, Chu NM, Liu HE, Deuson R, Lien J, Chen JS. Incidence of chemotherapy-induced nausea and vomiting in Taiwan: physicians' and nurses' estimation vs. patients' reported outcomes. Support Care Cancer. 2005;13:277–86.
9. MASCC Antiemesis Tool© (MAT) [http://www.mascc.org/mat]
10. Caracuel F, Muñoz N, Baños U, Ramirez G. Adherence to antiemetic guidelines and control of chemotherapy-induced nausea and vomiting (CINV) in a large hospital. J Oncol Pharm Pract. 2014. [Epub ahead of print].
11. Keat CH, Phua G, Abdul Kassim MS, Poh WK, Sriraman M. Can granisetron injection used as primary prophylaxis improve the control of nausea and vomiting with low-emetogenic chemotherapy? Asian Pac J Cancer Prev. 2013;14:469–73.
12. Jones JM, Qin R, Bardia A, Linquist B, Wolf S, Loprinzi CL. Antiemetics for chemotherapy-induced nausea and vomiting occurring despite prophylactic antiemetic therapy. J Palliat Med. 2011;14:810–4.
13. Bouganim N, Dranitsaris G, Hopkins S, Vandermeer L, Godbout L, Dent S, et al. Prospective validation of risk prediction indexes for acute and delayed chemotherapy-induced nausea and vomiting. Curr Oncol. 2012;19:e414–21.
14. Kris MG, Roila F, De Mulder PH, Marty M. Delayed emesis following anticancer chemotherapy. Support Care Cancer. 1998;6:228–32.
15. Kim HK, Hsieh R, Chan A, Yu S, Han B, Gao Y, et al. Impact of CINV in earlier cycles on CINV and chemotherapy regimen modification in subsequent cycles in Asia Pacific clinical practice. Support Care Cancer. 2014. [Epub ahead of print].
16. Molassiotis A, Stamataki Z, Kontopantelis E. Development and preliminary validation of a risk prediction model for chemotherapy-related nausea and vomiting. Support Care Cancer. 2013;21:2759–67.

18

Self-medication with antibiotics among non-medical university students of Karachi: a cross-sectional study

Syed Jawad Shah[1], Hamna Ahmad[1], Rija Binte Rehan[1], Sidra Najeeb[1], Mirrah Mumtaz[1], Muhammad Hashim Jilani[1], Muhammad Sharoz Rabbani[1], Muhammad Zakariya Alam[1], Saba Farooq[1] and M Masood Kadir[2]*

Abstract

Background: The prevalence of self -medication with antibiotics is quite high in developing countries as opposed to developed countries. Antibiotics are often taken erroneously for certain ailments, without having the appropriate knowledge of their use. This carries potential risks for the individual as well as the community, in form of several side effects such as antibiotic resistance. Therefore the prevalence of self-medicated antibiotics in developing countries needs to be studied.

Methods: A descriptive cross-sectional study was carried out at six different non-medical universities of Karachi. 431 students were included in the study. Data was collected using self-administered questionnaires and analyzed using SPSS version 19.

Results: 50.1% students reported having self-medicated themselves in the past 6 months and 205 (47.6%) reported self-medication with antibiotics. Amoxicillin was the most self-prescribed antibiotic (41.4%). Awareness of the adverse effects of antibiotics was demonstrated by 77.3% of the students and sleep disturbance was the most commonly known (46.5%) side effect. 63.1% denied having any knowledge about antibiotic resistance and only 19.9% correctly knew that indiscriminate use of antibiotics can lead to increased antibiotic resistance.

Conclusion: The prevalence of self-medication with antibiotics among the non-medical university students was high despite the awareness of adverse effects. Antibiotic resistance was a relatively unknown terminology.

Keywords: Self-medication, Antibiotics, Antibiotics resistance, Non-medical, Adverse effects

Background

Self-medication can be defined as the use of non-prescription medicines by people on their own initiative. The definition can be expanded to include treatment of family members and dependents, in particular children/minors and the elderly [1]. Self-medication is a component of self-care and is considered as primary public health resource in health care system.

Studies have revealed the burden of self-medication with antibiotics to be higher in developing countries than in developed countries [2]. The prevalence has been reported to be 3% in northern Europe as compared

to the 4-75% in Asia [3]. One study done in Karachi, Pakistan, showed the frequency of self-medication (as a whole) among university students to be as high as 80.4%. Frequency among non-medical students was 83.3% while for those in medical school, it was 77.7% [4].

World Health Organization has mentioned, according to a survey that self-medication, if administered appropriately and responsibly can help prevent and treat diseases economically and without medical consultation [5].

Although self-medication may prove useful when used judiciously, it is more often used erroneously, without proper guidance and rationale. This fact is highlighted by a study conducted in Jordan, which showed that 67.1% of adults believed that antibiotics cure common cold and cough [6]. Medications administered inappropriately not only leads to wastage of resources but also

* Correspondence: masood.kadir@aku.edu
[2]Department of Community Health Sciences, Aga Khan University, Karachi, Pakistan
Full list of author information is available at the end of the article

carries potential serious and life-threatening adverse effects for the users [3,6]. Research of health seeking attitudes in different parts of the world reveals that self-medication (with any drug) is higher among the literate, the young and people in low and middle income countries. The same study also highlights that 82.5% of the students are aware of some form of harm caused by self-medication [7-9].

The misuse of antibiotics is a serious problem in several respects. The medical community may be aware of the seriousness of this rising problem but this is not reflected in the non-medical community, which is still relatively unaware of any such issue. This was exhibited in one study in Italy, which showed that only 9.8% of the general public knew the definition of antibiotic resistance and only 21.2% knew when was it appropriate to use antibiotics [2]. Another study conducted in Yemen and Uzbekistan showed that 49% of respondents discontinued antibiotics as soon as they started feeling better [10].

The developing world is the hub for the emergence of rapidly mutating and resistant strains of several pathogens, including S. pnemoniae, S. typhi, and Shigella species [11-13]. Emergence of antibiotic resistant strains of several pathogens is linked directly to the use of antibiotics and with their unregulated use (or misuse) [11]. Secondly, unregulated use of antibiotics results in improper dosing (over and under dosing), which may adversely affect the person being administered the drug. Thirdly, antibiotics have their own side effects and hazards, which need to be considered, in particular, for people with other co-morbids.

Public education and enforcing and implementing laws about prescribed medications can help decrease the rate of self-medication as shown by previous researches in the developed world [3,14]. Therefore, ideally, antibiotics need to be regulated via prescription-only sales. Legally, the sale of antibiotics is regulated on a 'sold on prescription only' basis and this needs to be put into effect in reality as well [5,15]. So for implementation of such policies and carrying out general awareness programs, information should be available about how common the use of self-medicated antibiotics is. Therefore, we aimed to provide the prevalence of self-medication with antibiotics amongst the university students of Karachi, who are not associated with health care or medicine.

Methods
Study design and setting
This study was a descriptive cross-sectional study where the prevalence of self-medicated antibiotics among the university students of Karachi was investigated. The study was conducted in six different non-medical universities of Karachi, which included two engineering universities, one business and management university, one art university and two multi-disciplinary universities.

Sample size calculation
Previous studies in Karachi showed the prevalence of self-medication to be 75% - 80% [4]. Hence using 80% as a reference prevalence of use of self-medicated antibiotics in university students of Karachi, the sample size was calculated to be 246, at confidence level of 95%. For the second objective of this study, prevalence of each risk factor from previously conducted researches was used, which generated a sample size of 400. Lastly, prevalence of knowledge of adverse effects was taken to be 62%, and the aggregate sample size was calculated to be 423 after 10% inflation. Therefore, 425 individuals were planned to be approached and by the end, a total of 431 students answered the questionnaire (Additional file 1).

Inclusion and exclusion criteria
All male and female students enrolled in undergraduate or postgraduate programs in universities of Karachi who understood English were included. Medical, paramedical and pharmacology students were excluded from the study.

Self-medication was defined as use of any medication, in the past 6 months, with one's own accord, which was not prescribed by a doctor. A time period of 6 months was chosen to eliminate recall bias amongst those who had used antibiotics and were likely to recall it in this adequate time period, with those who had not used antibiotics and would also clearly remember not having used them.

Data collection procedure
A convenience sampling method was used to complete the required sample size. Students were approached in the areas specified by the respective university managements. Informed consent, both verbal and written, was taken from the study volunteers. The self-administered questionnaire was then filled by the students and returned back to our questionnaire administrators.

Date collection tool
A paper based questionnaire was used for data collection. The questionnaire was divided into three sections (A, B and C), each of which was preceded by statements to clarify the nature of questions that would follow, for the benefit of the subject. Details of this questionnaire are as follows: Section A, containing 6 items, assessed subject demographics, including age, sex, year in university, health insurance, household income. These were all close ended questions. Data is reflected in results Table 1, which is a summary of the data collected in this section. Section B, containing 7 items, assessed frequency of use of self-medicated antibiotics in the past 6 months along with the type of antibiotic used. A brief description of the definition of self-medication preceded the start of this section. Subjects were thence asked about self-medication in

Table 1 Distribution of demographic factors among non-medical students of Karachi

	Students using self-medication (n = 205)		Students not using self-medication (n = 226)		Odds ratio (95% confidence interval)
	Frequency (n)	Percentage (%)	Frequency (n)	Percentage (%)	
Gender					0.903(0.615-1.326)
• Male	123	60	130	57.5	
• Female	82	40	96	42.5	
TOTAL	205		226		
Year in university					
• 1st	116	56.6	132	58.4	
• 2nd	41	20	39	17.3	
• 3rd	16	7.8	21	9.3	
• 4th	29	14.1	29	12.8	
• 5th	1	0.5	3	1.3	
• >5th	2	1	2	0.9	
Marital status					
• Single	197	96.1	214	94.7	
• Married	3	1.5	8	3.5	
• Divorced	5	2.4	4	1.8	
Household income					
• <50,000	51	26.8	64	30.9	
• 50,000 to <100,000	73	38.4	66	31.9	
• 100,000-150,000	38	20	32	15.5	
• >150,000	28	14.7	45	21.7	
Healthcare expenses covered					1.186(0.804-1.750)
• Yes	116	57.4	136	61.5	
• No	86	42.6	85	38.5	

the past 6 months in general and then with respect to antibiotics alone. Subjects were given a list of generic along with market names of some of the most commonly used antibiotics. However, an additional option of 'other antibiotics used' was also presented for the ease of the subject and was the only open ended option in this section. Data is reflected in Table 2, which is a summary of the data collected in this section. Lastly, Section C assessed knowledge of adverse effects of antibiotics. This section

Table 2 Shows frequency of self-medicated antibiotics among non-medical university students of Karachi

	Used once (n = 127)	Used twice (n = 51)	More than twice (n = 54)
Ciprofloxacin	16(7.6%)	6(2.9%)	5(2.4%)
Cotrimoxazole	12(5.7%)	3(1.4%)	5(2.4%)
Amoxicillin	47(22.4%)	19(9%)	21(10%)
Ampiclox	7(3.3%)	3(1.4%)	3(1.4%)
Ampicillin	4(1.9%)	1(0.5%)	2(1.0%)
Erythromycin	8(3.8%)	3(1.4%)	3(1.4%)
Metronidazole	33(15.7%)	16(7.6%)	15(7.1%)

contained questions, where subjects were asked to check as many adverse effects they thought were possible, with the option 'others' as the only open ended question. Knowledge of the term antibiotic resistance and knowledge about effect of antibiotic use on resistance was assessed using close ended questions. The data from this section is reflected in Table 3.

The tool underwent a pilot phase where 30 subjects who met the inclusion criteria were asked to respond to the questionnaire. Data collected was analyzed and feedback was taken from the subjects about possible difficulties faced. No difficulties were faced by either subject or researcher. However, the data from these 30 subjects was not included in the study sample or result.

Data entry and analysis
Epidata 3.1 was used for data entry. Data analysis was performed using SPSS version 19. The software was used to run a descriptive analysis and the frequency tables generated were used to calculate the prevalence of self-medication. Frequency of use of different classes of antibiotics and frequency of the reasons which led to use of

Table 3 Knowledge of adverse effects caused by antibiotics

Symptoms	Frequency (n)	Percentage (%)
Diarrhea/abdominal pain	99	23.1
Nausea/Vomiting	127	29.7
Allergic Reactions	166	38.8
Yellow eyes/skin	51	11.9
Tiredness/Dizziness	128	29.9
Headache	143	33.4
Fever	79	18.5
Kidney problems	64	15
Liver problems	47	11
Teeth discoloration	36	8.4
Muscle/joint pain	65	15.2
Numbness/tingling	35	8.2
Sleep problems	199	46.5

self-medicated antibiotics was also calculated using descriptive analysis. Chi- square test of association was conducted for association of factors between self-medicated antibiotic users and non-users. We also calculated prevalence of awareness of side effects and frequency of most common adverse effects experienced by participants. Finally, frequency of knowledge regarding antibiotic resistance was also calculated.

Ethical consideration

Ethical clearance was given by Ethical Review Committee of Aga Khan University. Prior permission was sought from all 6 universities before conducting surveys among their students. Informed consent forms were signed by the study participants. Confidentiality was maintained by separating the filled questionnaires with the consent form.

Results
Study population

Four hundred and thirty one (431) non-medical University Students from Karachi, Pakistan were surveyed. Mean age of these students was 20.04(±1.74) years. The proportion of males was 58.7% while that of females was (41.3%). and majority (57.5%) was first year university students. Of the 431 University students surveyed, merely 397 gave information about their household income. About 64% of these respondents had a household income of <100,000 PKR.

Prevalence of self-medication and its association with demographic factors

205 respondents (47.6%) reported using antibiotics not prescribed by a doctor in the last six months. There was no statistical significance for frequency of self-medication

with antibiotics in relation to sex, marital status, year of university, household income and having healthcare expenses covered, as demonstrated by Table 1.

Trends in antibiotic usage

The most common antibiotic used for self-medication purposes was amoxicillin which was used by 81(41.4%) study participants. Amoxicillin was followed by Metronidazole (30.5%), Ciprofloxacin (12.7%) and Cotrimoxazole (9.5%). Erythromycin and Ampicillin/cloxacillin were used by 6.7% and 6.2% of the sample population respectively and other antibiotics were amongst the less frequently used antibiotics. The frequency of use of each antibiotic is depicted in Table 2.

Forty-three (10%) students mistook other classes of drugs for antibiotics. This was assessed using the 'Other antibiotics' option in Section B, where subjects were asked to enumerate any antibiotic other than the ones in the list provided by the researchers that they might have used. The most commonly mistaken drugs were analgesics and anti-allergy medications.

42.8% of students admitted to choosing the antibiotics themselves, 76% percent believed that they knew what antibiotics were and 77.3% of the population knew that antibiotics cause adverse effects.

Of the 217 students who reported using antibiotics, 83 used them to relieve fever (41.1%), 81 for pain relief (40.1%) while 80 students reported use of antibiotic for relief from respiratory symptoms (39.6%). Use for relief from gastrointestinal problems and from urinary symptoms was 15.8% and 6.9% respectively.

The reasons for choosing to self-medicate with antibiotics rather than visiting a certified healthcare professional for their ailments by students (N = 211) have been reported in Figure 1.

Out of the 427 people surveyed who answered the question about adverse effect awareness, 330 were aware that antibiotic use could lead to adverse effects (77.3%).

The most common adverse effects that the students knew could be caused by antibiotics were sleep problems (46.5%) and allergic reaction (38.8%). Other adverse effects that students showed most awareness about were headaches (33.4%), tiredness or dizziness (29.9%), nausea/ vomiting (29.7%), and diarrhea/ abdominal pain (23.1%). The complete list of adverse effects thought to be caused by antibiotics by University students is presented in Table 3.

However, only 21.8% of the students (93 out of 427) reported experiencing adverse effects after antibiotic usage. Of the 71 students who specified which adverse effects they had experienced, 19 reported presence of abdominal complaints after antibiotic usage (26.7%), 13 reported an allergic reaction (18.3%), 9 reported sleep disturbance (12.7%), and 8 reported weakness (11.3%).

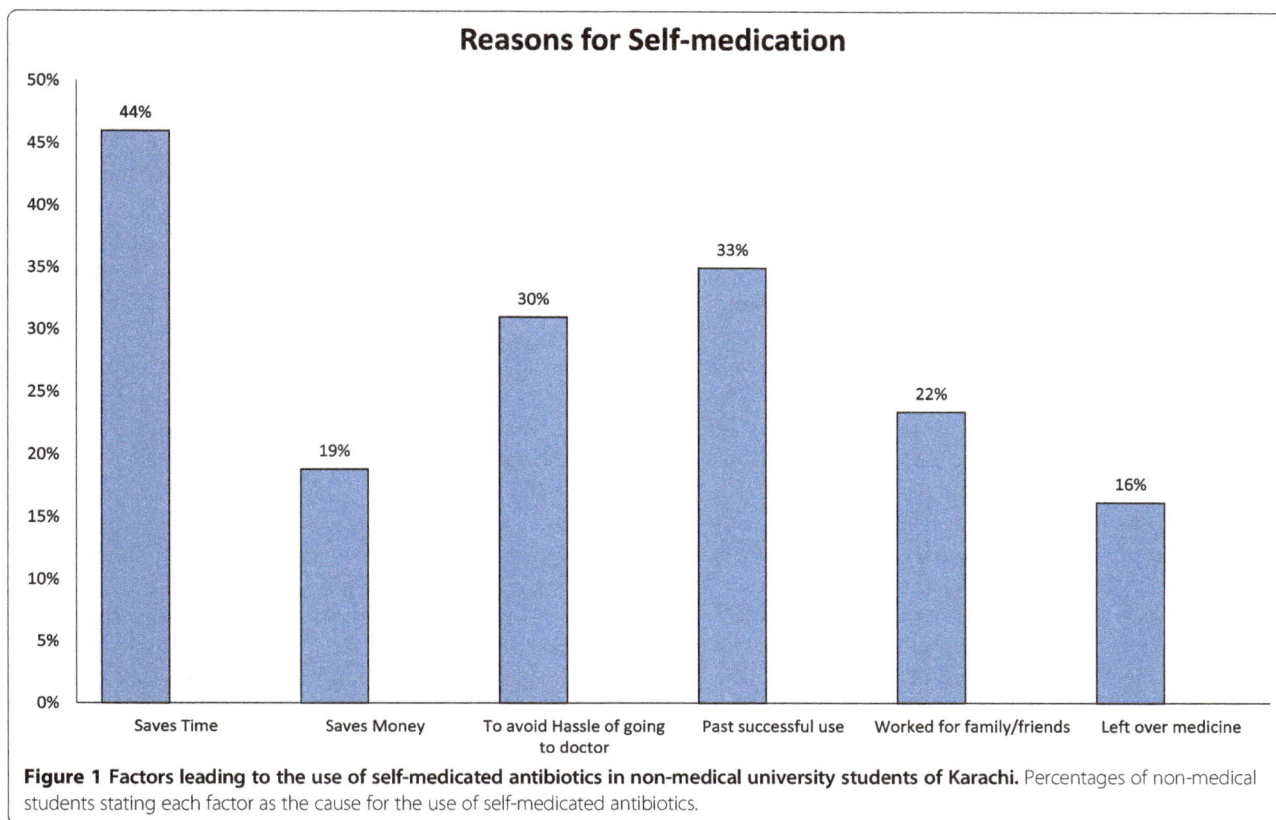

Figure 1 Factors leading to the use of self-medicated antibiotics in non-medical university students of Karachi. Percentages of non-medical students stating each factor as the cause for the use of self-medicated antibiotics.

When questioned regarding the term 'antibiotic resistance', 20.9% of the 425 students reported having heard of it while 63.1% denied having any knowledge about the term. However, as shown in Table 4, only 83 out of 423 students (19.9%) correctly knew that indiscriminate use of antibiotics can lead to increased antibiotic resistance. Majority (64.3%) admitted to having no idea about the relation of antibiotic resistance to indiscriminate antibiotic use.

An interesting fact to note is that 60.3% of the students (n = 123) who had self-medicated with antibiotics reported having heard of antibiotic resistance, showing a significant association between the two (χ^2 = 1.409, p = 0.494).

Discussion

The prevalence of self-medication with antibiotics, as previously mentioned, is much higher in developing countries

Table 4 Knowledge of effect of inadequate use of antibiotics on antibiotic resistance

Effect on antibiotic resistance	Frequency (n)	Percentage (%)
Increases	84	19.9
Decreases	45	10.6
Remains the same	22	5.2
I don't know	272	64.3

as compared to developed ones [2]. This study focused in particular on the non-medical university students.

Our study found out that almost half of our study population had self-medicated with antibiotics in the last 6 months. No study was available for comparison in Pakistan which had studied the prevalence of self-medication with antibiotics. However, in two studies, the prevalence of self-medication as a whole amongst university students of Karachi was found to be around 80% [4,9]. The possible reasons for this difference could be that our study included self-medication with antibiotics specifically and that too, within the last six months only, whereas the aforementioned studies did not restrict the time period for recall.

In other countries, studies have shown prevalence of self-medication with antibiotics to be 47.8% in Southern China, 79.5% in Sudan and 48% in Iran [16-18]. Similar trends for prevalence have also been found in studies conducted for general community in Middle Eastern countries [10].

Our study also assessed various factors that could be associated with the use of self-prescribed antibiotics amongst the study population. No association could be established between the demographic factors such as gender, year of study, marital status, monthly family income, health coverage and self-medication with antibiotics.

These findings are consistent with the previous studies which found no association between self-medication in general and socio-demographic factors [19].

Antibiotics carry several risks when used without physician advice. The exact burden of this problem is not known. The results indicate that the three most common reasons for self-prescription were to save time, previous successful experience and avoiding the hassle at clinics. These findings are not surprising considering the fact that most of the health care expenditure in our country is out-of-pocket and the healthcare facilities are already over-burdened; unable to satisfy the health related needs of the general population. For better understanding of this situation, further studies should be carried out to assess the satisfaction of patients with the health care services, especially the outpatient clinics.

Amongst the list of antibiotics given to the participants the most commonly used antibiotics were amoxicillin and metronidazole. This reflects in another study done in Karachi where the most common antibiotic used for self-medication was metronidazole, followed by co-amoxiclav and amoxicillin respectively [4]. In our study, fever, pain and respiratory complaints were the most common reasons for which the antibiotics were used. This finding matches the common reasons highlighted for self-medication with antibiotics in previous studies [10,17].

A large proportion (42.8%) of students admitted to choosing the antibiotics themselves. This high percentage might be due to our study subjects being educated university students who had access to online learning resources and may think of themselves as well equipped with knowledge of antibiotics. This is also reflected in our study results which showed that around 76% percent believed that they knew what antibiotics were. Further assessing knowledge about antibiotics, it was found that a vast majority (77.3%) of the population knew that antibiotics cause adverse effects and amongst the participants who had self-medicated with antibiotics, a similar proportion was aware of potential adverse effects.

A very small proportion of the total study population, however, had heard of the term antibiotic resistance and an even less had an idea that resistance increased with indiscriminate use of antibiotics. The rest denied having any knowledge of antibiotic resistance and its varying trend with indiscriminate use. Considering that our study subjects included students from non-medical background only, these findings were expected as antibiotic resistance is a technical term used in the field of medicine. These finding could be used as a basis to discourage self-medication with antibiotics.

Ideally, it is the government's responsibility to establish that any population uses self-medication responsibly. Drugs that are available without the need for prescription by physician or trained medical personnel should only be the ones which are safe to use. The government should also ensure that users are educated properly about not only the use of the drug but also the correct dosages, duration of use and potential side effects associated with them as antibiotics are tailored not only according to the disease but also according to the individual patient profile.

There are few limitations in our study. We did convenience sampling instead of systematic randomized approach. However, we tried to minimize the effect of this by taking a large sample size and selecting 6 different universities to ensure diversity among our study participants. The questions assessing the knowledge about antibiotics were very subjective so the true picture regarding this could not be determined.

Conclusion

This study was one of the few studies done in this part of the world to explore the prevalence and practices of self-medication with antibiotics and knowledge about the possible side effects of such practices among non-medical university students of Karachi. The results obtained can help in providing a framework for designing programs that will create awareness about the risks of self-prescribed antibiotics.

The prevalence of self-medication with antibiotics among the non-medical university student was high, with no variation based on gender, year of study, marital status, monthly family income and health. The majority of the study population was aware of potential adverse effects of antibiotics and yet the practice of using self-prescribed antibiotics was seen.

The study suggested that there is a necessity for educational programs emphasizing on the risks associated with indiscriminate antibiotic use in which health care providers, pharmacists and others, including parents, should be actively involved in health education that will help in inculcating the practice of responsible use of antibiotic amongst the general population at an early age. The study also showed that there is a need for strict law enforcement to limit the purchase of antibiotics without a prescription.

Additional file

Additional file 1: Frequency of self-medicated antibiotics, factors associated with their administration and knowledge of their adverse effects among university students of Karachi.

Competing interests
The authors declare that they have no competing interests.

Authors' contributions
All authors took part in data collection. SJS overlooked the process of data collection, did the analysis and discussion along with others and reviewed the whole manuscript. HA did the analysis, made the tables and contributed

towards discussion. RBR made a contribution towards methodology and did analysis as well. SNA contributed to the background. MM wrote the results portions and proofread it. MHJ was the major contributor towards discussion. MSR made an abstract and made few tables. ZA and SFA were involved in discussion as well. MMK supervised the whole process. All authors read and approved the final manuscript.

Author details
[1]Aga Khan University, Karachi, Pakistan. [2]Department of Community Health Sciences, Aga Khan University, Karachi, Pakistan.

References

1. Kiyingi K, Lauwo J (Eds): *Drugs in the Home: Danger and Waste*, World Health Forum. 1993.
2. Napolitano F, Izzo MT, Di Giuseppe G, Angelillo IF: **Public knowledge, attitudes, and experience regarding the use of antibiotics in Italy.** *PloS One* 2013, **8**(12):e84177.
3. Kafle KK, Gartoulla RP: *Self-Medication and its Impact on Essential Drugs Schemes in Nepal: A Socio-Cultural Research Project: Action Programme on Essential Drugs.* Geneva: World Health Organization; 1993.
4. Mumtaz Y, Jahangeer SA, Mujtaba T, Zafar S, Adnan S: **Self medication among university students of Karachi.** *JLUMHS* 2011, **10**(03):102–5.
5. World Health Organization: **The role of the pharmacist in self-care and self-medication.** In *Report of the 4th WHO Consultative Group on the Role of the Pharmacist in Health Care System.* Geneva: WHO; 1998.
6. Shehadeh M, Suaifan G, Darwish RM, Wazaify M, Zaru L, Alja'fari S: **Knowledge, attitudes and behavior regarding antibiotics use and misuse among adults in the community of Jordan. A pilot study.** *Saudi Pharmaceut J* 2012, **20**(2):125–33.
7. James H, Handu SS, Al Khaja KA, Otoom S, Sequeira RP: **Evaluation of the knowledge, attitude and practice of self-medication among first-year medical students.** *Medical Principles and Practice* 2006, **15**(4):270–5.
8. Shankar P, Partha P, Shenoy N: **Self-medication and non-doctor prescription practices in Pokhara valley, Western Nepal: a questionnaire-based study.** *BMC Family Practice* 2002, **3**(1):17.
9. Zafar SN, Syed R, Waqar S, Zubairi AJ, Vaqar T, Shaikh M: **Self-medication amongst university students of Karachi: prevalence, knowledge and attitudes.** *J Pakistan Med Ass* 2008, **58**(4):214.
10. Belkina T, Warafi AA, Eltom EH, Tadjieva N, Kubena A, Vlcek J: **Antibiotic use and knowledge in the community of Yemen, Saudi Arabia, and Uzbekistan.** *J Infect Dev Countries* 2014, **8**(4):424–429.
11. Appelbaum P, Scragg J, Bowen A, Bhamjee A, Hallett A, Cooper R: **Streptococcus pneumoniae resistant to penicillin and chloramphenicol.** *Lancet* 1977, **310**(8046):995–7.
12. Farrar WE, Eidson M: **R factors in strains of Shigella dysenteriae type 1 isolated in the western hemisphere during 1969–1970.** *J Infect Dis* 1971, **124**(3):327–9.
13. Olarte J, Galindo E: **Salmonella typhi resistant to chloramphenicol, ampicillin, and other antimicrobial agents: strains isolated during an extensive typhoid fever epidemic in Mexico.** *Antimicrob Agents Chemother* 1973, **4**(6):597–601.
14. Grigoryan L, Burgerhof JG, Degener JE, Deschepper R, Lundborg CS, Monnet DL, *et al*: **Determinants of self-medication with antibiotics in Europe: the impact of beliefs, country wealth and the healthcare system.** *J Antimicrob Chemother* 2008, **61**(5):1172–9.
15. stat Les Mimorandums, Memorandaare: **Control of antibiotic-resistant bacteria: memorandum from a WHO Meeting.** *Bull World Health Organ* 1983, **61**(3):423–433.
16. Awad AI, Eltayeb IB: **Self-medication practices with antibiotics and antimalarials among Sudanese undergraduate university students.** *Ann Pharmacother* 2007, **41**(7–8):1249–55.
17. Pan H, Cui B, Zhang D, Farrar J, Law F, Ba-Thein W: **Prior knowledge, older age, and higher allowance are risk factors for self-medication with antibiotics among university students in southern China.** *PloS One* 2012, **7**(7):e41314.
18. Sarahroodi S, Arzi A, Sawalha A, Ashtarinezhad A: **Antibiotics self-medication among Southern Iranian University students.** *Intern J Pharmacol* 2010, **6**(1):48–52.
19. Shehnaz SI, Khan N, Sreedharan J, Issa KJ, Arifulla M: **Self-medication and related health complaints among expatriate high school students in the United Arab Emirates.** *Pharmacy Pract* 2013, **11**(4):211–8.

19

Adverse drug events identified by triggers at a teaching hospital in Brazil

Fabíola Giordani[1*], Suely Rozenfeld[2†] and Mônica Martins[2†]

Abstract

Background: Adverse drug events (ADEs) are one of the most frequent causes of patient harm resulting from medical interventions, especially among inpatients. This study aimed to evaluate the incidence of ADEs and characterise them in terms of degree of harm, medication implicated and patient symptoms, at a Brazilian university hospital.

Methods: This is a retrospective study of chart review. The method, developed by the Institute for Healthcare Improvement, uses triggers to identify possible ADEs. The study population comprised adult inpatients at least 15 years old. Obstetric patients and those hospitalised for less than 48 hours were excluded. Time spent in the intensive care unit was not considered for the purposes of this study. Patients were selected on the basis of simple random sampling of records of patients discharged from January to July 2008. The records selected were reviewed by a multidisciplinary team. The indicators of ADE incidence were patients with ADEs and ADE rate per 100 patients. Patients with and without ADE were compared in the bivariate analysis. To identify the drugs classes most often associated with events, the number of prescriptions of each class of drug was related to the number of events assigned to it.

Results: The 240 inpatients studied were of mean age 50.8 (SD = 20.0) years, and mostly male (63.8%). A total of 44 ADEs were identified in 35 patient records, with 14.6% of patients presenting ADE and a rate of 18.3% ADEs per 100 patients. The most frequent were skin rash and nausea and vomiting, but severe ADEs were also identified. In the bivariate analysis long hospital stay and use of 10 or more drugs were associated with the occurrence of ADEs (p-value < 0.01). The drug classes associated with the highest number of events were anti-infective.

Conclusion: About 1/6 of the hospitalized patients in a teaching hospital showed adverse events what is, by itself, cause for concern. Increased number of prescribed drugs and greater period of hospitalization appear to favour the occurrence of these events. In the future studies with higher number of patients may offer evidences of the association.

Background

Adverse drug events (ADEs) are among the most frequent adverse events affecting hospital inpatients [1-3]. Percentages of hospital inpatients suffering ADEs range from 1.6% to 41.4% and the rate, from 1.7 to 51.8 events/100 admissions. A considerable proportion of such events are avoidable [4].

Despite a lack of consensus, important risk factors reported for ADEs include polypharmacy, female sex, administration of drugs with narrow therapeutic range, renal elimination of drug, age >65 years, and administration of anticoagulants or diuretics [5]. Other risk factors reported are acute diseases or metabolic disturbances, as well as use of drugs with low therapeutic indices and hepatic enzyme inhibitors or inducers [6].

Mechanisms for evaluating and monitoring the safety of drugs in clinical use are essential in order to prevent or reduce harm to patients [7]. There are various methods and techniques for identifying ADEs during hospital stay,

* Correspondence: fabiolagiordani@id.uff.br
†Equal contributors
[1]Department of Epidemiology and Biostatistics, Institute of Community Health, Fluminense Federal University, Marquês de Paraná Street 303, Annex HUAP 3rd floor, Niterói, RJ 24033-900, Brazil
Full list of author information is available at the end of the article

including voluntary notification of cases, retrospective or prospective patient record review, and analysis of administrative data. An approach to identifying, quantifying and monitoring ADEs is to use triggers. These correspond to signs found during patient record review that may relate to adverse events [8,9].

In Brazil this approach has been used in a few studies to identify events in general hospitals [10] and special units [11,12].

Accordingly, the trigger method was used in this study to evaluate the incidence of ADE and characterise them in terms of degree of harm, medication implicated and patient symptoms, at a Brazilian university hospital.

Methods
Study design and population
This is a retrospective study of chart review at a public teaching hospital in the west of Paraná State in southern Brazil. The 173-bed hospital offers care to acute patients in various specialities.

Ethical approval for the study was given by the Ethical Committee of the State University of West Paraná (039/2009-CEP).

The study population comprised adult patients at least 15 years old. Obstetric patients and those hospitalised for less than 48 hours were excluded. Time spent in the intensive care unit was not considered for the purposes of this study. Patients were selected on the basis of simple random sampling of records of patients discharged from January to July 2008 (n = 1302). The parameters for calculating sample size were an estimated 15% of patients with ADEs, 95% confidence level and 10% desired absolute precision. Sample size calculation was 242.

Review of patient charts was performed with a tool developed by the Institute of Health Care Improvement (IHI) which consists of a set of triggers used to identify possible ADEs. The method is useful to measure the overall level of harm from medications in a health care organization. The trigger tool provides instructions for conducting a retrospective review of patient records. The records selected were reviewed to identify the presence of at least one of the 19 triggers proposed by the IHI [13].

Definition of ADE
ADE was defined as any injury occurring during the patient's drug therapy and resulting either from appropriate care, or from unsuitable or suboptimal care. The definition encompasses adverse drug reactions and medication errors [14].

Data collection
The patient record review and evaluation were performed after training with the data collection instruments and instruction manuals. The reviewers discussed the methods

and procedures intensively. The definitions of each trigger and possible associated ADEs were standardised. A pretest of patient records not included in the sample helped standardise the data collection procedures. In addition, the reviewers were instructed to record any ADE identified during hospitalisation, even if the event was not associated with any trigger or was present on patient admission.

Evaluation of the adverse events was conducted in three stages:

- In the first stage, the following information was extracted from the patient records: social and demographic data; drug prescriptions; and characteristics of the clinical and hospitalisation histories. The patient records were reviewed in the following order: laboratory results, drug prescriptions, and doctors' and nurses' clinical progress notes. Two reviewers (one pharmacy student and one medical student), working independently, evaluated each patient record. Divergences were resolved by a pharmacist with a background in public health.
- The second stage was performed by a nurse and a pharmacist and comprised in-depth review of the records containing triggers. Those where at least one of these reviewers identified an ADE were selected for evaluation in the next stage.
- In the third stage, we decided whether ADEs had occurred. The possible ADE was evaluated by the participants of the preceding stages, plus a clinician, in a face-to-face meeting.

Possible associations between events and suspect drugs were examined according to the drugs' properties [15,16], the patient's clinical condition and the time until the occurrence of the event. The Naranjo algorithm [17] was applied to determine the strength of the causal relationship with the drugs used by the patient and implicated in the occurrence of each ADE. The total scores allowed us to classify the ADEs as doubtful (< 1), possible (1–4), probable (5–8) or definite (≥ 9).

The reviewers classified ADEs by degree of harm into five categories (E-I) [13]. The events were described using WHO Adverse Reaction Terminology (WHO-ART) [18].

Further information on the method and techniques employed can be found in a previous publication [19].

Study variables and statistical analysis
The outcome was the ADEs occurring during the hospital stay. The variables evaluated were: age in years; sex (female; male); type of admission (acute/emergency; elective); type of treatment (surgical; clinical); type of discharge (medical discharge; transfer; death); treatment in intensive care unit (yes; no); length of stay in days, cut-off point by

mean = 10.0 (SD = 12.2) days (2–10 days; 11 or more days); hospitalisation cost by tercile (low; middle; high); Charlson index (0; 1–2; and 3–9); number of drugs used (1–9; 10 or more); and medical diagnoses.

Drugs were coded according to the first and second levels of the Anatomical Therapeutic Chemical (ATC) classification [20]. The probability of association of each drug class with ADEs was calculated by dividing the number of times the class was positively related to an event by the number of prescriptions of each class, and multiplying by 100.

Co-morbidities – including the primary and secondary diagnosis from the cover sheet and coded according to the 10th International Classification of Diseases (ICD-10) [21], plus further co-morbidities identified from the progress sheets – were examined using the Charlson index [22]. The index evaluates patient severity by the presence of the following clinical conditions: AIDS, cerebrovascular disease, congestive heart failure, connective tissue disease, dementia, myocardial infarction, peripheral vascular disease, peptic ulcer disease, chronic obstructive pulmonary disease, hemiplegia, cancer, diabetes mellitus (with or without chronic complications); and liver and/or kidney disease.

The indicators of ADE frequency were: incidence of patients with ADEs (number of patients with at least one new ADE/number of patients) and ADE rate per 100 patients (number of new ADEs/number of patients) with their respective confidence intervals (95% CI). Patients with and without ADE were compared in the bivariate analysis. To identify the drugs classes most often associated with events, the number of prescriptions of each class of drug was related to the number of events assigned to it. To perform this the number of prescriptions of each drug class associated to an ADE was divided by the number of prescriptions of the drug class.

In the descriptive statistical analysis, the continuous variables were expressed by mean and standard deviation, and the categorical variables, by percentages. The continuous variables were subjected to the Kolmogorov-Smirnov test to examine the assumption of normal distribution. To test the differences between patients with and without ADEs, bivariate analysis was performed considering the independent variables. Where appropriate, the T-Student, Chi-square and Fisher's Exact tests were performed to compare sub-groups.

Data were processed using EpiData 3.0 and Microsoft Office Access 2003, and analysed using the statistical packages SPSS 15.0 for Windows ® (SPSS Inc., Chicago, IL, U.S.A.) and R version 2.11.1.

Results
Characteristics of participants
The sample calculated comprised 242 patients. Of these there were nine losses, seven of which were considered

replaceable (three patients received outpatient treatment and were not hospitalised; two remained in the ICU throughout their hospitalisation; one was an obstetric patient; and one spent less than 48 hours hospitalised). The other two losses were deemed irreplaceable (patient records not located). These hospitalisations comprised 238 patients, but two were re-admitted and these were considered independent events. Thus the final sample comprised 240 records of patients admitted between January and July 2008 (corresponding to 2408 patient-days), whose data were examined.

The primary diagnoses most often found included "injury, poisoning and certain other consequences of external causes", followed by "diseases of the digestive system" and "diseases of the circulatory system".

The patients' mean age was 50.8 years, very close to the median (50 years), and they were predominantly male (63.8%). In the study sample, most of the patients (79.6%) were acute or emergency admissions; approximately 62.0% received surgical treatment and 5.4% died. Seventy-five percent of the patients were hospitalised for less than 10 days and mean hospital stay was 10.0 (SD = 12.2) days. In the sample, 60.0% of the patients displayed no co-morbidities contributing to the Charlson index and 51.7% used, on average, 10 or more different drugs during their hospitalisation. In the bivariate analysis only long hospital stay and use of 10 or more drugs were associated with the occurrence of ADEs (p-value < 0.01) (Table 1).

Incidence and rate of ADEs
A total of 44 ADEs were identified in 35 patient records, with 14.6% (95% CI 10.1-19.1) of patients presenting ADE and a rate of 18.3% (95% CI 13.4-23.2) ADEs per 100 patients. Of the 35 patients with ADEs, seven showed two or more events, with two of them showing three. Among the ADEs identified, two were not associated with the triggers (one was increased transaminases from use of phenytoin and the other was urinary retention from use of chlorpromazine). Two other events led to patient hospitalisation and did not enter into the analyses. In nine ADEs, identification was made possible by the presence of two or more triggers. One ADE, a skin rash, was identified by three different triggers: "antiallergics", "skin rash" and "abrupt discontinuation of medication".

Characteristics of ADEs
Using the Naranjo algorithm, 23 (52.3%) of the ADEs were classified as "possible" and 20 (45.4%), as "probable". In one case (2.3%), it was not possible to apply the algorithm.

As regards patient harm produced, 37 events (84.1%) were classified in category E, as involving temporary harm requiring intervention, and 4 (9.1%) in category F, as causing temporary harm and more extended hospital stay. Three (6.8%) events were classified as H, where the

Table 1 In-patient characteristics by occurrence of Adverse Drug Events (ADEs) at a Brazilian hospital

Variable	Without ADE	With ADE	Total	P-value[a]
	N (%)	N (%)	N (%)	
Total	205	35	240	-
Age in years	50.6 (19.8)	51.6 (21.4)	50.8 (20.0)	0.788
Mean (standard deviation)				
Sex				
Female	71 (81.6)	16 (18.4)	87 (36.2)	0.208
Male	134 (87.6)	19 (12.4)	153 (63.8)	
Nature of the admission				
Urgency/emergency	162 (84.8)	29 (15.2)	191 (79.6)	0.603
Elective	43 (87.8)	6 (12.2)	49 (20.4)	
Type of treatment				0.09
Surgical	131 (88.5)	17 (11.5)	148 (61.7)	
Clinical	74 (80.4)	18 (19.6)	92 (38.3)	
Status of discharge				
Discharged/transferred	195 (85.9)	32 (14.1)	227 (94.6)	0.290
Death	10 (76.9)	3 (23.1)	13 (5.4)	
ICU				
Yes	11 (84.6)	2 (15.4)	13 (15.4)	0.933
No	194 (85.5)	33 (14.5)	225 (94.6)	
Length of stay[b]				
≤ 10 days	164 (91.1)	16 (8.9)	180 (75.0)	<0.001
> 10 days	41 (68.3)	19 (31.1)	60 (25.0)	
Cost of hospitalisation[c]				
Low	73 (90.1)	8 (9.9)	81 (33.8)	0.331
Medium	66 (82.5)	14 (17.5)	80 (33.8)	
High	66 (83.5)	13 (16.5)	79 (32.9)	
Charlson index				
0	126 (87.5)	18 (12.5)	144 (60.0)	0.084
1-2	55 (87.3)	8 (12.7)	63 (26.3)	
3-9	24 (72.7)	9 (27.3)	33 (13.8)	
Number of drugs				
1-9	117 (94.4)	7 (5.6)	124 (48.3)	<0.001
10 or more	88 (75.9)	28 (24.1)	116 (51.7)	
Total	205	35	240	-

[a]Using T-Student for comparing mean ages, Chi-square and Fisher's Exact tests for comparing categorical variables.
[b]Cut-off by mean (10.0).
[c]Categorised in tertiles.

harm demands intervention to keep the patient alive; these were hypoglycaemia, cardiac tamponade and over-sedation.

Table 2 describes the events. The most frequent were skin rash (8 events), where ranitidine figured prominently as the attributed drug, and nausea and vomiting (8 events)

associated mainly with the use of an opioid (nalbuphine) and anti-infectives. Severe events affecting other systems included prolonged hypoglycaemia, cardiac tamponade and bed fall.

The drug classes associated with the highest number of events were those used for the nervous system (15), anti-infectives for systemic use (13) and drugs used to treat problems of the alimentary tract and metabolism (10) and blood and blood forming organs (7), as a result of their being the most prescribed. The drug class most strongly associated with ADEs was antiparasitic products (12.5%). The drug sub classes most prescribed were analgesics, antibacterial for systemic use, antithrombotic agents and drugs for acid related disorders (Table 3). The drugs most commonly involved were nalbuphine (5), heparin (4), ranitidine (4), captopril (2), phenytoin (2), chlorpromazine (2), morphine (2), moxifloxacin (2), amphotericin B (2) and omeprazole (2).

Discussion

About on-sixth of inpatients were found to have experienced ADEs, at a mean rate of 18.3 ADEs per 100 patients. A meta-analysis of observational studies presented estimates of ADE according to the method of identification of events [23]. In two out of twenty five studies the events were identified by a similar set of triggers. One of them was conducted in the United States with six community hospitals and estimated a rate of 15.0 ADEs per 100 patients [24]. In the other study, researchers encountered in a Brazilian hospital a rate of 26.6 ADEs per 100 patients [10]. Although the event rate in the last study is higher than ours the proportion of people with ADE estimated by the authors [10] is similar, around 15%. Some characteristics of the study population and the hospital's profile may explain the differences. The differences in rates may be also attributed to staff education or case mix that may occur even when comparing data from a single country.

The characteristics of ADEs we focused on were patient symptoms and degree of harm. Rashes, nausea, vomiting, pruritus and dizziness accounted for almost half the events. The profile of ADEs identified in our study is similar to that identified in a study conducted in a tertiary care hospital in Northern Brazil, where skin was found to be the most commonly affected organ system. The gastrointestinal system was also among the three most affected of them [25].

As regards degree of harm, most of the events resulted in temporary patient harm that required some intervention. Other studies also used the same source to classify ADEs, which is the National Coordinating Council for Medication Error Reporting and Prevention Index. They obtained similar proportions of events of lower degree of severity, 87% [26] and 79.9% [8]. Life-threatening events were much less common, as in other studies [24].

Table 2 Adverse drug events (ADEs) and imputed drugs

Description ADE[a]	Number of cases (n = 44)	Drugs
Rash	8	Ranitidine. Metronidazole. Cefazolin. Omeprazole. Morphine. Drug undetermined
Nausea and/or vomiting	8	Nalbuphine. Amphotericin B. Omeprazole. Mannitol. Moxifloxacin
Pruritus, rash, and dizziness	4	Tenoxicam. Nalbuphine. Cefalotin
Bleeding (haemoptysis, bleeding or melena)	4	Warfarin. Heparin. Omeprazole. Amitriptyline. Simvastatin. Heparin
		Acetylsalicylic acid. Heparin
Somnolence	2	Chlorpromazine. Phenytoin
Diarrhoea	2	Ampicillin + sulbactam. Lactulose
Tremor	2	Metoclopramide. Moxifloxacin
Cardiac tamponade	1	Heparin
Fall (from bed)	1	Captopril. Hydrochlorothiazide
Seizure	1	Methylprednisolone
Pseudomembranous colitis	1	Cefepime. Clarithromycin
Hypoglycaemia	1	Insulin
Excessive sedation	1	Midazolam
Other	8	Captopril. Furosemide. Nalbuphine, Morphine. Amphotericin B. Sulfamethoxazole + trimethoprim. Cefepime. Fluconazole. Pentamidine. Phenytoin. Chlorpromazine.

[a]The events were described using WHO Adverse Reaction Terminology (WHO-ART).

We also identified events that required intervention to keep the patient alive, such as hypoglycemia, cardiac tamponade and over-sedation, related, respectively, to the use of insulin, heparin and midazolam.

In our sample, certain classes of drugs are intensively prescribed and also strongly associated with ADEs (i.e., return higher ratios of "related ADEs" to "number of prescriptions"), they were analgesics, antibacterials for systemic use, antithrombotic agents and drugs for acid-related disorders. Ranitidine is a drug from this last subclass, as it is a histamine H2 receptor antagonists, and serves to illustrate the problem.

Ranitidine was implicated in cases of rash. It was the most frequent event identified in our study. It was prescribed for 70% of patients, a value compatible with those found in the literature for use in therapy to suppress gastric acid production [27,28]. We observed that, in most patients, ranitidine was being used as prophylactic medication rather than to treat gastrointestinal diseases. Stress ulcer prophylaxis has become an increasingly common practice for clinical patients, although there is little or no clinical evidence to support it [27] and it can be considered unnecessary in 73% of cases [28]. According to figures from this hospital, more than 50% of the ranitidine dispensed is for intravenous administration, which exposes the patients to unnecessary risk, because the injection route can cause local burning, itching, skin rash and vasculitis [15].

The occurrence of ADEs is associated with the number of drugs used [5,25,29-31]. Our data corroborate that association: the likelihood of an ADE occurring was higher in users of 10 or more drugs than in those who used fewer drugs during their hospital stay (p value <0.001), although the analysis was not adjusted for confounders. When patients are seriously ill, it is often difficult to evaluate the degree of harm to be attributed to the number of prescribed drugs or to drug classes. In our study population, one patient suffered a bed fall during the hospital stay. Besides the fact that he was exposed to drugs likely to cause falls (captopril, hydrochlorothiazide), evaluation of the harm was jeopardised by the complexity of the patient's condition (serious traffic accident casualty).

Patients with longer hospital stays are exposed to greater likelihood of ADE than those hospitalised for up to nine days (p value <0.001). This finding is consistent with those of several previous studies [5]. Hence it is important draw attention to long-stay inpatients, because in addition to being prone to ADEs, the tendency is towards multiple events and more pronounced patient harm.

As longer hospital stays and use of more drugs are regarded as factors associated with ADEs, our findings may help physicians to identify at-risk patients and monitor them carefully. Moreover, to prevent ADES during hospital stay, the risk factors can be categorised according to opportunities for intervention, such as decreasing the number of drugs prescribed or adjusting the dose [32].

This study has limitations in terms of the internal validity. The results of specific events should be analysed with caution because the sample size was calculated considering the estimated global incidence of ADEs. Thus, the frequency of specific events may reflect random variations and may be skewed.

Table 3 Drug classes related to an adverse drug event (ADE), by anatomical therapeutic chemical classification (ATC)

ATC code[a]	Number of prescriptions of the drug class	Number of prescriptions of the drug class associated with an ADE[b]	Proportion (%)
A - Alimentary tract and metabolism	**478**	**10**	**2.09**
A02 - Drugs for acid related disorders	197	7	3.6
A03 - Drugs for functional gastrointestinal disorders	182	1	0.6
A06 – Laxatives	15	1	6.7
A10 - Drugs used in diabetes	59	1	1.7
B - Blood and blood forming organs	**354**	**7**	**2.0**
B01 - Antithrombotic agents	228	6	2.6
B05 - Plasma substitutes and perfusion solutions	102	1	1.0
C - Cardiovascular system	**277**	**5**	**1.8**
C03 – Diuretics	69	2	2.9
C09 - Agents acting on the renin-angiotensin system	79	2	2.5
C10 - Lipid modifying agents	28	1	3.6
H - Systemic hormonal prep, excluding sex hormones	**44**	**1**	**2.3**
H02 - Corticosteroids for systemic use	44	1	2.3
J - General antiinfectives for systemic use	**405**	**13**	**3.2**
J01 - Antibacterials for systemic use	387	10	2.6
J02 - Antimycotics for systemic use	7	3	42.9
M - Musculo-skeletal system	**177**	**1**	**0.6**
M01 - Antiinflammatory and antirheumatic products	168	1	0.6
N - Nervous system	**566**	**15**	**2.7**
N02 – Analgesics	419	9	1.7
N03 – Antiepileptics	40	2	5.0
N05 – Psycholeptics	82	3	6.1
N06 - Psychoanaleptics	11	1	9.1
P - Antiparasitic products	**8**	**1**	**12.5**
P01 – Antiprotozoals	2	1	50.0
Unclassified drug	**9**	**1**	**11.1**
Total	**2499**	**54**	**2.2**

[a]The first and second level of the Anatomical Therapeutic Chemical Classification (ATC) associated with at least one ADE.
[b]Number of ADE-drugs is greater (54) than number of ADEs (44), because one drug can be associated with several ADEs.

Although the study is not large, we did succeed in observing values of the estimates that differed with statistical significance between patients with or without ADEs for the variables length of stay and number of medications in the bivariate analysis. However studies with larger samples should test the hypothesis of association.

The study was conducted at only one hospital, which makes external validity troublesome and places limitations on how far the results can be generalised. Nonetheless, they may be applied to other tertiary hospitals in medical schools in Brazil and in other countries.

We endeavoured to increase internal validity by using double data collection and assembling a team of researchers and health professionals to evaluate the cases. In order to improve objectivity, the method was applied at all stages by two independent reviewers, using a specific manual containing definitions and detailed descriptions of the procedures. Nonetheless, some subjectivity in identifying and interpreting triggers and events cannot be ruled out, as demonstrated in other retrospective patient record review studies [33]. The double-blind evaluation performed here was not intended to assess inter-observer reliability, but rather to foster information completeness and improve validity of the information. The double evaluation process with two physicians of patient records to assess ADE is not more reliable than a record review process with one physician [34].

Poor quality of information in hospital records is a common problem in chart review-based research [35], but the choice of a teaching hospital possibly reduces information bias. There were concerns about data completeness, however. Conspicuous gaps in the recorded information included race/ethnicity and occupation, which were missing from about 20% of patient records.

During application of the method, two events unrelated to the triggers were identified, one of them a case of increased blood transaminase levels resulting from use of phenytoin. Studies have shown that laboratory test results for transaminases levels can be effective triggers for detecting ADEs. Aspartate aminotransferase (AST) screening returns a positive predictive value between 0.01 and 0.23, and alanine aminotransferase (ALT), a value from 0 to 0.31 [36]. The fact that, in our study, some ADEs were not found by triggers reinforces the idea that no single method captures every event that occurs in hospitals. This challenges managers and policy makers to test and harmonise different methods to address adverse events. The use of triggers to identify ADEs, when integrated with event monitoring, stimulated or unstimulated spontaneous reporting and other techniques, can be an important strategy for indicating possible shortcomings in the process of using medications for hospitalised patients.

According to Rozich [8] the trigger enables organisations to monitor longitudinally how ADE rates change in response to strategies designed to improve clinical safety [8]. However, this strategy is nowadays mainly theoretical, since there are several obstacles to be overcome, among them: scant evidence of impact of ongoing strategies; the existence of different subcategories of drug adverse events requiring different improvement interventions; the fact that many common adverse events require more complex detection strategies [37,38].

The concept of ADE we used included drug adverse reactions (ADR) and errors. It does not conflict with the concept of ADR that sustains the algorithm used to determine the strength of the causal relationship with the drugs in our study and others [39-41]. Steady conceptual advances in the field of pharmacoepidemiology are permitting studies focussing primarily on occurrences of patient harm, regardless of whether or not such harm is associated with errors in therapeutic indication or drug administration. Besides, examining carefully the patient charts we did not identified any case of error like non adherence and subtherapeutic doses.

In 2013 Brazil's Ministry of Health launched a national patient safety programme [42]. It hinges on engaging patients in health care, including the subject of 'patient safety' in undergraduate and postgraduate education, and increasing research. On this latter item, the programme specifies measuring harm, understanding the causes, identifying the solutions, assessing the impact and applying the evidence to assure safer patient care. Given that framework, we believe the results of this study can help to call attention to the need of develop researchs aiming to estimate and characterize ADE and medication involved as well as the role of number of drugs prescribed for inpatients.

Conclusion

This study draws attention to the problem of ADE in hospitalized patients and offers a methodological alternative for future research in Brazil as well as other underdeveloped countries. Our results suggests that trigger tool may be useful to identify ADE in hospitals.

About 1/6 of the hospitalized patients in a teaching hospital showed adverse events what is, by itself, cause for concern. Although the events were classified as less serious in over 80% of cases, we also identified additional and more severe events that required intervention to keep the patient alive.

Analgesics, antibacterials for systemic use, antithrombotic agents, drugs for acid-related disorders should be used sparingly, because they are very often prescribed and associated with the highest numbers of events. These results should be examined with caution, as the number of ADE is small (44/240 patients). Increased number of prescribed drugs and greater period of hospitalization appear to favour the occurrence of these events but additional research should test this hypothesis.

Competing interests
The authors declare that they have no competing interests.

Authors' contributions
FG, MM and SR conceived and designed the study. FG collected data. FG, RS and MM performed data analysis. FG wrote the first draft of the manuscript. All authors contributed to the final draft of the manuscript and have read and approved of the final draft.

Acknowledgements
Studies were conducted with financial support from National Counsel of Technological and Scientific Development - CNPq (n° 471685/2007-0).

Author details
[1]Department of Epidemiology and Biostatistics, Institute of Community Health, Fluminense Federal University, Marquês de Paraná Street 303, Annex HUAP 3rd floor, Niterói, RJ 24033-900, Brazil. [2]Sérgio Arouca National School of Public Health, Oswaldo Cruz Foundation, Rio de Janeiro, Brazil.

References
1. Davis P, Lay-Yee R, Schug S, Briant R, Scott A, Johnson S, Bingley W: **Adverse events regional feasibility study: indicative findings.** *N Z Med J* 2001, 114:203–205.
2. Baker GR, Norton PG, Flintoft V, Blais R, Brown A, Cox J, Etchells E, Ghali WA, Hébert P, Majumdar SR, O'Beirne M, Palacios-Derflingher L, Reid RJ, Sheps S, Tamblyn R: **The Canadian adverse events study: the incidence of adverse events among hospital patients in Canada.** *CMAJ* 2004, 170:1678–1686.
3. Mendes W, Martins M, Rozenfeld S, Travassos C: **The assessment of adverse events in hospitals in Brazil.** *Int J Qual Health Care* 2009, 21:279–284.
4. Cano FG, Rozenfeld S: **Adverse drug events in hospitals: a systematic review.** *Cad Saude Publica* 2009, 25(Suppl 3):S360–S372.

5. Krähenbühl-Melcher A, Schlienger R, Lampert M, Haschke M, Drewe J, Krähenbühl S: **Drug-related problems in hospitals: a review of the recent literature.** *Drug Saf* 2007, **30**:379–407.
6. Ajayi FO, Sun H, Perry J: **Adverse drug reactions: a review of relevant factors.** *J Clin Pharmacol* 2000, **40**:1093–1101.
7. World Health Organization: **Looking at the Pharmacovigilance: ensuring the safe use of medicines.** In *WHO Policy Perspectives on Medicines*; http://who-umc.org/DynPage.aspx?id=105892&mn1=7347&mn2=7259&mn3=7298&mn4=7509.
8. Rozich JD, Haraden CR, Resar RK: **Adverse drug event trigger tool: a practical methodology for measuring medication related harm.** *Qual Saf Health Care* 2003, **12**:194–200.
9. Resar RK, Rozich JD, Classen DC: **Methodology and rationale for the measurement of harm with trigger tools.** *Qual Saf Health Care* 2003, **12**(suppl 2):ii39–ii45.
10. Rozenfeld S, Giordani F, Coelho S: **Adverse drug events in hospital: pilot study with trigger tool.** *Rev Saude Publica* 2013, **47**:1102–1111.
11. Roque KE, Melo EC: **Adjustment of evaluation criteria of adverse drug events for use in a public hospital in the State of Rio de Janeiro.** *Rev Bras Epidemiol* 2010, **13**:607–619.
12. Reis AM, Cassiani SH: **Adverse drug events in an intensive care unit of a University Hospital.** *Eur J Clin Pharmacol* 2011, **67**:625–632.
13. **Trigger tool for measuring adverse drug events.** http://www.ihi.org/Pages/default.aspx.
14. Committee of Experts on Management of Safety and Quality in Health Care: **Glossary of terms related to patient and medication safety.** http://www.bvs.org.ar/pdf/seguridadpaciente.pdf.
15. **Micromedex® Healthcare Series: MICROMEDEX 2.0.** http://www.periodicos.capes.gov.br.
16. Aroson JK: *Meyler's Side Effects of Drugs: The International Encyclopedia of Adverse Drug Reactions and Interactions.* Oxford: Elsevier; 2006.
17. Naranjo CA, Busto U, Sellers EM, Sandor P, Ruiz I, Roberts EA, Janecek E, Domecq C, Greenblatt DJ: **A method for estimating the probability of adverse drug reactions.** *Clin Pharmacol Ther* 1981, **30**:239–245.
18. *Sistema de Notificações em Vigilância Sanitária*; http://www.anvisa.gov.br/hotsite/notivisa/index.htm.
19. Giordani F, Rozenfeld S, Oliveira DF, Versa GL, Terencio JS, Caldeira L d F, Andrade LC: **Vigilância de eventos adversos a medicamentos em hospitais: aplicação e desempenho de rastreadores.** *Rev Bras Epidemiol* 2012, **15**:455–467.
20. World Health Organization Collaborating Centre for Drug Statistics Methodology: **ATC classification index with DDD.** http://www.whocc.no/atc_ddd_index/.
21. **International statistical classification of disease and related health problems.** 10th rev. http://apps.who.int/classifications/apps/icd/icd10online/.
22. Charlson ME, Pompei P, Ales KL, MacKenzie CR: **A new method of classifying prognostic comorbidity in longitudinal studies: development and validation.** *J Chronic Dis* 1987, **40**:373–383.
23. Martins AC, Giordani F, Rozenfeld S: **Adverse drug events among adult inpatients: a meta-analysis of observational studies.** *J Clin Pharm Ther* 2014, **39**:609–620.
24. Hug BL, Witkowski DJ, Sox CM, Keohane CA, Seger DL, Yoon C, Matheny ME, Bates DW: **Adverse drug event rates in six community hospitals and the potential impact of computerized physician order entry for prevention.** *J Gen Intern Med* 2010, **25**:31–38.
25. Lobo MG, Pinheiro SM, Castro JG, Momenté VG, Pranchevicius MC: **Adverse drug reaction monitoring: support for pharmacovigilance at a tertiary care hospital in Northern Brazil.** *BMC Pharmacol Toxicol* 2013, **14**:5.
26. Nebeker JR, Hoffman JM, Weir CR, Bennett CL, Hurdle JF: **High rates of adverse drug events in a highly computerized hospital.** *Arch Intern Med* 2005, **165**:1111–1116.
27. Grube RR, May DB: **Stress ulcer prophylaxis in hospitalized patients not in intensive care units.** *Am J Health Syst Pharm* 2007, **64**:1396–1400.
28. Gupta R, Garg P, Kottoor R, Munoz JC, Jamal MM, Lambiase LR, Vega KJ: **Overuse of acid suppression therapy in hospitalized patients.** *South Med J* 2010, **103**:207–211.
29. Van DenBemt PM, Egberts AC, Lenderink AW, Verzijl JM, Simons KA, Van Der Pol WS, Leufkens HG: **Risk factors for the development of adverse drug events in hospitalized patients.** *Pharm World Sci* 2000, **22**:62–66.
30. Sánchez Muñoz-Torrero JF, Barquilla P, Velasco R, Fernández Capitan Mdel C, Pacheco N, Vicente L, Chicón JL, Trejo S, Zamorano J, Lorenzo Hernandez A: **Adverse drug reactions in internal medicine units and associated risk factors.** *Eur J Clin Pharmacol* 2010, **66**:1257–1264.
31. Davies EC, Green CF, Taylor S, Williamson PR, Mottram DR, Pirmohamed M: **Adverse drug reactions in hospital in-patients: a prospective analysis of 3695 patient-episodes.** *PLoS One* 2009, **4**:e4439.
32. Kane-Gill SL, Kirisci L, Verrico MM, Rothschild JM: **Analysis of risk factors for adverse drug events in critically ill patients.** *Crit Care Med* 2012, **40**:823–828.
33. Thomas EJ, Lipsitz SR, Studdert DM, Brennan TA: **The reliability of medical record review for estimating adverse event rates.** *Ann Intern Med* 2002, **136**:812–816.
34. Zegers M, de Bruijne MC, Wagner C, Groenewegen PP, van der Wal G, de Vet HC: **The inter-rater agreement of retrospective assessments of adverse events does not improve with two reviewers per patient record.** *J Clin Epidemiol* 2010, **63**:94–102.
35. Lau HS, Florax C, Porsius AJ, De Boer A: **The completeness of medication histories in hospital medical records of patients admitted to general internal medicine wards.** *Br J Clin Pharmacol* 2000, **49**:597–603.
36. Handler SM, Altman RL, Perera S, Hanlon JT, Studenski SA, Bost JE, Saul MI, Fridsma DB: **A systematic review of the performance characteristics of clinical event monitor signals used to detect adverse drug events in the hospital setting.** *J Am Med Inform Assoc* 2007, **14**:451–458.
37. Classen DC, Metzger J: **Improving medication safety: the measurement conundrum and where to start.** *Int J Qual Health Care* 2003, **15**(Suppl 1):i41–i47.
38. Shojania KG, Thomas EJ: **Trends in adverse events over time: why are we not improving?** *BMJ Qual Saf* 2013, **22**:273–277.
39. Mycyk MB, McDaniel MR, Fotis MA, Regalado J: **Hospital wide adverse drug events before and after limiting weekly work hours of medical residents to 80.** *Am J Health Syst Pharm* 2005, **62**:1592–1595.
40. Kilbridge PM, Campbell UC, Cozart HB, Mojarrad MG: **Automated surveillance for adverse drug events at a community hospital and an academic medical center.** *J Am Med Inform Assoc* 2006, **13**:372–377.
41. Chen YC, Fan JS, Chen MH, Hsu TF, Huang HH, Cheng KW, Yen DH, Huang CI, Chen LK, Yang CC: **Risk factors associated with adverse drug events among older adults in emergency department.** *Eur J Intern Med* 2014, **25**:49–55.
42. **Documento de referência para o Programa Nacional de Segurança do Paciente.** http://bvsms.saude.gov.br/bvs/publicacoes/documento_referencia_programa_nacional_seguranca.pdf.

20

Modeling skin sensitization potential of mechanistically hard-to-be-classified aniline and phenol compounds with quantum mechanistic properties

Qin Ouyang[1,4†], Lirong Wang[1†], Ying Mu[3] and Xiang-Qun Xie[1,2*]

Abstract

Background: Advanced structure-activity relationship (SAR) modeling can be used as an alternative tool for identification of skin sensitizers and in improvement of the medical diagnosis and more effective practical measures to reduce the causative chemical exposures. It can also circumvent ethical concern of using animals in toxicological tests, and reduce time and cost. Compounds with aniline or phenol moieties represent two large classes of frequently skin sensitizing chemicals but exhibiting very variable, and difficult to predict, potency. The mechanisms of action are not well-understood.

Methods: A group of mechanistically hard-to-be-classified aniline and phenol chemicals were collected. An *in silico* model was established by statistical analysis of quantum descriptors for the determination of the relationship between their chemical structures and skin sensitization potential. The sensitization mechanisms were investigated based on the features of the established model. Then the model was utilized to analyze a subset of FDA approved drugs containing aniline and/or phenol groups for prediction of their skin sensitization potential.

Results and discussion: A linear discriminant model using the energy of the highest occupied molecular orbital (ϵ_{HOMO}) as the descriptor yielded high prediction accuracy. The contribution of ϵ_{HOMO} as a major determinant may suggest that autoxidation or free radical binding could be involved. The model was further applied to predict allergic potential of a subset of FDA approved drugs containing aniline and/or phenol moiety. The predictions imply that similar mechanisms (autoxidation or free radical binding) may also play a role in the skin sensitization caused by these drugs.

Conclusions: An accurate and simple quantum mechanistic model has been developed to predict the skin sensitization potential of mechanistically hard-to-be-classified aniline and phenol chemicals. The model could be useful for the skin sensitization potential predictions of a subset of FDA approved drugs.

Keywords: Chemical mechanisms, Structure-activity relationship, Skin sensitizer, Anilines, Phenols, Quantum mechanism

* Correspondence: xix15@pitt.edu
†Equal contributors
[1]Department of Pharmaceutical Sciences, Computational Chemical Genomics Screening Center, School of Pharmacy, NIH National Center, of Excellence for Computational Drug Abuse Research, Drug Discovery Institute, Pittsburgh, PA 15261, USA
[2]Department of Computational and Systems Biology, University of Pittsburgh, Pittsburgh, PA 15261, USA
Full list of author information is available at the end of the article

Background

Skin sensitization related dermatitis and rash represents the most common manifestation of chemical immunotoxicity in humans, which results in a cost estimated $1 billion annually due to lost work, reduced productivity, medical care, and disability payments in USA [1,2]. In addition, as part of the regulatory review process, an increase in the incidence of skin allergies and hypersensitivity-related adverse events associated with the use of FDA regulated products or approved drugs has been observed, suggesting a safety gap between premarket review and the post market surveillance [2].

Common testing methods to assess skin sensitization potential of materials include: (1) guinea pig maximization test (GPMT); (2) murine-based local lymph node assay (LLNA). In GPMT tests, hazard identification is done by visual observations of erythema and edema reactions, which are subjective, are difficult to differentiate between contact allergens and strong irritants, and is time consuming [3]. The LLNA is recommended by international regulatory agencies; however, inconsistencies between LLNA and clinical observations have been documented [4]. Considering the existence of vast compounds around today, developing rapid and effective methods for chemical sensitizer identification/risk assessment is still a challenge [2].

In silico approaches are an attractive alternative to animal testing through analyzing the structural features of sensitizers/non-sensitizers to derive predictive rules or models [5]. The risks of thousands of commercially available chemicals could be assessed in a cost effective manner. Among these approaches, mechanism based rules, which investigate the structural characteristics of sensitizers, are promising [6].

Historically, the first study of chemical reactivity and skin sensitization was reported in 1936 [7]. A mechanism of small organic molecules to form an immunogenic complex by reacting with macromolecules (proteins or others) in the skin to cause sensitization was postulated. Currently, a more plausible mechanism reported involves a formation of covalent bonding between electrophilic allergens and nucleophilic moieties of amino acids from skin proteins (usually side chains) [8]. Such amino acids include cysteine thiol (mainly) and lysine (amino), and to a lesser extent arginine, histidine, methionine and tyrosine [9]. Based on the well-established principles of mechanistic organic chemistry, the skin sensitization potential of a chemical in many cases was predicted by its reactivity with these residues [9,10]. However, some compounds need to be activated via either autoxidation outside the skin (prehaptens) or bioactivation inside the skin (prohaptens) to be able to form immunogenic complexes with skin proteins [11].

Structure-activity relationship (SAR) studies of skin sensitization potential have been successfully carried out for epoxyaldehydes [12], enone [13], halogenated aromatics [14], benzaldehydes [15], dienes [16], oximes [17], aldehydes [18] and epoxides [19]. Aniline/aromatic amine and/or phenol derivatives are two large classes of frequently sensitizing chemicals. Quite a few pilot studies have been conducted [20-23]. Roberts *et al.* specifically investigated the sensitization mechanisms of diaminobenzenes or dihydroxylbenzenes [24]. However, the predictability of the skin sensitization potential for these two classes of chemicals is unsatisfactory [6,25]. Further exploration of novel sensitization mechanisms will be informative for constructing better SAR models/rules. In addition, aniline and phenol moieties that are often present in approved drugs can also cause skin sensitization. For example, contact dermatitis occurs in one individual following prolonged subcutaneous infusion of hydromorphone [26], a cancer pain treatment agent which contains one phenol moiety.

Drug-induced skin reactions may be associated with several biological mechanisms, but in many cases the precise mechanism is unclear [27]. It is well-known that Type IV allergic reaction induced by many chemicals and drugs is a T-cell mediated delay type hypersensitivity which can cause skin sensitization/dermatitis [27].

In this study, we intended to establish an *in silico* model for a class of mechanistically hard-to-classify anilines and phenols to study the relationship between their chemical reactivity and biological allergic response. We then investigated sensitization mechanisms of action associated with these compounds based on the features of this model. The model was further utilized to analyze a subset of FDA approved drugs containing aniline and/or phenol groups in skin sensitization potential. The predicted skin sensitization potential for these drugs was validated according to relevant literatures and adverse event reports.

Methods

Data sets

A data set of 63 chemicals, including 30 anilines and 33 phenols, was collected from published literature [11,23,28-36]. Chemicals with well-known allergic mechanisms, *i.e.* Michael acceptors (MA), SN_2 electrophiles, S_NAr electrophiles, Schiff base formers, and acylation agents, were excluded from the data set. For example, pentachlorophenol (CAS: 87-86-5) belongs to S_NAr electrophiles; benzyl salicylate (CAS: 118-58-1) and 3,3′,4′,5-tetrachlorosalicylanilide (CAS: 1154-59-2) are acylation agents. In addition, chemicals having two OH and NH_2 substituents at aromatic rings were also excluded from the data set because these compounds are known to easily form a benzoquinone (a Michael acceptor) or a nitrogen analogue of benzoquinone (also a Michael acceptor) [24]. Finally, a list of 30 chemicals was obtained (Table 1). They

Table 1 Summary of the ϵ_{HOMO}, predicted values of the 30 chemicals and their experimentally determined data [11,23,28-36]

ID	Cas #	Name	Sensitizer	EC3	Ref.	ϵ_{HOMO} (hartree)	P
1	101-80-4	4,4-diaminodiphenylether	Y		30	−0.262	1.0694
2	106-47-8	4-Chloroaniline	Y	6.5	33,35	−0.289	0.6563
3	150-13-0	4-Aminobenzoic acid	N		31	−0.306	0.3962
4	369-36-8	2-Fluoro-5-nitroaniline	N		34	−0.325	0.1055
5	538-41-0	4,4-diaminoazobenzene	Y		30	−0.258	1.1306
6	62-53-3	Aniline	Y	89	31,36	−0.286	0.7022
7	79456-26-1	3-Chloro-5-(trifluoromethyl)-2-pyridinamine	N		23	−0.326	0.0902
8	2050-14-8	2,2'-Azodiphenol	Y	27.9	34	−0.294	0.5798
9	55845-90-4	(N-Benzyl-N-ethylamino)-3'-hydroxyacetophenone hydrochloride	N		23	−0.316	0.2432
10	69-72-7	Salicylic acid	N		31	−0.343	−0.1699
11	90-15-3	1-Naphthol	Y	1.3	11,29.33	−0.274	0.8858
12	94-13-3	Propylparaben	N		11	−0.329	0.0443
13	97-54-1	Isoeugenol	Y	3.5	31,33,32	−0.277	0.8399
14	99-96-7	4-Hydrobenzoic acid	N		11	−0.341	−0.1393
15	186743-26-0	3-Methyleugenol	Y	32	33,36	−0.294	0.5798
16	101-77-9*	4,4-diaminodiphenylmethane	Y		30	−0.266	1.0082
17	121-57-3*	Sulphanilic acid	N		11	−0.322	0.1514
18	537-65-5*	4,4-diaminodiphenylamine	Y		30	−0.243	1.3601
19	60-09-3*	4-aminophenylazobenzene	Y		30	−0.276	0.8552
20	63-74-1*	Sulfanilamide	N		11	−0.307	0.3809
21	94-09-7*	Benzocaine	N		33	−0.303	0.4421
22	15128-82-2*	3-Hydroxy-2-nitropyridine	N		31	−0.362	−0.4606
23	2785-87-7*	Dihydroeugenol	Y	12.45	11,29,32	−0.288	0.6716
24	619-14-7*	3-Hydroxy-4-nitrobenzoic acid	N		31	−0.371	−0.5983
25	80-05-7*	bisphenol A	Y		30	−0.287	0.6869
26	93-51-6*	2-Methoxy-4-methyl-phenol	Y	5.8	11,29,32	−0.288	0.6716
27	97-53-0*	Eugenol	Y	13.95	31,32,33	−0.296	0.5492
28	99-76-3*	Methyl 4-hydroxybenzoate	N		11	−0.329	0.0443
29	119-36-8*	Methyl salicylate	N		28	−0.326	0.0902
30	831-82-3*	4-Phenoxyphenol	Y		33	−0.293	0.5951

*Test set.

represent a class of mechanistically hard-to-be-classified compounds because they can't be classified into any of the abovementioned five categories. These compounds were then randomly split into a training set of 15 compounds and a test set of 15 compounds. As shown in Table 1, the training set includes 7 anilines and 8 phenols, while the test set includes 6 anilines and 9 phenols. The detailed information including initial screening of the 63 selected chemicals is available as Additional file 1.

Quantum mechanics calculations

All chemical optimization and subsequent orbital analysis were performed by using the Gaussian 03 suite of programs [37]. Chemicals were optimized using the AM1 Hamiltonian with the default optimization criteria [38,39]. Calculations of the frontier molecular orbital, charge distribution and other quantum properties were carried out by using the 6-31Gd basis set. The quantum descriptors used in this study include the energies of the highest occupied molecular orbital (ϵ_{HOMO}), the lowest unoccupied molecular orbital (ϵ_{LUMO}), the second lowest unoccupied molecular orbital (ϵ_{LUMO+1}), the second highest occupied molecular orbital (ϵ_{HOMO-1}), the Mulliken atomic charges of the most negative (Q_{min}) and most positive atoms (Q_{max}), the Mulliken atomic charges of the N atom (Q_N) in anilines or O atom (Q_O) in phenols, the average of the absolute values of the charges on all atoms (Q_m), and molecular dipole moment (μ). The shapes of the resulting orbitals were visualized using the GaussView application within Gaussian 03. All structures were either drawn or converted from SMILES (Simplified molecular-input line-entry system) strings, using Chembiodraw Ultra V12.0 (PerkinElmer Informatics Desktop Software).

Statistical analysis

The skin sensitization potency of a compound was symbolized by 1 (Yes) and 0 (No). The values of each quantum descriptor were linearly normalized to the same range (0 to 1), stepwise linear regressions between the quantum properties and experimental outputs of the training set were performed by the statistical package of R program version 3.0.0 [40]. The properties with lower weighting factors were abandoned in the second step of linear regression.

Results and discussion

The compounds with aniline and/or phenol moieties can be classified into a single subclass for consideration of skin sensitizers. However, not all of the compounds possessing aniline or phenol groups are sensitizers, suggesting some compounds can form covalent bonds with skin proteins whereas others cannot. In this study, the sensitization potential of anilines and phenols were modeled using quantum mechanical descriptors.

Modeling the skin sensitization potential by quantum properties of anilines and phenols

The coefficient constant of ϵ_{HOMO} was determined as the highest weighting factor based on the results of linear regression analysis. The skin sensitization potential of anilines and phenols can be formulated as:

$$\text{Predicted Value}(P) = 15.30 * \epsilon_{HOMO}(\text{Hartree}) + 5.08(1) \quad (1)$$

The median of the symbolized skin sensitization potency, 0.50, was considered as the threshold for prediction of sensitizers and non-sensitizers. An aniline or phenol is predicted as a sensitizer if P is greater than 0.50, and as a non-sensitizer if P is below 0.5. With a threshold of $P = 0.50$, Equation 1 implies that a chemical within the applicability domain is predicted to be a skin sensitizer if the HOMO energy is greater than −0.30 Hartree $((0.5-5.08)/15.30 = -0.299 \approx -0.30)$. The experimental allergenicity categories (sensitizer or non-sensitizer) and predicted results of the training set are shown in Figure 1, where red-open circle dots indicate well-known sensitizers at 1 and non-sensitizers at 0, respectively. The blue-solid-diamond dots indicate the predicted values. All of the training compounds were correctly predicted by Formula 1. The same model was applied to the test set. Interestingly, all test compounds were correctly predicted (Figure 2). The total prediction accuracy of chemicals in training and test sets was 100% (30/30). The model shows very high accuracy and only depends on the value of ϵ_{HOMO}, suggesting that ϵ_{HOMO} is a key factor for the assessment of skin sensitization potential of those aniline and phenol containing compounds.

The linear relationship between the predicted values and ϵ_{HOMO} also suggests that a chemical with higher predicted value implies a higher reactivity for oxidation consequently resulting in higher skin sensitization potential. The LLNA data as a quantitative endpoint, posed

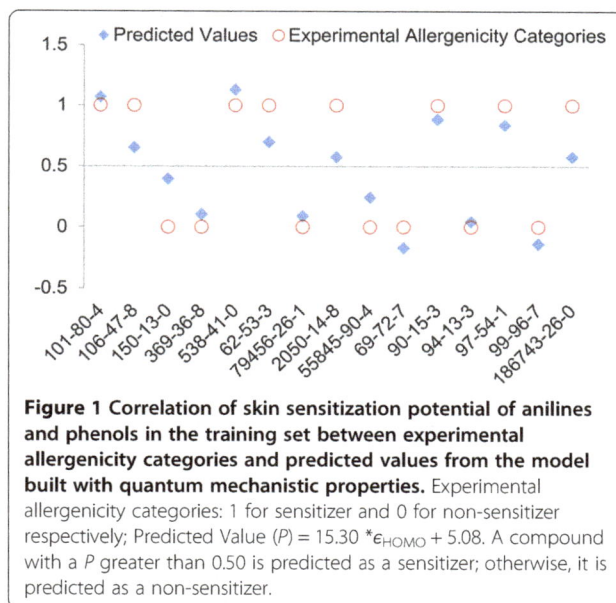

Figure 1 Correlation of skin sensitization potential of anilines and phenols in the training set between experimental allergenicity categories and predicted values from the model built with quantum mechanistic properties. Experimental allergenicity categories: 1 for sensitizer and 0 for non-sensitizer respectively; Predicted Value $(P) = 15.30 * \epsilon_{HOMO} + 5.08$. A compound with a P greater than 0.50 is predicted as a sensitizer; otherwise, it is predicted as a non-sensitizer.

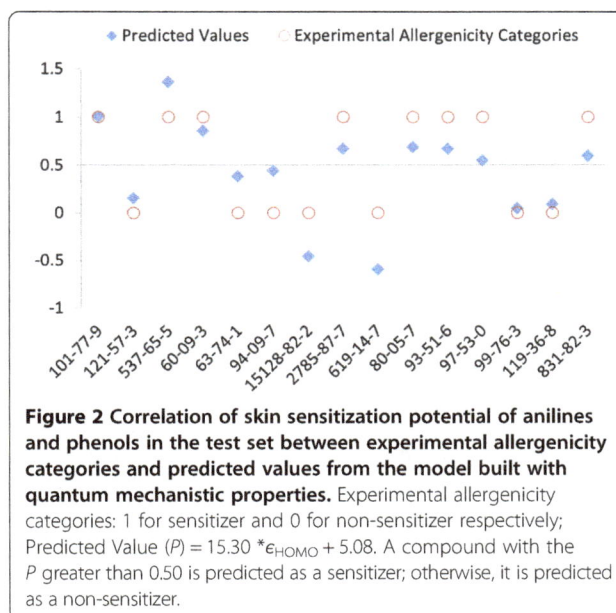

Figure 2 Correlation of skin sensitization potential of anilines and phenols in the test set between experimental allergenicity categories and predicted values from the model built with quantum mechanistic properties. Experimental allergenicity categories: 1 for sensitizer and 0 for non-sensitizer respectively; Predicted Value $(P) = 15.30 * \epsilon_{HOMO} + 5.08$. A compound with the P greater than 0.50 is predicted as a sensitizer; otherwise, it is predicted as a non-sensitizer.

a semi-dose-dependent manner, allows for prediction of potency. The EC3 values (effective concentration for a three-fold proliferation of lymph node cells) from the reported LLNA experiments of most allergen phenols were also collected as shown in Table 1. Weak sensitizers with higher EC3 values (meaning lower sensitization potential) have smaller P values. For example, P values of five weak sensitizers with 100 > EC3 > 10 i.e., eugenol (CAS: 97-53-0, EC3 = 13.95), Dihydroeugenol (CAS: 2785-87-7, EC3 = 12.45), 2,2'-azodiphenol (CAS: 2050-14-8, EC3 = 27.90), 3-methyleugenol (CAS: 186743-26-0, EC3 = 32), and aniline (CAS: 62-53-3, EC3 = 89) were 0.549, 0.672, 0.580, 0.580, and 0.702, respectively. On the other hand, two moderate sensitizers, 2-Methoxy-4-methyl-phenol (CAS: 93-51-6, EC3 = 5.8), 4-Chloroaniline (CAS: 106-47-8, EC3 = 6.5), have a slightly higher P value 0.672, 0.656, respectively. Another two moderate sensitizers with smaller EC3 value, isoeugenol (CAS: 97-54-1, EC3 = 3.5) and 1-naphthol (CAS: 90-15-3, EC3 = 1.3) have greater P values, 0.840 and 0.886, respectively. For most chemicals, their -logEC3 values correlate with P values quite well, but for aniline, its −logEC3 value is much less potent than its P value predicted. This may indicate that the initial oxidation of aniline, which is quite fast, is not in this case the rate-determining step for protein haptenation. The analysis of the relationship between EC3 and ϵ_{HOMO} for these nine chemicals was reported in the Additional file 1.

Possible reaction mechanisms of aromatic anilines and phenols

Occurrence of electrophilic–nucleophilic reactions between chemical and skin proteins is a primary reason of chemical induced skin sensitization [8]. Most chemicals with high skin sensitization potential can be classified as Michael acceptors (MA), SN_2 electrophiles, S_NAr electrophiles, Schiff base formers, or acylation agents. The reaction mechanisms of anilines and phenols, however, are poorly understood and very few of them can be classified into the aforementioned five categories. One proposed mechanism is that sensitization occurs via oxygen attack ortho to an amino group or via oxidative quinone-methide formation [25,41]. For example, Roberts et al. reported the mechanistic chemistry of aromatic diamino-, dihydroxy-, and amino-hydroxy compounds [24] where two parallel chemical mechanisms were described as the most possible processes: oxidation to electrophilic (protein reactive) quinones, quinone imines, or quinone di-imines or formation of protein reactive free radicals. These mechanisms, unfortunately, are not applicable to the all single NH/OH substituted anilines and phenols. For instance, aniline and 4-butylaniline are sensitizers whereas 4-aminobenzoic acid, 4-aminobenzenesulfonamide, and 4-aminobenzenesulfonic acid are non-sensitizers. Beside the

solubility effects and the formation of ions/zwitterions, the reactivity variety of chemical entities by substituent effects play an important role in reducing dermal penetration and immunogenicity of protein conjugates.

By analyzing the relationship between quantum properties and chemical reactivity, we successfully modeled the skin sensitization potential of two groups of chemicals (aromatic anilines and phenols) with a single coefficient of ϵ_{HOMO}, while the energy of the lowest unoccupied molecular orbital (ϵ_{LUMO}), considered as the critical factor for most electrophilic reactions [8,11], was poorly correlated with sensitization potential. These results suggest the skin sensitization mechanism of those compounds may result from several steps but not a directly electrophilic reaction.

The ϵ_{HOMO} dependent results implied that a process of losing electron may be involved in the activation of those sensitizers. Those compounds may be activated via an autoxidation mechanism to further interact with skin proteins as prehaptens. In addition, the mechanisms where these chemicals directly react with free radical of skin proteins also should be considered [42]. In the present study, we proposed that two potential pathways could lead these compounds to cause skin sensitization as shown in Scheme 1 [42]. In the first pathway (Scheme 1a), an aniline (or a phenol) is readily oxidized to a radical cation through loss of an electron at the aromatic ring [43] and forms two possible reactive intermediates. A protein-associated sulfhydryl radical then attacks the aromatic of the radical cation to form a covalent bond at the orth- or para-position. Or, the reactive intermediates bind to nucleophilic moieties on proteins through the Michael addition. The second pathway corresponds to what Lepoittevin defined as a direct haptenation route [44], whereby attack of a protein associated sulfhydryl radical on the ring gives an intermediate radical (Scheme 1b).

A compound with lower energy of HOMO appears either more stable or less reactive when reacting with a protein associated sulfhydryl radical [24]. Therefore, as shown in Figure 3, the sensitizers e.g., the aniline (CAS: 62-53-3) and the eugenol (CAS: 97-53-0) equipped with higher ϵ_{HOMO} values can lose electron(s) more easily to form radical cation intermediates than non-sensitizers (e.g., 2-fluoro-5-nitroaniline (CAS: 369-36-8), 4-aminobenzoic acid (CAS: 150-13-0), salicylic acid (CAS: 69-72-7), and 3-hydroxy-4-nitrobenzoic acid (CAS: 619-14-7)). We noted that the non-sensitizers of anilines and phenols are those that have the electron withdrawing groups attached to the aromatic ring, such as −F, −NO$_2$, −COOH. This implies that introduction of electron withdrawing groups to the aromatic ring of anilines or phenols may be one of the effective ways to reduce the potency of skin sensitizers.

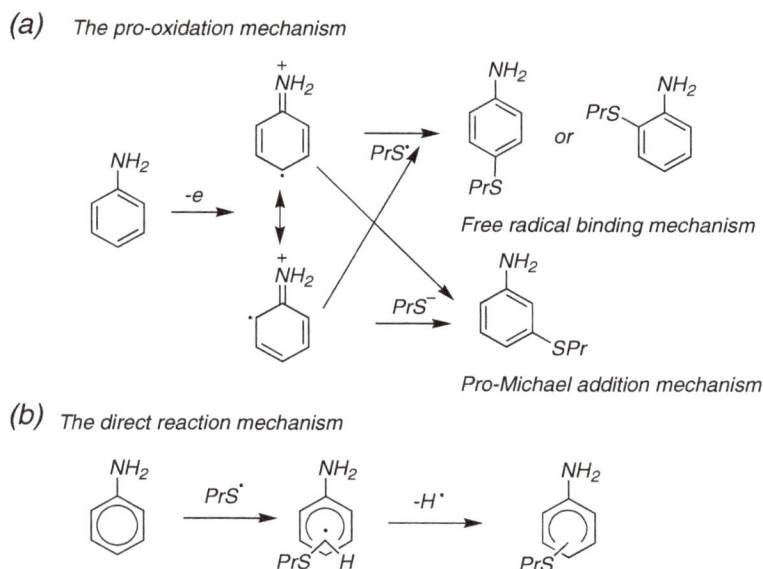

Scheme 1 Reaction mechanisms of anilines binding to protein. (a) The pro-oxidation mechanism. **(b)** The direct reaction mechanism.

Predicting skin sensitization potentials of a subset of FDA approved drugs with aniline and phenol groups

There are no effective tools to predict the skin sensitization potential of drugs, because drug-induced skin reactions may be caused by several mechanisms either single or mixed [27]. The skin sensitization, in the context, refers to T-cell mediated sensitization (type IV allergy). The reaction of chemicals with proteins was recognized as one of the necessary process of the T-cell mediated sensitization [23]. The *in silico* mechanistic models may offer valuable insights into better understanding the initiation of drug induced allergies.

We collected 53 drugs containing aniline and/or phenol moieties from the DrugBank database. The information of these 53 compounds is also available in the Additional file 1. These FDA approved drugs were then analyzed to filter out those with structural alerts of skin sensitization. The sulfonamide drugs were also removed due to they have different mechanisms of action. For example, sulfamethoxazole (DrugBank ID: DB01015) can

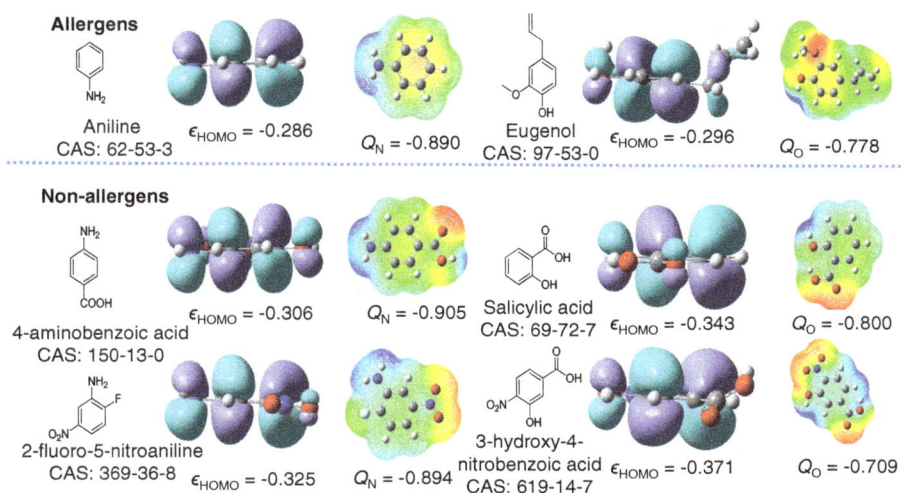

Figure 3 The structures, energies and shapes of HOMO, and charge density of representative anilines and phenols. Anilines (left column: aniline, 4-aminobenzoic acid, and 2-fluoro-5-nitroaniline); Phenols (right column: eugenol, salicylic acid, and 3-hydroxy-4-nitrobenzoic acid). The unit of the energy is hartree.

Table 2 Prediction of skin sensitization potential for 6 FDA approved drugs that have side effect of allergic dermatitis reported in MetaADEDB database

	DrugBank ID	Name	P	Prediction[a]	MetaADEDB[b]
1	DB00279	Liothyronine	−0.001	N	Y
2	DB01407	Clenbuterol	0.589	Y	Y
3	DB00250	Dapsone	0.700	Y	Y
4	DB00295	Morphine	0.580	Y	Y
5	DB00327	Hydromorphone	0.595	Y	Y
6	DB00481	Raloxifene	0.977	Y	Y

[a]A drug is predicted as an sensitizer if its P value is greater than 0.50; Otherwise, as a non-sensitizer. [b]Compounds having the keywords "allergic dermatitis" in their side effect reports in the MetaADEDB database are indicated as sensitizers. Y: Sensitizer; N: Non-sensitizer.

be oxidized to a hydroxylamine metabolite and subsequently form a reactive nitroso intermediate by autooxidation that enables it to react with skin proteins [45]. Finally, twenty six compounds were obtained and their skin sensitization potential was predicted by our model. Among these 26 compounds, six of them were reported to be able to induce "allergic dermatitis" according to the side effect information in MetaADEDB database (Table 2). Interestingly, our results showed that five of them, e.g. Clenbuterol, Dapsone, Morphine, Hydromorphone and Raloxifene were correctly predicted as sensitizers (Table 2) as their P values are greater than the threshold 0.50. In addition, allergic dermatitis is a rare side effect of Liothyronine according to the information from https://www.universaldrugstore.com/medications/Liothyronine/side-effects. However, users should be cautious that there is no label for drugs not causing "allergic dermatitis", thus it is hard to find a negative set in FDA approved drugs to further evaluate our model.

Conclusion

This study has demonstrated how quantum chemical calculations can be utilized to predict skin sensitization potential and to infer the reaction mechanism for a class of mechanistically hard-to-be-classified chemicals containing aniline and phenol moieties. The outcomes emphasized that the energy of highest occupied molecular orbital plays an important role for predicting skin sensitization potential of these compounds, indicating the activation process occurred via either autoxidation or direct reaction with free radical. Our model was further applied to predict the allergenic potential of the approved drugs containing aniline and/or phenol moieties. Several of these drugs were identified as sensitizers and the prediction agreed well with their "allergic dermatitis" side effect. Thus, the data indicate that our newly developed *in silico* algorithm shows promise as a preclinical risk assessment tool for screening allergenic potential.

Again, we should point out that skin allergic reactions are not commonly seen for drugs given via the oral route. Though they may share similar mechanisms, caution should be taken when extrapolating our model from skin sensitization potential for topically applied chemicals to predict "allergic potential" of drugs.

Additional file

Additional file 1: Predicted values and experimental data of reported chemicals and FDA approved drugs that contain aniline and/or phenol moieties.

Abbreviations

ACD: Allergic contact dermatitis; AM1: Austin model 1; CAS: Chemical abstracts service; EC3: Effective concentration for a three-fold proliferation of lymph node cells; FDA: Food and drug administration; GPMT: Guinea pig maximization test; HOMO: Highest occupied molecular orbital; LLNA: The murine-based local lymph node assay; LUMO: Lowest unoccupied molecular orbital; MA: Michael acceptors; SAR: Structure-activity relationship; SMILES: Simplified molecular-input line-entry system; SN_2: A kind of nucleophilic substitution reaction mechanism; S_NAr: Nucleophilic aromatic substitution.

Competing interests

The authors declare that they have no competing interests.

Authors' contributions

OQ and LW carried out the experiments; OQ, LW and X-QX designed the study and carried out the analysis. OQ, LW, YM and X-QX interpreted the data and drafted the manuscript. X-QX supervised the progress and critically revised the manuscript. All authors read and approved the final manuscript.

Acknowledgements

OQ would like to acknowledge the support from the National Natural Science Foundation of China (NSFC21202201).

Disclaimer

The mention of commercial products, their sources, or their use in connection with material reported herein is not to be construed as either an actual or implied endorsement of such products by the Department of Health and Human Services. The findings and conclusions in this article have not been formally disseminated by the Food and Drug Administration and should not be considered to represent any agency determination or policy.

Author details

[1]Department of Pharmaceutical Sciences, Computational Chemical Genomics Screening Center, School of Pharmacy, NIH National Center, of Excellence for Computational Drug Abuse Research, Drug Discovery Institute, Pittsburgh, PA 15261, USA. [2]Department of Computational and Systems Biology, University of Pittsburgh, Pittsburgh, PA 15261, USA. [3]Division of Biology, Office of Science and Engineering Laboratories, Center for Devices and Radiobiological Health, US Food and Drug Administration, Silver Spring, MD 20993, USA. [4]College of Pharmacy, Third Military Medical University, Chongqing 400038, China.

References

1. Lushniak BD: Occupational contact dermatitis. *Dermatol Ther* 2004, **17**(3):272–277.

2. Wizemann T: *Public Health Effectiveness of the FDA 510(k) Clearance Process: Measuring Postmarket Performance and Other Select Topics: Workshop Report (2011)*; 2011.

3. Basketter DA, Scholes EW: Comparison of the local lymph-node assay with the guinea-pig maximization test for the detection of a range of contact allergens. *Food Chem Toxicol* 1992, **30**(1):65–69.

4. Uter W, Johansen JD, Borje A, Karlberg AT, Liden C, Rastogi S, Roberts D, White IR: Categorization of fragrance contact allergens for prioritization of preventive measures: clinical and experimental data and consideration of structure-activity relationships. *Contact Dermatitis* 2013, **69**(4):196–230.

5. Teubner W, Mehling A, Schuster PX, Guth K, Worth A, Burton J, van Ravenzwaay B, Landsiedel R: Computer models versus reality: how well do in silico models currently predict the sensitization potential of a substance. *Regul Toxicol Pharmacol* 2013, **67**(3):468–485.

6. Enoch SJ, Cronin MT, Schultz TW, Madden JC: An evaluation of global QSAR models for the prediction of the toxicity of phenols to Tetrahymena pyriformis. *Chemosphere* 2008, **71**(7):1225–1232.

7. Landsteiner K, Jacobs J: Studies on the sensitization of animals with simple chemicals compounds. II. *J Exp Med* 1936, **64**:625–639.

8. Aptula AO, Roberts DW: Mechanistic applicability domains for nonanimal-based prediction of toxicological end points: general principles and application to reactive toxicity. *Chem Res Toxicol* 2006, **19**(8):1097–1105.

9. Divkovic M, Pease CK, Gerberick GF, Basketter DA: Hapten–protein binding: from theory to practical application in the in vitro prediction of skin sensitization. *Contact Dermatitis* 2005, **53**(4):189–200.

10. Aleksic M, Thain E, Roger D, Saib O, Davies M, Li J, Aptula A, Zazzeroni R: Reactivity profiling: covalent modification of single nucleophile peptides for skin sensitization risk assessment. *Toxicol Sci* 2009, **108**(2):401–411.

11. Enoch SJ, Madden JC, Cronin MTD: Identification of mechanisms of toxic action for skin sensitisation using a SMARTS pattern based approach. *Sar Qsar Environ Res* 2008, **19**(5–6):555–578.

12. Delaine T, Hagvall L, Rudbäck J, Luthman K, Karlberg A-T: Skin sensitization of epoxyaldehydes: importance of conjugation. *Chem Res Toxicol* 2013, **26**(674):684.

13. Enoch SJ, Roberts DW: Predicting skin sensitization potency for michael acceptors in the LLNA using quantum mechanics calculations. *Chem Res Toxicol* 2013, **26**(5):767–774.

14. Roberts DW, Aptula AO, Patlewicz GY: Chemistry-based risk assessment for skin sensitization: quantitative mechanistic modeling for the SNAr domain. *Chem Res Toxicol* 2011, **24**(7):1003–1011.

15. Natsch A, Gfeller H, Haupt T, Brunner G: Chemical reactivity and skin sensitization potential for Benzaldehydes: can schiff base formation explain everything? *Chem Res Toxicol* 2012, **25**(10):2203–2215.

16. Bergström MA, Luthman K, Nilsson JLG, Karlberg A-T: Conjugated dienes as prohaptens in contact allergy: in Vivo and in Vitro studies of structure–activity relationships, sensitizing capacity, and metabolic activation. *Chem Res Toxicol* 2006, **19**(6):760–769.

17. Bergström MA, Andersson SI, Broo K, Luthman K, Karlberg A-T: Oximes: metabolic activation and structure – allergenic activity relationships. *J Med Chem* 2008, **51**(8):2541–2550.

18. Patlewicz GY, Basketter DA, Smith Pease CK, Wilson K, Wright ZM, Roberts DW, Bernard G, Arnau EG, Lepoittevin J-P: Further evaluation of quantitative structure–activity relationship models for the prediction of the skin sensitization potency of selected fragrance allergens. *Contact Dermatitis* 2004, **50**(2):91–97.

19. Niklasson IB, Delaine T, Luthman K, Karlberg A-T: Impact of a heteroatom in a structure – activity relationship study on analogues of Phenyl Glycidyl Ether (PGE) from epoxy resin systems. *Chem Res Toxicol* 2011, **24**(4):542–548.

20. Itoh M: Sensitization potency of some phenolic compounds–with special emphasis on the relationship between chemical structure and allergenicity. *J Dermatol* 1982, **9**(3):223–233.

21. Malkowski J, Klenieswka D, Maibach H: Relationship between chemical structure and allergenicity: aromatic amines. *Derm Beruf Umwelt* 1983, **31**(2):48–50.

22. Kleniewska D, Maibach H: Allergenicity of aminobenzene compounds: structure-function relationships. *Derm Beruf Umwelt* 1980, **28**(1):11–13.

23. Payne MP, Walsh PT: Structure-activity-relationships for skin sensitization potential - development of structural alerts for use in knowledge-based toxicity prediction systems. *J Chem Inf Comput Sci* 1994, **34**(1):154–161.

24. Aptula AO, Enoch SJ, Roberts DW: Chemical mechanisms for skin sensitization by aromatic compounds with hydroxy and amino groups. *Chem Res Toxicol* 2009, **22**(9):1541–1547.

25. Patlewicz G, Roberts DW, Uriarte E: A comparison of reactivity schemes for the prediction skin sensitization potential. *Chem Res Toxicol* 2008, **21**(2):521–541.

26. Cuyper C, Goeteyn M: Systemic contact dermatitis from subcutaneous hydromorphone. *Contact Dermatitis* 1992, **27**(4):220–223.

27. Lee A, Thomson J: Drug-induced skin reactions. *Pharmaceut J 1999* 2006, **262**:357–362.

28. Gerberick GF, Vassallo JD, Bailey RE, Chaney JG, Morrall SW, Lepoittevin JP: Development of a peptide reactivity assay for screening contact allergens. *Toxicol Sci* 2004, **81**(2):332–343.

29. Estrada E, Patlewicz G, Gutierrez Y: From knowledge generation to knowledge archive. a general strategy using TOPS-MODE with DEREK to formulate new alerts for skin sensitization. *J Chem Inf Comput Sci* 2004, **44**(2):688–698.

30. Barratt MD, Langowski JJ: Validation and subsequent development of the DEREK skin sensitization rulebase by analysis of the BgVV list of contact allergens. *J Chem Inf Comput Sci* 1999, **39**(2):294–298.

31. Schneider K, Akkan Z: Quantitative relationship between the local lymph node assay and human skin sensitization assays. *Regul Toxicol Pharmacol* 2004, **39**(3):245–255.

32. Roberts DW, Patlewicz G, Kern PS, Gerberick F, Kimber I, Dearman RJ, Ryan CA, Basketter DA, Aptula AO: Mechanistic applicability domain classification of a local lymph node assay dataset for skin sensitization. *Chem Res Toxicol* 2007, **20**(7):1019–1030.

33. Miller MD, Yourtee DM, Glaros AG, Chappelow CC, Eick JD, Holder AJ: Quantum mechanical structure-activity relationship analyses for skin sensitization. *J Chem Inf Model* 2005, **45**(4):924–929.

34. Kern PS, Gerberick GF, Ryan CA, Kimber I, Aptula A, Basketter DA: Local lymph node data for the evaluation of skin sensitization alternatives: a second compilation. *Dermatitis* 2010, **21**(1):8–32.

35. Estrada E, Patlewicz G, Chamberlain M, Basketter D, Larbey S: Computer-aided knowledge generation for understanding skin sensitization mechanisms: the TOPS-MODE approach. *Chem Res Toxicol* 2003, **16**(10):1226–1235.

36. Basketter DA: Skin sensitization: strategies for the assessment and management of risk. *Br J Dermatol* 2008, **159**(2):267–273.

37. Frisch MJ, Trucks GW, Schlegel HB, Scuseria GE, Robb MA, Cheeseman JR, Montgomery JA Jr, Vreven T, Kudin KN, Burant JC, Millam JM, Iyengar SS, Tomasi J, Barone V, Mennucci B, Cossi M, Scalmani G, Rega N, Petersson GA, Nakatsuji H, Hada M, Ehara M, Toyota K, Fukuda R, Hasegawa JIM, Nakajima T, Honda Y, Kitao O, Nakai H: *Gaussian 03. In., Revision C.02.* Wallingford, CT: Gaussian, Inc; 2003.

38. Dewar MJS, Zoebisch EG, Healy EF, Stewart JJP: Development and use of quantum mechanical molecular models. 76. AM1: a new general purpose quantum mechanical molecular model. *J Am Chem Soc* 1985, **107**(13):3902–3909.

39. Enoch SJ, Roberts DW, Cronin MTD: Mechanistic category formation for the prediction of respiratory sensitization. *Chem Res Toxicol* 2010, **23**(10):1547–1555.

40. R Development Core Team: *R: A Language and Environment for Statistical Computing*. Vienna, Austria: R Foundation for Statistical Computing; 2010. Retrieved from http://www.R-project.org

41. Enoch SJ, Cronin MT, Schultz TW, Madden JC: **Quantitative and mechanistic read across for predicting the skin sensitization potential of alkenes acting via Michael addition.** *Chem Res Toxicol* 2008, **21**(2):513–520.

42. Karlberg AT, Bergstrom MA, Borje A, Luthman K, Nilsson JLG: **Allergic contact dermatitis-formation, structural requirements, and reactivity of skin sensitizers.** *Chem Res Toxicol* 2008, **21**(1):53–69.

43. Storle C, Eyer P: **Reactions of the wurster blue radical cation with thiols, and some properties of the reaction-products.** *Chem Biol Interact* 1991, **78**(3):333–346.

44. Lepoittevin JP: **Metabolism versus chemical transformation or pro- versus prehaptens?** *Contact Dermatitis* 2006, **54**(2):73–74.

45. Choquet-Kastylevsky G, Vial T, Descotes J: **Allergic adverse reactions to sulfonamides.** *Curr Allergy Asthma Rep* 2002, **2**(1):16–25.

21

Phenotypic expression and prevalence of ESBL-producing *Enterobacteriaceae* in samples collected from patients in various wards of Mulago Hospital, Uganda

John N Kateregga[*], Ronah Kantume, Collins Atuhaire, Musisi Nathan Lubowa and James G Ndukui

Abstract

Background: Resistance to extended-spectrum cephalosporins among Enterobacteriaceae has been reported yet they serve as the last line treatment for severe infections in Uganda and other countries. This resistance often leads to nosocomial infection outbreaks and therapeutic failures from multidrug resistant bacteria. The main objective of this study was to determine the prevalence of extended-spectrum beta-lactamase (ESBL)-producing Enterobacteriaceae in clinical samples of patients in various wards of Mulago Hospital; Uganda's main national referral and teaching hospital.

Methods: This cross-sectional study was conducted between January-April, 2014. Purposive consecutive sampling was used to collect pus swab, urine, blood and CSF samples from patients in the various wards. A total of 245 consecutive, non-repetitive, clinical samples were obtained and tested for phenotypic ESBL production using the Double Disc Synergy Test using cefotaxime, ceftazidime, cefotaxime-clavulanic acid and ceftazidime-clavulanic acid.

Results: Results show that 47 % of the 245 samples had *Enterobacteriaceae* isolates. Of these isolates 62 % were ESBL producers while 38 % were of non-ESBL phenotype. *E. coli* was the most isolated organism (53.9 %), followed by *K. pneumoniae* (28.7 %). Majority of Enterobacteriaceae organisms were isolated from urine samples, followed by pus samples and of these 64.9 % and 47.4 % were ESBL-producers respectively. *Klebsiella pneumoniae* had the highest percentage of ESBL producers (72.7 %). There was a higher percentage of isolates showing resistance to ceftazidime (73 %) compared to cefotaxime (57.5 %). All *Enterobacter cloacae* isolates showed resistance to ceftazidime. There were no statistically significant association between phenotype (ESBL/non-ESBL) and patients' age or gender or Enterobacteriaceae spp.

Conclusions: This study reveals a high prevalence of ESBL producing organisms in Mulago Hospital and high levels of resistance to third generation cephalosporins. In addition to undertaking appropriate infection control measures, there is urgent need for formulation of an antibiotic policy in Uganda to prevent spread of these organisms. This also calls for continuous monitoring and reporting of the presence of such organisms in order to ensure rational and judicious use of antibiotics by clinicians.

Keywords: ESBL, Enterobacteriaceae, Cefotaxime, Ceftazidime, Clavulanic acid

* Correspondence: katereggaj@covab.mak.ac.ug
College of Veterinary Medicine, Animal Resources & Biosecurity, Makerere University, P.O Box 7062, Kampala, Uganda

Table 1 Criteria for determining the potency of the test antibiotics

ESBLS	E. coli ATCC 25922	K. pneumoniae ATCC 700603
Ceftazidime 30 µg	(25-32 mm)	(22-29 mm)
Cefotaxime 30 µg	(29-35 mm)	(18-22 mm)

The antibiotics had to show inhibition zone diameters in the above ranges in order to be used in the study

Background

Production of β-lactamase enzymes that hydrolyze the β-lactam ring is a predominant resistance mechanism for many Gram-negative bacteria including *Enterobacteriaceae* such as *E. coli, Klebsiella pneumoniae, Klebsiella oxytoca, Pseudomonas aeruginosa, Proteus mirabilis, Enterobacter cloacae* and *Aeromonas spp.* [1]. Extended-Spectrum β-Lactamase (ESBL)-producing bacteria are capable of expressing these enzymes and this confers bacterial resistance to penicillins; first, second, and third-generation cephalosporins and aztreonam. ESBL-producing bacteria have been isolated in many parts of North America and Europe [2] and in Africa. In one South African hospital, 36 % of *K. pneumoniae* isolates were ESBL-producers and outbreaks of infections due to *Klebsiella* strains resistant to third-generation cephalosporins have also been reported in Nigeria and Kenya [3, 4]. In Uganda there has been lack of published information about ESBL-producers among organisms isolated from patients.

ESBL producers have a wide clinical significance and potential impact in healthcare settings especially in low income countries such as Uganda. The selection pressure and overuse of new antibiotics in the treatment of patients leads to selection for new variants of β-lactamase producers. ESBL producers are associated with various infections in virtually all body organs leading to meningitis, pneumonia, urinary tract infections, septicaemia and intra-abdominal infections [5, 6]. Other conditions include osteomyelitis, endophthalmitis, pyomyositis and wound infections [7].

The possible spread of ESBL-producing organisms in a clinical setting is real. ESBL-associated antibiotic resistance causes increased morbidity and mortality; and hampers the control of infectious diseases. This in turn leads to increase in durations of illness and hospital stay; increase in health-care costs and more economic burden

Table 3 Enterobacteriaceae species isolated from patient samples

Isolates	Frequency	Percent
E. coli	62	53.9
Klebsiella pneumoniae	33	28.7
Proteus mirabilis	16	13.9
Enterobacter cloacae	4	3.5
Total	115	100.0

E. coli was the predominant isolate

to families. This study sought to determine the prevalence of ESBL-producing bacteria among isolates from samples in various wards of Mulago Hospital, the main national referral hospital in Uganda with a bed-capacity of 1,600.

Methods

Study design

This was a cross-sectional study conducted between January-April 2014 to determine the prevalence of ESBL-producing Enterobacteriaceae in clinical samples collected from in-patient and out-patient wards of Mulago Hospital. The samples collected included urine, swabs (oral, HVS, wound), blood and CSF. *Escherichia coli, Klebsiella pneumoniae, Proteus mirabilis* and *Enterobacter cloacae* bacteria were isolated from the samples. The number of samples containing ESBL-producing *Enterobacteriaceae* was recorded. The prevalence of ESBL phenotypes among the isolates was determined.

Sample size

The sample size was determined using the formula advanced by Kish and Leslie [8]. Basing on results of a previous study in a similar setting, a prevalence of 20 % [9] and confidence interval of 95 % were used in the formula. The sample size was estimated to be about 245 samples.

Sample collection and bacterial isolation

Samples from 25 wards of Mulago Hospital were aseptically collected by purposive consecutive sampling from patients who gave informed written consent; properly

Table 2 Baseline characteristics of patients whose samples had Enterobacteriaceae isolates

	ESBL n = 71 (61.7 %)	Non-ESBL n = 44 (38.3 %)	Total	p value
Sex				
Female	37 (52.1 %)	30 (68.2 %)	67 (58.3 %)	0.089
Male	34 (47.9 %)	14 (31.8 %)	48 (41.7 %)	
Age			Overall mean	
Mean	42 (SD 22)	38 (SD 19)	40	0.355

The Chi-square and independent t-tests showed that sex and age were not significantly associated with ESBL phenotype
Chi-square and independent t-test

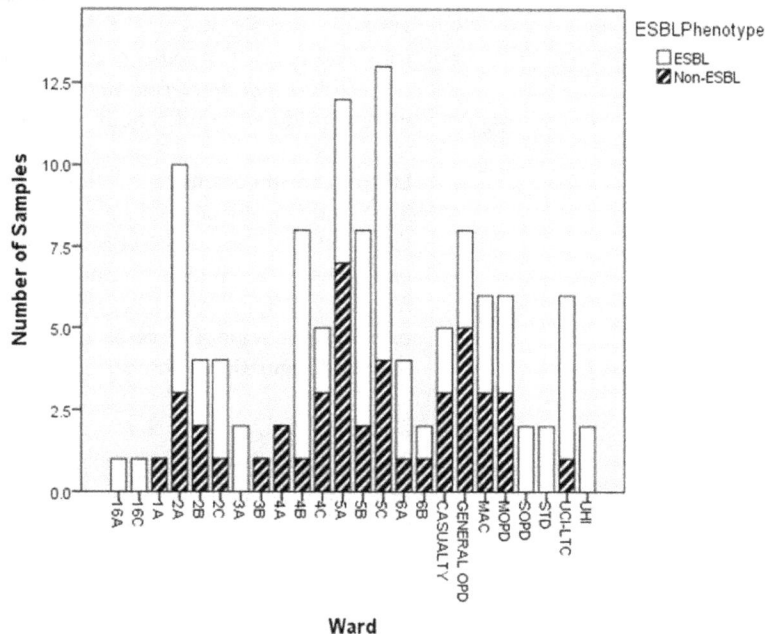

Fig. 1 Distribution of samples from the various wards. Surgical wards contributed the highest number of samples in the Microbiology laboratory during the study period. Surgical wards – 1A, 2A, 2B, 2C, 3A, 5A, 5B, 5C and SOPD; Medical wards – 3B, 4A, 4B, 4C, 6A, 6B, MOPD, MAC, UCI-LTC and UHI; Pediatric wards – 16A and 16C; General - OPD, MOPD, STD. Key: SOPD = Surgical Outpatients Dept; UCI-LTC = Uganda Cancer Institute-Liquid Tumor Cancer, MAC = Medical assessment Centre; MOPD = Medical outpatients Dept; OPD = Outpatients Dept; STD = Sexually Transmitted Diseases Dept; UHI = Uganda Heart Institute

labelled and taken to the Microbiology Laboratory for Enterobacteriaceae culture and isolation. The originating ward, patient's gender and age were recorded. The samples were inoculated by streaking on Blood agar (Oxoid, UK), MacConkey agar (Oxoid, UK) and CLED agar (Oxoid, UK) plates. The plates were incubated aerobically at 37 °C for 18–24 h to allow development of bacterial colonies. Preliminary identification of the isolates was done using phenotypic colonial characteristics. Confirmatory identification of the suspect colonies was carried out by conventional biochemical tests as described by Cheesbrough [10]. These were: indole, Methyl red, Voges-Proskauer, citrate utilization and urease production tests as well as triple sugar iron and oxidase tests.

Detection of ESBL-producing Enterobacteriaceae

ESBL detection was based on the Double Disc Synergy Test and interpretation of the results done using the CLSI M100-S20 (2010) [11]. Briefly; 3–5 colonies of each isolate were picked from the growth plates with sterile wire loop, and suspended in 1 ml of physiological saline. The resultant bacterial suspension was matched to the 0.5 McFarland turbidity standard so as to approximate the seeding density of the respective organisms. 100 µl the bacterial suspension/broth culture were then surface-spread on Muller Hinton Agar (Oxoid, UK) plates using a

sterile spreader. Antibiotic discs containing ceftazidime (CTC), cefotaxime (CTZ), ceftazidime-clavulanic acid (CFC) and cefotaxime-clavulanic acid (CTX) were placed on the plates which were incubated overnight at 37 °C. The zones of clearance (mm) for the respective antibiotics were measured for each isolate using a divider and ruler. Organisms were considered to be ESBL-producers if the difference in zone of clearance between ceftazidime and ceftazidime-clavulanic acid or cefotaxime and cefotaxime-clavulanic acid was ≥5 mm. The prevalence of ESBL-producing bacteria was determined using the formula:

$$\text{Prevalence (P)} = \frac{\text{Number of ESBL producing organisms}}{245} \times 100$$

Quality control

Standard organisms (*E. coli* ATCC 25922 and *K. pneumoniae* ATCC 700603) were used to test for the potency of the antimicrobial discs (Table 1).

Data analysis

Clinical and socio-demographic data were entered into Epi Info[TM] v7 and exported to SPSSv21. Pearson Chi-square test was used to assess for any differences between the two ESBL phenotype categories with respect to clinical and demographic parameters. The means of the continuous variables, age and zones of clearance were

Table 4 Association between ESBL phenotype and Enterobacteriaceae isolated, sample type and susceptibility pattern

	ESBL (%)	Non-ESBL (%)	P value
Isolate			
E. coli	36 (58.1)	26 (41.9)	0.924
Klebsiella pneumoniae	24 (72.7)	9 (27.3)	0.908
Enterobacter cloacae	1 (25)	3 (75)	0.695
Proteus mirabilis	10 (62.5)	6 (37.5)	0.999
Sample type			
Urine	46 (63.9)	26 (36.1)	0.980
HVS	6 (54.5)	5 (45.5)	0.999
CSF	1 (100)	0 (0)	0.999
Urethral swab	1 (100)	0 (0)	1.000
Wound swab	2 (100)	0 (0)	1.000
Blood	2 (40)	3 (60)	1.000
Pus swab	9 (47.4)	10 (52.6)	0.999
Surgical wound swab	4 (100)	0 (0)	0.999
Ceftazidime Susceptibility			
Resistant	62 (73.8)	22 (26.2)	0.408
Intermediate	4 (36.4)	7 (63.6)	0.187
Susceptible	5 (25)	15 (75)	0.480
Cefotaxime Susceptibility			
Resistant	54 (81.8)	12 (18.2)	0.013
Intermediate	4 (30.8)	9 (69.2)	0.067
Susceptible	13 (36.1)	23 (63.9)	0.430
Binomial logistic regression			

When analysed using binomial logistic regression, ESBL phenotype was significantly associated with resistance to cefotaxime but not with resistance to ceftadizime, bacterial species or sample type

compared using the Independent *t*-test. Crude logistic regression analysis was used to explore clinical and laboratory features of the ESBL phenotype for comparison with non-ESBL *Enterobacteriaceae* phenotypes. The differences were considered significant at p < 0.05.

Ethical considerations

The study protocol was approved by the Ethics Review Committee of the School of Biomedical Sciences of Makerere University Medical School. Permission was sought from the hospital and laboratory authorities. The ethical principles of scientific research as well as related national laws and regulations were strictly adhered to.

Results

The mean age of the participants was 40 years as shown in Table 2. Results indicated that 115 of the 245 samples (47 %) had *Enterobacteriaceae* isolates. Of these isolates, 58.3 % were from female patients while 41.7 % were from males (Table 2). Statistical analysis of patient data using Chi-square and independent t-test indicated that gender and age were not significantly associated with ESBL phenotype. *E. coli* was the most isolated organism (53.9 %, n = 62), followed by *K. pneumoniae* (28.7 %) as shown in Table 3. Most samples with Enterobacteriaceae isolates were from Obstetrics and Gynaecology wards i.e. 5A (10.4 %, n = 12) and 5C (11.3 %, n = 13) (Fig. 1).

Results further showed that 62 % of Enterobacteriaceae isolates were of the ESBL phenotype while 38 % were of non-ESBL phenotype (Table 2). Most of the Enterobacteriaceae were isolated from the urine samples followed by pus samples as shown in Table 4 and Fig. 2. However, just 64.9 % and 47.4 % of urine and pus isolates respectively were ESBL-producers. On the other hand,

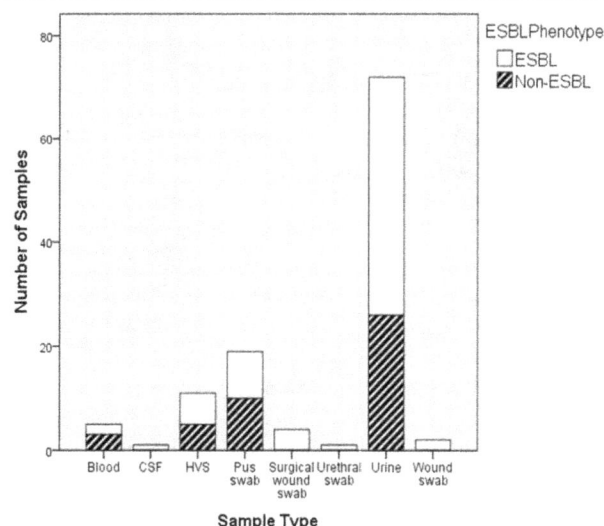

Fig. 2 Distribution of Enterobacteriaceae-positive samples. Most of the Enterobacteriaceae were isolated from urine samples

Table 5 Mean zone of clearance (± SD) of Enterobacteriaceae segregated by ESBL phenotype

Antibiotic	ESBL	Non-ESBL	P value
Ceftazidime	10.1 ± 6.2	18.1 ± 7	0.000
Cefotaxime	13.4 ± 8.3	21.6 ± 8.3	0.000
Ceftazidime-Clavulanic acid	22.3 ± 6	20.7 ± 6.8	0.198
Cefotaxime-Clavulanic acid	25.1 ± 6.6	22.3 ± 8.3	0.051

The zones of clearance of ceftazidime and cefotaxime were statistically significantly associated with ESBL phenotype (Independent samples t-test)

albeit their small number, all isolates from CSF, wound and urethral swabs were ESBL producers (Fig. 2).

The mean zones of clearance for ESBL and non-ESBL phenotypes were lowest for ceftazidime (10.1 ± 6.2 mm; 18.1 ± 7 mm respectively) and highest for cefotaxime-clavulanic acid (25.1 ± 6.6 mm; 22.3 ± 8.3 mm respectively) as shown in Table 5. The zones of clearance of ceftazidime and cefotaxime were significantly associated with ESBL phenotype (p = 0.000; 0.000 respectively) while those of ceftazidime-clavulanic acid and cefotaxime-clavulanic acid were not (p = 0.198, 0.051 respectively).

There was a higher percentage of isolates showing resistance to ceftazidime (73 %) compared to cefotaxime (57.5 %) as shown in Table 6. All *Enterobacter cloacae* isolates were resistant to both cefotaxime and ceftazidime. Table 4 shows that *Klebsiella pneumoniae* had the highest percentage of ESBL producers (72.7 %). There were no statistically significant association between phenotype (ESBL/non-ESBL) and patients' age or gender (Table 4). Similarly, there were no significant association between phenotype (ESBL/non-ESBL) and species of Enterobacteriaceae (*E. coli, Klebsiella pneumoniae, Enterobacter cloacae, Proteus mirabilis*) or sample type (Table 4).

Discussion

The 3rd and 4th generation cephalosporins are often reserved for severe infections [12] but resistance to these drugs has been strikingly rapid worldwide [4]. Consequently, therapeutic options for the infections caused by the ESBL producers are becoming increasingly limited and; if available, expensive for low and middle income countries. The study revealed a slight female preponderance for ESBL-producing Enterobacteriaceae among the patients though gender was not statistically significant (p = 0.089) as a factor. Kiratisin *et al.*, [13] also revealed a female preponderance.

Urine samples constituted the greatest number of clinical samples in this study. According to Wilson and Gaido [14], urinary tract infections constitute the commonest bacterial infections and urine samples account for a significant percentage of samples in clinical microbiology laboratories worldwide. Most Enterobacteriaceae isolates were *E. coli*. Wilson and Gaido [14] indicates that *E. coli* is the most frequent cause of urinary tract infections and this could probably explain the high prevalence of *E. coli* isolates in our study. Similarly, studies in Tanzania [15] indicate that *E. coli* and *Klebsiella pneumoniae* are the most prevalent Enterobacteriaceae species in clinical samples. Furthermore, Maina *et al.*, [16] in a study in Kenya reported higher prevalence for *E. coli* (53.8 %). Similar findings were reported in Bahrain [17].

In our study, the highest numbers of ESBL-producing isolates were from gynaecological and surgical wards. Many studies associate ESBL-producing Enterobacteriaceae with surgical wards. Studies by Seni *et al.*, [9] show that most isolates from surgical wards are ESBL-producers. Prolonged hospital stay; inappropriate therapy; use of indwelling catheters, endotracheal/nasogastric tubes and severe illnesses are all possible drivers of their dissemination. Significantly, there is also movement of health workers between wards in the hospital and can migrate ESBL-producers from ward to ward leading to dissemination throughout the hospital.

The prevalence of ESBL producers among Enterobacteriaceae (62 %) was quite high compared to that reported by Moyo *et al.*, [15] in Tanzania (45.2 %). This wide variation in prevalence is probably due to differences in types of samples analysed and the extent of antibiotic use in the various wards. The present study reveals that *K. pneumoniae* and *E. coli* are major ESBL producers. Moyo *et al.*, [15] showed 51.5 % and 39.1 % ESBL positivity among *Klebsiella* spp and *E. coli* respectively. On the other hand,

Table 6 Susceptibility pattern of Enterobacteriaceae to ceftazidime and cefotaxime

	Ceftazidime (%)			Cefotaxime (%)		
	Resistant	Intermediate	Susceptible	Resistant	Intermediate	Susceptible
E. coli	41 (66.1)	7 (11.3)	14 (22.6)	32 (51.6)	9 (14.5)	21 (33.9)
E. cloacae	4 (100)	0 (0)	0 (0)	3 (75)	0 (0)	1 (25)
K. pneumoniae	27 (81.8)	1 (3)	5 (15.2)	21 (63.6)	3 (9.1)	9 (27.3)
Proteus mirabilis	12 (75)	3 (18.8)	1 (6.3)	10 (62.5)	1 (6.3)	5 (31.2)
%	73.0	9.6	17.4	57.5	11.3	31.3

There was a higher percentage of Enterobacteriaceae isolates showing resistance to ceftazidime than to cefotaxime. The interpretative criteria used was based on CLSI M100-S20 (2010) [11] where for ceftazidime (Resistant ≤17 mm; Intermediate 18-20 mm; Susceptible ≥ 21 mm) and for cefotaxime (Resistant ≤22 mm; Intermediate 23-25 mm; Susceptible ≥ 26 mm)

Seni *et al.*, [9] reported that 79.2 % and 92.3 % of *E. coli* and *K. pneumoniae* isolates are ESBL producers; further evidence that these two organisms account for most ESBL producers in the region. Our study showed a higher resistance to ceftazidime than to cefotaxime. On the other hand, Maina *et al.*, [16] reported 21.2 % resistance to ceftazidime and 65.4 % resistance to cefotaxime. The differences seen in this study could be due to regional differences and the type of samples collected.

Conclusions

This study has demonstrated high prevalence of ESBL-producing Enterobacteriaceae in Mulago Hospital. The spread of these organisms reduces the antibiotic alternatives for the treatment of infections by these pathogens to mainly carbapenems; which are often reserved for life-threatening infections. The study underscores the need for routine detection and reporting of ESBL-producers in Ugandan medical facilities so that measures are taken to avoid their uncontrolled spread and possible therapeutic failures. Clinicians need to be rational and judicious in use of antibiotics. An antibiotic use policy is also imperative to limit the dissemination of these organisms.

Abbreviations
ATCC: American type culture collection; CI: Confidence interval; CLED: Cystine Lactose-Electrolyte-Deficient (agar); CSF: Cerebro-spinal fluid; ESBL: Extended spectrum beta-lactamase; HVS: High vaginal swab.

Competing interests
The authors declare that they have no competing interests.

Authors' contributions
JNK, MLN and RK conceptualized the project, performed most of the lab experiments and wrote the manuscript. MLN contributed specific knowledge in conduction of the microbiological assays. CA assisted in statistically analysing the data. JGN assisted in finalizing the manuscript. All authors read and approved the final manuscript.

Acknowledgements
Special thanks go staff of Central Public Health Laboratory for their assistance during collection of the samples. We also like to acknowledge the Clinical Microbiology Laboratory of Mulago Hospital for their support in laboratory analysis of the samples. This study was financed by funds internally generated by the Pharmacology and Toxicology Research Lab of Makerere University.

References
1. Toth A, Juhasz-Kaszanyitzky E, Mag T, Hajbel-Vekony G, Paszti J, Damjanova I. Characterization of extended-spectrum beta-lactamase (ESBL) producing *Escherichia coli* strains isolated from animal and human clinical samples in Hungary in 2006–2007. Acta Microbiol Immunol Hung. 2013;60:175–85.
2. Hoban DJ, Lascols C, Nicolle LE, Badal R, Bouchillon S, Hackel M, et al. Antimicrobial susceptibility of Enterobacteriaceae, including molecular characterization of extended-spectrum beta-lactamase-producing species, in urinary tract isolates from hospitalized patients in North America and Europe: results from the SMART study 2009–2010. Diag Microbiol Infect Dis. 2012;74:62–7.
3. Akindele JA, Rotilu IO. Outbreak of neonatal *Klebsiella* septicaemia: a review of antimicrobial sensitivities. Afr J Med Med Sci. 1997;26:51–3.
4. Musoke RN, Revathi G. Emergence of multidrug-resistant gram-negative organisms in a neonatal unit and the therapeutic implications. J Trop Pediatr. 2000;46:86–91.
5. Dayan NH, Dabbah I, Weissman I, Aga I, Even L, Glikman D. Urinary Tract Infections Caused by Community-Acquired Extended-Spectrum beta-Lactamase-Producing and Nonproducing Bacteria: A Comparative Study. J Pediatr. 2013;163:1417–21.
6. Badal RE, Bouchillon SK, Lob SH, Hackel MA, Hawser S, Hoban DJ. Etiology, Extended-Spectrum Beta-Lactamase Rates and Antimicrobial Susceptibility of Gram-negative Bacilli causing Intra-abdominal Infections in Patients in General Pediatric and Pediatric Intensive Care Units - Global Data from the Study for Monitoring Antimicrobial Resistance Trends 2008–2010. Pediatr Infect Dis J. 2013;32:636–40.
7. Agostinho A, Renzi G, Haustein T, Jourdan G, Bonfillon C, Rougemont M, et al. Epidemiology and acquisition of extended-spectrum beta-lactamase-producing in a septic orthopedic ward. Springerplus. 2013;2:91.
8. Kish L. Sampling Organizations and Groups of Unequal Sizes. Am Sociol Rev. 1965;30:564–72.
9. Seni J, Najjuka CF, Kateete DP, Makobore P, Joloba ML, Kajumbula H, et al. Antimicrobial resistance in hospitalized surgical patients: a silently emerging public health concern in Uganda. BMC Research Notes. 2013;6:298.
10. Cheesebrough M: [District Laboratory Practice in Tropical Countries Part II]. Second Edition, Cambridge University Press 2006. p. 62. http://www.cambridge.org/us/academic/subjects/medicine/medicine-general-interest/district-laboratorypractice-tropical-countries-part-2-2nd-edition.
11. Clinical and Laboratory Standards Institute. Performance Standards for Antimicrobial Susceptibility Testing: Twentieth Informational Supplement M100-S20. Wayne, PA, USA: CLSI; 2010.
12. Trivedi M, Patel V, Soman R, Rodriguez C, Singhal T. The Outcome of Treating ESBL Infections with Carbapenems vs. Non Carbapenem Antimicrobials. J Assoc Physicians India. 2012;60:28–30.
13. Kiratisin P, Apisarnthanarak A, Laesripa C, Saifon P. Molecular characterization and epidemiology of extended spectrum-beta-lactamase-producing *Escherichia coli* and *Klebsiella pneumoniae* isolates causing health care associated infection in Thailand, where the CTX-M family is endemic. Antimicrob Agents Chemother. 2008;52:2818–24.
14. Wilson ML, Gaido L. Laboratory diagnosis of urinary tract infections in adult patients. Clinical Infectious Diseases. 2004;38:1150–8.
15. Moyo SJ, Aboud S, Kasubi M, Lyamuya EF, Maselle SY. Antimicrobial resistance among producers and non-producers of extended spectrum beta-lactamases in urinary isolates at a tertiary Hospital in Tanzania. BMC Research Notes. 2010;3:348.
16. Maina D, Revathi G, Kariuki S, Ozwara H. Genotypes and cephalosporin susceptibility in extended-spectrum β-lactamase producing enterobacteriaceae in the community. The Journal of Infection in Developing Countries. 2011;6:470–7.
17. Bindayna KM, Senok AC, Jamsheer AE. Prevalence of extended-spectrum beta-lactamase-producing Enterobacteriaceae in Bahrain. Journal of Infection and Public Health. 2009;2:129–35.

22

Comparing antibiotic self-medication in two socio-economic groups in Guatemala City: a descriptive cross-sectional study

Brooke M Ramay[1*†], Paola Lambour[1†] and Alejandro Cerón[2]

Abstract

Background: Self-medication with antibiotics may result in antimicrobial resistance and its high prevalence is of particular concern in Low to Middle Income Countries (LMIC) like Guatemala. A better understanding of self-medication with antibiotics may represent an opportunity to develop interventions guiding the rational use of antibiotics. We aimed to compare the magnitude of antibiotic self-medication and the characteristics of those who self-medicate in two pharmacies serving disparate socio-economic communities in Guatemala City.

Methods: We conducted a descriptive, cross-sectional study in one Suburban pharmacy and one City Center pharmacy in Guatemala City. We used a questionnaire to gather information about frequency of self-medication, income and education of those who self-medicate. We compared proportions between the two pharmacies, using two-sample z-test as appropriate.

Results: Four hundred and eighteen respondents completed the survey (221 in the Suburban pharmacy and 197 in the City Center pharmacy). Most respondents in both pharmacies were female (70%). The reported monthly income in the suburban pharmacy was between $1,250.00-$2,500.00, the city-center pharmacy reported a monthly income between $125.00- $625.00 (p < 0.01). Twenty three percent of Suburban pharmacy respondents and 3% in the City Center pharmacy completed high school (p < 0.01). Proportion of self-medication was 79% in the Suburban pharmacy and 77% in City Center pharmacy. In both settings, amoxicillin was reported as the antibiotic most commonly used.

Conclusions: High proportions of self-medication with antibiotics were reported in two pharmacies serving disparate socio-economic groups in Guatemala City. Additionally, self-medicating respondents were most often women and most commonly self-medicated with amoxicillin. Our findings support future public health interventions centered on the regulation of antibiotic sales and on the potential role of the pharmacist in guiding prescription with antibiotics in Guatemala.

Keywords: Self-medication, Guatemala, Antibiotic use, Socio-economic factors, Role of the pharmacist

Background

Self-medication with antibiotics occurs worldwide, fostering antibiotic misuse and antimicrobial resistance. The World Health Organization (WHO) recently reported alarming levels of resistance to penicillin, fluoroquinolones and third generation cephalosporins in member countries [1]. The misuse of antibiotics poses a serious risk to infectious disease control and public health in general [1,2]. In Low to Middle Income Countries (LMIC) like Guatemala antibiotics are sold essentially as over-the-counter medications. In addition to easy access of antibiotics, self-medication is highly prevalent in LMIC and Organization for Economic Co-operation and Development (OECD) countries although no patterns in the characteristics of those who self-medicate have been established [3,4]. What is clear, is that patients practicing self-medication in LMIC are often unaware of potential problems that may arise [5] including side

* Correspondence: bramay@uvg.edu.gt
†Equal contributors
[1]Department of Pharmaceutical Chemistry, Universidad del Valle de Guatemala, Guatemala City, Guatemala
Full list of author information is available at the end of the article

effects, antimicrobial resistance, or worsening of symptoms. [6-9] Additionally, self-medicating individuals don't have pertinent information regarding medications' side effects and dosing instructions [10,11]. These problems are to be expected in self-medicating patients given that patients often obtain medication advice from non-professionals [3], family and friends [12]. In these cases self-medication may lead to irrational use, poor adherence to regimens, side-effects and overuse of antibiotics.

Evidence shows excessive self-medication practice in Latin America [6,7,13,14] but data indicating types of drugs and factors associated with self-medication is limited and often contradictory. In Argentina, Brazil, Chile, Colombia, Costa Rica, and Nicaragua, authors attributed the high prevalence of self-medication to poor access to health care services [13]. In Peru there were no significant differences in self-medication practices associated with gender, occupation, educational level or being head of the household [14]. In Honduras, higher proportions of self-medicating patients have been reported among those living in urban areas, but socio-economic status was not associated with self-medication [6].

Evidence regarding self-medication and its relationship to educational level and socio-economic status is mixed. In Peru, authors found that education had no significant effect on self-medication [14], while two studies in Sudan and one in Jordan found that self-medication was associated with higher literacy levels [15-17]. In one European study, higher educational level predicted higher self-medication rates [4]. Educational level does not clearly predict proportions of those who self-medicate, the same is true for socio-economic status where data is inconsistent among groups. In Jordan, one study showed positive association between self-medication and low income [17]; in Syria, patients with a middle income more frequently self-medicated [8], whereas in the United Arab Emirates there was no association to income but rather self-medication was related to ethnicity [18].

In addition to the varying data surrounding characteristics of those who self-medicate, the official health system has been ambiguous and contradictory about self-medication, recommending it in some cases while challenging it in others [19]. Multiple factors facilitate high prevalence of self-medication, such as poor access to health care providers, low quality of health services, high costs of medications, absence of regulations regarding the promotion and sale of medications, easy access in pharmacy outlets without a prescription, and publicity of pharmacy chains [20].

In Latin America pharmacists have shown interest in participating in patient-care to aid in safe medication practice [21], which may be more effective in curbing antibiotic misuse when the characteristics of self-medication with antibiotics are better understood. In order to design these types of educational interventions in the community it is important to understand the environment surrounding the practice of self-medication: motives for self-medicating, ways of self-medicating, and characteristics of those who self-medicate.

In this study we aimed to compare the magnitude of antibiotic self-medication and the characteristics of those who self-medicate with antibiotics in two pharmacies serving disparate socio-economic communities in Guatemala City.

Methods

From May to August of 2013 we carried out a descriptive cross-sectional study in two pharmacies in Guatemala City. We used purposeful sampling to select two private pharmacies serving different segments of the population according to key informants from pharmacy staff members. The first pharmacy was located in San Cristobal (zone 8 of Mixco, according to the local nomenclature), a suburb that is part of the city's metropolitan area serving clients characterized as professional or executive employees with higher levels of education and higher purchasing power. The second pharmacy, located in historical City Center (zone 1, using the local nomenclature), serves clients generally characterized as being working class and with lower levels of education and lower purchasing power.

Sample size was calculated for each pharmacy using Epidat 4.0 based on a population of 350 patients arriving to the pharmacy weekly, assuming that 50% of the population self-medicates, a precision of 5% and a 95% confidence level. Customers who purchased antibiotics without a prescription were invited to participate in the study. Written informed consent was obtained and participants were given a brief verbal definition of the practice of self-medication and the opportunity to ask any questions regarding the study or self-medication with antibiotics. Participants were asked to complete the questionnaire, which consisted of a brief introduction of study objectives and a definition of self-medication: "Self-medication occurs when patients obtain and use medications without a prescription from a doctor, meaning that patients make a personal decision to seek treatment for their illness." We determined which antibiotics were being used for self-medication by documenting the generic name of the antibiotic at the time the participant purchased the medication. Potential participants were excluded from the study if they were less than 16 years old, had seen a doctor that day, were already taking antibiotics, belonged to a vulnerable population (HIV positive, elderly or underage), were under the influence of alcohol or drugs, and/or did not understand Spanish.

Data was collected by a questionnaire [1] that was designed based on instruments used in previous studies

[10,22,23]. The questionnaire was validated by interviewing approximately 20 customers with the aim of detecting comprehension problems and to assess if the questions responded to the research aims. The instrument consisted of 22 questions: 21 multiple choice and 1 open ended question. Multiple responses were allowed for the following items: 1) Respondent symptoms provoking self-medication, 2) Reasons for self-medicating, and 3) Locations where respondents purchased antibiotics for self-medicating. We gathered information about frequency of self-medication, symptoms that provoked self-medication, with which antibiotics patients self-medicated, whom they went to for advice upon self-medicating, and if they read the antibiotic information handout. We defined antibiotics as the following: medications that treat bacterial and protozoal infections, and that are found on the World Health Organization's (WHO) Model list of Essential medicines and on the Guatemalan national "basic list" of medications [24,25]. The questionnaire was administered in a private area of the pharmacy from May to August of 2013, Monday through Friday between the hours of 9 am and 4 pm (until the target number of questionnaires were obtained). Participants were given the option of self-administering the questionnaire or having the researcher register their responses through verbal response.

Data analysis compared proportions of self-medication between the two pharmacies, using two-sample z-test as appropriate. The Research Ethics Committee at the Universidad del Valle de Guatemala approved all research materials before the study began.

Results

Socio-demographic characteristics

A total of 418 people responded to the survey, 221 in the Suburban pharmacy and 197 in the City Center pharmacy, with approximately 70% of participants self-administering the questionnaire. The majority of participants in the Suburban pharmacy and City Center pharmacy were female (70%) and between the ages of 20-29 years old (28%, 39% respectively).

Although the majority of study participants were salaried employees (62% Suburban pharmacy, 55% City Center), there was a marked difference between pharmacies when looking at the monthly income and educational level. In the Suburban pharmacy the monthly income of participants was between \$1,334.00-\$2,666.00, whereas in the City-Center pharmacy the monthly income was between \$0.00- \$667.00 (p < 0.01). The proportion of respondents who had completed a high school education was 27% in the Suburban pharmacy and 3% in the City Center pharmacy (p < 0.01). The demographic characteristics of the respondents are shown in Table 1.

Magnitude of self-medication

The proportion of self-medication with antibiotics was high in both pharmacies: 79% in the Suburban pharmacy and 77% in City Center pharmacy. The two primary reasons for self-medicating in both pharmacies were time constraints for doctors' visits (38% Suburb, 56% City Center p < 0.01) and purchasing convenience (27% Suburb, 17% City Center). Frequency of self-medication differed between pharmacies. Suburban pharmacy participants reported self-medicating once a month (35%) or once a year (30%). In contrast City Center pharmacy respondents reported self-medicating once a week (33%) or once a year (34%). Although many respondents claimed to buy medications several times a year, most reported seeing a doctor only once a year (City Center 48%, Suburban pharmacy 51%).

In both settings, amoxicillin was most commonly purchased for self-medication, followed by tetracycline and sulfamethoxazole/trimethoprim, as it is detailed in Table 2. Flu-like symptoms were the most common reason for self-medicating in the Suburban and City Center pharmacy (33%, 32%, respectively), followed by fever and pain as shown in Table 3.

Characteristics of self-medication

In the Suburban pharmacy, respondents purchased self-medicating products in pharmacies (77%) and supermarkets (9%). In the City Center pharmacy, the majority of respondents purchased antibiotics in pharmacies (70%) followed by neighborhood stores (or "tiendas" in Spanish) (29%).

Participants were asked to rate, on a scale of 1-10, the effect self-medication could have on one's health (1 being a negative effect and 10 being a positive effect). The majority of respondents, 63% of Suburban and 65% of City Center participants, responded marking 6 and above, perceiving little or no negative effect in self-medication (see Table 3).

Participants from both pharmacies obtained information regarding self-medication with antibiotics through advice rather than by reading patient handouts. In the Suburban pharmacy, respondents sought advice from pharmacy technicians (38%), followed by family (36%) and friends (23%). In contrast, City Center respondents spoke with family members (65%) or friends (30%) while only 4% went to pharmacy employees for advice. A large majority of respondents in both the Suburban and City Center pharmacies indicated that they did not read the instructions or the patient handout accompanying the antibiotic before self-medicating (80% and 95%, respectively). These findings are summarized in Table 3.

Discussion

High proportions of self-medication were similar in both pharmacies, despite the differences in monthly income

Table 1 Demographics of self-medication survey respondents visiting two pharmacies in the Guatemala City area

Basic demographics	# Suburb n = 221, (%)	# City center n = 197, (%)
Age		
16-19	14 (6%)	15 (7%)
20-29	63 (29%)	77 (39%)
30-39	59 (27%)	45 (23%)
40-49	43 (19%)	25 (13%)
50 and above	42 (19%)	35 (18%)
Gender		
Female	155 (70%)	137 (70%)
Male	66 (30%)	60 (30%)
Marital Status		
Married	124 (56%)	88 (45%)
Single	28 (13%)*	53 (27%)*
Other	69 (31%)	56 (28%)
Educational level		
Less than Middle School	60 (27%)*	131 (66%)*
Middle School Education	55 (25%)	52 (26%)
High School Education	59 (27%)*	6 (3%)*
College Education	47 (21%)*	8 (4%)*
Income		
$0-$667	95 (43%)*	153 (77%)*
$668-$1,333	38 (17%)*	9 (5%)*
$1,334-$2,666	88 (40%)*	35 (18%)*
Occupation		
House wife	45 (20%)	49 (25%)
Salaried employee	138 (62%)	108 (55%)
Independent worker	22 (10%)	17 (8%)
Other	16 (7%)	23 (12%)

*Significant difference between suburb and city center pharmacies, p < 0.01.

and educational level. This differs with findings in other studies. One comparative study in Brazil documented a higher prevalence of self-medication in higher socio-economic classes versus lower socio-economic classes; higher socio-economic patients paid out of pocket for their medications and lower socio-economic patients had free access to medication. In this Brazilian study, paying for medications was a positive factor associated to self-medication [26]. Another study in Mexico showed that low socio-economic status and lower educational level were positively associated to self-medication [11]. Practices in self-medication and their relation to socio-economic status have been defined in these settings, but to our knowledge this has not been previously established in Guatemala. Our findings suggest that self-medication

with antibiotics in this urban Guatemala City setting is high despite differences in monthly income and educational level.

More women came to pharmacies to self-medicate with antibiotics than men in both settings. This is similar to a recent study carried out in Chile whose findings indicated that 73% of those who self-medicated were female [10]. The high proportion of females who self-medicate has also been reported in several LMIC, OECD and European countries [3] with the exception of Nepal, Syria and the United Arab Emirates [8,18,27]. In Mexico women have been reported to self-medicate themselves or their children more often than men, in this context, authors agreed that women should be targeted in health-education campaigns [7]. One study in rural Peru interviewed heads of the household in order to understand characteristics surrounding those who self-medicate. The head of the household was predominately male and responded more frequently to the questionnaire, however, there was no significant association found between gender and self-medicating practices [14]. The patterns of women who self-medicate are unknown in rural areas of Guatemala, in other urban areas outside of Guatemala City, and in areas with high proportions of indigenous people who do not use Spanish as their first language. These factors may affect the proportion of men and women who obtain medications from the pharmacy in order to self-medicate. Further investigation regarding gender and self-medication is warranted in Guatemala given that the gender of those who self-medicate may vary based on pharmacy and socio-cultural practices of each region.

We found that participants of a lower socio-economic status go to family or friends for advice when self-medicating, whereas those of a higher socio-economic status more frequently talk to a pharmacy technician although they also rely on family. In a recent review of 70 studies looking at self-medication, 8 studies cited family as the major source of information for those who self-medicate. Seven studies cited friends and only 6 studies recorded pharmacists as the primary source of drug-information [3]. A recent study in older Mexican participants showed that respondents seek out advice first from family (30%), followed by a pharmacist (27%) [11]. In Guatemala we see a significant difference in whom participants are willing to approach for advice based on their socio-economic status. These findings would likely be important when designing educational programs aiding participants in the selection of self-medication.

The majority of respondents in both pharmacies indicated that self-medication has a positive effect on their health. Previous studies have emphasized the dangers in self-medicating with antibiotics. Side effects, incorrect

Table 2 Number of respondents purchasing antibiotics when self medicating

Antibiotic purchased for use in self-medication	Suburb (n = 221)		City center (n = 197)	
	Number of respondents	%	Number of respondents	%
Amoxicillin	114	51.58	82	41.62
Tetracycline	34	15.38	55	27.92
Trimethoprim-sulfamethoxazol	13	5.88	20	10.15
Erythromycin	11	4.98	18	9.14
Ciprofloxacin	9	4.07	9	4.57
Cefadroxil	0	0.00	4	2.03
Cefixime	0	0.00	4	2.03
Amoxicilin/Clavulanic Acid	9	4.07	3	1.52
Azithromycin	5	2.26	2	1.02
Secnidazol	8	3.62	0	0.00
Albendazol	6	2.71	0	0.00
Metronidazol	6	2.71	0	0.00
Levofloxacin	3	1.36	0	0.00
Ceftriaxone	2	0.90	0	0.00
Clarithromycin	1	0.45	0	0.00
Total	221	100	197	100

drugs or dosages and antibiotic resistances are all factors that make the practice problematic [1,7,28]. Patient awareness surrounding the "how", "why" and "when" to use antibiotics as well as the risks involved in self-medication with antibiotics may be created through educational initiatives. One study reviewed LMIC pharmacy interventions and placed an emphasis on the educational services pharmacists may provide in order to improve outcomes [9]. These types of services must go beyond classifying medication use as "good or bad" [29]. If educational services are to be implemented, they must be all-inclusive resulting in a comprehensive educational plan for those who self-medicate [6,9,13]. There must be support within the local health-system giving incentive to form sustainable educational programs in the community. The gender of those who self medicate, how the socio-economic status influences self-medication, with whom respondents are willing to go to for advice, and techniques by which participants receive information about self-medicating all contribute to developing educational and political movements to ensure the safety and efficacy of antibiotic use.

Participants in this study did not read the antibiotic information handout associated with the medications they purchased, regardless of their socio-economic status and educational level. Educational level plays an important role when deciding how to effectively design drug information for participants [9]. Informing patients about a medication's indications, posology and side effects using means other than patient handouts that accompany medications is an important challenge if antibiotic use is to be

addressed. Although all participants had some level of schooling, patient handouts accompanying medications may be inadequate in Guatemala given that the majority of self-medicators did not have a secondary school education. Combining the risks of self-medication with the demographic data we have gathered, we provide a basis for initiating educational policies surrounding medication use in the urban setting of Guatemala.

The majority of respondents purchased antibiotics from pharmacies where antibiotics are sold in the absence of any medical regulation, contributing to irrational use and antimicrobial resistance. In most LMIC, the debate of antibiotic regulation skews towards authorization of unregulated vendors selling antibiotics in order to maintain reasonable access to medications [30,31]. Additionally, competing interests of the pharmaceutical industry and pharmacy chains promote unregulated use of antibiotics [30]. Nevertheless, restricted and regulated use of antibiotics is of public health concern both locally and for many globally recognized organizations [2,28].

There is currently no law in Guatemala requiring the continual presence of a pharmacist in the pharmacy. Trained health care professionals do not monitor the sale and dispensing of antibiotics in Guatemala in community pharmacies, and there is no law requiring a prescription for antibiotic use; prescriptions are only required for controlled substances. Both factors -absence of health care professionals in the pharmacy and lack of regulations- lead to irrational use of antibiotics and antimicrobial resistance. This presents an opportunity for

Table 3 Characteristics of self-medication in two Guatemala City pharmacies

	Number of respondents in Suburb (n = 221)	Number of respondents in City Center (n = 197)
Symptoms resulting in self-medication[+]		
Cold/flu	74 (33%)	65 (33%)
Pain	66 (30%)	54 (27%)
Fever	39 (18%)	41 (21%)
Stomach ache	22 (10%)	26 (13%)
Diarrhea	10 (5%)	5 (3%)
Allergy	10 (4%)	6 (3%)
Reasons for self-medicating[+]		
Lack of time and to save time	84 (38%)*	110 (56%)*
Easily purchasable medications from pharmacies	60 (27%)	34 (17%)
Economic reasons (High costs of visits to doctor/Low cost of purchasing drugs)	34 (15%)	29 (15%)
Simple sign and symptom of a disease	20 (9%)	18 (9%)
Convenient (ease of curing perceived symptoms)	18 (8%)	3 (2%)
Lack of trust toward doctors	4 (2%)	3 (2%)
Locations for obtaining medications[+]		
Pharmacies	172 (77%)	139 (70%)
Supermarket	20 (9%)*	0 (0%)*
Corner stores	19 (8%)*	58 (29%)*
From home (previously purchased)	9 (4%)*	0*
Frequency of self-medication		
One time per week	42(19%)*	65(33%)*
One time per month	77(35%)*	12(6%)*
Two times per month	1(0.5%)	6(3%)
Every two months	1(0.5%)	2(1%)
Every three months	5(2%)	8(4%)
Every six months	16(7%)	21(11%)
Two times per year	2(1%)	0
One time per year	66(30%)	67(34%)
Never	11(5%)	16 (8%)
Regarding the antibiotic information handout		
Do not read antibiotic information handout	176 (80%)*	188 (95%)*
Read antibiotic information handout	45 (20%)*	9 (5%)*
How it can effect one's health, 1 negative effect 10 positive effect		
1 on a scale of 10	0 (0%)*	0 (0%)*
2-4 on a scale of 10	37 (17%)	24 (12%)
5 on a scale of 10	45 (20%)	35 (18%)
6 on a scale of 10	67 (30%)	40 (20%)
7 on a scale of 10	42 (19%)	46 (23%)
8-10 on a scale of 10	30 (14%)	44 (22%)
Who respondents go to for advice		
Pharmacy employee	84 (38%)*	8 (4%)*
Family	81 (37%)*	129 (65%)*
Friend	52 (23%)	60 (30%)
Other	4 (2%)	0 (0%)

*Significant difference between suburb and city center pharmacies, p < 0.01.
[+]Multiple responses were allowed for these items.

developing the role of the pharmacist in guiding the rational use of antibiotics in Guatemala where we have shown that a proportion of respondents seek advice from pharmacists. Fundamental to the policy development surrounding the role of a pharmacist is the establishment of associated laws regulating the dispensing of medications [14]. Relationships with other health care professionals, social pressures and conflicts of business and professional roles must be taken into account in this type of policy development [9]. Restructuring and eventual development of the role of the pharmacist may improve safe and rational use, affordability and accessibility of antibiotics in Guatemala [9,12].

Limitations of this study include those inherent to the cross-sectional research design, as well as the use of purposeful sampling for selecting the pharmacies. The study is not population-based and therefore its results cannot be assumed to be generalizable to all pharmacies in Guatemala City or to Guatemala City. The study did not ask qualitative questions that allowed participants to provide their own explanations and meanings around self-medication.

The results of our study contribute to a better understanding of why people self-medicate, the characteristics of those who self-medicate and how people self-medicate in Guatemala and should be complemented with further investigations that include pharmacies located in other urban and rural settings. It is also important to determine which, if any, side effects participants may experience as a result of self-medicating with antibiotics and if their perceived risk of self-medication changes across rural versus urban settings. Also, it may be important to know if participants perceive self-medication as "curative" or, if as a result of their practice, they have to see a physician to improve health outcomes. Additionally, further studies may focus on health literacy and the health systems dimensions of this problem.

Conclusions

The high proportion and factors contributing to self-medication with antibiotics in Guatemala City are similar in two disparate socio-economic pharmacies. In this setting, women come to the pharmacy more often than men in order to self-medicate and perceive little risk in its practice. Those of higher socio-economic status in Guatemala City are willing to speak to pharmacy personnel for advice regarding self-medication and, although future studies are necessary, this study sets the stage for future policy development regarding the role of the pharmacist in addressing self-medication with antibiotics. This type of role, however, may have a limited public health impact if there are no changes in the regulation of antibiotic promotion, sale and use in Guatemala.

Additional file

Additional file 1: Antibiotic self-medication questionnaire_Spanish.

Competing interests
The authors declare that they have no competing interests.

Authors' contributions
BR supervised study design and data interpretation, conceptualized the article, drafted the manuscript, and coordinated review of co-authors. PL designed the study, conducted interviews, processed and analyzed data, and reviewed and revised the manuscript. AC contributed to the conceptualization of the article and data interpretation, and advised the development of the manuscript. All authors read and approved the final manuscript.

Acknowledgements
BR and PL covered research costs, with logistic support from Universidad del Valle de Guatemala. Dr. Elfego Rolando Lopez gave input to early versions of this manuscript. Dr. Carrie Coates and Rochelle Ramay, MA, edited final versions of the manuscript. Institutional support from the Center for the Study of Equity and Governance in Health Systems (CEGSS) was fundamental for developing the collaboration between BR and AC that led to the completion of this manuscript.

Author details
[1]Department of Pharmaceutical Chemistry, Universidad del Valle de Guatemala, Guatemala City, Guatemala. [2]Department of Anthropology, University of Denver, Denver, Colorado, USA.

References
1. World Health Organization. Antimicrobial Resistance Global Report on Surveillance. Geneva, Switzerland: World Health Press; 2014.
2. World Health Organization, Health Action International global. The World Medicines Situation 2011 Rational Use of Medicines, 3rd edition. Geneva Switzerland: WHO Press; 2011.
3. Ahaghaghi A, Asadi M, Allahverdipour H. Predictors of Self-Medication Behavior: A Systematic Review. Iran J Publ Health. 2014;43:136–46.
4. Grigoryan L, Haaijer-Ruskamp FM, Burgerhof JGM, Mechtler R, Deschepper R, Tambic-Andrasevic A, et al. Self-medication with Antimicrobial Drugs in Europe. Emerg Infect Dis. 2006;12:452–9.
5. Stosic R, Fiona D, Hazel P, Fowler T, Adams I. Responsible self-medication: perceived risks and benefits of over-the-counter analgesic use. Int J Pharm Pract. 2011;19:236–45.
6. Crigger NJ, Grogan RL. Development of the choices and acquisition of antibiotics model from a descriptive study of a lay Honduran population. Int J Nurs Stud. 2004;41:745–53.
7. Angeles P, Maria Luisa M, Juan Francisco M. Automedicacion en poblacion urbana de Cuernavaca. Salud Publica Mex. 1992;34:554–61.
8. Barah F, Morris J, Gonçalves V. Irrational use and poor public beliefs regarding antibiotics in developing countries: a pessimistic example of Syria. Int J Clin Pract. 2009;63:1263–4.
9. Smith F. Private local pharmacies in low- and middle-income countries: a review of interventions to enhance their role in public health. Trop Med Int Health. 2009;14:362–72.
10. Fuentes Albarrán K, Villa Zapata L. Analysis and quantification of self-medication patterns of customers in community pharmacies in southern Chile. Pharm World Sci. 2008;6:863–8.
11. Balbuena FR, Aranda AB, Figueras A. Self-Medication in Older Urban Mexicans: An Observational, Descriptive, Cross-Sectional Study. Drugs Aging. 2009;26:51–60.
12. Sonam J, Reetesh M, Jeetendra Kumar P. Concept of Self Medication: A review. Int J Pharm Biol Arch. 2011;2:831–6.
13. Drug Utilization Research Group, Latin America WHO. Multicenter study on self-medication and self-prescription in six Latin American Countries. Clin Pharmacol Ther. 1996;61:488–93 [4].

14. Llamos Zavalaga LF, Contreras Rios C, Velasquez Hurtado J, Mayca Perez J, Lecca Garcia L, Reyes Lecca R, et al. Automedicacion en cinco provincias de Cajamarca. Rev Med Hered Online. 2001;12:127–33.

15. Awad AI, Eltayeb IB, Capps PA. Self-medication practices in Khartoum State, Sudan. Eur J Clin Pharmacol. 2006;62:317–24.

16. Abdelmoneim A, Idris E, Lloyd M. Self-medication with Antibiotics and Antimalarials in the community of Khartoum State, Sudan. J Pharm Pharm Sci. 2005;8:326–31.

17. Al-Azzam S, Al-Husein B, Alzoubi F, Masadeh M, Al-Horani MA. Self-Medication with Antibiotics in Jordanian Population. Int J Occup Med Environ Health. 2007;20:1232–087.

18. Abasaeed A, Vlcek J, Abuelkhair M, Kubena A. Self-medication with antibiotics by the community of Abu Dhabi Emirate, United Arab Emirates. J Infect Dev Ctries. 2009;3:491–7.

19. Mendez E. Modelos de atención de los padecimientos: de exclusiones teóricas y articulaciones prácticas. Cienc Saude Colect. 2003;8:185–207.

20. Versporten A, Bolokhovets G, Ghazaryan L, Abilova V, Pyshnik G, Spasojevic T, et al. Antibiotic use in eastern Europe: a cross-national database study in coordination with the WHO Regional Office for Europe. Lancet Infect Dis. 2014;14(5):381–7.

21. Dupotey Varela NM, Oliveira DR D, Sedeño Argilagos C, Oliveros Castro K, Mosqueda Pérez E, Hidalgo Clavel Y, et al. What is the role of the pharmacist?: physicians' and nurses' perspectives in community and hospital settings of Santiago de Cuba. Braz J Pharm Sci. 2011;47:709–18.

22. Fuentes Albarrán K, Viila I, Mller C. Análisis y cuantificación de los patrones de automedicación en usuarios de farmacias Salcobrand de Valdivia. Undergraduate Thesis Universidad Austral de Chile; 2006. p. 1-66.

23. Tobon Marulanda FA. Estudio sobre la automediaccion en La Universidad de Antioquia, Medellin Colombia. Iatreia. 2002;15:242–7.

24. WHO. Model List of Essential Medicines, 18th list. Geneva Switzerland: WHO Press; 2013.

25. Ministerio de Salud Publica y Asistencia Social, Viallavicencio JA, Galvan MG, Sandoval WE, Arevalo MV, et al. Lista basica de medicamentos. Guatemala: MSPAS; 2013.

26. Schmid B, Bernal R, Silva NN. Self-medication in low-income adults in Southeastern Brazil. Rev Saúde Pública. 2010;44:2–6.

27. Shankar PR, Partha P, Shenoy N: Self-medication and non-doctor prescription practices in Pokhara valley, Western Nepal: a questionnaire-based study. BMC Fam Pr 2002, 3

28. Kelley PW. Antimicrobial resistance in the age of noncommunicable diseases. Rev Panam Salud Publica. 2011;30(6):515–8.

29. Fainzang S. Managing Medicinal Risks in Self-Medication. Drug Saf. 2014;37:333–42.

30. Dreser A, Vázquez-Vélez E, Treviño S, Wirtz VJ. Regulation of antibiotic sales in Mexico: an analysis of printed media coverage and stakeholder participation. BMC Public Health. 2012;12:1051.

31. Carlet J, Pittet D. Access to antibiotics: a safety and equity challenge for the next decade. Antimicrob Resist Infect Control. 2013;2:1.

23

Differences between murine arylamine N-acetyltransferase type 1 and human arylamine N-acetyltransferase type 2 defined by substrate specificity and inhibitor binding

Nicola Laurieri[1], Akane Kawamura[2], Isaac M Westwood[1,3], Amy Varney[1], Elizabeth Morris[1], Angela J Russell[1,2], Lesley A Stanley[4] and Edith Sim[1,5]*

Abstract

Background: The mouse has three arylamine N-acetyltransferase genes, (MOUSE)Nat1, (MOUSE)Nat2 and (MOUSE)Nat3. These are believed to correspond to (HUMAN)NAT1, (HUMAN)NAT2 and NATP in humans. (MOUSE)Nat3 encodes an enzyme with poor activity and human NATP is a pseudogene. (MOUSE)Nat2 is orthologous to (HUMAN)NAT1 and their corresponding proteins are functionally similar, but the relationship between (MOUSE)Nat1 and (HUMAN)NAT2 is less clear-cut.

Methods: To determine whether the (MOUSE)NAT1 and (HUMAN)NAT2 enzymes are functionally equivalent, we expressed and purified (MOUSE)NAT1*1 and analysed its substrate specificity using a panel of arylamines and hydrazines. To understand how specific residues contribute to substrate selectivity, three site-directed mutants of (MOUSE)NAT2*1 were prepared: these were (MOUSE)NAT2_F125S, (MOUSE)NAT2_R127G and (MOUSE)NAT2_R127L. All three exhibited diminished activity towards "(MOUSE)NAT2-specific" arylamines but were more active against hydrazines than (MOUSE)NAT1*1. The inhibitory and colorimetric properties of a selective naphthoquinone inhibitor of (HUMAN)NAT1 and (MOUSE)NAT2 were investigated.

Results: Comparing (MOUSE)NAT1*1 with other mammalian NAT enzymes demonstrated that the substrate profiles of (MOUSE)NAT1 and (HUMAN)NAT2 are less similar than previously believed. Three key residues (F125, R127 and Y129) in (HUMAN)NAT1*4 and (MOUSE)NAT2*1 were required for enzyme inhibition and the associated colour change on naphthoquinone binding. In silico modelling of selective ligands into the appropriate NAT active sites further implicated these residues in substrate and inhibitor specificity in mouse and human NAT isoenzymes.

Conclusions: Three non-catalytic residues within (HUMAN)NAT1*4 (F125, R127 and Y129) contribute both to substrate recognition and inhibitor binding by participating in distinctive intermolecular interactions and maintaining the steric conformation of the catalytic pocket. These active site residues contribute to the definition of substrate and inhibitor selectivity, an understanding of which is essential for facilitating the design of second generation (HUMAN)NAT1-selective inhibitors for diagnostic, prognostic and therapeutic purposes. In particular, since the expression of (HUMAN)NAT1 is related to the development and progression of oestrogen-receptor-positive breast cancer, these structure-based tools will facilitate the ongoing design of candidate compounds for use in (HUMAN)NAT1-positive breast tumours.

Keywords: Arylamine N-acetyltransferase, (MOUSE)NAT1, (MOUSE)NAT2, Substrate specificity, Inhibitor selectivity, Structural docking

* Correspondence: edith.sim@pharm.ox.ac.uk
[1]Department of Pharmacology, University of Oxford, Oxford, UK
[5]Faculty of Science, Engineering and Computing, Kingston University, Kingston on Thames, UK
Full list of author information is available at the end of the article

Background

Arylamine *N*-acetyltransferases (NATs, EC. 2.3.1.5) [1] are drug metabolising enzymes which catalyse the conjugation of an acetyl group from acetyl Coenzyme A (AcCoA) to arylamines, hydrazines and *N*-hydroxyarylamines. They participate in the detoxification and metabolic activation of xenobiotics and are found in a wide variety of prokaryotic and eukaryotic species [2].

The human genome contains two polymorphic *NAT* genes, *(HUMAN)NAT1* and *(HUMAN)NAT2* [3,4], which play important pharmacogenetic roles in cancer susceptibility and have the potential to contribute to personalised medicine [5,6]. The corresponding enzymes possess distinct substrate profiles: HUMAN(NAT1) preferentially *N*-acetylates the arylamines 4-aminobenzoic acid (4ABA), 4-aminobenzoyl glutamate (4ABglu) and 4-aminosalicylate (4AS), whereas (HUMAN)NAT2 has higher activity towards the hydrazines isoniazid (INH) and hydralazine (HDZ) and the arylamine sulfamethazine (SMZ) [7,8]. The crystal structures of human NATs [9] resemble the three-domain conformation observed in prokaryotic NATs [10]. Like their prokaryotic counterparts, each has a catalytic triad comprising cysteine (C), histidine (H) and aspartic acid (D) at the active site; they also contain an additional loop of 17 residues which many prokaryotic enzymes lack. These observations helped to lay the foundations for studies addressing the structural determinants of their catalytic selectivity [11].

Human NATs are characterised by differing tissue distributions and patterns of gene expression during development [12-14]. In particular, while (HUMAN)NAT2 appears to be a well-established drug metabolising enzyme and is mainly expressed in the liver [15], the selective *N*-acetylation of the folate catabolites 4ABglu and 4ABA by (HUMAN)NAT1 suggests that this isoform may have an endogenous role in folate homeostasis [16,17]. Furthermore, recent studies indicate that (HUMAN)NAT1 has a novel catalytic function as a folate-dependent AcCoA hydrolase [18].

Rodents also have multiple NAT isoforms which have been investigated as animal models for the corresponding human enzymes. Mice, for example, have three *NAT* genes, *(MOUSE)Nat1*, *(MOUSE)Nat2* and *(MOUSE)Nat3*. All of these are polymorphic; the *(MOUSE)Nat3* gene exhibits the greatest extent of polymorphism and may effectively be considered a pseudogene like *(HUMAN)NAT3* [19], although it does have enzymatic activity [20,21].

Historically, (MOUSE)NAT2 has been considered to correspond to (HUMAN)NAT1 because their primary sequences are 82% homologous and they exhibit similarities in terms of expression profile, tissue distribution and substrate preference [8,22-24]. Furthermore, inhibition studies have identified a (HUMAN)NAT1/(MOUSE)NAT2 selective inhibitor, naphthoquinone **1** (*N*-(3-(3,5-dimethylphenylamino)-1,4-dioxo-1,4-dihydronaphthalen-

2-yl)benzenesulphonamide; Additional file 1: Figure S1), which undergoes a distinctive colour change from red to blue upon binding to either of these two enzymes but not to other mammalian NAT isoenzymes [24,25]. Virtual modelling studies [25,26] indicate that the interaction between naphthoquinone **1** and (HUMAN)NAT1 or (MOUSE)NAT2 depends on selective ionic interactions between the conjugate base of compound **1** and the guanidinium moiety of an active site residue, arginine 127 (R127). This is part of a group of active site residues which had previously been identified as being involved, together with phenylalanine 125 (F125) and tyrosine 129 (Y129), in substrate specificity [27,28]. These residues differ between (HUMAN)NAT1*4 and (HUMAN)NAT2*4 and between (MOUSE)NAT1*1 and (MOUSE)NAT2*1, while the catalytic triad of C, H and D is identical.

The (MOUSE)NAT1 enzyme is commonly assumed to be functionally equivalent to (HUMAN)NAT2 because both can metabolise isoniazid (INH) and sulfamethazine (SMZ) [29-31]. In order to determine whether these enzymes are true functional equivalents, we used a previously reported *(MOUSE)Nat1*1* clone [32] to express and purify the (MOUSE)NAT1*1 enzyme and compared its substrate profile with those of other rodent and human NAT enzymes using a broad panel of aromatic amines and hydrazines. In addition, we used three site-directed mutants ((MOUSE)NAT2_F125S, (MOUSE)NAT2_R127G and (MOUSE)NAT2_R127L) to investigate the effects of key active site residues on the substrate specificity of (MOUSE)NAT2. In the present study we focused on residues 125 and 127; the role of the Y129 residue found in (HUMAN)NAT1 and (MOUSE)NAT2, at least with respect to inhibitor binding, has previously been investigated using (MESAU)NAT2, which has identical active site residues except for a leucine (L) at location 129 [33]. The results of this earlier study [26] suggest that Y129 is functionally important, at least in inhibitor recognition, and illustrate the value of (MESAU)NAT2 as a protein model for comparative studies with (HUMAN)NAT1 and (MOUSE)NAT2.

Finally, we modelled the binding of representative arylamine substrates within the active sites of reference and mutant mammalian NATs in order to elucidate key interactions within the NAT/substrate complex. The identification of (HUMAN)NAT1 as a potential therapeutic target in cancer means that understanding the molecular details of this series of enzymes in humans and potential animal models is important for their potential exploitation in both diagnostics [24] and therapy [34].

Methods

Chemicals and reagents

All chemicals were purchased from Sigma-Aldrich unless otherwise stated. Molecular biology reagents were obtained from Promega.

Expression of pure recombinant NATs
Expression and purification of (MOUSE)NAT1*1

The open reading frame of *(MOUSE)Nat1*1* [32] was subcloned into the *Nde*I and *Eco*RI sites of pET28b(+) (Novagen) and transformed into *Escherichia coli* BL21 (DE3)CodonPlus-RIL (Stratagene). BL21 cells carrying the expression plasmid were grown in auto-induction medium at 27°C in the presence of kanamycin (30 µg. mL^{-1}) and chloramphenicol (34 µg.mL^{-1}) and harvested after 24 hrs by centrifugation (5,000 g, 4°C, 20 min). The cell pellet was resuspended in lysis buffer (300 mM NaCl, 20 mM Tris–HCl (pH 8.0), 1 × EDTA-free Complete Protease Inhibitor (Roche)) and stored at –80°C. Cells were thawed, lysed by sonication and the soluble protein fraction was separated from cell debris by centrifugation (12,000 *g*, 4°C, 20 min). The soluble fraction was incubated with pre-equilibrated Ni-NTA resin (Qiagen) for 5 min, loaded on a chromatography column and washed with buffer solutions containing increasing imidazole concentrations at 4°C (two washes each of 0 mM, 10 mM, 20 mM, 50 mM and 100 mM imidazole). Fractions containing (MOUSE)NAT1*1 were identified by sodium dodecyl sulphate-polyacrylamide gel electrophoresis and NAT activity assays using 5-aminosalicylate (5AS) [35]. The hexa-His tag was removed by thrombin cleavage (5 U thrombin/mg of protein, 16 h incubation, 4°C) and the cleaved protein was dialysed against 20 mM Tris–HCl (pH 8.0), 1 mM DTT, 1 mM EDTA buffer. Glycerol was added to 5%. Samples were concentrated by centrifugal ultrafiltration (Amicon), snap frozen in liquid nitrogen and stored at –80°C (1 mg. mL^{-1} in 20 mM Tris–HCl (pH 7.0), 5 mM DTT, 5% glycerol).

Site-directed mutagenesis, expression and purification of (MOUSE)NAT2_F125S

QuikChange II (Stratagene) was used to mutate codon 125 (TTT; F125) of *(MOUSE)Nat2*1* [22] to TCT, which encodes serine (F125S) (Additional file 2: Figure S2). The resulting mutant was expressed in Rosetta(DE3) pLysS as described previously [22,25]. (MOUSE)NAT2_ F125S was purified by Ni-NTA affinity chromatography and thrombin cleavage, as described. Fractions containing mutant (MOUSE)NAT2_F125S protein were identified by sodium dodecyl sulphate-polyacrylamide gel electrophoresis and NAT activity assays using 4ABA [35].

Preparation of pure recombinant mammalian NATs

The preparation of pure recombinant (MOUSE)NAT2*1, (MOUSE)NAT2_R127G, (MOUSE)NAT2_R127L, (MESAU) NAT2*1, (HUMAN)NAT1*4 and (HUMAN)NAT2*4 was performed as described previously [8,22,25].

Substrate and inhibitor selectivity and spectrometry of (MOUSE)NAT1*1 and three (MOUSE)NAT2 mutants

Substrate specific *N*-acetylation profiles were determined according to published methods with minor modifications [8,36]. Recombinant proteins were used immediately after purification. The quantity of each protein used in assay mixes (100 µL) was: (MOUSE)NAT1*1, 0.633 µg; (MOUSE)NAT2*1, 1.4 µg; (MOUSE)NAT2_ F125S, 1 µg; (MOUSE)NAT2_R127G, 0.8 µg; and (MOUSE)NAT2_R127L, 5.5 µg. The substrates used were 4ABglu, 4ABA, 4AS, 5AS, 4-chloroaniline (4CA), 4-bromoaniline (4BA), 4-iodoaniline (4IA), 4-methoxyaniline (ANS), 4-aminoveratrole (4AV), 4-hexyloxyaniline (HOA), 4-phenoxyaniline (POA), SMZ, INH and HDZ. In each case the final concentration in the reaction mix was 500 µM. All measurements were performed in triplicate and are expressed as mean ± standard deviation. For each enzyme tested, average measures of specific activity were calculated relative to the substrate exhibiting the highest specific activity (100%) for that enzyme.

In order to highlight differences in substrate preference among murine NAT proteins, the substrate profiles of (MOUSE)NAT2*1, (MOUSE)NAT1*1, (MOUSE)NAT2_ F125S, (MOUSE)NAT2_R127G and (MOUSE)NAT2_ R127L were compared by ANOVA (confidence limit 95%) using the Shapiro-Wilk test to verify normal distribution and Cochran's test to check the equality of variances. Statistical significance was evaluated using Student's t-test with a Bonferroni adjustment if required.

Inhibition of NAT activity was determined as the ratio of specific activity in the presence and absence of the inhibitor naphthoquinone **1** using the preferred substrate for the enzyme under investigation. The final concentration of dimethyl sulphoxide (DMSO) in reaction mixes was 5% (v/v). IC$_{50}$ values were estimated using a dose–response-based regression model in Kyplot® software. Curves were fitted by least squares analysis with confidence limits of 95%. Visible spectra (λ = 800 to 326 nm) of naphthoquinone **1** in the presence of pure recombinant NATs were recorded with a U-2001 spectrophotometer (Hitachi) using 50 µL UVettes® (Eppendorf).

Structural modelling and docking simulations

Structural models of wild type (MOUSE)NAT2*1, (MOUSE) NAT2 mutants and (MESAU)NAT2*1 were generated based on the structure of (HUMAN)NAT1*4 [PDB:2PQT] [9] using SwissModel software (http://swissmodel.expasy. org/) in automated mode [37-39]. Each substrate was drawn in 3D using ChemBio3D Ultra 12.0 and its ground state conformation predicted before it was docked into the catalytic pocket of the appropriate NAT structure ((HUMAN)NAT1*4: 2PQT, (HUMAN)NAT2*4: 2PFR [9]) or NAT model ((MOUSE)NAT2*1, (MOUSE)NAT2 mutants and (MESAU)NAT2*1). Protein and substrate structures were defined as pdbqt files and protein-structure interactions were analysed using Autodock Vina [40]. After adding polar hydrogen atoms to the NAT target and defining the rotatable bonds of the ligand, a docking site was defined within the active site pocket and possible solutions were ranked according to affinity energy (lowest to highest; kcal.mol^{-1}). The docking results were visualised in 3D using PyMOL [41].

Results

Substrate selectivity of (MOUSE)NAT1*1 and (MOUSE)NAT2*1

We expressed (MOUSE)NAT1*1 in *E. coli* Rosetta (DE3) pLysS and used the resulting recombinant protein to determine the activity of (MOUSE)NAT1*1 towards a panel of chemicals commonly used as NAT substrates (Additional file 3: Table S1). The highest specific activities were with the hydrazines INH and HDZ and the arylamine SMZ (Figure 1). A parallel screening experiment with (MOUSE)NAT2*1 yielded results corresponding to those published previously [22]. The differences between (MOUSE)NAT1*1 and (MOUSE)NAT2*1 for most substrates were statistically significant. (MOUSE)NAT1*1 did, however, have low but measurable activity towards certain arylamine substrates which are usually considered to be (MOUSE)NAT2-specific (4ABA and 4AS but not 4ABglu) and towards halogenated arylamines and alkyloxy- and aryloxy-substituted arylamines.

Site-directed mutagenesis of (MOUSE)NAT2

Three (MOUSE)NAT2 mutants ((MOUSE)NAT2_F125S, (MOUSE)NAT2_R127G and (MOUSE)NAT2_R127L) were used to explore the effects of mutating a single residue within the active site on the substrate specificity of (MOUSE)NAT2. Two of these, (MOUSE)NAT2_R127G and (MOUSE)NAT2_R127L, were reported previously [8,22]. The third, (MOUSE)NAT2_F125S was generated by site-directed mutagenesis, as described above and illustrated in Additional file 2: Figure S2.

The substrate panel listed in Additional file 3: Table S1 was used to characterise the activity profiles of the three mutants in comparison with that of (MOUSE)NAT2*1. The maximum specific activity of (MOUSE)NAT2_F125S (observed with EOA) was around 7.5 times lower than the maximal value of (MOUSE)NAT2*1 (observed with 4ABA), but the substrate preferences of (MOUSE)NAT2_F125S and (MOUSE)NAT2*1 were similar. Some discrepancies were, however, observed: the main differences observed were marked reductions in the relative rate of *N*-acetylation of the arylamines 4ABglu and 4ABA and an augmentation of activities towards the hydrazines INH and HDZ.

Substituting R127 with glycine (R127G) or leucine (R127L) caused a dramatic loss of *N*-acetylation activity towards 4ABA and 4ABglu (Figure 2). Aminosalicylic acids were differentially *N*-acetylated by (MOUSE)NAT2*1 and its R127 mutants: (MOUSE)NAT2_R127G and (MOUSE)NAT2_R127L had significantly lower *N*-acetylation activity towards the (MOUSE)NAT2-specific substrate 4AS, but higher catalytic activity with 5AS compared with (MOUSE)NAT2*1. These mutations had no marked effects on the *N*-acetylation of halogenated arylamines and alkyloxy-substituted arylamines with small alkyl chains (ANS, 4AV), but those with extended alkyloxy or bulkier aryloxy substituents (hexyloxy in HOA and phenoxy in POA) were strongly preferred by both R127 mutants compared with (MOUSE)NAT2*1. The mutants also had

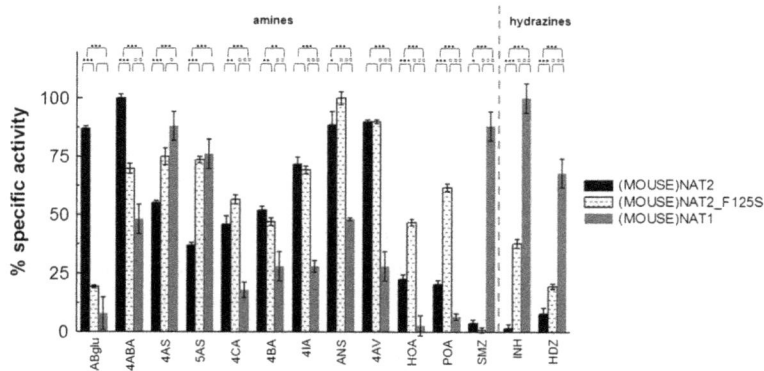

Figure 1 Substrate profiles of (MOUSE)NAT2*1, (MOUSE)NAT2_F125S and (MOUSE)NAT1*1. Substrate specific activity profiles of (MOUSE) NAT2*1 (black columns), (MOUSE)NAT2_F125S (dashed white columns) and (MOUSE)NAT1*1 (gray columns) are shown. Maximal specific activity values (normalised as 100% relative specific activity) were: 196 μM.sec^{-1}.mg^{-1} for (MOUSE)NAT2*1 with 4ABA, 25 μM.sec^{-1}.mg^{-1} for (MOUSE) NAT2_F125S with ANS and 104 μM.sec^{-1}.mg^{-1} for (MOUSE)NAT1*1 with INH. A dashed line separates aromatic amines from hydrazines. The circles above the bars show the significance of the differences between (MOUSE)NAT2_F125S or (MOUSE)NAT1*1 and (MOUSE)NAT2*1 (●) and between (MOUSE)NAT2_F125S and (MOUSE)NAT1*1 (○) using ANOVA with Student's t-test; ● or ○: $p \leq 0.05$; ●● or ○○: $p \leq 0.01$; ●●● or ○○○: $p \leq 0.001$.

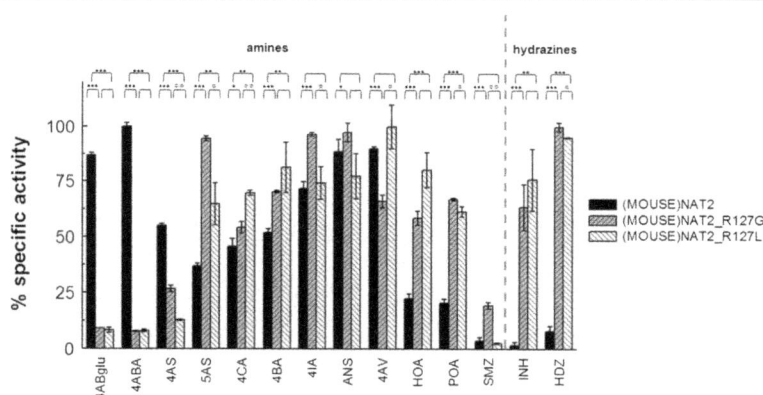

Figure 2 Substrate profiles of (MOUSE)NAT2*1, (MOUSE)NAT2_R127G and (MOUSE)NAT2_R127L. Substrate specific activity profiles of (MOUSE)NAT2*1 (black columns), (MOUSE)NAT2_R127G (dashed gray columns), (MOUSE)NAT2_R127L (dashed white columns) are shown. Maximal specific activity values (normalised as 100% relative specific activity) are: 196 $\mu M.sec^{-1}.mg^{-1}$ for (MOUSE)NAT2*1 with 4ABA, 1385 $\mu M.sec^{-1}.mg^{-1}$ for (MOUSE)NAT2_R127G with HDZ and 82.5 $\mu M.sec^{-1}.mg^{-1}$ for (MOUSE)NAT2_R127L with 4AV. A dashed line separates aromatic amines from hydrazines. The circles above the bars show the significance of the differences between (MOUSE)NAT2_R127G or (MOUSE)NAT2_R127L and (MOUSE)NAT2*1 (●) and between (MOUSE)NAT2_R127G and (MOUSE)NAT2_R127L (o) using ANOVA with Student's t-test; ● or o: $p \leq 0.05$; ●● or oo: $p \leq 0.01$; ●●● or ooo: $p \leq 0.001$.

much higher N-acetylation activity towards hydrazines such as HDZ.

Comparison of the substrate profiles of the two R127 mutants did not identify significant differences in their activity profiles. Overall, the best substrate for (MOUSE)NAT2_R127G was HDZ. The observed specific activity (1,385 $\mu M.sec^{-1}.mg^{-1}$) was 7 fold higher than the maximum specific activity of (MOUSE)NAT2*1 with 4ABA (196 $\mu M.sec^{-1}.mg^{-1}$), suggesting that (MOUSE)NAT2_R127G mutant had greater catalytic efficiency than (MOUSE)NAT2*1. In contrast, comparing the maximum specific activity value of (MOUSE)NAT2*1 (196 $\mu M.sec^{-1}.mg^{-1}$ with 4ABA) with that of (MOUSE)NAT2_R127L (82.5 $\mu M.sec^{-1}.mg^{-1}$ with 4AV) indicated that the maximum catalytic turnover of (MOUSE)NAT2_R127L was ~2.5 fold lower than that of (MOUSE)NAT2*1.

Comparison of substrate selectivity among mammalian NATs

The assays described here were performed under the conditions described in our previous publications [8,22]. We were therefore able to compare previously published substrate selectivity profiles of (HUMAN)NAT1*4, (HUMAN)NAT2*4 and (MESAU)NAT2*1 with those of (MOUSE)NAT1*1, (MOUSE)NAT2*1 and the three engineered (MOUSE)NAT2 mutants reported here (Table 1). In Table 1, the NAT enzymes are arranged according to divergence of the active site sequence from that of (HUMAN)NAT1*4 (Figure 3) [9] and plotted against arylamine and hydrazine substrates organised according to their chemical functionalities and physicochemical properties. Overall, as the active site diverged further from that of (HUMAN)NAT1*4, substrate preference moved from

arylamines with negatively charged *para*-substituents towards aromatic amines and hydrazines without ionised, polar or *para*-substituents around the aromatic core. In particular, 4ABglu, 4ABA and 4AS have an acetyl acceptor amine with $pK_{aH} < 3$ (Additional file 3: Table S1) and are subject to N-acetylation by (HUMAN)NAT1*4 and its homologues (MOUSE)NAT2*1 and (MESAU)NAT2*1. The other substrates have an acceptor amine with $pK_{aH} \geq 3$. These are better substrates for (HUMAN)NAT2*4, (MOUSE)NAT1*1 and the two R127-mutated (MOUSE)NAT2 enzymes.

In general, the results obtained corresponded with previous reports of functional similarities between (HUMAN)NAT1*4, (MOUSE)NAT2*1 and (MESAU)NAT2*1 [8,22]; however, the substrate profile of (MOUSE)NAT1*1 did not, as expected, correspond to that of (HUMAN)NAT2*4 [29,31]. Indeed, (MOUSE)NAT1*1 was able to N-acetylate substrates characteristic of both (HUMAN)NAT1*4 (4ABA and 4AS) and (HUMAN)NAT2*4 (SMZ, INH and HDZ).

Inhibition studies

The inhibitory potency and colorimetric properties of the (HUMAN)NAT1-selective inhibitor naphthoquinone **1** were also explored in relation to alterations at positions 125, 127 and 129 using (MOUSE)NAT2_F125S, (MOUSE)NAT1*1 and (HUMAN)NAT2*4, comparing the results with those of previous studies using (HUMAN)NAT1*4, (MESAU)NAT2*1, (MOUSE)NAT2*1, (MOUSE)NAT2_R127G and (MOUSE)NAT2_R127L [24-26] (Table 2). The lowest IC_{50} values for naphthoquinone **1** were exhibited by (HUMAN)NAT1*4 and (MOUSE)NAT2*1 enzymes, both of which possess the triad F125, R127 and Y129. Naphthoquinone **1** was at least an order of magnitude

Table 1 Arylamine activity profiles of native and engineered NATs in relation to substrate physicochemical properties

			NAT enzymes: % specific activity values							
			(HUMAN) NAT1*4	(MOUSE) NAT2*1	(MESAU) NAT2*1	(MOUSE) NAT2 F125S	(MOUSE) NAT2 R127G	(MOUSE) NAT2 R127L	(MOUSE) NAT1*1	(HUMAN) NAT2*4
		F125		-	-	S	-	-	Y	S
	NAT substrates	R127		-	-	-	G	L	G	S
		Y129		-	L	-	-	-	-	S
Negatively charged arylamines at pH 8.0	Folate catabolites	4AB glu	20 ± 1	87 ± 1	57 ± 3	19 ± 1	9 ± 1	8 ± 1	8 ± 7	3 ± 1
		4ABA	**100 ± 2**	**100 ± 2**	**100 ± 6**	70 ± 2	8 ± 1	8 ± 1	48 ± 6	6 ± 1
	Salicylic acids	4AS	67 ± 2	55 ± 1	74 ± 3	75 ± 3	27 ± 1	13 ± 1	88 ± 6	7 ± 1
		5AS	64 ± 3	37 ± 1	30 ± 1	74 ± 1	94 ± 1	65 ± 9	76 ± 6	64 ± 2
Neutral electron-rich arylamines at pH 8.0	Halogenated anilines	4CA	36 ± 2	46 ± 4	61 ± 2	56 ± 2	54 ± 3	70 ± 1	18 ± 3	71 ± 3
		4BA	50 ± 1	52 ± 2	72 ± 1	47 ± 2	70 ± 1	81 ± 11	28 ± 6	72 ± 1
		4IA	63 ± 1	72 ± 3	81 ± 1	69 ± 2	**97 ± 1**	74 ± 8	28 ± 3	65 ± 2
	Alkyl- and aryl-oxyanilines	ANS	56 ± 2	88 ± 6	89 ± 1	**100 ± 3**	**97 ± 4**	77 ± 10	48 ± 1	9 ± 2
		4AV	25 ± 2	90 ± 1	32 ± 1	90 ± 1	66 ± 3	**100 ± 10**	28 ± 6	57 ± 3
		HOA	12 ± 4	23 ± 2	35 ± 1	47 ± 1	59 ± 3	80 ± 8	3 ± 4	51 ± 2
		POA	17 ± 7	20 ± 2	22 ± 1	62 ± 2	67 ± 1	61 ± 2	6 ± 1	62 ± 11
	Other aniline	SMZ	1 ± 1	4 ± 1	1 ± 1	1 ± 1	19 ± 2	3 ± 1	88 ± 6	46 ± 1
Arylhydrazines		INH	0 ± 2	2 ± 2	1 ± 1	38 ± 2	63 ± 10	76 ± 14	**100 ± 6**	62 ± 2
		HDZ	2 ± 1	8 ± 2	3 ± 1	19 ± 1	**100 ± 2**	**95 ± 1**	68 ± 6	**100 ± 1**

Percentage specific activity values of native and engineered mammalian NAT proteins are shown. A value of 100% is attributed to the substrate towards which the isoform in question has the highest specific activity. All results shown are the mean of 3 measurements ± standard deviation. Percentages ≥90% for each isoenzyme were compared by ANOVA using a Student's t-test and statistically similar values are emboldened. Isoforms are ordered according to increasing number of residue differences within the active site in relation to (HUMAN)NAT1*4. Residues identical to those in (HUMAN)NAT1*4 are labelled with a hyphen; residues different from the corresponding residue of (HUMAN)NAT1*4 are specified. Substrates are ordered according to the number of negative charges at pH 8.0, then to electron-richness and increasing size of aromatic substituents. The chemical structures and physicochemical properties of the chemicals used as substrates for NAT in this study are shown in Additional file 3: Table S1.

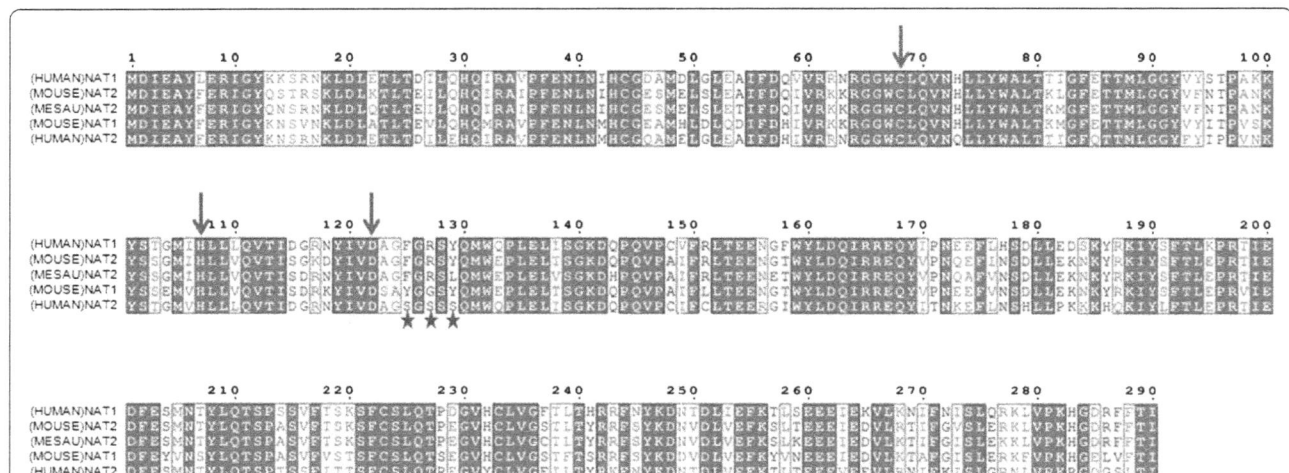

Figure 3 Sequence alignment of five mammalian NAT proteins. The primary sequences of human, mouse and Syrian hamster NAT proteins are aligned. Similar amino acids are highlighted by dark grey lettering in pale grey boxes; completely conserved residues are indicated by white lettering on a dark grey background. The residues of the catalytic triad are indicated by a blue arrow. Each residue putatively involved in substrate selectivity is indicated by a star. Alignments were generated using Clustal W [42] and the figure was prepared using ESPript 2.2 [43].

Table 2 Effects of naphthoquinone 1 on the activity of mammalian NATs and their colorimetric detection

Enzyme		(HUMAN) NAT1*4	(MOUSE) NAT2*1	(MESAU) NAT2*1	(MOUSE) NAT2_F125S	(MOUSE) NAT2_R127G	(MOUSE) NAT2_R127L	(MOUSE) NAT1*1	(HUMAN) NAT2*4
Primary sequence identity *versus* (HUMAN)NAT1*4		100	82	81	82	82	82	74	71
Active site residues	125	F	F	F	**S**	F	F	**Y**	**S**
	127	R	R	R	R	**G**	**L**	**G**	**S**
	129	Y	Y	**L**	Y	Y	Y	Y	**S**
IC_{50} with naphthoquinone 1 (μM)		5.3[a]	1.3[a,b]	89.0[c]	68.7	51.7[a]	102.5[a]	129.7	>100
λ_{max} of naphthoquinone 1 (nm)		585[a,b]	625[a,b]	525[c]	498	498[a]	498[a]	498[b]	498[a]

IC_{50} values were calculated using decreasing concentrations of naphthoquinone 1. NAT activity was measured following the hydrolysis rate of AcCoA (400 μM) in the presence of 4ABA for (HUMAN)NAT1*4, (MOUSE)NAT2*1 and (MESAU)NAT2*1; 5AS for (MOUSE)NAT2 mutants and (MOUSE)NAT1*1; and 2-aminofluorene for (HUMAN)NAT2*4. [a]adapted from [25] [b]adapted from [24] [c]adapted from [26]. Residues which are different from the corresponding residues in (HUMAN)NAT1*4 are labeled in bold.

more potent against (HUMAN)NAT1*4 and (MOUSE) NAT2*1 (IC_{50} values of 5.3 and 1.3 μM, respectively) than the other NATs used in this study. When pure recombinant (MOUSE)NAT2_F125S was incubated with naphthoquinone 1 under the conditions reported previously, it did not shift the λ_{max} of naphthoquinone 1 towards longer wavelengths (585–625 nm), in contrast to previous observations with (HUMAN)NAT1*4 and (MOUSE)NAT2*1 (Additional file 4: Figure S3, Table 2).

In silico analysis of substrate selectivity in mammalian NATs

The structural features underlying substrate selectivity were investigated by *in silico* analysis of interactions between the NAT proteins and their arylamine substrates.

Structural models of (MOUSE)NAT2*1 and (MESAU) NAT2*1 were generated using the crystal structure of (HUMAN)NAT1*4 [PDB:2PQT] [9] because these three isoforms have >80% amino acid identity (Additional file 5: Table S2). Swiss-Model simulations generated models of (MOUSE)NAT2*1 and (MESAU)NAT2*1 which were of high quality according to their scoring functions and background noise, thus confirming the reliability of the template used. The mutations (MOUSE)NAT2_F125S, (MOUSE)NAT2_R127G and (MOUSE)NAT2_R127L did not abolish the catalytic reactivity compared with the reference enzyme, so each individual residue modification was considered unlikely to have altered overall protein folding. The same modelling procedure was therefore used to create structural models of (MOUSE)NAT2_F125S, (MOUSE)NAT2_R127G and (MOUSE)NAT2_R127L. However, attempts to model (MOUSE)NAT1*1 (64% identity; Additional file 5: Table S2) based on the structure of (HUMAN)NAT2*4 [PDB:2PFR] [9] did not yield reliable results.

Substrates were docked into the catalytic site of each enzyme as shown in the selectivity profile summarised in Table 1. 4ABglu was docked in the active sites of (HUMAN)NAT1*4, (MOUSE)NAT2*1, (MESAU)NAT2*1

and (MOUSE)NAT2_F125S (Figure 4). The affinity energies of all these simulations were low (−8.0/−7.0 kcal. mol^{-1}) and probable polar and hydrophobic interactions were revealed within the enzyme-substrate complexes. For example, the amide functionality of 4ABglu could point towards the guanidinium of R127 *via* hydrogen bonds (<3.2 Å); the Cγ carboxylic group of glutamate could form a hydrogen bridge with the hydroxyl tail of Y129 (<3.1 Å) in (HUMAN)NAT1*4, (MOUSE)NAT2*1 and (MOUSE)NAT2_F125S; and/or the aromatic substrate core could interact *via* π-π stacking (<3.8 Å) with the hydrophobic plane defined by the isopropyl moiety of valine 93 (V93) and the phenyl ring of F125 in all the reference enzymes. The results obtained with 4ABA support the postulated interactions inferred from 4ABglu, suggesting a polar interaction between the carboxylate of 4ABA and the guanidinium of R127 at pH 8.0 (~3.6 Å) and hydrophobic stacking of the aromatic portion of 4ABA on the apolar flat surface defined by the side chains of V93 and F125 (~4 Å) (Additional file 6: Figure S4).

We also attempted to model the selective hydrazine substrates INH and HDZ within the active site of (HUMAN)NAT2*4 and the (MOUSE)NAT2 mutants. No proximity between the hydrazine functionality and C68 thiolate compatible with the NAT catalytic mechanism [44] was observed, possibly because of the smaller steric size of the substrate docked. However, when a bulkier selective arylamine substrate such as POA was docked into (HUMAN)NAT2*4 and the three (MOUSE) NAT2 mutants, the results indicated proximity between the primary amine of the substrate and the key active site residues C68 and H106 (<4 Å) (Figure 5). These simulations indicated that the 4-aminoarene of POA could be sandwiched between the benzyl ring of F217 and the apolar side chain of F93 in (HUMAN)NAT2*4 and F125 in (MOUSE)NAT2_R127G and (MOUSE)NAT2_ R127L *via* hydrophobic interactions. In the (MOUSE) NAT2 mutants, the phenoxy group of POA was predicted to make further π-stacking interactions with the side

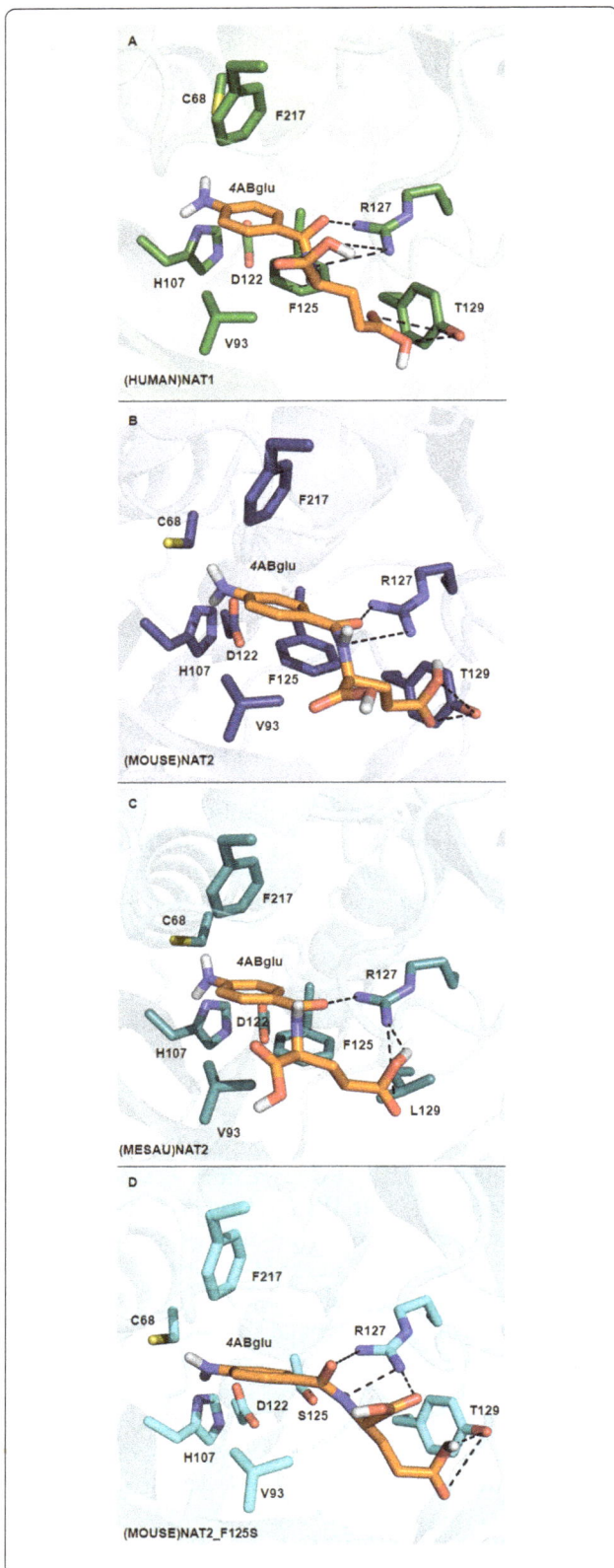

Figure 4 Substrate binding pockets of (HUMAN)NAT1*4, (MOUSE)NAT2*1, (MESAU)NAT2*1 and (MOUSE)NAT2_F125S with 4ABglu docked. Maximised view of the active sites of (**A**): (HUMAN)NAT1*4; (**B**): (MOUSE)NAT2*1; (**C**): (MESAU)NAT2*1; (**D**): (MOUSE)NAT2_F125S with the arylamine substrate 4ABglu docked. The overall structure of each NAT enzyme is drawn as a ribbon diagram: (HUMAN)NAT1*4 is coloured in green [PDB:2PQT] [9] (MOUSE)NAT2*1 model in dark blue, (MESAU)NAT2*1 model in cyan and (MOUSE)NAT2_F125S model in pale blue. The side chains of the key residues involved in substrate binding within the active site are drawn in stick representation and labelled with carbon atoms in the corresponding colour of the enzyme, nitrogen in blue, oxygen in red and sulphur in yellow. The arylamine substrate 4ABglu is labelled with carbon atoms in orange, nitrogen in blue, oxygen in red and polar hydrogen in gray. The figures were generated using PyMOL [41].

chain of Y129 (~3.9 Å), whereas the equivalent residue in (HUMAN)NAT2*4, S129, is incapable of this interaction.

Discussion

The present study has extended our understanding of (MOUSE)NAT1 by demonstrating that it is functionally different from (HUMAN)NAT2. In addition to its known activity in N-acetylating the hydrazine INH and the arylamine SMZ [29,30], (MOUSE)NAT1*1 was shown to have significant activity towards the hydrazine HDZ and two arylamine substrates which were previously considered to be (HUMAN)NAT1 and (MOUSE)NAT2-specific (4ABA and 4AS).

The substrate-binding interactions involved in N-acetylation were previously characterised using nuclear magnetic resonance [33,45], demonstrating that an arylamine or hydrazine could bind to a non-acetylated NAT active site. In the present study, arylamine substrates were docked within the catalytic pockets of different non-acetylated NATs in silico in order to identify possible selective interactions underlying the formation of the enzyme-substrate complex.

In (HUMAN)NAT1*4, the positively charged guanidinium (at pH 8.0) of R127 plays an essential role in recognising the negatively charged carboxylate of 4ABA, as illustrated by modelling 4ABA (Additional file 6: Figure S4) or 4AS [9] within the active site. The significant N-acetylation activity of (MOUSE)NAT1*1 towards 4ABA, 4AS and ANS in the present study was difficult to reconcile with the presence of an apolar G127 instead of an R127. However, it is possible that the presence of a sterically smaller residue (G) at this position in (MOUSE)NAT1*1 permits bulky or highly polar substrates to enter and allows their charged para-substituents to interact with other polar side chains in the active site (e.g. Y125 and Y129). Similarly, essential π-π stacking interactions observed between the aromatic core of 4ABA and F125, as seen in (HUMAN)NAT1*4, may be permitted by the side chain arene of Y125 within the

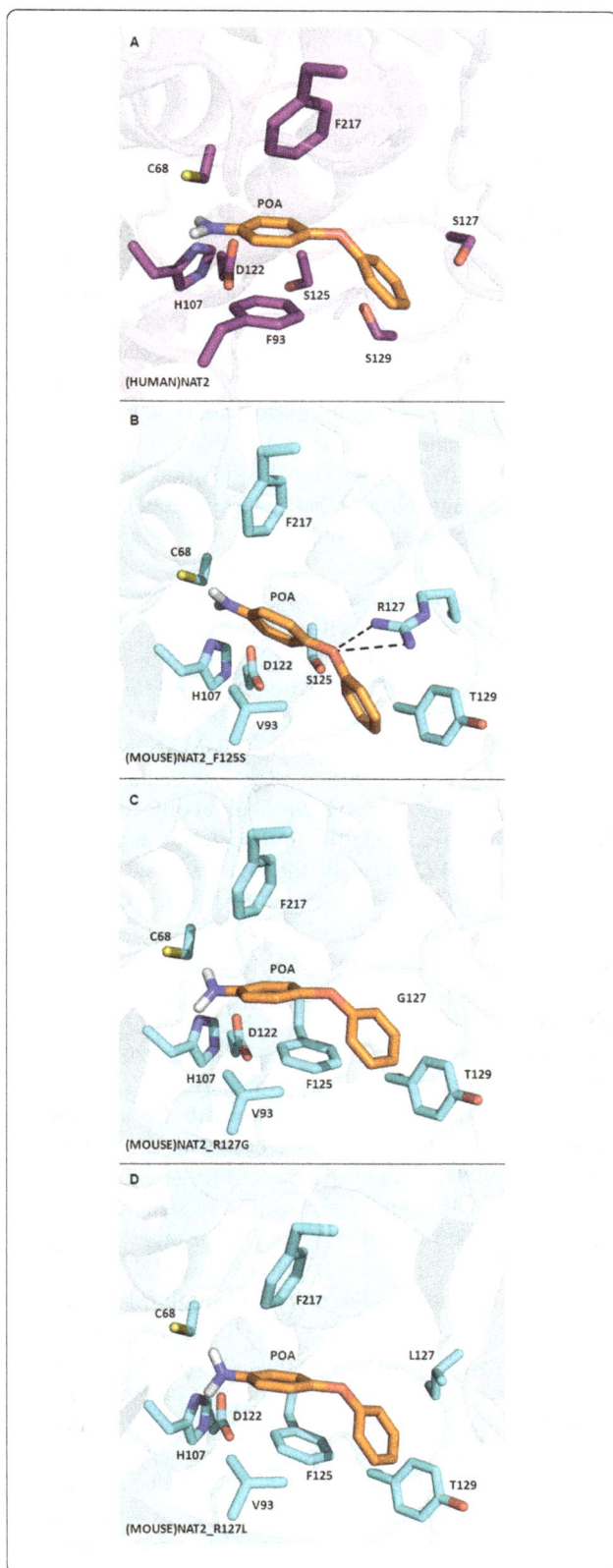

Figure 5 Substrate binding pockets of (HUMAN)NAT2*4, (MOUSE)NAT2_F125S, (MOUSE)NAT2_R127G and (MOUSE) NAT2_R127L with POA docked. Maximised view of the active sites of **(A)**: (HUMAN)NAT2*4; **(B)**: (MOUSE)NAT2_F125S; **(C)**: (MOUSE) NAT2_R127G; **(D)**: (MOUSE)NAT2_R127L with the arylamine substrate POA docked. The overall structure of each NAT enzyme is drawn as a ribbon diagram: (HUMAN)NAT2*4 is coloured in mauve [PDB:2PFR] [9] and (MOUSE)NAT2 mutants in light blue. The side chains of the key residues involved in substrate binding within the active site are drawn in stick representation and labelled with carbon atoms in the corresponding colour of the enzyme, nitrogen in blue, oxygen in red and sulphur in yellow. The arylamine substrate POA is labelled with carbon atoms in orange, nitrogen in blue, oxygen in red and polar hydrogen in gray. The figures were generated using PyMOL [41].

active site of (MOUSE)NAT1*1. The lack of a structural model suitable for docking studies and the restricted commonality of substrate selectivity between (MOUSE) NAT1*1 and either of the two human NATs precluded the construction of a structural model for (MOUSE) NAT1*1, so this hypothesis could not be tested.

When 4ABglu was docked into the structure of (HUMAN)NAT1*4 and models of (MOUSE)NAT2*1 and (MESAU)NAT2*1, the essential role of R127 in forming ionic interactions with the electron-negative *para*-substituent of the substrate was evident; this may explain why a bulky charged arylamine such as 4ABglu can enter a small, very hydrophobic microenvironment such as the active site crevice of (HUMAN)NAT1*4 [9]. The preference of (HUMAN)NAT1*4 and its homologues (MOUSE) NAT2*1 and (MESAU)NAT2*1 for arylamine substrates with a negatively charged *para*-substituent (e.g. 4ABA and 4AS) may therefore be due to the positively charged guanidinium moiety of R127.

Previous studies have shown that mutation of F125 to S125 modifies the catalytic preference of (HUMAN) NAT1*4 from the conventional probe substrate 4AS to SMZ [27]. When we examined the effect of the equivalent mutation on (MOUSE)NAT2, no such shift in substrate preference was observed; neither did the general substrate preferences of (MOUSE)NAT2 change to resemble those of (MOUSE)NAT1*1. The higher reactivity of (MOUSE)NAT2_F125S with conformationally flexible hydrazines than with planar arylamines could be associated with increased active site space in (MOUSE) NAT2*1 after the substitution of the bulky benzyl group of F with the less hindering hydroxymethyl of S.

Site-directed mutagenesis of R127 to G127 or L127 within (MOUSE)NAT2 markedly altered the enzyme's substrate selectivity. Overall, the non-polar side chains of G and L appeared to have similar effects in terms of modifying the substrate preferences of (MOUSE)NAT2: the metabolism of 4ABglu and 4ABA was dramatically decreased whereas *N*-acetylation of the hydrazines INH and HDZ, which are commonly used as probe substrates for (MOUSE)NAT1 and (HUMAN)NAT2, was augmented. R127 seemed to play a crucial role in discriminating between arylamines with highly hydrophilic substituents and hydrazines with less polar aromatic functional groups. Moreover, the (MOUSE)NAT2_R127G mutation improved the overall catalytic activity of the enzyme, possibly due to the larger size of the active site cavity generated after substitution. Similarly, when the arylamine POA was docked into the active sites of (MOUSE)NAT2_F125S, (MOUSE)NAT2_R127G and (MOUSE)NAT2_R127L, the results suggested that accommodation of this substrate *via* stacking interactions is facilitated by the larger cavity created by these single substitutions. When POA was docked into the active pocket of (HUMAN)NAT2*4, the results of substrate fitting were very similar to previous modelling results obtained with SMZ [9], consistent with the preference of (HUMAN)NAT2*4 for apolar and flexible substrates [11].

The individual (MOUSE)NAT2 mutants tested did not affect the specificity of (MOUSE)NAT2 for SMZ, which is a very poor substrate for this isoform. This may be related to the need for a larger active site to accommodate SMZ, which is a bulky arylamine; a single amino acid change may not be sufficient to permit access to the active site. Further 3D structural data and thermal stability studies on the mutants would help to ascertain the extent of the folding perturbations produced by each mutation. However, it is also intriguing that small hydrazines such as INH and phenylhydrazine are poor substrates for (HUMAN)NAT1 and its rodent homologues [8,22], whereas arylamines of similar steric size such as 4ABA, 4AS and ANS are good substrates.

While the amine nitrogen and the aromatic carbons of an arylamine substrate are on the same plane, crystallographic studies of INH, HDZ and phenylhydrazine as single molecules [46-50] and protein co-crystallised ligands [51,52], showed that the hydrazine bond could also be off the plane defined by the remaining aryl and acyl carbon atoms, thereby giving the hydrazine substrate a non-planar conformation. Our docking simulations using the crystal structure of (HUMAN)NAT1*4 and the model of (MOUSE)NAT2*1 show that the bulky side chain of R127, the benzyl ring of F125 and the 4-hydroxybenzyl of Y129 create a characteristic constrained microenvironment which appears to allow preferable accommodation of planar arylamines rather than conformationally flexible hydrazines in the active site of (HUMAN)NAT1*4. This is consistent with the volumes of the active sites in human NAT structures: the (HUMAN)NAT1*4 cavity has a volume of 162 Å^3, whereas (HUMAN)NAT2*4 (with S at positions 125, 127 and 129) has a larger active pocket (257 Å^3). In this context it is also noteworthy that the crystal structures of prokaryotic NATs from *Mycobacterium tuberculosis*, *M. marinum* and *M. smegmatis*,

which preferentially *N*-acetylate conformationally flexible hydrazine substrates, have much larger active sites (>200 Å^3) than (HUMAN)NAT1*4 [53-55].

Recent studies have suggested that F125, R127 and Y129 in the active sites of (HUMAN)NAT1*4 and (MOUSE)NAT2*1 are essential for selective recognition and binding of the potent inhibitor naphthoquinone **1** [24-26]. In particular, ionic recognition between the conjugate base of naphthoquinone **1** and the guanidinium moiety of R127 is known to be essential for inhibitor binding. The results shown here confirm that these key residues are required for the interaction with naphthoquinone **1**, since the absence of any of them results in a protein which is resistant to inhibition and colour shifting in response to naphthoquinone **1** (Table 2).

Overall, our results suggest that the substrate selectivity of the mammalian NATs investigated in this study is influenced by two major factors; firstly, the planarity of the acceptor arylamine and the polarity of its *para* substituent (which appear to affect both the type of the intermolecular interactions within the enzyme and the pK_{aH} strength and nucleophilicity of the acceptor amine); and secondly, the size of the catalytic cavity and its overall polarity, as determined by the residues at positions 125, 127 and 129. In particular, F125 in (HUMAN)NAT1*4 and (MOUSE)NAT2*1 appears to play a key role in discriminating between planar arylamines and conformationally flexible hydrazines, while the ionised (at physiological pH) side chain of R127 perturbs the characteristic hydrophobicity of the NAT active site and, in cooperation with the 4-hydroxybenzyl side chain of Y129, contributes to the narrowness of the (HUMAN)NAT1*4 active site.

Conclusions

In conclusion, this evaluation of the substrate profiles of various native and engineered mammalian NATs in the context of their structures has highlighted the features which influence NAT substrate selectivity in mammals. The virtual models of mammalian NATs generated in this study, used in conjunction with X-ray structures of human NATs, constitute a rich resource for investigating the roles of particular residues within the NAT active site in relation to both NAT activity and inhibitor selectivity. Three non-catalytic residues within (HUMAN)NAT1*4 (F125, R127 and Y129) contribute both to substrate recognition and inhibitor binding by participating in distinctive intermolecular interactions and maintaining the steric conformation of the catalytic pocket. These active site residues contribute to the definition of substrate and inhibitor selectivity, an understanding of which is essential for facilitating the design of second generation (HUMAN)NAT1-selective inhibitors for diagnostic, prognostic and therapeutic purposes. In particular, since the expression of (HUMAN)NAT1 is related to the development and progression of oestrogen-receptor-positive breast cancer, these structure-based tools will facilitate the ongoing design of candidate compounds for use in (HUMAN)NAT1-positive breast tumours.

Chemical compounds studied in this article

Aminobenzoyl glutamate (PubChem CID: 5103842), 4-aminobenzoic acid (PubChem CID: 978), 4-aminosalicylate (PubChem CID: 4649), 5-aminosalicylate (PubChem CID: 4075), 4-chloroaniline (PubChem CID: 7812), 4-methoxyaniline (PubChem CID: 7732), 4-phenoxyaniline (PubChem CID: 8764), hydralazine (PubChem CID: 3637), isoniazid (PubChem CID: 3767), sulfamethazine (PubChem CID: 5327).

Additional files

Additional file 1: Figure S1. Selective functionality of (HUMAN)NAT1*4 and (MOUSE)NAT2*1. Two catalytic reactions are selective to (HUMAN) NAT1*4 and (MOUSE)NAT2*1 amongst mammalian NATs: the N-acetylation of the folate catabolite 4ABglu and the folate-dependent hydrolysis of AcCoA. Both reactions are selectively inhibited by naphthoquinone **1** (shown in red).

Additional file 2: Figure S2. Multiple sequence alignment of *(MOUSE) Nat2*1* gene and *(MOUSE)Nat2_F125S* gene. Alignment of *(MOUSE)Nat2*1* sequence and the forward and reverse sequences obtained after mutagenesis was conducted by ClustalW [42]. The single mutated nucleotide is highlighted in red. *indicates nucleotide identity among all three genetic sequences. No additional mutations were generated during the process of site directed mutagenesis.

Additional file 3: Table S1. Chemical NAT substrates used in this study. Ionic charges of substrates at assay pH 8.0 are shown according to their $pK_{a(H)}$ values [56-61].

Additional file 4: Figure S3. Visible spectra of naphthoquinone **1** in the presence of different mammalian NAT variants. Naphthoquinone **1** (15 μM) was incubated with 20 mM Tris–HCl, pH 8.0, 5% DMSO (v/v) (red line) or NAT variants (30 μM): (MOUSE)NAT2*1 (blue line); (MOUSE)NAT2_F125S (yellow line)). Wavelength scans from 800 to 350 nm were recorded against the appropriate blank (20 mM Tris–HCl, pH 8.0, 5% DMSO (v/v)).

Additional file 5: Table S2. Comparison of eukaryotic NAT sequence identity and similarity. Percentage identity (no shade) and similarity (grey shade) values were calculated amongst five mammalian NATs using BLAST2 sequences.

Additional file 6: Figure S4. Substrate binding pockets of (HUMAN) NAT1*4 with 4ABA docked. Maximised view of the active sites of (HUMAN)NAT1*4 with the arylamine substrate 4ABA docked. The overall structure of (HUMAN)NAT1*4 is drawn in ribbon diagram (green) [PDB:2PQT]. The side chain of the key residues involved in substrate binding within the active site are drawn in stick representation and labelled with carbon atoms in the colour of the enzyme, nitrogen in blue, oxygen in red and sulphur in yellow. The arylamine substrate 4ABA is labelled with carbon atoms in orange, nitrogen in blue, oxygen in red and polar hydrogen in gray. The figures were generated using PyMOL [41].

Abbreviations

4ABA: 4-aminobenzoic acid; 4ABglu: 4-aminobenzoylglutamate; 4AS: 4-aminosalicylate; 5AS: 5-aminosalicylate; 4AV: 4-aminoveratrole; 4BA: 4-bromoaniline; 4CA: 4-chloroaniline; 4IA: 4-iodoaniline; ANS: 4-methoxyaniline; AcCoA: Acetyl coenzyme A; DMSO: Dimethyl sulphoxide; HOA: 4-hexyloxyaniline; HDZ: Hydralazine; INH: Isoniazid; NAT: Arylamine N-acetyltransferase; POA: 4-phenoxyaniline; SMZ: Sulfamethazine.

Competing interests
The authors declare that they have no competing interests.

Authors' contributions
The authors contributed to this manuscript as follows: NL, AK, IMW and ES conceived and designed the experiments; NL, AK, IMW, AV and EM performed the experiments; NL, AK, IMW, AM, EM, AJR, LAS and ES analyzed the data; AJR and ES contributed reagents, materials and/or analysis tools; and NL, LAS and ES wrote the manuscript. All authors read and approved the final manuscript.

Acknowledgements
Financial support for this work was provided by Servier. NL held a Cancer Research UK Cancer Medicinal Chemistry Studentship and AJR was the recipient of a Research Councils UK fellowship. The authors thank Dr. Ali Ryan and Hilary Long for technical support and helpful discussions.

Author details
[1]Department of Pharmacology, University of Oxford, Oxford, UK. [2]Department of Chemistry, Chemistry Research Laboratory, University of Oxford, Oxford, UK. [3]Current address: Divisions of Structural Biology and Cancer Therapeutics, The Institute of Cancer Research, Chester Beatty Laboratories, London, UK. [4]Consultant in Investigative Toxicology, Linlithgow, West Lothian, Scotland. [5]Faculty of Science, Engineering and Computing, Kingston University, Kingston on Thames, UK.

References
1. Weber WW, Hein DW: N-acetylation pharmacogenetics. *Pharmacol Rev* 1985, **37**:25–79.
2. Sim E, Abuhammad A, Ryan A: Arylamine N-acetyltransferases: from drug metabolism and pharmacogenetics to drug discovery. *Br J Pharmacol* 2014, **171**:2705–2725.
3. Blum M, Grant DM, McBride W, Heim M, Meyer UA: Human arylamine N-acetyltransferase genes: isolation, chromosomal localization, and functional expression. *DNA Cell Biol* 1990, **9**:193–203.
4. Hickman D, Risch A, Buckle V, Spurr NK, Jeremiah SJ, McCarthy A, Sim E: Chromosomal localization of human genes for arylamine N-acetyltransferase. *Biochem J* 1994, **297**(Pt 3):441–445.
5. Hein DW: N-acetyltransferase SNPs: emerging concepts serve as a paradigm for understanding complexities of personalized medicine. *Expert Opin Drug Metab Toxicol* 2009, **5**:353–366.
6. Hein DW, Doll MA, Fretland AJ, Leff MA, Webb SJ, Xiao GH, Devanaboyina US, Nangju NA, Feng Y: Molecular genetics and epidemiology of the NAT1 and NAT2 acetylation polymorphisms. *Cancer Epidemiol Biomarkers Prev* 2000, **9**:29–42.
7. Ohsako S, Deguchi T: Cloning and expression of cDNAs for polymorphic and monomorphic arylamine N-acetyltransferases from human liver. *J Biol Chem* 1990, **265**:4630–4634.
8. Kawamura A, Graham J, Mushtaq A, Tsiftsoglou SA, Vath GM, Hanna PE, Wagner CR, Sim E: Eukaryotic arylamine N-acetyltransferase: investigation of substrate specificity by high-throughput screening. *Biochem Pharmacol* 2005, **69**:347–359.
9. Wu H, Dombrovsky L, Tempel W, Martin F, Loppnau P, Goodfellow GH, Grant DM, Plotnikov AN: Structural basis of substrate-binding specificity of human arylamine N-acetyltransferases. *J Biol Chem* 2007, **282**:30189–30197.
10. Sim E, Lack N, Wang CJ, Long H, Westwood I, Fullam E, Kawamura A: Arylamine N-acetyltransferases: structural and functional implications of polymorphisms. *Toxicology* 2008, **254**:170–183.
11. Zhou X, Ma Z, Dong D, Wu B: Arylamine N-acetyltransferases: a structural perspective. *Br J Pharmacol* 2013, **169**:748–760.
12. Butcher NJ, Arulpragasam A, Pope C, Minchin RF: Identification of a minimal promoter sequence for the human N-acetyltransferase type I gene that binds AP-1 (activator protein 1) and YY-1 (Yin and Yang 1). *Biochem J* 2003, **376**:441–448.
13. Minchin RF, Hanna PE, Dupret JM, Wagner CR, Rodrigues-Lima F, Butcher NJ: Arylamine N-acetyltransferase I. *Int J Biochem Cell Biol* 2007, **39**:1999–2005.

14. Sim E, Walters K, Boukouvala S: **Arylamine *N*-acetyltransferases: from structure to function.** *Drug Metab Rev* 2008, 40:479–510.

15. Boukouvala S, Fakis G: **Arylamine *N*-acetyltransferases: what we learn from genes and genomes.** *Drug Metab Rev* 2005, 37:511–564.

16. Minchin RF: **Acetylation of *p*-aminobenzoylglutamate, a folic acid catabolite, by recombinant human arylamine *N*-acetyltransferase and U937 cells.** *Biochem J* 1995, 307(Pt 1):1–3.

17. Ward A, Summers MJ, Sim E: **Purification of recombinant human *N*-acetyltransferase type 1 (NAT1) expressed in *E. coli* and characterization of its potential role in folate metabolism.** *Biochem Pharmacol* 1995, 49:1759–1767.

18. Laurieri N, Dairou J, Egleton JE, Stanley LA, Russell AJ, Dupret JM, Sim E, Rodrigues-Lima F: **From arylamine *N*-Acetyltransferase to folate-dependent acetyl CoA hydrolase: impact of folic acid on the activity of (HUMAN)NAT1 and its homologue (MOUSE)NAT2.** *PLoS One* 2014, 9:e96370.

19. Sugamori KS, Brenneman D, Wong S, Gaedigk A, Yu V, Abramovici H, Rozmahel R, Grant DM: **Effect of arylamine acetyltransferase *Nat3* gene knockout on *N*-acetylation in the mouse.** *Drug Metab Dispos* 2007, 35:1064–1070.

20. Boukouvala S, Price N, Sim E: **Identification and functional characterization of novel polymorphisms associated with the genes for arylamine *N*-acetyltransferases in mice.** *Pharmacogenetics* 2002, 12:385–394.

21. Fretland AJ, Doll MA, Gray K, Feng Y, Hein DW: **Cloning, sequencing, and recombinant expression of NAT1, NAT2, and NAT3 derived from the C3H/HeJ (rapid) and A/HeJ (slow) acetylator inbred mouse: functional characterization of the activation and deactivation of aromatic amine carcinogens.** *Toxicol Appl Pharmacol* 1997, 142:360–366.

22. Kawamura A, Westwood I, Wakefield L, Long H, Zhang N, Walters K, Redfield C, Sim E: **Mouse *N*-acetyltransferase type 2, the homologue of human *N*-acetyltransferase type 1.** *Biochem Pharmacol* 2008, 75:1550–1560.

23. Stanley LA, Mills IG, Sim E: **Localization of polymorphic *N*-acetyltransferase (NAT2) in tissues of inbred mice.** *Pharmacogenetics* 1997, 7(2):121–130.

24. Laurieri N, Crawford MH, Kawamura A, Westwood IM, Robinson J, Fletcher AM, Davies SG, Sim E, Russell AJ: **Small molecule colorimetric probes for specific detection of human arylamine *N*-acetyltransferase 1, a potential breast cancer biomarker.** *J Am Chem Soc* 2010, 132:3238–3239.

25. Laurieri N, Egleton JE, Varney A, Thinnes CC, Quevedo CE, Seden PT, Thompson S, Rodrigues-Lima F, Dairou J, Dupret JM, Russell AJ, Sim E: **A novel color change mechanism for breast cancer biomarker detection: naphthoquinones as specific ligands of human arylamine *N*-acetyltransferase 1.** *PLoS One* 2013, 8:e70600.

26. Egleton JE, Thinnes CC, Seden PT, Laurieri N, Lee SP, Hadavizadeh KS, Measures AR, Jones AM, Thompson S, Varney A, Wynne GM, Ryan A, Sim E, Russell AJ: **Structure–activity relationships and colorimetric properties of specific probes for the putative cancer biomarker human arylamine *N*-acetyltransferase 1.** *Bioorg Med Chem* 2014, 22:3030–3054.

27. Goodfellow GH, Dupret JM, Grant DM: **Identification of amino acids imparting acceptor substrate selectivity to human arylamine acetyltransferases NAT1 and NAT2.** *Biochem J* 2000, 348(Pt 1):159–166.

28. Dupret JM, Goodfellow GH, Janezic SA, Grant DM: **Structure-function studies of human arylamine *N*-acetyltransferases NAT1 and NAT2. Functional analysis of recombinant NAT1/NAT2 chimeras expressed in *Escherichia coli*.** *J Biol Chem* 1994, 269:26830–26835.

29. Estrada-Rodgers L, Levy GN, Weber WW: **Substrate selectivity of mouse *N*-acetyltransferases 1, 2, and 3 expressed in COS-1 cells.** *Drug Metab Dispos* 1998, 26:502–505.

30. Martell KJ, Levy GN, Weber WW: **Cloned mouse *N*-acetyltransferases: enzymatic properties of expressed *Nat-1* and *Nat-2* gene products.** *Mol Pharmacol* 1992, 42:265–272.

31. Sugamori KS, Wong S, Gaedigk A, Yu V, Abramovici H, Rozmahel R, Grant DM: **Generation and functional characterization of arylamine *N*-acetyltransferase *Nat1/Nat2* double-knockout mice.** *Mol Pharmacol* 2003, 64:170–179.

32. Kelly SL, Sim E: **Arylamine *N*-acetyltransferase in Balb/c mice: identification of a novel mouse isoenzyme by cloning and expression *in vitro*.** *Biochem J* 1994, 302(Pt 2):347–353.

33. Zhang N, Liu L, Liu F, Wagner CR, Hanna PE, Walters KJ: **NMR-based model reveals the structural determinants of mammalian arylamine *N*-acetyltransferase substrate specificity.** *J Mol Biol* 2006, 363:188–200.

34. Butcher NJ, Minchin RF: **Arylamine *N*-acetyltransferase 1: a novel drug target in cancer development.** *Pharmacol Rev* 2012, 64:147–165.

35. Andres HH, Klem AJ, Szabo SM, Weber WW: **New spectrophotometric and radiochemical assays for acetyl-CoA: arylamine *N*-acetyltransferase applicable to a variety of arylamines.** *Anal Biochem* 1985, 145:367–375.

36. Brooke EW, Davies SG, Mulvaney AW, Pompeo F, Sim E, Vickers RJ: **An approach to identifying novel substrates of bacterial arylamine *N*-acetyltransferases.** *Bioorg Med Chem* 2003, 11:1227–1234.

37. Arnold K, Bordoli L, Kopp J, Schwede T: **The SWISS-MODEL workspace: a web-based environment for protein structure homology modelling.** *Bioinformatics* 2006, 22:195–201.

38. Kiefer F, Arnold K, Kunzli M, Bordoli L, Schwede T: **The SWISS-MODEL repository and associated resources.** *Nucleic Acids Res* 2009, 37:D387–D392.

39. Peitsch MC: **Protein modeling by E-Mail.** *Bio-Technol* 1995, 13:658–660.

40. Trott O, Olson AJ: **AutoDock Vina: improving the speed and accuracy of docking with a new scoring function, efficient optimization, and multithreading.** *J Comput Chem* 2010, 31:455–461.

41. DeLano WL: **PyMOL: An open-source molecular graphics tool.** In *DeLano Scientific, San Carlos, California, USA*; 2002. http://www.ccp4.ac.uk/newsletters/newsletter40/11_pymol.pdf.

42. Thompson JD, Higgins DG, Gibson TJ: **CLUSTAL W: improving the sensitivity of progressive multiple sequence alignment through sequence weighting, position-specific gap penalties and weight matrix choice.** *Nucleic Acids Res* 1994, 22:4673–4680.

43. Gouet P, Courcelle E, Stuart DI, Metoz F: **ESPript: analysis of multiple sequence alignments in PostScript.** *Bioinformatics* 1999, 15:305–308.

44. Westwood IM, Kawamura A, Fullam E, Russell AJ, Davies SG, Sim E: **Structure and mechanism of arylamine *N*-acetyltransferases.** *Curr Top Med Chem* 2006, 6:1641–1654.

45. Delgoda R, Lian LY, Sandy J, Sim E: **NMR investigation of the catalytic mechanism of arylamine *N*-acetyltransferase from *Salmonella typhimurium*.** *Biochim Biophys Acta* 2003, 1620:8–14.

46. Abboud KA, Smith DW Jnr, Wagener KB: **Structure of cyclo-1,1',4,4'-bis (1,1,3,3-tetramethyl-1,3-disiloxanediyl)dibenzene.** *Acta Crystallogr C* 1993, 49:1845–1848.

47. Borba A, Gomez-Zavaglia A, Fausto R: **Molecular structure, infrared spectra, and photochemistry of isoniazid under cryogenic conditions.** *J Phys Chem A* 2009, 113:9220–9230.

48. Srinivasan S, Swaminathan S: **The crystal structure of phenyl hydrazine, C6H5 · NH · NH2.** *Zeitschrift für Kristallographie* 1968, 127:442–449.

49. Okabe N, Fukuda H, Nakamura T: **Structure of hydralazine hydrochloride.** *Acta Crystallogr C* 1993, 49:1844–1845.

50. Lemmerer A: **Covalent assistance to supramolecular synthesis: modifying the drug functionality of the antituberculosis API isoniazid *in situ* during co-crystallization with GRAS and API compounds.** *Cryst Eng Comm* 2012, 14:2465–2478.

51. Abuhammad AM, Lowe ED, Fullam E, Noble M, Garman EF, Sim E: **Probing the architecture of the *Mycobacterium marinum* arylamine *N*-acetyltransferase active site.** *Protein Cell* 2010, 1:384–392.

52. Sandy J, Mushtaq A, Kawamura A, Sinclair J, Sim E, Noble M: **The structure of arylamine *N*-acetyltransferase from *Mycobacterium smegmatis*–an enzyme which inactivates the anti-tubercular drug, isoniazid.** *J Mol Biol* 2002, 318:1071–1083.

53. Sinclair JC, Sandy J, Delgoda R, Sim E, Noble ME: **Structure of arylamine *N*-acetyltransferase reveals a catalytic triad.** *Nat Struct Biol* 2000, 7:560–564.

54. Fullam E, Westwood IM, Anderton MC, Lowe ED, Sim E, Noble ME: **Divergence of cofactor recognition across evolution: coenzyme A binding in a prokaryotic arylamine *N*-acetyltransferase.** *J Mol Biol* 2008, 375:178–191.

55. Abuhammad A, Lowe ED, McDonough MA, Shaw Stewart PD, Kolek SA, Sim E, Garman EF: **Structure of arylamine *N*-acetyltransferase from *Mycobacterium tuberculosis* determined by cross-seeding with the homologous protein from *M. marinum*: triumph over adversity.** *Acta Crystallogr D Biol Crystallogr* 2013, 69:1433–1446.

56. Szakacs Z, Noszal B: **Determination of dissociation constants of folic acid, methotrexate, and other photolabile pteridines by pressure-assisted capillary electrophoresis.** *Electrophoresis* 2006, 27:3399–3409.

57. Brown HC, McDaniel DH, Haflinger P: *Determination of Organic Structures by Physical Methods.* New York: Academic Press; 1955.

58. Nobilis M, Vybiralova Z, Sladkova K, Lisa M, Holcapek M, Kvetina J: **High-performance liquid-chromatographic determination of 5-aminosalicylic**

acid and its metabolites in blood plasma. *J Chromatogr A* 2006, 1119:299–308.

59. Lukács M, Barcsa G, Kovács-Hadady K: The effects of pH, ionic strength and buffer concentration of mobile phase on R F of acidic compounds in ion-pair TLC. *Chromatographia* 1998, **48**:511–516.

60. Machado JD, Gomez JF, Betancor G, Camacho M, Brioso MA, Borges R: Hydralazine reduces the quantal size of secretory events by displacement of catecholamines from adrenomedullary chromaffin secretory vesicles. *Circ Res* 2002, **91**:830–836.

61. Becker C, Dressman JB, Amidon GL, Junginger HE, Kopp S, Midha KK, Shah VP, Stavchansky S, Barends DM: Biowaiver monographs for immediate release solid oral dosage forms: isoniazid. *J Pharm Sci* 2007, **96**:522–531.

24

Deprescribing benzodiazepines and Z-drugs in community-dwelling adults: a scoping review

André S. Pollmann[1]*, Andrea L. Murphy[2], Joel C. Bergman[2] and David M. Gardner[3]

Abstract

Background: Long-term sedative use is prevalent and associated with significant morbidity, including adverse events such as falls, cognitive impairment, and sedation. The development of dependence can pose significant challenges when discontinuation is attempted as withdrawal symptoms often develop. We conducted a scoping review to map and characterize the literature and determine opportunities for future research regarding deprescribing strategies for long-term benzodiazepine and Z-drug (zopiclone, zolpidem, and zaleplon) use in community-dwelling adults.

Methods: We searched PubMed, Cochrane Central Register of Controlled Trials, EMBASE, PsycINFO, CINAHL, TRIP, and JBI Ovid databases and conducted a grey literature search. Articles discussing methods for deprescribing benzodiazepines or Z-drugs in community-dwelling adults were selected.

Results: Following removal of duplicates, 2797 articles were reviewed for eligibility. Of these, 367 were retrieved for full-text assessment and 139 were subsequently included for review. Seventy-four (53 %) articles were original research, predominantly randomized controlled trials (n = 52 [37 %]), whereas 58 (42 %) were narrative reviews and seven (5 %) were guidelines. Amongst original studies, pharmacologic strategies were the most commonly studied intervention (n = 42 [57 %]). Additional deprescribing strategies included psychological therapies (n = 10 [14 %]), mixed interventions (n = 12 [16 %]), and others (n = 10 [14 %]). Behaviour change interventions were commonly combined and included enablement (n = 56 [76 %]), education (n = 36 [47 %]), and training (n = 29 [39 %]). Gradual dose reduction was frequently a component of studies, reviews, and guidelines, but methods varied widely.

Conclusions: Approaches proposed for deprescribing benzodiazepines and Z-drugs are numerous and heterogeneous. Current research in this area using methods such as randomized trials and meta-analyses may too narrowly encompass potential strategies available to target this phenomenon. Realist synthesis methods would be well suited to understand the mechanisms by which deprescribing interventions work and why they fail.

Keywords: Benzodiazepines, Z-drugs, Deprescribing, Clinical pharmacology, Behaviour change wheel, Scoping review

Background

Benzodiazepines and similar sedative hypnotics, including zopiclone, zaleplon, and zolpidem ("Z-drugs"), are extensively prescribed medications in the community setting [1–7]. The annual incidence of long-term benzodiazepine use across North America and Europe is estimated to be between 0.4 % to 6 %, with higher rates of chronic use in patients older than 65 years [5, 8–10]. The prevalence of benzodiazepine use in adults aged 18 to 64 years has remained relatively stable over the past

decade, suggesting potential issues with long-term use beyond what is normally indicated [3, 5, 11]. Recent data from Canada suggest important changes in prescribing practices. New prescriptions for benzodiazepines are declining, especially in older adults, while Z-drug use has steadily increased [5]. These trends mirror similar findings from other international studies [8, 12–18].

While indicated only for short-term management of anxiety and insomnia, reasons for acute benzodiazepine and Z-drug therapy transforming into chronic use are complex. Several prescriber related factors are believed to influence this process. These factors may include the prescriber's attitudes toward these medications and toward

* Correspondence: andre.p@dal.ca
[1]Faculty of Medicine, Dalhousie University, Mail Box #259, 5849 University Avenue, Room C-125, PO Box 15000, Halifax, NS B3H 4R2, Canada
Full list of author information is available at the end of the article

the 'deserving' patient, deficits in specialized knowledge about sedative prescribing, the clinical work environment, conflicting patient health priorities, and the prescribing practices of others involved in the patient's care [19, 20]. The perceived or real inaccessibility to alternative treatment modalities may further encourage the renewal of benzodiazepine and Z-drug prescriptions in favor of initiating other interventions that are perceived as less effective [21]. Patient factors including disagreement with appropriateness of cessation, fears of symptom return, withdrawal experiences, and the impression of unsuitability of alternatives also act to promote continued use [22, 23]. Considering the highly varied contributing factors that lead to long-term benzodiazepine and Z-drug use, deprescribing strategies need to be flexible and acceptable to both patients and clinicians.

Deprescribing is the collaborative and supportive process of identifying, modifying, and discontinuing therapies that are no longer indicated or may be causing harm to patients [24, 25]. Research and clinical programs for deprescribing typically focus on elderly patients due to high rates of medication-related morbidity and mortality, such as falls, fractures, motor vehicle collisions, daytime sedation, and cognitive impairment [26–31]. However, stable prevalence of benzodiazepine use and increasing Z-drug use in adults will also require that best-practice deprescribing strategies in this population be identified.

Numerous pharmacologic and nonpharmacologic deprescribing strategies have been reported in the literature with significant heterogeneity in the range and scope of psychological therapies, pharmacotherapy substitution approaches, and gradual dose reduction (GDR) schedules. We conducted a scoping review to map and characterize the literature, identify potential research gaps, and determine opportunities for future systematic syntheses regarding strategies and behaviour change interventions for deprescribing benzodiazepines and Z-drugs in community-dwelling adults who are long-term users (i.e., eight weeks or longer).

Methods

Scoping review methods are appropriate for our topic area given the complexity and heterogeneity of existing research [32]. The intention is to characterize and map the literature, identify research gaps, and prioritize targeted areas for future reviews and research [33]. We also aimed to explicate various interventions used in the literature and characterize them according to the Behaviour Change Wheel based on the work of Michie et al. [34]. We followed scoping review procedures slightly modified, but as outlined by Arskey and O'Malley [35] and further explicated by Levac et al. [32] and others [33, 36–39]. Our review was conducted in six iterative stages including

developing the research question, identifying relevant articles, selecting articles, extracting data, collating results, and engaging stakeholders through consultation (e.g., presentations on the topic) (Additional file 1).

Definitions and search strategies

As a research team we met and reached consensus on population, intervention, comparator, and outcome definitions (Additional file 1). We limited our target population to patients taking benzodiazepines and Z-drugs in the community or outpatient settings as individuals receiving care in inpatient, long-term care, or residential aged care facilities can differ systematically with respect to numerous factors. These factors include, but are not limited to, the context of the environment, frailty, nature and number of illnesses, and treatment goals. Long-term use was defined as regular use beyond an eight-week period. The target medications for this review included all benzodiazepines and Z-drugs, defined as "zopiclone", "eszopiclone", "zolpidem", or "zaleplon".

Due to the broad nature of scoping reviews, we did not limit our research question to a particular type of intervention or comparator and included studies investigating pharmacologic, psychological, and various mixed methods of discontinuing benzodiazepine or Z-drug therapy. We classified pharmacologic interventions as those adding additional drug therapy (non-benzodiazepine or Z-drug) to facilitate discontinuation of the sedative or mitigate withdrawal symptoms. Psychological interventions were those utilizing behavioural techniques, such as cognitive behavioural therapy (CBT), to reduce benzodiazepine or Z-drug use. We categorized studies as mixed interventions if they compared various pharmacologic, psychological, or other interventions with each other. GDR included employing a taper regimen or switching between sedatives to facilitate benzodiazepine or Z-drug withdrawal. The remaining intervention types not falling within these categories were classified as 'other' (i.e., letter or brief consultation).

We collaborated with a medical science librarian to develop search methods for each database and to identify key terms and relevant medical subject headings. Our searches were developed to model the PICO (Population, Intervention, Comparator, Outcome) format for clinical questions [40].We searched PubMed, EMBASE, PsycINFO, the Cochrane Central Register of Controlled Trials (CENTRAL), CINAHL, and JBI Ovid databases from inception to December 19, 2013. Systematic combinations of the medical subject headings "benzodiazepine", "hypnotics and sedatives", "substance withdrawal syndrome", "dependency", "sleep disorders", and "anxiety disorders" were used together with the keywords "hypnotic", "sedative", "zopiclone", "eszopiclone", "zolpidem", "zaleplon", "withdraw*", "deprescrib*", "taper", "stop", and "discontinu*". Search terms were translated as appropriate for each database.

To identify further references not captured in the published medical literature, we used relevant sections of the Canadian Agency for Drugs and Technologies in Health's (CADTH) "Grey Matters: a practical search tool for evidence-based medicine" [41] to search 69 international grey literature sources from the earliest available date through January 30, 2014. We also searched Opengrey (SIGLE), Google Advanced, screening the first 100 results for relevance to our clinical question, and the Turning Research Into Practice (TRIP) database for clinical practice guidelines concerning deprescribing of benzodiazepines and Z-drugs. Additional articles potentially relevant to our objectives were identified through reviewing reference lists of articles captured in our initial searches and by engaging with experts and colleagues.

Study selection
We used pre-defined inclusion criteria to select articles identified through the search strategy that were relevant to our study objectives. We included those studies that were published in English and investigated or discussed methods for discontinuing benzodiazepines and sedative hypnotics in community-dwelling individuals aged 18 years and older. Based on our pre-determined criteria, we did not include studies that exclusively investigated benzodiazepine and Z-drug use in patients with conditions other than anxiety or insomnia disorders. We excluded studies in animals, pediatric patients (<18 years old), and short-term users of benzodiazepines or Z-drugs (less than eight weeks). We did not include studies investigating non-clinical outcomes (e.g., electroencephalography and brain imaging studies), and articles not investigating benzodiazepine and Z-drug discontinuation as a primary focus. With the exception of case-reports, case-series, and commentaries, articles were not excluded based on methodology or publication type as we sought to identify trends across the wide spectrum of research and publications in the area [35]. Original investigations, research syntheses, guidelines, and narrative review articles were all eligible for inclusion in order to capture potential differences amongst these publications with respect to benzodiazepine and Z-drug deprescribing recommendations. Indicators of study quality were broadly assessed as a means to understand the nature of research methods used and reported, but study quality was not used as an inclusion criterion.

The list of article titles and abstracts resulting from the database and grey literature searches were scanned independently by two reviewers (AP and JB), who assigned a value of "include", "exclude", or "assess further" to each reference. After the initial screening phase, full-text articles were retrieved and independently assessed by AP and JB for inclusion in the review using forms for determining eligibility criteria. Disagreements between the two assessors were discussed, and a third author (AM) was consulted if agreement could not be reached.

Collating, summarizing, and reporting results
The data abstraction tool was drafted and revised through meetings throughout the stages of the review (Additional file 1). The standardized form was designed to capture information about the year of publication, country of origin, study type, target medication investigated, types of interventions, GDR protocol if used, duration of intervention, and information about the participants. Behaviour change interventions used in original research trials were categorized according to the Behaviour Change Wheel as enablement ("increasing means/reducing barriers to increase capability or opportunity"), training ("imparting skills"), persuasion ("using communication to induce positive or negative feelings or stimulate action"), environmental restructuring ("changing the physical or social context"), modeling ("providing an example for people to aspire to"), education ("increasing knowledge or understanding"), incentivisation ("creating expectation of reward"), coercion ("creating expectation of punishment or cost"), and restriction ("using rules to reduce opportunity to engage in target behaviour") [34]. Study methodology was characterized according to the Agency for Healthcare Research and Quality's (AHRQ) "Assessing Risk of Bias and Confounding in Observational Studies of Interventions or Exposures: Further Development of the RTI Item Bank" [42] with the addition of systematic reviews and narrative review articles. We categorized general data regarding the direction of effect of endpoints related to benzodiazepine and Z-drug discontinuation as a formal evaluation of the effect size of specific interventions is beyond the objective of a scoping review.

Prior to beginning the abstractions, an abstraction meeting was held to outline the process and model how to characterize intervention functions to establish consistency among team members. Initial articles were abstracted in a group environment so that discussion could occur surrounding issues or uncertainties regarding intervention function categorization. Following the initial abstractions one investigator (AP) reviewed all article abstractions for consistency in terminology, accuracy, and comprehensiveness. The PRISMA checklist form is provided as Additional file 2.

Results
Search
Our literature search yielded 2797 articles after duplicates were removed. Review of titles and abstracts led to retrieval of 367 full-text articles for assessment (Fig. 1). Of these, 74 original research studies and 65 review

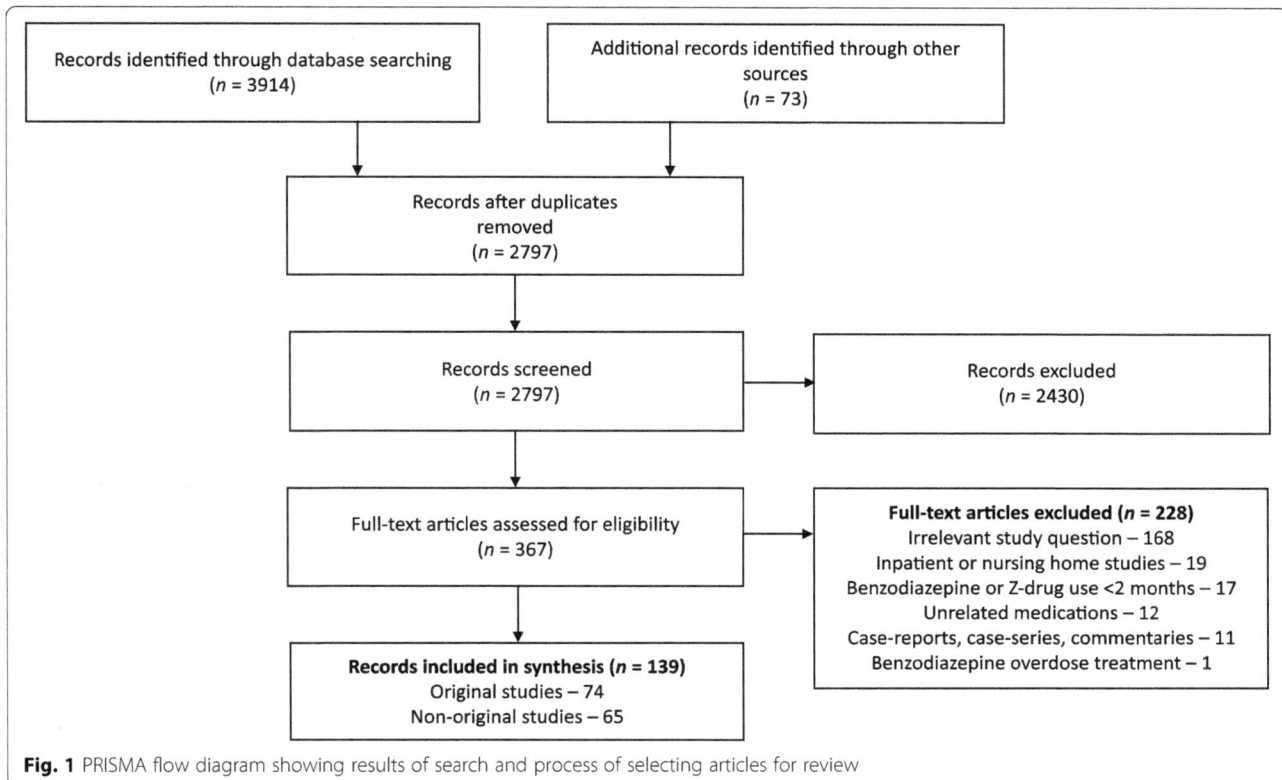

Fig. 1 PRISMA flow diagram showing results of search and process of selecting articles for review

articles or guidelines were included (Additional file 3) [8, 43–180]. The absence of benzodiazepine or Z-drug discontinuation strategies as a major focus of the intervention or outcome was the most frequent reason for excluding articles.

Description of articles

Deprescribing articles for benzodiazepines and Z-drugs were published between 1982 and 2014 with no apparent trend towards growing publications in this field over the past 30 years (Table 1). Research was primarily conducted in the United States (27 %) and United Kingdom (24 %). Articles were published in a variety of journals with scopes including psychiatry (n = 43 [31 %]), general/primary care (n = 37 [27 %]), pharmacology (n = 28 [20 %]), psychology and behavioural sciences (n = 11 [8 %]), and addiction (n = 11 [8 %]). Most original research studies were randomized controlled trials (RCTs) (n = 52 [37 %]), but nearly 50 % of all included articles were non-original research (Table 1). The majority of studies were relatively small, with less than 100 participants in total (n = 51 [69 %]). The setting of original research included primary care and outpatient clinics (n = 45 [61 %]), specialty clinics (n = 14 [19 %]), and university research units (n = 8 [11 %]), while seven studies did not report setting details (10 %).

Amongst research trials, most (n = 36 [49 %]) investigated patient populations taking benzodiazepines for multiple reasons. Insomnia or anxiety disorders were the primary diagnosis in 16 studies each (22 %). Fewer (n = 6 [8 %]) trials focused on patients with panic disorder. In contrast, 57 % (n = 37) of review articles examined mixed conditions, 11 % (n = 7) insomnia, 17 % (n = 11) anxiety disorders, and 15 % (n = 10) panic disorders. The distribution of studies reporting a mean age of 40 to 49 years, 50 to 59 years and 60 to 69 years, was 43 % (n = 32), 18 % (n = 13), and 19 % (n = 14), respectively. The duration of prior benzodiazepine or Z-drug use varied widely among studies and details concerning the length of therapy were not reported in 41 % (n = 30). The mean duration of benzodiazepine or Z-drug use was typically less than a decade (n = 30 [41 %]). The majority of original trials (n = 41 [55 %]) investigated the discontinuation of any benzodiazepine, whereas 16 % (n = 12) examined both benzodiazepine and Z-drug discontinuation. Only three (4 %) of 74 original studies exclusively examined strategies for stopping Z-drugs. The remaining studies enrolled patients only if they were taking specific benzodiazepines, most frequently alprazolam (n = 11), diazepam (n = 7), and lorazepam (n = 6).

The general direction of effect for the endpoint of discontinuation of benzodiazepine or Z-drug therapy was

Table 1 Characteristics of publications on benzodiazepine and Z-drug discontinuation in community dwelling adults

Characteristic	No.	% of 139 articles
Type of article		
Original research		
Randomized-controlled trial	52	37.4 %
Before-after study	8	5.8 %
Nonrandomized controlled trial	6	4.3 %
Systematic review/meta-analysis	3	2.2 %
Prospective cohort study	2	1.4 %
Non-comparative study	2	1.4 %
Retrospective cohort study	1	0.7 %
Non-original research		
Narrative review	58	41.7 %
Guideline	7	5.0 %
Country of origin		
United States	38	27.3 %
United Kingdom	33	23.7 %
Europe	24	17.3 %
Canada	20	14.4 %
Australia	13	9.4 %
Asia	2	1.4 %
Other	9	6.5 %
Year of publication		
<1985	4	2.9 %
1985–1994	50	36.0 %
1995–2004	40	28.8 %
2005–2015	45	32.4 %
Primary medical condition		
Mixed	73	52.5 %
Anxiety disorders	27	19.4 %
Insomnia	23	16.5 %
Panic disorders	16	11.5 %

Table 2 Benzodiazepine and Z-drug deprescribing strategies studied or discussed in publications

Strategies researched in original studies	No.	% of 74
Pharmacologic therapy	42	56.8 %
Psychological therapy	10	13.5 %
Mixed	12	16.2 %
Other	10	13.5 %
Strategies discussed in non-original articles	No.	% of 65
Pharmacologic therapy	24	36.9 %
Psychological therapy	30	46.2 %
GDR	60	92.3 %
Other	21	32.3 %

three studies investigated the addition of pharmacologic therapies to facilitate benzodiazepine or Z-drug discontinuation. Amongst these, buspirone was the most frequently studied therapy in RCTs (n = 4) and nonrandomized controlled trials (n = 3), with a total of 275 subjects. Melatonin was studied in five trials, of which four were RCTs with 244 subjects. Sixteen other additive pharmacologic agents were studied, which included beta-adrenergic receptor antagonists (n = 3), anti-seizure drugs such as carbamazepine, pregabalin, and valproate (n = 5), and antidepressants such as imipramine, paroxetine, and trazodone (n = 5). Other medications investigated were ondansetron (n = 1) and progesterone (n = 1).

Gradual dose reduction

Original research investigations of pharmacologic, psychological, mixed, and other interventions frequently included GDR as a component of the discontinuation method (60 of 74 [80 %]). However, the types of GDR regimens employed varied dramatically among trials and 15 studies did not report details about their GDR methods. Stabilization (i.e., establishing a consistent daily dose) of benzodiazepine or Z-drug dose prior to the initiation of tapering was a strategy employed in 28 % of studies. As part of the GDR regimen, 31 (42 %) trials established flexible taper plans, which involved altering the rate of taper based on patient symptoms. The remaining trials established a uniform tapering regimen that was applied to all subjects. In 13 trials (18 %), participants were switched to another agent, most frequently diazepam (n = 10), but also Z-drugs including zopiclone (n = 2) and zolpidem (n = 1). The time frame over which GDR was conducted ranged from one to more than 16 weeks with the most common (n = 11) being four weeks (median 6 weeks, interquartile range 4–8 weeks). Twenty studies employing GDR did not report the time frame of their taper regimen. The most common taper rate among studies (n = 16) was decreasing the original dose by 25 % weekly (i.e., 75 % of original

noted for each research trial, regardless of the type of intervention studied. Of original research studies, 41 % (n = 30) of studies demonstrated a negative (or nonsignificant) effect of the intervention being investigated. A positive effect was demonstrated in 47 % (n = 35) of studies, while 12 % (n = 9) of research studies did not provide sufficient data to clearly assess the direction of the effect (Additional file 3).

Deprescribing strategies
Pharmacologic

Among original research studies, pharmacologic interventions were the most common types of interventions assessed for their impact on reducing benzodiazepine and Z-drug exposure (n = 42 [57 %]) (Table 2). Thirty-

dose for one week, then 50 % of original dose for one week, then 25 % of original dose for one week, then stop). Seven studies outlined a slower approach, decreasing the dose by 25 % every two to four weeks. Shorter tapers were also reported in seven studies, with the dose reduced by half for one to two weeks before the benzodiazepine or Z-drug was discontinued.

The majority of review articles and clinical practice guidelines (60 of 65 [92 %]) recommended GDR as part of a discontinuation strategy (Table 2). Recommendations concerning GDR strategy varied widely but a flexible approach and substitution of a long-acting benzodiazepine were frequent suggestions.

Psychological therapies
Psychological therapies to facilitate discontinuation of benzodiazepines and Z-drugs were studied in 10 trials (14 %), with 60 % of these trials utilizing CBT (Table 2). Other strategies employed via both group and individualized therapies included anxiety management, stress management, and psychotherapy. Nine of these 10 trials were RCTs with a total of 408 patients.

Mixed and other interventions
Mixed interventions comparing various pharmacologic, psychological, or other interventions were the focus of 12 (16 %) studies (Table 2). Five of these 12 trials compared more than two types of interventions. Common interventions included psychological therapy (most frequently CBT), GDR alone, and usual care. Other interventions that were investigated in 14 % of original research studies included interventions such as sending a letter or detailed information to patients and brief counseling by clinicians.

Intervention functions
Six of the nine intervention types described by Michie et al., [34] were used in the research studies included. The majority of original studies included a single intervention function (n = 39 [53 %]), while the remainder combined two (n = 12 [16 %]), three (n = 21 [28 %]), or four (n = 2 [3 %]) distinct functions (Additional file 3). The most common method employed was enablement, which was used in 76 % (n = 56) of studies. The majority of studies using enablement techniques attempted to achieve benzodiazepine or Z-drug cessation by testing the effect of GDR, additional pharmacotherapy, or psychological therapies. Education and training were also frequent elements assessed by research studies, being a component of 47 % (n = 35) and 38 % (n = 28) of studies, respectively. A total of 11 studies investigated persuasion interventions (15 %), which frequently involved the physician sending a letter to patients to explain the harms of benzodiazepines or Z-drugs and

encouraging discontinuation. Three trials tested environmental restructuring techniques to facilitate discontinuation. In addition to other strategies, one trial evaluated modeling as a component of a patient information package [8].

Discussion
We identified 139 articles for deprescribing benzodiazepines and Z-drugs in community-dwelling adults that included a range of different strategies and behaviour change interventions. This is in contrast to recent meta-analyses that included 32 studies or fewer [117, 136, 138]. While meta-analyses of data can offer valuable answers to specific research and clinical questions, the strict inclusion criteria based on study methodology and quality can limit the amount of information they provide on the research area as a whole. Research and publications that would be characterized as lower levels of evidence in hierarchies [181–183] (e.g., non-randomized trials, guidelines, narrative reviews) can be captured in scoping reviews, which is important in many clinical questions given the kinds of evidence that inform clinicians and patients in decision-making [184]. In our scoping review, we included systematic reviews, individual RCTs, practice guidelines, reviews, and other study designs to characterize the literature, identify research gaps and future research priorities, and determine opportunities for future systematic syntheses regarding deprescribing strategies. This more inclusive approach reflects the sources of information utilized by clinicians, especially for therapeutic decisions that require individualized and flexible care plans, such as benzodiazepine and Z-drug discontinuation [185].

Pharmacologic interventions have been the primary discontinuation strategy reported on in the majority of studies within previous meta-analyses [117, 136, 138]. Likewise, our scoping review found that the addition of pharmacologic agents to facilitate discontinuation has been the most commonly studied type of intervention in RCTs (31 trials, totaling 2273 patients). This method of discontinuation may be counterintuitive to both prescribers and patients as risks for different adverse events and increased costs are inherent within this approach. Despite the majority of trials studying this method, non-original review articles and guidelines included in our scoping review did not discuss this approach as frequently. This is especially important to consider given the large degree of variability and tensions that can exist with the use of different forms of evidence in clinical decision-making [186–188]. Depending on the practitioner, guidelines and narrative reviews may be significantly influential in decision-making. Patients will also inherently use various forms of information about medications in their decision-making, much of which will not necessarily include information from clinical trials but that is readily accessible on the internet [189].

Our review revealed that benzodiazepine and Z-drug deprescribing interventions are numerous, largely heterogeneous, and poorly described. The pace of publication annually remained stable, indicating maintained interest in this field. Estimates of effect size direction, while not attributable to a specific intervention or intervention type, were mixed with 47 % of trials being positive, 41 % negative, and 12 % undetermined, suggesting a lack of clarity regarding how to best deprescribe benzodiazepines and Z-drugs. Replication of strategies in the clinical practice setting with fidelity to interventions that were studied is nearly impossible owing to the large number of approaches examined and the lack of details provided in some reports. Guidelines such as the Template for Intervention Description and Replication (TIDieR) [190] and the checklist by the Workgroup for Intervention Development and Evaluation Research (WIDER) [191] should be used to describe interventions in sufficient detail to allow for their replication not only for subsequent research but in clinical practice. It would also allow investigators to better develop implementation strategies for various interventions in a range of settings using implementation frameworks [192].

Limited theoretical underpinnings of interventions combined with the significant heterogeneity and complexity of strategies as found in our review, presents challenges in helping to understand and explain the mechanisms by which interventions work, why they work, for whom, and in which contexts. Furthermore, with rising use of Z-drugs and other psychotropics for insomnia (e.g., quetiapine) [193] we need to understand whether strategies that work for benzodiazepines are in fact those that work for discontinuing other types of hypnotics. We recommend that a realist synthesis [194] approach be used in future syntheses given the complexity of these issues and the need to better understand the mechanisms by which deprescribing interventions for benzodiazepines and Z-drugs work and why they fail [195].

The generalizability of results from available studies is problematic due to the risk of sample distortion bias and selection bias affecting the findings. Across several studies, subjects participated because they were already motivated to stop their benzodiazepine or Z-drug. For many existing users, there is significant reluctance or refusal to discontinue benzodiazepines and Z-drugs when given the opportunity [22, 196, 197]. Additionally, long-term users of benzodiazepines and Z-drugs may have comorbidities that would exclude them from participating in many deprescribing clinical trials. The goals of care in patients with ongoing comorbidities may be quite different and benzodiazepine and Z-drug deprescribing may not be an immediate priority. Participants in trials

were often of younger age (i.e., 40 to 50 years), which does not match with the older population targeted by deprescribing initiatives that aim to reduce harm. Research in the area of deprescribing benzodiazepines and Z-drugs should focus on older people with a wide range of comorbidities.

To date, the outcome of interest in benzodiazepine and Z-drug deprescribing research has largely been whether or not treatment was successfully stopped. Clinical outcomes such as impact on reducing falls, fractures, quality of life, and mortality have been evaluated less frequently [108, 198]. Future research should determine the specific harms associated with long term sedative use, especially in vulnerable groups (e.g., frail adults, patients with multiple comorbidities), and aim to identify which patients benefit from benzodiazepine and Z-drug discontinuation in terms of quality of life, morbidity, and mortality.

There are limitations to this review. First, our search may not have been exhaustive, despite the search of multiple databases and grey literature sources. The lack of standardized medical subject headings in the developing area of deprescribing may have partially contributed to this. Second, we did not extract specific information about interventions studied and reviewed within the literature to determine which strategies are optimal for facilitating benzodiazepine and Z-drug discontinuation, as this is not the intended purpose of a scoping review. Third, although a predefined abstraction tool and classification scheme can minimize subjectivity among abstractors, there may be variability among investigators.

Conclusions

Long-term and inappropriate use of benzodiazepines and Z-drugs remains a problem in community dwelling adults. Numerous pharmacologic, psychological, and other interventions have been used to support long-term benzodiazepine and Z-drug discontinuation, yet strategies are diverse and often poorly reported in sufficient detail to allow replication in future research or clinical practice. Using scoping review methods for this complex problem allowed for inclusion of a greater breadth of literature and the freedom to characterize and identify existing gaps in research, whereas traditional syntheses methods restrict clinicians to mostly RCT data of pharmacologic augmentation of GDR. Our results indicate that the current research in this area using methods such as RCTs and meta-analysis may too narrowly encompass the potential strategies available to target this phenomenon. Future studies in this area should describe interventions in sufficient detail, including information on various behaviour change techniques, to allow for their replication in research and clinical practice. This process could be facilitated by the use of standardized reporting guidelines and various checklists that currently exist [190, 191]. More research regarding the impact of deprescribing strategies on patient-centered outcomes in real-word settings is required. Realist synthesis methods would be well suited to understand the mechanisms by which deprescribing interventions for benzodiazepines and Z-drugs work and why they fail.

Additional files

Additional file 1: Table S1. Research stages and methods for scoping review. *Summarizes the methods used for this scoping review, outlining the various stages and contributions of each author.*

Additional file 2: Table S2. PRISMA checklist.

Additional file 3: Table S3. Description of articles included in review. *This table displays information about the studies selected for inclusion in the review, including author, date of publication, study design, discontinuation strategies, age of participants studied, medication discontinued, key study outcomes, and Behaviour Change Wheel intervention functions employed.*

Abbreviations
CBT: Cognitive behavioural therapy; GDR: Gradual dose reduction; RCT: Randomized controlled trial.

Competing interests
AP, AM, and JB declare that they have no competing interests. DG is a developer of Sleepwell Nova Scotia (http://sleepwellns.ca/).

Authors' contributions
AP and AM conceptualized, designed, and coordinated the project. AP, AM, and DG prepared the search and data collection protocol, with input from JB. AP conducted the literature searches. AP, JB, and AM were responsible for data acquisition and analysis, in collaboration with DG. AP and AM drafted the manuscript and all authors contributed critical review and feedback. AP, AM, JB, and DG had full access to all the data in the study and take responsibility for the integrity of the data and accuracy of the data analysis. AP, the corresponding author, had the final responsibility to submit for publication. All authors read and approved the final manuscript.

Acknowledgments
Melissa Helwig, Information Services Librarian, W.K. Kellogg Health Sciences Library, Dalhousie University, assisted with the literature search strategy. Chad Purcell, Luiza Radu, Scott Haslam, Melanie McIvor, and Heather Phelan, from the College of Pharmacy, Dalhousie University assisted with the parts of the research process. The Drug Evaluation Alliance of Nova Scotia (DEANS) provided funding support for this publication through Dr. Andrea Murphy. The views represented in this publication are those of the authors and not the funder.

Author details
[1]Faculty of Medicine, Dalhousie University, Mail Box #259, 5849 University Avenue, Room C-125, PO Box 15000, Halifax, NS B3H 4R2, Canada. [2]College of Pharmacy and Department of Psychiatry, Dalhousie University, 5968 College St, PO Box 15000, Halifax, NS B3H 4R2, Canada. [3]Department of Psychiatry and College of Pharmacy, Dalhousie University, QEII HSC, AJLB 7517, 5909 Veterans' Memorial Lane, Halifax, NS B3H 2E2, Canada.

References
1. Ohayon MM, Lader MH. Use of psychotropic medication in the general population of France, Germany, Italy, and the United Kingdom. J Clin Psychiatry. 2002;63:817–25.
2. Olfson M, Pincus HA. Use of benzodiazepines in the community. Arch Intern Med. 1994;154:1235–40.
3. Neutel CI. The epidemiology of long-term benzodiazepine use. Int Rev Psychiatry. 2005;17:189–97.
4. Paulose-Ram R, Safran MA, Jonas BS, Gu Q, Orwig D. Trends in psychotropic medication use among U.S. adults. Pharmacoepidemiol Drug Saf. 2007;16:560–70.
5. Alessi-Severini S, Boulton JM, Enns MW, Dahl M, Collins DM, Chateau D, et al. Use of benzodiazepines and related drugs in Manitoba: a population-based study. CMAJ Open. 2014;2:e208–16.
6. Mamdani M, Rapoport M, Shulman KI, Herrmann N, Rochon PA. Mental health-related drug utilization among older adults: prevalence, trends, and costs. Am J Geriatr Psychiatry. 2005;13:892–900.
7. Hogan DB, Maxwell CJ, Fung TS, Ebly EM. Canadian Study of Health and Aging. Prevalence and potential consequences of benzodiazepine use in senior citizens: results from the Canadian study of health and aging. Can J Clin Pharmacol. 2003;10:72–7.
8. Tannenbaum C, Martin P, Tamblyn R, Benedetti A, Ahmed S. Reduction of inappropriate benzodiazepine prescriptions among older adults through direct patient education: the EMPOWER cluster randomized trial. JAMA Intern Med. 2014;174:890–8.
9. Cunningham CM, Hanley GE, Morgan S. Patterns in the use of benzodiazepines in British Columbia: examining the impact of increasing research and guideline cautions against long-term use. Health Policy. 2010;97:122–9.
10. Lagnaoui R, Depont F, Fourrier A, Abouelfath A, Begaud B, Verdoux H, et al. Patterns and correlates of benzodiazepine use in the French general population. Eur J Clin Pharmacol. 2004;60:523–9.
11. van Hulten R, Isacson D, Bakker A, Leufkens HG. Comparing patterns of long-term benzodiazepine use between a Dutch and a Swedish community. Pharmacoepidemiol Drug Saf. 2003;12:49–53.
12. Patten SB, Williams JV, Lavorato DH, Kassam A, Sabapathy CD. Pharmacoepidemiology of benzodiazepine and sedative-hypnotic use in a Canadian general population cohort during 12 years of follow-up. Can J Psychiatry. 2010;55:792–9.
13. Esposito E, Barbui C, Patten SB. Patterns of benzodiazepine use in a Canadian population sample. Epidemiol Psichiatr Soc. 2009;18:248–54.
14. De Wilde S, Carey IM, Harris T, Richards N, Victor C, Hilton SR, et al. Trends in potentially inappropriate prescribing amongst older UK primary care patients. Pharmacoepidemiol Drug Saf. 2007;16:658–67.
15. Lai HY, Hwang SJ, Chen YC, Chen TJ, Lin MH, Chen LK. Prevalence of the prescribing of potentially inappropriate medications at ambulatory care visits by elderly patients covered by the Taiwanese national health insurance program. Clin Ther. 2009;31:1859–70.
16. Smolders M, Laurant M, van Rijswijk E, Mulder J, Braspenning J, Verhaak P, et al. The impact of co-morbidity on GPs' pharmacological treatment decisions for patients with an anxiety disorder. Fam Pract. 2007;24:538–46.
17. Ford ES, Wheaton AG, Cunningham TJ, Giles WH, Chapman DP, Croft JB. Trends in outpatient visits for insomnia, sleep apnea, and prescriptions for sleep medications among US adults: findings from the national ambulatory medical care survey 1999–2010. Sleep. 2014;37:1283–93.
18. Olfson M, King M, Schoenbaum M. Benzodiazepine Use in the United States. JAMA Psychiatry. 2015;72:136–42.
19. Sirdifield C, Anthierens S, Creupelandt H, Chipchase SY, Christiaens T, Siriwardena AN. General practitioners' experiences and perceptions of benzodiazepine prescribing: systematic review and meta-synthesis. BMC Fam Pract. 2013;14:191.
20. Martinsson G, Fagerberg I, Wiklund-Gustin L, Lindholm C. Specialist prescribing of psychotropic drugs to older persons in Sweden—register-based study of 188,024 older persons. BMC Psychiatry. 2012;12:197.
21. Everitt H, McDermott L, Leydon G, Yules H, Baldwin D, Little P. GPs' management strategies for patients with insomnia: a survey and qualitative interview study. Br J Gen Pract. 2014;64:e112–9.
22. Reeve E, To J, Hendrix I, Shakib S, Roberts MS, Wiese MD. Patient barriers to and enablers of deprescribing: a systematic review. Drugs Aging. 2013;30:793–807.
23. Cook JM, Biyanova T, Masci C, Coyne JC. Older patient perspectives on long-term anxiolytic benzodiazepine use and discontinuation: a qualitative study. J Gen Intern Med. 2007;22:1094–100.
24. Frank C. Deprescribing: a new word to guide medication review. CMAJ. 2014;186:407–8.
25. Woodward MC. Deprescribing: achieving better health outcomes for older people through reducing medications. J Pharm Pract Res. 2003;33:323–8.

26. Holbrook AM, Crowther R, Lotter A, Cheng C, King D. Meta-analysis of benzodiazepine use in the treatment of insomnia. CMAJ. 2000;162:225–33.

27. Glass J, Lanctot KL, Herrmann N, Sproule BA, Busto UE. Sedative hypnotics in older people with insomnia: meta-analysis of risks and benefits. BMJ. 2005;331:1169.

28. Neutel CI, Perry S, Maxwell C. Medication use and risk of falls. Pharmacoepidemiol Drug Saf. 2002;11:97–104.

29. Wagner AK, Zhang F, Soumerai SB, Walker AM, Gurwitz JH, Glynn RJ, et al. Benzodiazepine use and hip fractures in the elderly: who is at greatest risk? Arch Intern Med. 2004;164:1567–72.

30. Barbone F, McMahon AD, Davey PG, Morris AD, Reid IC, McDevitt DG, et al. Association of road-traffic accidents with benzodiazepine use. Lancet. 1998;352:1331–6.

31. McIntosh B, Clark M, Spry C. Benzodiazepines in older adults: a review of clinical effectiveness, cost-effectiveness, and guidelines. Canadian Agency for Drugs and Technologies in Health. 2011. http://www.ncbi.nlm.nih.gov/books/NBK174561/. Accessed 16 Nov 2014.

32. Levac D, Colquhoun H, O'Brien KK. Scoping studies: advancing the methodology. Implement Sci. 2010;5:69.

33. Kastner M, Tricco AC, Soobiah C, Lillie E, Perrier L, Horsley T, et al. What is the most appropriate knowledge synthesis method to conduct a review? Protocol for a scoping review BMC Med Res Methodol. 2012;12:114.

34. Michie S, van Stralen MM, West R. The behaviour change wheel: a new method for characterising and designing behaviour change interventions. Implement Sci. 2011;6:42.

35. Arskey H, O'Malley L. Scoping studies: towards a methodological framework. Int J Soc Res Methodol. 2005;8:19–32.

36. Valaitis R, Martin-Misener R, Wong ST, MacDonald M, Meagher-Stewart D, Austin P, et al. Methods, strategies and technologies used to conduct a scoping literature review of collaboration between primary care and public health. Prim Health Care Res Dev. 2012;13:219–36.

37. Bragge P, Clavisi O, Turner T, Tavender E, Collie A, Gruen RL. The global evidence mapping initiative: scoping research in broad topic areas. BMC Med Res Methodol. 2011;11:92.

38. Brien SE, Lorenzetti DL, Lewis S, Kennedy J, Ghali WA. Overview of a formal scoping review on health system report cards. Implement Sci. 2010;5:2.

39. Rumrill PD, Fitzgerald SM, Merchant WR. Using scoping literature reviews as a means of understanding and interpreting existing literature. Work. 2010;35:399–404.

40. Richardson WS, Wilson MC, Nishikawa J, Hayward RS. The well-built clinical question: a key to evidence-based decisions. ACP J Club. 1995;123:A12–3.

41. Grey matters: a practical search tool for evidence-based medicine. Canadian Agency for Drugs and Technologies in Health. 2013. http://www.cadth.ca/en/resources/finding-evidence-is/grey-matters. Accessed 19 Jan 2014.

42. Viswanathan M, Berkman ND, Dryden DM, Hartling L. Assessing risk of bias and confounding in observational studies of interventions or exposures: further development of the RTI item bank. Agency for Healthcare Research and Quality. 2013. http://www.ncbi.nlm.nih.gov/books/NBK154461/. Accessed 15 Mar 2014.

43. Abelson JL, Curtis GC. Discontinuation of alprazolam after successful treatment of panic disorder: a naturalistic follow-up study. J Anxiety Disord. 1993;7:107–17.

44. Ahmed M, Westra HA, Stewart SH. A self-help handout for benzodiazepine discontinuation using cognitive behavioral therapy. Cong Behav Pract. 2008;15:317–24.

45. Allain H, Le Coz F, Borderies P, Schuck S, Giclais DL, Patat A, et al. Use of zolpidem 10 mg as a benzodiazepine substitute in 84 patients with insomnia. Hum Psychopharmacol. 1998;13:551–9.

46. Ashton H. The treatment of benzodiazepine dependence. Addiction. 1994;89:1535–41.

47. Ashton CH, Rawlins MD, Tyrer SP. A double-blind placebo-controlled study of buspirone in diazepam withdrawal in chronic benzodiazepine users. Br J Psychiatry. 1990;157:232–8.

48. Baillargeon L, Landreville P, Verreault R, Beauchemin JP, Grégoire JP, Morin CM. Discontinuation of benzodiazepines among older insomniac adults treated with cognitive-behavioural therapy combined with gradual tapering: a randomized trial. CMAJ. 2003;169:1015–20.

49. Ballenger JC. Long-term pharmacologic treatment of panic disorder. J Clin Psychiatry. 1991;52 Suppl 2:18–23.

50. Ballenger JC, Pecknold J, Rickels K, Sellers EM. Medication discontinuation in panic disorder. J Clin Psychiatry. 1993;54 Suppl 10:15–21.

51. Bartholomew S. Benzodiazepine dependence in the elderly. J Am Acad Phys Assist. 1990;3:535–9.

52. Bashir K, King M, Ashworth M. Controlled evaluation of brief intervention by general practitioners to reduce chronic use of benzodiazepines. Br J Gen Pract. 1994;44:408–12.

53. Belanger L, Belleville G, Morin C. Management of hypnotic discontinuation in chronic insomnia. Sleep Med Clin. 2009;4:583–92.

54. Belleville G, Guay C, Guay B, Morin CM. Hypnotic taper with or without self-help treatment of insomnia: a randomized clinical trial. J Consult Clin Psychol. 2007;75:325–35.

55. Blais D, Petit L. Benzodiazepines: dependence and a therapeutic approach to gradual withdrawal. Can Fam Physician. 1990;36:1779–82.

56. Bobes J, Rubio G, Teran A, Cervera G, Lopez-Gomez V, Vilardaga I, et al. Pregabalin for the discontinuation of long-term benzodiazepines use: an assessment of its effectiveness in daily clinical practice. Eur Psychiatry. 2012;27:301–7.

57. Burrows GD. Managing long-term therapy for panic disorder. J Clin Psychiatry. 1990;51 Suppl 11:9–12.

58. Burrows GD, Norman TR, Judd FK, Marriott PF. Short-acting versus long-acting benzodiazepines: discontinuation effects in panic disorders. J Psychiatr Res. 1990;24 Suppl 2:65–72.

59. Cantopher T, Olivieri S, Cleave N, Edwards JG. Chronic benzodiazepine dependence: a comparative study of abrupt withdrawal under propranolol cover versus gradual withdrawal. Br J Psychiatry. 1990;156:406–11.

60. Chang F. Strategies for benzodiazepine withdrawal in seniors. Can Pharm J. 2005;138:38–40.

61. Choy Y. Managing side effects of anxiolytics. Primary Psychiatry. 2007;14:68–76.

62. Chung KF, Cheung RCH, Tam JWY. Long-term benzodiazepine users - characteristics, views and effectiveness of benzodiazepine reduction information leaflet. Singapore Med J. 1999;40:138–43.

63. Cormack MA, Sinnott A. Psychological alternatives to long-term benzodiazepine use. J R Coll Gen Pract. 1983;33:279–81.

64. Cormack MA, Sweeney KG, Hughes-Jones H, Foot GA. Evaluation of an easy, cost-effective strategy for cutting benzodiazepine use in general practice. Br J Gen Pract. 1994;44:5–8.

65. Crouch G, Robson M, Hallstrom C. Benzodiazepine dependent patients and their psychological treatment. Prog Neuropsychopharmacol Biol Psychiatry. 1988;12:503–10.

66. Davidson JR. Continuation treatment of panic disorder with high-potency benzodiazepines. J Clin Psychiatry. 1990;51 Suppl 12:31–7.

67. Dell'osso B, Lader M. Do benzodiazepines still deserve a major role in the treatment of psychiatric disorders? A critical reappraisal. Eur Psychiatry. 2013;28:7–20.

68. Benzodiazepines: good practice guidelines for clinicians. Department of Health and Children, Ireland. 2002. http://hdl.handle.net/10147/46748. Accessed 19 Jan 2014.

69. Drug misuse and dependence: UK guidelines on clinical management. Department of Health (England), the Scottish Government, Welsh Assembly Government, and Northern Ireland Executive. 2007. http://www.nta.nhs.uk/guidelines.aspx. Accessed 31 Mar 2014.

70. Drake J. Temazepam 'planpak': a multicentre general practice trial in planned benzodiazepine hypnotic withdrawal. Curr Med Res Opin. 1991;12:390–3.

71. Dubovsky SL. Generalized anxiety disorder: new concepts and psychopharmacologic therapies. J Clin Psychiatry. 1990;51 Suppl 1:3–10.

72. DuPont RL. Thinking about stopping treatment for panic disorder. J Clin Psychiatry. 1990;51:38–45.

73. DuPont RL. A practical approach to benzodiazepine discontinuation. J Psychiatr Res. 1990;24 Suppl 2:81–90.

74. El-Guebaly N, Sareen J, Stein MB. Are there guidelines for the responsible prescription of benzodiazepines? Can J Psychiatry. 2010;55:709–14.

75. Elsesser K, Sartory G, Maurer J. The efficacy of complaints management training in facilitating benzodiazepine withdrawal. Behav Res Ther. 1996;34:149–56.

76. Office-based outpatient withdrawal techniques: a guide–anxiolytic/sedative/hypnotic drugs. Federation of Texas Psychiatry. 2002. http://www.txpsych.org/guidelinesanxiolyticsedativehypnotic.htm. Accessed 31 Mar 2014.

77. Fraser D, Peterkin GS, Gamsu CV, Baldwin PJ. Benzodiazepine withdrawal: a pilot comparison of three methods. Br J Clin Psychol. 1990;29:231–3.

78. Fyer AJ, Liebowitz MR, Gorman JM, Campeas R, Levin A, Davies SO, et al. Discontinuation of alprazolam treatment in panic patients. Am J Psychiatry. 1987;144:303–8.

79. Garfinkel D, Zisapel N, Wainstein J, Laudon M. Facilitation of benzodiazepine discontinuation by melatonin: a new clinical approach. Arch Intern Med. 1999;159:2456–60.

80. Gilhooly TC, Webster MG, Poole NW, Ross S. What happens when doctors stop prescribing temazepam? Use of alternative therapies. Br J Gen Pract. 1998;48:1601–2.

81. Clinical comparison of paroxetine and placebo on the symptoms emerging during the taper phase of a chronic benzodiazepine treatment, in patients suffering from a variety of anxiety disorders. GlaxoSmithKline. 2008. http://www.gsk-clinicalstudyregister.com/study/29060/730#rs. Accessed 31 Mar 2014.

82. Gosselin P, Ladouceur R, Morin CM, Dugas MJ, Baillargeon L. Benzodiazepine discontinuation among adults with GAD: a randomized trial of cognitive-behavioral therapy. J Consult Clin Psychol. 2006;74:908–19.

83. Hadley SJ, Mandel FS, Schweizer E. Switching from long-term benzodiazepine therapy to pregabalin in patients with generalized anxiety disorder: a double-blind, placebo-controlled trial. J Psychopharmacol. 2012;26:461–70.

84. Hallström C, Crouch G, Robson M, Shine P. The treatment of tranquilizer dependence by propranolol. Postgrad Med J. 1988;64 Suppl 2:40–4.

85. Harangozo J, Magyar I, Faludy G. Use of benzodiazepines in psychiatry. Ther Hung. 1991;39:103–11.

86. Hayward P, Wardle J, Higgitt A. Benzodiazepine research: current findings and practical consequences. Br J Clin Psychol. 1989;28:307–27.

87. Heather N, Bowie A, Ashton H, McAvoy B, Spencer I, Brodie J, et al. Randomised controlled trial of two brief interventions against long-term benzodiazepine use: outcome of intervention. Addict Res Theory. 2004;12:141–54.

88. Higgitt AC, Lader MH, Fonagy P. Clinical management of benzodiazepine dependence. BMJ. 1985;91:688–90.

89. Hofmann SG, Spiegel DA. Panic control treatment and its applications. J Psychother Pract Res. 1999;8:3–11.

90. Holm KJ, Goa KL. Zolpidem: an update of its pharmacology, therapeutic efficacy and tolerability in the treatment of insomnia. Drugs. 2000;59:865–89.

91. Hopkins DR, Sethi KB, Mucklow JC. Benzodiazepine withdrawal in general practice. J R Coll Gen Pract. 1982;32:758–62.

92. Huston PG. Moderating benzodiazepine use in the elderly. Can Fam Phys. 1992;38:2459–67.

93. Jensen B. Benzodiazepine comparison chart. In: Jensen B, Regier L, editors. RxFiles Drug Comparison Charts. 9th ed. Saskatoon: Saskatoon Health Region; 2013. p. 101.

94. Keck Jr PE, McElroy SL, Friedman LM. Valproate and carbamazepine in the treatment of panic and posttraumatic stress disorders, withdrawal states, and behavioral dyscontrol syndromes. J Clin Psychopharmacol. 1992;12 Suppl 1:36S–41S.

95. Alcohol and other drug withdrawal practice guidelines. Drug and Alcohol Clinical Advisory Service. 2009. http://www.dacas.org.au/Clinical_Resources/Clinical_Guidelines.aspx. Accessed 31 Mar 2014.

96. Klein E. The role of extended-release benzodiazepines in the treatment of anxiety: a risk-benefit evaluation with a focus on extended-release alprazolam. J Clin Psychiatry. 2002;63 Suppl 14:27–33.

97. Klein E, Colin V, Stolk J, Lenox RH. Alprazolam withdrawal in patients with panic disorder and generalized anxiety disorder: vulnerability and effect of carbamazepine. Am J Psychiatry. 1994;151:1760–6.

98. Kunz D, Bineau S, Maman K, Milea D, Toumi M. Benzodiazepine discontinuation with prolonged-release melatonin: hints from a German longitudinal prescription database. Expert Opin Pharmacother. 2012;13:9–16.

99. Lader M. Benzodiazepines revisited–will we ever learn? Addiction. 2011;106:2086–109.

100. Lader M. Long-term anxiolytic therapy: the issue of drug withdrawal. J Clin Psychiatry. 1987;48 Suppl 12:12–6.

101. Lader M, Farr I, Morton S. A comparison of alpidem and placebo in relieving benzodiazepine withdrawal symptoms. Int Clin Psychopharmacol. 1993;8:31–6.

102. Lader M, Olajide D. A comparison of buspirone and placebo in relieving benzodiazepine withdrawal symptoms. J Clin Psychopharmacol. 1987;7:11–5.

103. Lader M, Tylee A, Donoghue J. Withdrawing benzodiazepines in primary care. CNS Drugs. 2009;23:19–34.

104. Lähteenmäki R, Puustinen J, Vahlberg T, Lyles A, Neuvonen PJ, Partinen M, et al. Melatonin for sedative withdrawal in older patients with primary insomnia: a randomised double-blind placebo-controlled trial. Br J Clin Pharmacol. 2013;77:975–85.

105. Landry MJ, Smith DE, McDuff DR, Baughman 3rd OL. Benzodiazepine dependence and withdrawal: identification and medical management. J Am Board Fam Pract. 1992;5:167–75.

106. Lemoine P, Allain H, Janus C, Sutet P. Gradual withdrawal of zopiclone (7.5 mg) and zolpidem (10 mg) in insomniacs treated for at least 3 months. Eur Psychiatry. 1995;10(3):161S–5S.

107. Lemoine P, Kermadi I, Garcia-Acosta S, Garay RP, Dib M. Double-blind, comparative study of cyamemazine vs. bromazepam in the benzodiazepine withdrawal syndrome. Prog Neuropsychopharmacol Biol Psychiatry. 2006;30:131–7.

108. Lopez-Peig C, Mundet X, Casabella B, del Val JL, Lacasta D, Diogene E. Analysis of benzodiazepine withdrawal program managed by primary care nurses in Spain. BMC Res Notes. 2012;5:684.

109. MacKinnon GL, Parker WA. Benzodiazepine withdrawal syndrome: a literature review and evaluation. Am J Drug Alcohol Abuse. 1982;9:19–33.

110. Insomnia: benzodiazepines, complementary medicines and non-drug treatments. National Prescribing Service. 2002. http://www.nps.org.au/publications/health-professional/nps-news/2006/nps-news-24. Accessed 31 Mar 2014.

111. Marriott S, Tyrer P. Benzodiazepine dependence: avoidance and withdrawal. Drug Saf. 1993;9:93–103.

112. Mercier-Guyon C, Chabannes JP, Saviuc P. The role of captodiamine in the withdrawal from long-term benzodiazepine treatment. Curr Med Res Opin. 2004;20:1347–55.

113. Michelini S, Cassano GB, Frare F, Perugi G. Long-term use of benzodiazepines: tolerance, dependence and clinical problems in anxiety and mood disorders. Pharmacopsychiatry. 1996;29:127–34.

114. Morin CM, Bastien C, Guay B, Radouco-Thomas M, Leblanc J, Vallières A. Randomized clinical trial of supervised tapering and cognitive behavior therapy to facilitate benzodiazepine discontinuation in older adults with chronic insomnia. Am J Psychiatry. 2004;161:332–42.

115. Morin CM, Colecchi CA, Ling WD, Sood RK. Cognitive behavior therapy to facilitate benzodiazepine discontinuation among hypnotic-dependent patients with insomnia. Behav Ther. 1995;26:733–45.

116. Morton S, Lader M. Buspirone treatment as an aid to benzodiazepine withdrawal. J Psychopharmacol. 1995;9:331–5.

117. Mugunthan K, McGuire T, Glasziou P. Minimal interventions to decrease long-term use of benzodiazepines in primary care: a systematic review and meta-analysis. Br J Gen Pract. 2011;61:e573–8.

118. Murphy SM, Tyrer P. A double-blind comparison of the effects of gradual withdrawal of lorazepam, diazepam and bromazepam in benzodiazepine dependence. Br J Psychiatry. 1991;158:511–6.

119. Nakao M, Takeuchi T, Nomura K, Teramoto T, Yano E. Clinical application of paroxetine for tapering benzodiazepine use in non-major-depressive outpatients visiting an internal medicine clinic. Psychiatry Clin Neurosci. 2006;60:605–10.

120. Nardi AE, Freire RC, Valenca AM, Amrein R, de Cerqueira AC, Lopes FL, et al. Tapering clonazepam in patients with panic disorder after at least 3 years of treatment. J Clin Psychopharmacol. 2010;30:290–3.

121. Nathan RG, Robinson D, Cherek DR, Sebastian CS, Hack M, Davison S. Alternative treatments for withdrawing the long-term benzodiazepine user: a pilot study. Int J Addict. 1986;21:195–211.

122. Management options for improving sleep. National Prescribing Service. 2010. http://www.nps.org.au/publications/health-professional/prescribing-practice-review/2010/prescribing-practice-review-49. Accessed 31 Mar 2014.

123. Benzodiazepines: managing withdrawal. National Prescribing Service. 1999. http://www.nps.org.au/publications/health-professional/nps-news/2006/nps-news-4. Accessed 31 Mar 2014.

124. Benzodiazepine and z-drug withdrawal. National Health Service. 2013. http://cks.nice.org.uk/benzodiazepine-and-z-drug-withdrawal. Accessed 31 Mar 2014.

125. What's wrong with prescribing hypnotics? Drug Ther Bull. http://dtb.bmj.com/content/42/12/89.abstract (http://dtb.bmj.com/content/42/12/89.abstract) 2004;42:89–93.

126. Appendix B-6: Benzodiazepine tapering. In: Canadian guideline for safe and effective use of opioids for chronic non-cancer pain. National Opioid Use Guideline Group. 2010. http://nationalpaincentre.mcmaster.ca/opioid/cgop_b_app_b06.html. Accessed 31 Mar 2014.

127. Noyes Jr R, Garvey MJ, Cook BL, Perry PJ. Benzodiazepine withdrawal: a review of the evidence. J Clin Psychiatry. 1988;49:382–9.

128. Drug and alcohol withdrawal clinical practice guidelines. NSW Government. 2008. http://www.health.nsw.gov.au/mhdao/Pages/pubs-guidelines.aspx. Accessed 31 Mar 2014.

129. O'Connor K, Marchand A, Brousseau L, Aardema F, Mainguy N, Landry P, et al. Cognitive-behavioural, pharmacological and psychosocial predictors of outcome during tapered discontinuation of benzodiazepine. Clin Psychol Psychother. 2008;15:1–14.

130. Onyett SR. The benzodiazepine withdrawal syndrome and its management. J R Coll Gen Pract. 1989;39:160–3.

131. Onyett SR, Turpin G. Benzodiazepine withdrawal in primary care: a comparison of behavioural group training and individual sessions. Behav Psychother. 1988;16:297–312.

132. Otto MW, Hong JJ, Safren SA. Benzodiazepine discontinuation difficulties in panic disorder: conceptual model and outcome for cognitive-behavior therapy. Curr Pharm Des. 2002;8:75–80.

133. Otto MW, McHugh RK, Simon NM, Farach FJ, Worthington JJ, Pollack MH. Efficacy of CBT for benzodiazepine discontinuation in patients with panic disorder: further evaluation. Behav Res Ther. 2010;48:720–7.

134. Otto MW, Pollack MH, Meltzer-Brody S, Rosenbaum JF. Cognitive-behavioral therapy for benzodiazepine discontinuation in panic disorder patients. Psychopharmacol Bull. 1992;28:123–30.

135. Otto MW, Pollack MH, Sachs GS, Reiter SR, Meltzer-Brody S, Rosenbaum JF. Discontinuation of benzodiazepine treatment: efficacy of cognitive-behavioral therapy for patients with panic disorder. Am J Psychiatry. 1993;150:1485–90.

136. Oude Voshaar RC, Couvee JE, Balkom AJ, Mulder PG, Zitman FG. Strategies for discontinuing long-term benzodiazepine use: meta-analysis. Br J Psychiatry. 2006;189:213–20.

137. Oude Voshaar RC, Gorgels WJ, Mol AJ, Balkom AJ, Lisdonk EH, Breteler MH, et al. Tapering off long-term benzodiazepine use with or without group cognitive-behavioural therapy: three-condition, randomised controlled trial. Br J Psychiatry. 2003;182:498–504.

138. Parr JM, Kavanagh DJ, Cahill L, Mitchell G, Young RM. Effectiveness of current treatment approaches for benzodiazepine discontinuation: a meta-analysis. Addiction. 2009;104:13–24.

139. Pat-Horenczyk R, Hacohen D, Herer P, Lavie P. The effects of substituting zopiclone in withdrawal from chronic use of benzodiazepine hypnotics. Psychopharmacology (Berl). 1998;140:450–7.

140. Pecknold JC. Discontinuation reactions to alprazolam in panic disorder. J Psychiatr Res. 1993;27 Suppl 1:155–70.

141. Peles E, Hetzroni T, Bar-Hamburger R, Adelson M, Schreiber S. Melatonin for perceived sleep disturbances associated with benzodiazepine withdrawal among patients in methadone maintenance treatment: a double-blind randomized clinical trial. Addiction. 2007;102:1947–53.

142. Petrovic M, Mariman A, Warie H, Afschrift M, Pevernagie D. Is there a rationale for prescription of benzodiazepines in the elderly? Review of the literature. Acta Clin Belg. 2003;58:27–36.

143. Poyares DR, Guilleminault C, Ohayon MM, Tufik S. Can valerian improve the sleep of insomniacs after benzodiazepine withdrawal? Prog Neuropsychopharmacol Biol Psychiatry. 2002;26:539–45.

144. Raju B, Meagher D. Patient-controlled benzodiazepine dose reduction in a community mental health service. Ir J Psychol Med. 2005;22:42–5.

145. Rickels K, DeMartinis N, García-España F, Greenblatt DJ, Mandos LA, Rynn M. Imipramine and buspirone in treatment of patients with generalized anxiety disorder who are discontinuing long-term benzodiazepine therapy. Am J Psychiatry. 2000;157:1973–9.

146. Rickels K, Schweizer E, García-España F, Case G, DeMartinis N, Greenblatt D. Trazodone and valproate in patients discontinuing long-term benzodiazepine therapy: effects on withdrawal symptoms and taper outcome. Psychopharmacology (Berl). 1999;141:1–5.

147. Rickels K, DeMartinis N, Rynn M, Mandos L. Pharmacologic strategies for discontinuing benzodiazepine treatment. J Clin Psychopharmacol. 1999;19 Suppl 2:12S–6S.

148. Romach MK, Kaplan HL, Busto UE, Somer G, Sellers EM. A controlled trial of ondansetron, a 5-HT3 antagonist, in benzodiazepine discontinuation. J Clin Psychopharmacol. 1998;18:121–31.

149. Roth SM. Anxiety disorders and the use and abuse of drugs. J Clin Psychiatry. 1989;50 Suppl 11:30–5.

150. Roy-Byrne PP, Sullivan MD, Cowley DS, Ries RK. Adjunctive treatment of benzodiazepine discontinuation syndromes: a review. J Psychiatr Res. 1993;27 Suppl 1:143–53.

151. Roy-Byrne PP, Cowley DS. The use of benzodiazepines in the workplace. J Psychoactive Drugs. 1990;22:461–5.

152. Roy-Byrne PP, Hommer D. Benzodiazepine withdrawal: overview and implications for the treatment of anxiety. Am J Med. 1988;84:1041–52.

153. Rynn M, García-España F, Greenblatt DJ, Mandos LA, Schweizer E, Rickels K. Imipramine and buspirone in patients with panic disorder who are discontinuing long-term benzodiazepine therapy. J Clin Psychopharmacol. 2003;23:505–8.

154. Sanchez-Craig M, Cappell H, Busto U, Kay G. Cognitive-behavioural treatment for benzodiazepine dependence: a comparison of gradual versus abrupt cessation of drug intake. Br J Addict. 1987;82:1317–27.

155. Saul PA, Korlipara K, Presley P. A randomised, multicentre, double-blind, comparison of atenolol and placebo in the control of benzodiazepine withdrawal symptoms. Acta Ther. 1989;15:117–23.

156. Schweizer E, Rickels K. Benzodiazepine dependence and withdrawal: a review of the syndrome and its clinical management. Acta Psychiatr Scand Suppl. 1998;393:95–101.

157. Schweizer E, Rickels K. Failure of buspirone to manage benzodiazepine withdrawal. Am J Psychiatry. 1986;143:1590–2.

158. Schweizer E, Rickels K, Case WG, Greenblatt DJ. Carbamazepine treatment in patients discontinuing long-term benzodiazepine therapy: effects on withdrawal severity and outcome. Arch Gen Psychiatry. 1991;48:448–52.

159. Schweizer E, Rickels K, Case WG, Greenblatt DJ. Long-term therapeutic use of benzodiazepines II: effects of gradual taper. Arch Gen Psychiatry. 1990;47:908–15.

160. Schweizer E, Case WG, García-España F, Greenblatt DJ, Rickels K. Progesterone co-administration in patients discontinuing long-term benzodiazepine therapy: effects on withdrawal severity and taper outcome. Psychopharmacology (Berl). 1995;117:424–9.

161. Shapiro CM, Sherman D, Peck DF. Withdrawal from benzodiazepines by initially switching to zopiclone. Eur Psychiatry. 1995;10 Suppl 3:145S–51S.

162. Sloan E. Medication and substance use: keeping insomnia treatment safe. Insomnia Rounds. 2013;2:1–6.

163. Smith AJ, Tett SE. Improving the use of benzodiazepines–is it possible? A non-systematic review of interventions tried in the last 20 years. BMC Health Serv Res. 2010;10:321.

164. Spiegel DA. Psychological strategies for discontinuing benzodiazepine treatment. J Clin Psychopharmacol. 1999;19 Suppl 2:17S–22S.

165. Stewart R, Niessen WJ, Broer J, Snijders TA, Haaijer-Ruskamp FM, Meyboom-De JB. General practitioners reduced benzodiazepine prescriptions in an intervention study: a multilevel application. J Clin Epidemiol. 2007;60:1076–84.

166. Taylor DJ, Schmidt-Nowara W, Jessop CA, Ahearn J. Sleep restriction therapy and hypnotic withdrawal versus sleep hygiene education in hypnotic using patients with insomnia. J Clin Sleep Med. 2010;6:169–75.

167. Management of anxiety disorders in primary care. Therapeutics Initiative. 1997. http://www.ti.ubc.ca/newsletter/management-anxiety-disorders-primary-care. Accessed 31 Mar 2014.

168. Thirtala T, Kaur K, Karlapati SK, Lippmann S. Consider this slow-taper program for benzodiazepines. Curr Psychiatr. 2013;12:55–6.

169. Addressing hypnotic medicines use in primary care. National Prescribing Service. 2010. http://www.nps.org.au/publications/health-professional/nps-news/2010/nps-news-67. Accessed 31 Mar 2014.

170. Tyrer P, Ferguson B, Hallström C, Michie M, Tyrer S, Cooper S, et al. A controlled trial of dothiepin and placebo in treating benzodiazepine withdrawal symptoms. Br J Psychiatry. 1996;168:457–61.

171. Tyrer PJ, Seivewright N. Identification and management of benzodiazepine dependence. Postgrad Med J. 1984;60 Suppl 2:41–6.

172. Udelman HD, Udelman DL. Concurrent use of buspirone in anxious patients during withdrawal from alprazolam therapy. J Clin Psychiatry. 1990;51:46–50.

173. van de Steeg-van Gompel CH, Wensing M, De Smet PA. Implementation of a discontinuation letter to reduce long-term benzodiazepine use: a cluster randomized trial. Drug Alcohol Depend. 2009;99:105–14.

174. Vicens C, Fiol F, Llobera J, Campoamor F, Mateu C, Alegret S, et al. Withdrawal from long-term benzodiazepine use: randomised trial in family practice. Br J Gen Pract. 2006;56:958–63.

175. Vicens C, Bejarano F, Sempere E, Mateu C, Fiol F, Socías I, et al. Comparative efficacy of two interventions to discontinue long-term benzodiazepine use: cluster randomised controlled trial in primary care. Br J Psychiatry. 2014;204:471–9.

176. Vissers FH, Knipschild PG, Crebolder HF. Is melatonin helpful in stopping the long-term use of hypnotics? a discontinuation trial. Pharm World Sci. 2007;29:641–6.

177. Vorma H, Naukkarinen H, Sarna S, Kuoppasalmi K. Treatment of out-patients with complicated benzodiazepine dependence: comparison of two approaches. Addiction. 2002;97:851–9.

178. Woodward M. Hypnotics: options to help your patients stop. Aust Fam Physician. 2000;29:939–44.

179. Woodward M. Hypnosedatives in the elderly: a guide to appropriate use. CNS Drugs. 1999;11:263–79.

180. Zee P, Wang-Weigand S, Roth T. Facilitation of zolpidem discontinuation using ramelteon in subjects with chronic insomnia. Am J Addict. 2011;20:380–1.

181. Atkins D, Best D, Briss PA, Mrukowicz J, O'Connell D, Oxman AD, et al. Grading quality of evidence and strength of recommendations. BMJ. 2004;328:1490.

182. Guyatt GH, Haynes RB, Jaeschke RZ, Cook DJ, Green L, Naylor CD, et al. Users' Guides to the Medical Literature: XXV. Evidence-based medicine: principles for applying the Users' Guides to patient care. Evidence-Based Medicine Working Group. JAMA. 2000;284:1290–6.

183. Guyatt GH, Sackett DL, Sinclair JC, Hayward R, Cook DJ, Cook RJ. Users' Guides to the medical literature. IX. A method for grading health care recommendations. Evidence-Based Medicine Working Group. JAMA. 1995;274:1800–4.

184. Oxford levels of evidence 2. Centre for Evidence Based Medicine. 2011. http://www.cebm.net/index.aspx?o=5653. Accessed 28 Nov 2014.

185. Coumou HC, Meijman FJ. How do primary care physicians seek answers to clinical questions? A literature review. J Med Libr Assoc. 2006;94:55–60.

186. Lewis PJ, Tully MP. The discomfort of an evidence-based prescribing decision. J Eval Clin Pract. 2009;15:1152–8.

187. Swennen MH, van der Heijden GJ, Boeije HR, van Rheenen N, Verheul FJ, van der Graaf Y, et al. Doctors' perceptions and use of evidence-based medicine: a systematic review and thematic synthesis of qualitative studies. Acad Med. 2013;88:1384–96.

188. Murphy AL, Fleming M, Martin-Misener R, Sketris IS, MacCara M, Gass D. Drug information resources used by nurse practitioners and collaborating physicians at the point of care in Nova Scotia. Canada: a survey and review of the literature BMC Nurs. 2006;5:5.

189. Kravitz RL, Bell RA. Media, messages, and medication: strategies to reconcile what patients hear, what they want, and what they need from medications. BMC Med Inform Decis Mak. 2013;13 Suppl 3:S5.

190. Hoffmann TC, Glasziou PP, Boutron I, Milne R, Perera R, Moher D, et al. Better reporting of interventions: template for intervention description and replication (TIDieR) checklist and guide. BMJ. 2014;348:g1687.

191. Albrecht L, Archibald M, Arseneau D, Scott SD. Development of a checklist to assess the quality of reporting of knowledge translation interventions using the workgroup for intervention development and evaluation research (WIDER) recommendations. Implement Sci. 2013;8:52.

192. Damschroder LJ, Aron DC, Keith RE, Kirsh SR, Alexander JA, Lowery JC. Fostering implementation of health services research findings into practice: a consolidated framework for advancing implementation science. Implement Sci. 2009;4:50.

193. Pringsheim T, Gardner DM. Dispensed prescriptions for quetiapine and other second-generation antipsychotics in Canada from 2005 to 2012: a descriptive study. CMAJ Open. 2014;2:E225–32.

194. Pawson R, Greenhalgh T, Harvey G, Walshe K. Realist review–a new method of systematic review designed for complex policy interventions. J Health Serv Res Policy. 2005;10:21–34.

195. Rycroft-Malone J, McCormack B, Hutchinson AM, DeCorby K, Bucknall TK, Kent B, et al. Realist synthesis: illustrating the method for implementation research. Implement Sci. 2012;7:33.

196. Reeve E, Shakib S, Hendrix I, Roberts MS, Wiese MD. Review of deprescribing processes and development of an evidence-based, patient-centred deprescribing process. Br J Clin Pharmacol. 2014;78:738–47.

197. Reeve E, Shakib S, Hendrix I, Roberts MS, Wiese MD. The benefits and harms of deprescribing. Med J Aust. 2014;201:386–9.

198. Curran HV, Collins R, Fletcher S, Kee SC, Woods B, Iliffe S. Older adults and withdrawal from benzodiazepine hypnotics in general practice: effects on cognitive function, sleep, mood and quality of life. Psychol Med. 2003;33:1223–37.

25

Analgesic use in a Norwegian general population: change over time and high-risk use - The Tromsø Study

Per-Jostein Samuelsen[1,2*], Lars Slørdal[3,4], Ulla Dorte Mathisen[5] and Anne Elise Eggen[2]

Abstract

Background: Increased use of analgesics in the population is a cause for concern in terms of drug safety. There is a paucity of population-based studies monitoring the change in use over time of both non-prescription (OTC) analgesics and prescription (Rx) analgesics. Although much is known about the risks associated with analgesic use, we are lacking knowledge on high-risk use at a population level. The purpose of this study was to estimate the prevalence of non-prescription and prescription analgesic use, change over time and the prevalence in the presence of potential contraindications and drug interactions in a general population.

Methods: A repeated cross-sectional study with data from participants (30–89 years) of the Tromsø Study in 2001–02 (Tromsø 5; $N = 8039$) and in 2007–08 (Tromsø 6; $N = 12,981$). Participants reported use of OTC and Rx analgesics and regular use of all drugs in the preceding four weeks. Change over the time period was analyzed with generalized estimating equations. The prevalence of regular analgesic use in persons with or without a clinically significant contraindication or drug interaction was determined in the Tromsø 6 population, and differences were tested with logistic regression.

Results: Analgesic use increased from 54 to 60 % in women (OR = 1.24, 95 % CI 1.15–1.32) and from 29 to 37 % in men (OR = 1.39, 95 % CI 1.27–1.52) in the time period; the increase was due to sporadic use of OTC analgesics. There was substantial regular use of analgesics in several of the contraindication categories examined; the prevalence of non-steroidal anti-inflammatory drugs was more than eight per cent among persons with chronic kidney disease, gastrointestinal ulcers, or high primary cardiovascular risk. About four per cent of the study population demonstrated at least one potential drug interaction with an analgesic drug.

Conclusions: The use of analgesics increased in the time period due to an increase in the use of OTC analgesics. Analgesic exposure in the presence of contraindications or drug interactions may put patients at risk. Public and prescriber awareness about clinically relevant contraindications and drug interactions with analgesics need to be increased.

Keywords: Analgesics, NSAIDs, Drug interactions, Contraindications, Prevalence, Pharmacoepidemiology

* Correspondence: per-jostein.samuelsen@unn.no
[1]Regional Medicines Information and Pharmacovigilance Center (RELIS),
University Hospital of North Norway, N-9038 Tromsø, Norway
[2]Department of Community Medicine, UiT-The Arctic University of Norway,
Tromsø, Norway
Full list of author information is available at the end of the article

Background

The availability of analgesics has increased in Norway due to a major rise in the number of pharmacies since 2001 and the release of ibuprofen and paracetamol to general sales in supermarkets, grocery stores and petrol stations in 2003 [1]. The sales of analgesics has increased considerably in Norway over the last decades [2]. The prevalence of analgesic use has been examined in several international cross-sectional studies [3–10]. However, there is a paucity of population-based studies monitoring the change in use over time of both OTC analgesics and prescription (Rx) analgesics.

Increased use of analgesics in the population is a cause for concern in terms of drug safety. Paracetamol and in particular non-steroidal anti-inflammatory drugs (NSAIDs) and opioids are among the drugs that are most often implicated in serious or fatal medication errors [11]. NSAID use is associated with increased risk of cardiovascular disease (CVD) [12–14], gastrointestinal damage [15], renal disease [16, 17] and a number of drug interactions [15, 18]. Opioids have an abuse potential but few adverse effects when used correctly. They can, however, produce respiratory depression [15, 19] and increase the risk of falls and subsequent injuries [20], particularly in combinations with other central nervous system (CNS) depressant drugs [19]. Paracetamol, although considered safe in recommended doses, is hepatotoxic in high doses and can give rise to drug induced liver injury [21]; there is some concern about a possible association with increased CVD risk [22]. The potential inappropriate use of analgesics in the general population has previously been reported in smaller studies of variable rigor, most of them focusing on OTC analgesics [7, 23–27].

This study aimed to estimate the prevalence of OTC and Rx analgesic use, change over time and the prevalence of use in the presence of potential contraindications and pharmacodynamic drug interactions.

Methods

Study population

The Tromsø Study is a population-based study of various health issues and diseases. It consists of six surveys (Tromsø 1–6) carried out in the municipality of Tromsø, Norway, from 1974 to 2008 [28]. Eligible for the present study were participants from Tromsø 5 (2001–02, $N = 8039$) and Tromsø 6 (2007–08, $N = 12,981$), aged 30–89 years (Fig. 1). The participants in Tromsø 5 and Tromsø 6 consisted of persons who attended a second visit in Tromsø 4 in 1994–5 (i.e. all Tromsø inhabitants aged 55–74 years, and a 5–10 % random sample of those 25–50 and 75–85 years of age were invited), in addition to whole birth cohorts or random samples of birth cohorts (see [28, 29] for further explanation). A total of 4630 individuals participated in both Tromsø 5 and Tromsø 6. The data collection is described elsewhere [29]. An English translation of the questionnaires is available at the Tromsø Study homepage (www.tromsostudy.com).

Definition of analgesic use

Analgesic use was assessed through questionnaire based on the question "How often have you used painkillers [with]/[without] prescription during the last four weeks?" (Fig. 1). Analgesic users were defined as persons reporting any use. This variable was recoded into use of OTC analgesics only ("OTC"), use of prescribed analgesics only ("Rx") and use of concomitantly OTC and prescribed analgesics ("OTC + Rx"; Fig. 1).

Participants in Tromsø 6 also reported drugs used regularly the preceding four weeks; this was coded according to the Anatomical Therapeutic Chemical (ATC) classification system version 2007 (www.whocc.no). Analgesics were defined as belonging to ATC groups N02B (other antipyretic and analgesic drugs), N02A (opioids) and M01A (NSAIDs, excluding glucosamine).

Criteria for contraindications and drug interactions

The analyses of potential contraindications and drug interactions were done among participants in Tromsø 6 (Fig. 1). A contraindication was defined as a condition that indicates that a drug should not be used. The criteria were developed a priori, based on literature and available variables:

Chronic kidney disease: estimated glomerular filtration rate (eGFR) < 60 ml/min per 1.73 m^2 or ≥ 60 ml/min per 1.73 m^2 and either macroalbuminuria or persistent microalbuminuria [30]. EGFR was estimated by the CKD-EPI equation [31]. *Gastrointestinal ulcers*: self-reported stomach or duodenal ulcer or ulcer surgery. A secondary measure was use of H2 antagonists, misoprostol or proton pump inhibitors (ATC codes A02B A, A02B B, A02B C, respectively). *CVD*: NORRISK cardiovascular risk score estimates the 10-year risk of fatal CVD, using sex, age, systolic blood pressure, total cholesterol and smoking [32]. The primary CVD risk group was defined as individuals with no prior myocardial infarction (MI), angina pectoris or stroke, aged 40–49 years and with a NORRISK score > 1 %; 50–59 years and NORRISK score ≥ 5 %; or 60–69 years and NORRISK score ≥ 10 % according to national guidelines [33]. The secondary CVD risk group consisted of those with a history of stroke, MI or angina pectoris. *Hypertension*: systolic blood pressure ≥ 140 mmHg or diastolic blood pressure ≥ 90 mmHg or self-reported current use of antihypertensive drugs. *Interacting drugs*: warfarin (B01A A03), low-dose acetylsalicylic acid (ASA; B01A C06), selective serotonin reuptake inhibitors (SSRI; N06A B), glucocorticoids (H02A B), angiotensin converting enzyme (ACE) inhibitors (C09A, C09B), angiotensin II (AT II) antagonists (C09C, C09D), other antihypertensive drugs

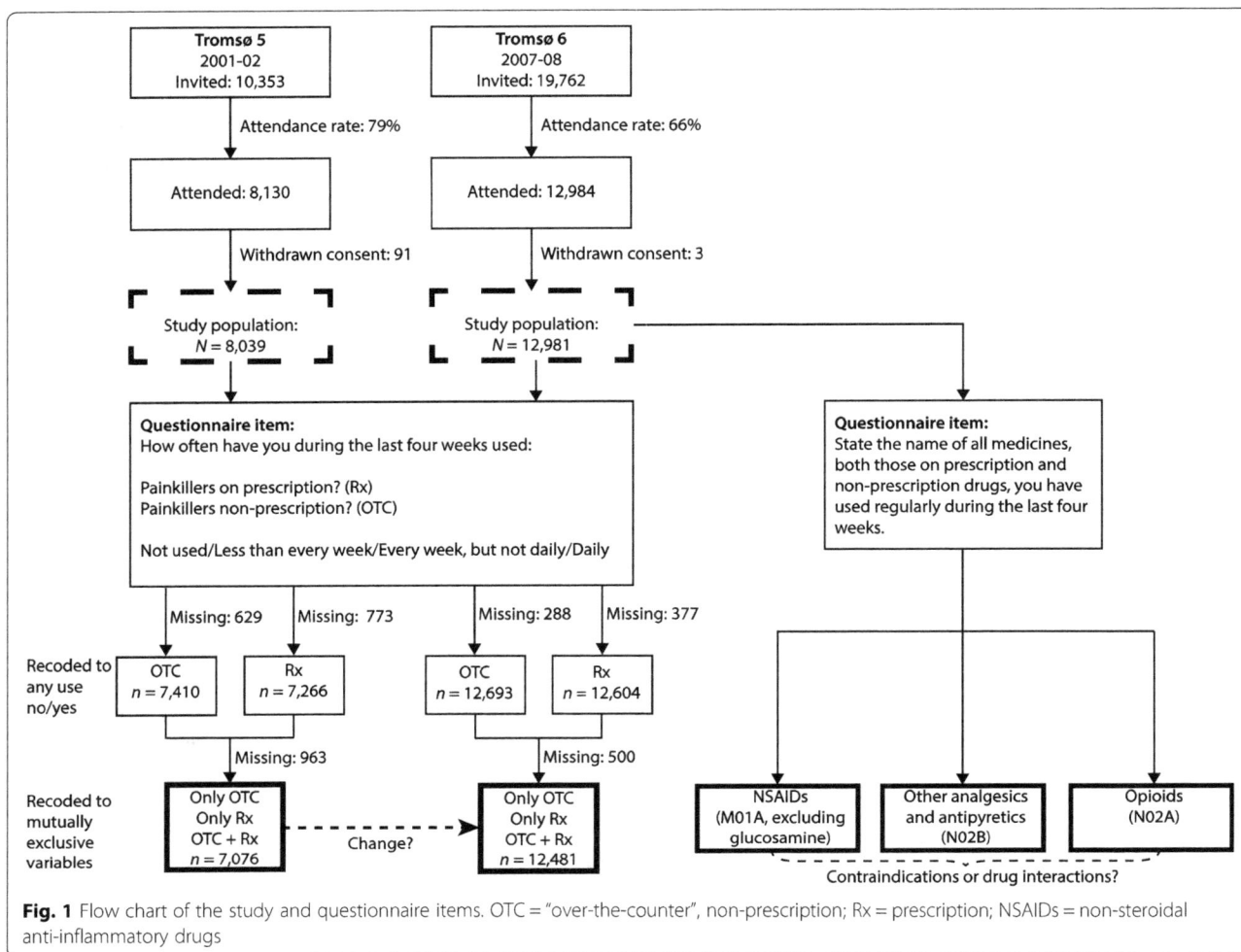

Fig. 1 Flow chart of the study and questionnaire items. OTC = "over-the-counter", non-prescription; Rx = prescription; NSAIDs = non-steroidal anti-inflammatory drugs

(C02, C03, C07, C08) and CNS depressant drugs (N05C A-F, N05B A, N03A E, N03A A). *Use of multiple analgesics*: regular use of more than one analgesic drug within the same pharmacological group: NSAIDs, opioids and paracetamol-containing drugs (N02B E01 and N02A A59).

Statistical analysis

Descriptive statistics were age-adjusted with logistic regression (*adjprop* command). The changes in prevalences between Tromsø 5 and Tromsø 6 were tested with generalized estimating equations (GEE) and estimated as odds ratios (ORs) with 95 % confidence intervals (CI) using a logit link function, exchangeable covariance matrix and robust standard errors; separate binary GEE models were fitted for each prescription category with non-users of both OTC and Rx as the reference group. The prevalence measures were age-adjusted by the direct method, with the Norwegian population per 01.01.2008 as standard population [34]. Linear age trends across age groups were tested with logistic regression. Sex differences in age-adjusted prevalences were

tested with two-sample proportion test (Z test) and crude prevalences with Fisher's exact test. Differences in analgesic use in the absence or presence of contraindications or drug interactions were tested with logistic regression and likelihood ratio test, adjusted for age and sex (*adjprop*). All analyses were complete case analyses. The overall proportion of missing data in the dependent variables in the GEE analyses was 12.0 % in Tromsø 5 and 3.9 % in Tromsø 6 (Fig. 1). Sensitivity analyses by imputing missing values as non-user or user, were generally consistent with the main results. All analyses were conducted in Stata 13.1 (Stata Corp, College Station, Texas).

Ethics

This study has been approved by the Regional Committee for Medical and Health Research Ethics, North Norway (2012/1636), and was performed in accordance with the 1964 Helsinki declaration and its later amendments. Informed consent was obtained from all individual participants included in the study.

Results

There was a tendency of worsening health, more pain and less education across the analgesic user groups, from non-users to users of OTC + Rx analgesics (Table 1).

Women used more analgesics than men, both in total and in all prescription categories, in both surveys (Table 2). The total analgesic use decreased with age in both sexes and in both surveys ($p < .001$). The use of OTC decreased, whereas Rx increased with age in both sexes and in both surveys.

The total use of analgesics and the use of OTC increased in the time period (Table 2). Total use increased from 53.7 to 59.6 % in women and from 29.1 to 36.7 % in men, corresponding to OR = 1.24, 95 % CI 1.15–1.32 and OR = 1.39, 95 % CI 1.27–1.52, respectively. The use of Rx analgesics did not show any change, while the use of OTC + Rx analgesics increased in both women and men. When the analyses were restricted to frequent users, defined as daily or weekly users, there was no change in total use (data not shown).

The crude prevalences of regular use of NSAIDs, other analgesics and antipyretics, and opioids were 12.7 % ($n =$ 1646), 12.5 % ($n = 1624$) and 3.7 % ($n = 475$), respectively. The prevalences of cyclooxygenase 2 (COX-2) inhibitors and high-dose ASA use were 0.1 % ($n = 13$) and 0.2 % ($n = 31$), respectively. The use of NSAIDs and other analgesics decreased with age in both sexes ($p < .001$), while opioid use increased in women ($p = .048$) and decreased in men ($p = .027$; Fig. 2). More women than men used analgesics regularly ($p < .001$). The sex difference for opioids was only apparent in the highest age groups (≥ 60 years).

Table 3 shows the prevalence of regular analgesic use in the absence or presence of contraindications. The prevalence was high in several of the contraindication groups; for the important contraindications chronic kidney disease, gastrointestinal ulcer diseases and high

Table 1 Charactheristics of non-users and users of OTC, Rx, or combined OTC + Rx analgesics

	Non-users		OTC		Rx		OTC + Rx	
	% (n)		% (n)		% (n)		% (n)	
Analgesic use (n = 12,481)[a]	53.8	(6719)	31.7	(3957)	5.1	(641)	9.3	(1164)
Sex, % women (n = 12,481)	41.8	(2818)	65.1	(2561)	58.6	(378)	70.8	(824)
Age (n = 12,481)								
30–39	3.2	(213)	6.2	(247)	1.2	(8)	3.3	(38)
40–49	23.1	(1549)	37.4	(1479)	20.7	(133)	31.4	(365)
50–59	18.4	(1236)	20.5	(813)	16.8	(108)	18.1	(211)
60–69	35.5	(2388)	24.7	(979)	35.7	(229)	28.4	(330)
70–79	15.5	(1041)	8.8	(347)	20.1	(129)	14.8	(172)
80–87	4.3	(292)	2.3	(92)	5.3	(34)	4.1	(48)
Mean (SD), 30–87 years	58.9	(12.3)	53.6	(12.3)	60.8	(12.0)	57.1	(12.8)
Bad or very bad self-reported health (n = 12,390)	3.2	(226)	4.3	(162)	10.1	(70)	15.9	(185)
Education below college or university (n = 12,341)	59.9	(4029)	63.0	(2278)	69.4	(451)	74.3	(827)
Smoking, current daily (n = 12,329)	18.1	(1194)	21.1	(873)	24.1	(146)	27.5	(318)
Pain lasting three months or more (n = 12,462)	19.9	(1344)	35.6	(1393)	63.1	(404)	74.7	(868)
Headache, last year (n = 11,472)	18.5	(1156)	50.0	(1928)	46.7	(257)	61.3	(645)
Severe pain or stiffness in muscles, last four weeks								
Neck (n = 10,665)	4.2	(243)	9.6	(326)	20.1	(104)	29.5	(289)
Hip/leg (n = 10,531)	3.8	(237)	7.8	(249)	20.5	(122)	28.9	(280)
Psychological distress[b] (n = 11,941)	5.4	(343)	8.7	(340)	11.4	(67)	20.9	(230)
Frequent GP consultations, last 12 months[c] (n = 9335)	10.9	(538)	11.6	(343)	19.7	(105)	25.2	(243)
Drug use, last four weeks								
Antidepressants (n = 12,195)	1.6	(116)	2.9	(106)	4.3	(29)	9.0	(97)
Sleeping pills or tranquilizers (n = 12,164)	5.7	(476)	12.0	(445)	14.8	(112)	27.3	(297)

Age-adjusted. The Tromsø Study: Tromsø 6 (2007–8, n = 12,481)

OTC "over-the-counter", non-prescription, Rx prescription, SD standard deviation, GP general practitioner

[a] Crude prevalence

[b] Hopkins Symptoms Checklist 10-item version > 1.85

[c] ≥ 6 visits per year (>90th percentile)

Table 2 Prevalence of analgesic use and change over time

Survey		Population		OTC only			Rx only			OTC + Rx			Total		
Age (years)		T5 n (%)	T6 n (%)	T5 %	T6 %	OR (95 % CI)[a]	T5 %	T6 %	OR (95 % CI)[a]	T5 %	T6 %	OR (95 % CI)[a]	T5 %	T6 %	OR (95 % CI)[a]
Women															
30–39		408 (10.4)	295 (4.5)	46.3	55.6	1.45 (1.05–1.99)	2.2	1.4	0.75 (0.23–2.48)	10.3	9.2	1.09 (0.63–1.86)	58.8	66.1	1.37 (1.00–1.86)
40–49		710 (18.1)	1880 (28.6)	44.9	49.3	1.29 (1.07–1.56)	5.2	3.8	0.87 (0.57–1.31)	10.9	13.6	1.41 (1.08–1.84)	61.0	66.6	1.29 (1.08–1.53)
50–59		637 (16.2)	1245 (18.9)	32.2	43.6	1.68 (1.36–2.07)	6.0	5.1	1.05 (0.68–1.61)	12.7	11.7	1.85 (0.71–4.80)	50.9	60.4	1.49 (1.23–1.79)
60–69		1187 (30.2)	1987 (30.2)	29.0	31.4	1.11 (0.96–1.29)	7.6	7.1	0.96 (0.74–1.24)	11.2	11.5	1.01 (0.83–1.22)	47.8	50.0	1.06 (0.94–1.21)
70–79		871 (22.2)	886 (13.5)	23.7	26.1	1.16 (0.94–1.43)	9.5	8.5	0.95 (0.69–1.31)	11.5	14.3	1.25 (1.00–1.56)	44.7	48.9	1.14 (0.96–1.36)
80+		118 (3.0)	288 (4.4)	25.4	25.7	1.15 (0.68–1.92)	5.9	8.3	1.18 (0.80–1.77)	15.3	13.9	0.98 (0.53–1.82)	46.6	47.9	1.15 (0.76–1.74)
30–89		3931 (100)	6581 (100)	32.9	38.9	1.26 (1.17–1.36)	6.7	5.7	0.98 (0.84–1.14)	11.5	12.5	1.19 (1.08–1.30)	51.1	57.2	1.21 (1.13–1.30)
Age-adjusted[b]				36.7	42.9	1.30 (1.20–1.41)	5.5	4.8	0.98 (0.84–1.14)	11.5	11.9	1.20 (1.09–1.32)	53.7	59.6	1.24 (1.15–1.32)
p, age trend				<.001	<.001		<.001	<.001		.370	.471		<.001	<.001	
Men															
30–39		273 (8.7)	211 (3.6)	30.4	39.3	1.58 (1.08–2.30)	1.8	1.9	1.23 (0.32–4.64)	4.4	5.2	1.40 (0.60–3.29)	36.6	46.5	1.55 (1.08–2.22)
40–49		569 (18.1)	1646 (27.9)	27.2	33.6	1.45 (1.18–1.78)	2.6	3.8	1.69 (0.97–2.95)	3.3	6.7	2.39 (1.45–3.94)	33.2	44.1	1.56 (1.29–1.89)
50–59		332 (10.6)	1123 (19.0)	18.4	24.0	1.34 (1.01–1.79)	6.3	4.0	0.68 (0.42–1.13)	2.4	5.8	2.63 (1.25–5.51)	27.1	33.8	1.29 (1.01–1.65)
60–69		1108 (35.2)	1939 (32.9)	14.0	18.4	1.37 (1.13–1.66)	5.7	4.5	0.84 (0.61–1.15)	4.5	5.2	1.19 (0.87–1.63)	24.2	28.1	1.21 (1.04–1.41)
70–79		769 (24.5)	803 (13.6)	10.4	14.5	1.52 (1.13–2.06)	5.6	6.7	1.31 (0.88–1.94)	4.3	5.6	1.43 (0.91–2.24)	20.3	26.8	1.46 (1.17–1.83)
80+		94 (3.0)	178 (3.0)	10.6	10.1	0.93 (0.42–2.05)	7.5	5.6	0.75 (0.28–2.05)	1.1	4.5	4.27 (0.53–34.60)	19.2	20.2	1.05 (0.56–1.96)
30–89		3145 (100)	5900 (100)	17.3	23.7	1.46 (1.32–1.61)	4.9	4.5	1.02 (0.84–1.23)	3.9	5.8	1.59 (1.31–1.92)	26.1	33.9	1.38 (1.27–1.50)
Age-adjusted[b]				21.3	27.1	1.48 (1.33–1.65)	4.3	3.9	1.03 (0.85–1.24)	3.5	5.7	1.57 (1.29–1.91)	29.1	36.7	1.39 (1.27–1.52)
p, age trend				<.001	<.001		.001	.001		.727	.127		<.001	<.001	
p, sex				<.001	<.001		.037	.046		<.001	<.001		<.001	<.001	

The proportion of analgesic users last four weeks and odds ratios for use of analgesics in Tromsø 6 compared to Tromsø 5, according to age, sex and prescription category. The Tromsø Study: Tromsø 5 (2001–02, n = 7076) and Tromsø 6 (2007–08, n = 12,481)

OTC "over-the-counter", non-prescription, Rx prescription, T5 Tromsø 5, T6 Tromsø 6, CI confidence interval, OR odds ratio

[a]Reference category: non-users of both OTC and Rx

[b]Prevalence estimates age-adjusted with the Norwegian population 01.01.2008 as standard population

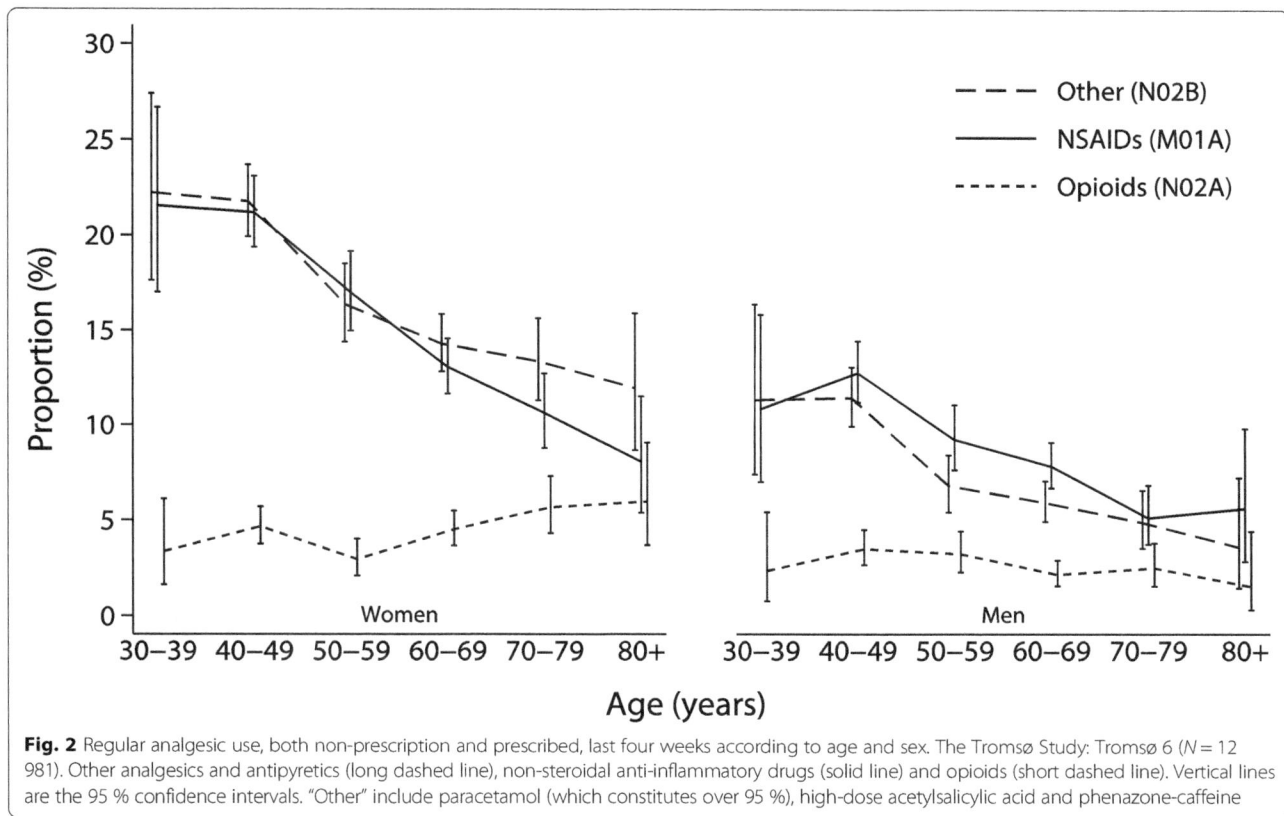

Fig. 2 Regular analgesic use, both non-prescription and prescribed, last four weeks according to age and sex. The Tromsø Study: Tromsø 6 (N = 12 981). Other analgesics and antipyretics (long dashed line), non-steroidal anti-inflammatory drugs (solid line) and opioids (short dashed line). Vertical lines are the 95 % confidence intervals. "Other" include paracetamol (which constitutes over 95 %), high-dose acetylsalicylic acid and phenazone-caffeine

Table 3 Regular use of analgesics in the absence or presence of contraindications

Contraindication[a]	Unadjusted		Age- and sex-adjusted			Potential clinical consequence
	Absent	Present	Absent	Present	p value	
	% (n)	% (n)	%	%		
Non-steroidal anti-inflammatory drugs						
Chronic kidney disease (6834/10.1)	11.2 (686)	8.6 (59)	11.6	12.0	.802	Acute renal failure, disease progression
GI ulcers						
Ulcers (11,516/7.4)	12.8 (1365)	12.0 (102)	11.8	12.6	.509	GI ulceration and complications
Ulcers or use of GI-protective drugs (11,516/10.7)	12.7 (1301)	13.4 (166)	11.6	14.1	.014	GI ulceration and complications
CVD						
High primary CVD risk (9000/13.0)	14.4 (1125)	11.1 (129)	12.1	13.5	.220	Increased risk of CVD
Stroke, MI, angina pectoris (12,540/9.6)	13.3 (1506)	6.7 (80)	12.1	8.8	.003	Increased risk of CVD
Hypertension (12,725/49.1)	14.2 (922)	11.3 (705)	11.5	12.5	.122	Increased blood pressure
Paracetamol						
CVD						
High primary CVD risk (9000/13.0)	14.5 (1139)	9.7 (113)	11.6	12.6	.401	Possible increased risk of CVD
Stroke, MI, angina pectoris (12,540/9.6)	13.8 (1565)	9.9 (119)	12.3	12.8	.712	Possible increased risk of CVD

The Tromsø Study: Tromsø 6 (N = 12,981)
GI gastrointestinal, *CVD* cardiovascular disease, *MI* myocardial infarction
[a]Numbers in parentheses are total n in variable and prevalence (%) in the study population

primary cardiovascular risk there were no differences in regular NSAID use between those with and without the contraindication, when adjusting for age and sex differences. Among the categories examined, only persons with a history of CVD had a lower prevalence of NSAID use compared to those without a CVD history.

Four hundred and sixteen instances of use of multiple analgesics were found in 384 persons; the proportions were 11.2 % (n = 184) in NSAID users, 12.0 % (n = 209) in users of paracetamol-containing analgesics and 4.8 % (n = 23) in opioid users.

Table 4 shows the prevalence of regular analgesic use in the absence or presence of interacting drugs. In total 4.1 % (n = 538) of the population presented at least one of the identified potential drug interactions. One percent presented more than one potential drug interaction. For interactions potentially increasing the bleeding risk, the use of NSAIDs was the same or higher among users of glucocorticoids or SSRIs, respectively. The use of NSAIDs was comparatively lower for patients using the anticoagulant warfarin and low-dose ASA.

Discussion

The use of analgesics increased from 2001–02 to 2007–08, due to an increase in the use of OTC analgesics. The prevalence of regular analgesic use in the contraindication categories examined was more than six per cent, and about four per cent of the study population presented at least one potential drug interaction with an analgesic drug. In particular, the use of NSAIDs in the presence of chronic kidney disease, gastrointestinal

ulcers, high primary risk of CVD and interacting drugs increasing the bleeding risk was a cause for concern.

The sales of NSAIDs more than doubled, paracetamol tripled, while high-dose ASA declined substantially in Norway from 1990 to 2013 [2]. A comparison of our data with data from the 1980s and 1990s [3–5, 10], and studies on changes in Rx analgesic use [35–37] points towards an increase in analgesic use from the 1980s to the present. However, a US study employing data from around 1990 shows much higher use of OTC analgesics in corresponding age groups compared to our findings, whereas the use of Rx analgesics was lower in women and comparable in men [6], suggestive of a different usage pattern in the US. We found no increase in frequent analgesic use in the time period, reflecting that the increase was due to sporadic use of OTC analgesics. Possible hypotheses for the trend in analgesic use include increased prevalence of pain, a shift in the attitude towards perceived pain and/or drug use, and increased availability. It has been previously shown that a switch to OTC status leads to an initial increase in total sales of the drug [38], while the release to general sales may increase the use of NSAIDs [26]. However, the possible link between increased availability and increased use warrants further research.

Users of OTC NSAIDs are generally unaware of or unconcerned with the potential harmful effects, as OTC drugs are perceived to be relatively safe [27]. The recommended doses of OTC NSAIDs are lower than the recommended prescription doses. However, use of OTC analgesics in doses exceeding the maximum has been reported [27].

Table 4 Regular use of analgesics in the absence or presence of interacting drugs

Interacting drug[a]	Unadjusted		Age- and sex-adjusted			Potential clinical consequence
	Absent	Present	Absent	Present	p value	
	% (n)	% (n)	%	%		
Non-steroidal anti-inflammatory drugs						
Warfarin (2.5)	12.9 (1637)	2.8 (9)	12.1	3.9	<.001	Increased bleeding risk
ASA, low dose (11.7)	13.6 (1558)	5.8 (88)	12.5	7.4	<.001	Increased bleeding risk
SSRI (1.5)	12.5 (1602)	22.0 (44)	11.8	19.5	.001	Increased bleeding risk
Glucocorticoids (1.3)	12.7 (1625)	12.6 (21)	11.9	13.0	.672	Increased bleeding risk
ACE inhibitors (3.8)	12.9 (1614)	6.5 (32)	12.0	7.8	.007	Diminished effect, renal impairment, hyperkalemia
AT II antagonists (9.2)	12.8 (1508)	11.5 (138)	11.8	12.8	.326	Diminished effect, renal impairment, hyperkalemia
Other antihypertensives (18.8)[b]	13.3 (1397)	10.2 (249)	11.8	12.1	.693	Diminished effect
Opioids						
CNS depressants (4.9)[c]	2.9 (359)	18.1 (116)	2.9	17.5	<.001	CNS depression, respiratory depression, falls
Paracetamol						
Warfarin (2.5)	13.6 (1719)	7.1 (23)	12.5	9.5	.154	Increased bleeding risk

The Tromsø Study: Tromsø 6 (N = 12,981)
ASA acetylsalicylic acid, *SSRI* selective serotonin reuptake inhibitors, *ACE* angiotensin converting enzyme, *AT II* angiotensin II, *CNS* central nervous system
[a]The number in parentheses is the prevalence (%) in the study population
[b]ATC-groups C02, C03, C07, C08
[c]Benzodiazepines, z hypnotics and barbiturates (ATC-groups N05C A-F, N05B A, N03A E, N03A A)

For most of the contraindications examined, the prevalence of analgesic use was not different between persons with and without the condition when adjusted for age and sex differences. This suggests lack of awareness about the contraindications. We demonstrated frequent use of multiple analgesics within the same pharmacological group, in line with previous studies [25, 26], and frequent combined use of OTC and Rx analgesics; this would be expected to increase the risk of dose-dependent adverse effects.

NSAID use is associated with further renal impairment in individuals with underlying kidney disease [15], acute renal failure [16] and progression of chronic kidney disease [17]. We found no difference in regular use of NSAIDs among those with and without chronic kidney disease, in line with previous research [39]. Some eight percent ($n = 59$) of subjects reported using NSAIDs regularly despite having chronic kidney disease, putting them at risk of disease progression and acute renal failure.

The use of NSAIDs was not affected by a history of gastrointestinal ulcers. However, the prevalence of NSAID use was higher in patients using gastroprotective agents than in non-users. The use of gastroprotective agents may be considered either as a marker of gastrointestinal disease, i.e. a risk factor, or as a prudent precautionary measure, i.e. the prophylactic use of gastroprotective agents in persons at increased risk.

The prevalence of NSAID use was lower in persons with a history of CVD compared with those with no CVD. The risk of CVD is increased by most NSAIDs, even as short-term treatment and both in healthy individuals and in those with known CVD [12, 14] or high CVD risk [13]. There were almost no users of COX-2 inhibitors in our study population. However, diclofenac is comparable to the COX-2 inhibitors in terms of CVD risk [12]. Diclofenac is the second most sold NSAID in Norway [2] and has been available as an OTC drug from 2001.

If our data are applied to the entire Norwegian population per 2008 [34], approximately 25,000 persons aged 40–69 years with high primary CVD risk would be regular NSAID users. The NORRISK equation overestimates the prevalence of high primary CVD risk, but nevertheless our results suggest that being at high primary CVD risk does not lead to lower NSAID use. This constitutes an important problem even when the absolute risks in the population decrease.

Low-dose ASA, glucocorticoids, SSRIs, and in particular warfarin increase the gastrointestinal bleeding risk when combined with NSAIDs [15]. The much lower prevalence of NSAID use among warfarin users may be due to prescriber diligence and frequent consultations with this group of patients. Our results do however suggest that the concomitant use of glucocorticoids or SSRIs with NSAIDs is not perceived as problematic.

The prevalence of NSAID use was lower among patients taking ACE inhibitors compared to non-users, while no such difference was found for the AT II antagonists. This is somewhat surprising, as the combination of either ACE inhibitors or AT II antagonists with NSAIDs is associated with both diminished antihypertensive efficacy as well as an increased risk of renal impairment and hyperkalemia [18].

Our results show a high degree of co-medication with CNS depressant drugs among opioid users, in agreement with previous research [40]. The combination with other CNS depressant drugs increases respiratory depression [15, 19] and the risk of fractures [20], and can be suggestive of substance abuse [19], as well as be detrimental on activities requiring alertness, i.e. driving.

This observational study has some limitations. Our analyses included data from two cross-sections of the Tromsø study; inferences on causality are difficult if not impossible due to the lack of temporality between exposure and effect.

The agreement between self-reported analgesic use and prescription records is moderate [41]. The rate of underreporting of self-reported use of ibuprofen and paracetamol is approximately 15 % or more [42]. Recall of NSAID use declines over time, and particularly among infrequent users of OTC NSAIDs [43]. Higher use of strong analgesics among non-participants compared to participants has been reported [9]. This all points toward an underestimation of the prevalence of analgesic use in the present study.

Participants reported the use of "painkillers", leading to possible ambiguity and misclassification. We could not separate OTC and Rx use in the analyses on high-risk use. The contraindications and drug interactions identified may have been dealt with in an adequate manner by the prescribing physician or other health personnel. The most severe cases may have been missed due to non-participation, leading to an underestimation of high-risk analgesic use.

Study strengths include the use of a large, repeated population-based survey and self-reported data on both OTC analgesics and Rx analgesics. A comprehensive estimate of the use of analgesics cannot be done without the use of interview or questionnaires.

The Tromsø population may be regarded as representative of a Northern European, white, urban population [29], and the results may be generalizable to such populations.

Conclusions

The use of analgesics increased in the time period, in line with other studies and gross sales statistics, mainly due to an increase in sporadic use of OTC analgesics. We have identified several areas of high risk use of analgesics where a known contraindication or drug interaction do not seem to lead to lower use at a population level. This could put people at risk and pose a threat to public health. Public and prescriber awareness about important contraindications, such as chronic kidney disease, gastrointestinal ulcers and risk of CVD, as well as clinically relevant drug interactions with analgesics, need to be increased.

Abbreviations
ACE: Angiotensin-converting enzyme; ASA: Acetylsalicylic acid; ATC: Anatomical therapeutic chemical classification system; AT II: Angiotensin II; CI: Confidence interval; CKD-EPI: Chronic Kidney Disease Epidemiology collaboration; CNS: Central nervous system; COX-2: Cyclooxygenase 2; CVD: Cardiovascular disease; eGFR: Estimated glomerular filtration rate; GEE: Generalized estimating equations; NSAIDs: Non-steroidal anti-inflammatory drugs; OR: Odds ratio; OTC: "Over-the-counter", non-prescription; Rx: Prescription; SSRI: Selective serotonin reuptake inhibitors.

Competing interests
The authors declare that they have no competing interests.

Authors' contributions
PJS planned the study, conducted the analyses, and wrote the draft and the final manuscript. AEE planned the study, aided in the analyses and interpretation of the data and revised the manuscript. PJS, AEE and LS developed the contraindication and drug interactions criteria. LS aided in the interpretation of data and revised the manuscript. UDM aided in the analyses and interpretation of the renal function data, and revised the manuscript. All authors approved the final manuscript.

Acknowledgements
This study was funded by the Northern Norway Regional Health Authority (project ID: 8709/SFP1092-13). We wish to thank Randi Selmer for aiding in the calculation of the NORRISK score, Frode Skjold for aiding in data management and Tom Wilsgaard and Tonje Braaten for aiding in the statistical analysis.

Author details
[1]Regional Medicines Information and Pharmacovigilance Center (RELIS), University Hospital of North Norway, N-9038 Tromsø, Norway. [2]Department of Community Medicine, UiT-The Arctic University of Norway, Tromsø, Norway. [3]Department of Laboratory Medicine, Children's and Women's Health, Norwegian University of Science and Technology, Trondheim, Norway. [4]Department of Clinical Pharmacology, St. Olav University Hospital, Trondheim, Norway. [5]Section of Nephrology, University Hospital of North Norway, Tromsø, Norway.

References
1. Association TNP. Facts and figures - pharmacies and pharmaceuticals in Norway 2012. Oslo. 2012. Available at: http://www.apotek.no/.
2. Sakshaug S, editor. Drug consumption in Norway 2009–2013. Oslo: Norwegian Institute of Public Health; 2014. Available at: http://www.drugconsumption.no/.
3. Eggen AE. The Tromso study: frequency and predicting factors of analgesic drug use in a free-living population (12–56 years). J Clin Epidemiol. 1993;46(11):1297–304.
4. Antonov K, Isacson D. Use of analgesics in Sweden - the importance of sociodemographic factors, physical fitness, health and health-related factors, and working conditions. Soc Sci Med. 1996;42(11):1473–81.
5. Isacson D, Bingefors K. Epidemiology of analgesic use: a gender perspective. Eur J Anaesthesiol. 2002;19:5–15.
6. Paulose-Ram R, Hirsch R, Dillon C, Losonczy K, Cooper M, Ostchega Y. Prescription and non-prescription analgesic use among the US adult population: results from the third National health and nutrition examination survey (NHANES III). Pharmacoepidemiol Drug Saf. 2003;12(4):315–26.
7. Porteous T, Bond C, Hannaford P, Sinclair H. How and why are non-prescription analgesics used in Scotland? Fam Pract. 2005;22(1):78–85.
8. Hargreave M, Andersen TV, Nielsen A, Munk C, Liaw KL, Kjaer SK. Factors associated with a continuous regular analgesic use - a population-based study of more than 45,000 Danish women and men 18–45 years of age. Pharmacoepidemiol Drug Saf. 2010;19(1):65–74.
9. Eggen AE. The use of controlled analgesics in a general population (15–59 years)- the influence of age, gender, morbidity, lifestyle and sociodemographic factors. Pharmacoepidemiol Drug Saf. 1996;5(2):101–11.
10. Antonov KI, Isacson DG. Prescription and nonprescription analgesic use in Sweden. Ann Pharmacother. 1998;32(4):485–94.
11. Saedder E, Brock B, Nielsen L, Bonnerup D, Lisby M. Identifying high-risk medication: a systematic literature review. Eur J Clin Pharmacol. 2014;70(6):637–45.
12. Schjerning Olsen A-M, Fosbøl EL, Gislason GH. The impact of NSAID treatment on cardiovascular risk – insight from Danish observational data. Basic Clin Pharmacol Toxicol. 2014;115(2):179–84.
13. de Abajo FJ, Gil MJ, Garcia Poza P, Bryant V, Oliva B, Timoner J, et al. Risk of nonfatal acute myocardial infarction associated with non-steroidal antiinflammatory drugs, non-narcotic analgesics and other drugs used in osteoarthritis: a nested case-control study. Pharmacoepidemiol Drug Saf. 2014;23(11):1128–38.
14. Schjerning Olsen A-M, Fosbøl EL, Lindhardsen J, Folke F, Charlot M, Selmer C, et al. Duration of treatment with nonsteroidal anti-inflammatory drugs and impact on risk of death and recurrent myocardial infarction in patients with prior myocardial infarction: a nationwide cohort study. Circulation. 2011;123(20):2226–35.
15. Aronson JK. Meyler's side effects of analgesics and anti-inflammatory drugs. Amsterdam; Boston; London: Elsevier Science; 2010.
16. Huerta C, Castellsague J, Varas-Lorenzo C, García Rodríguez LA. Nonsteroidal anti-inflammatory drugs and risk of ARF in the general population. Am J Kidney Dis. 2005;45(3):531–9.
17. Gooch K, Culleton BF, Manns BJ, Zhang J, Alfonso H, Tonelli M, et al. NSAID use and progression of chronic kidney disease. Am J Med. 2007;120(3):280e1–e7.
18. Baxter K, Preston C, editors. Stockley's drug interactions. [online] London: Pharmaceutical Press; 2014
19. Gudin JA, Mogali S, Jones JD, Comer SD. Risks, management, and monitoring of combination opioid, benzodiazepines, and/or alcohol use. Postgrad Med. 2013;125(4):115–30.
20. Li L, Setoguchi S, Cabral H, Jick S. Opioid use for noncancer pain and risk of fracture in adults: a nested case-control study using the General practice research database. Am J Epidemiol. 2013;178(4):559–69.
21. Tarantino G, Di Minno MND, Capone D. Drug-induced liver injury: is it somehow foreseeable? World J Gastroenterol. 2009;15(23):2817–33.
22. Roberts E, Delgado Nunes V, Buckner S, Latchem S, Constanti M, Miller P, et al. Paracetamol: not as safe as we thought? A systematic literature review of observational studies. Ann Rheum Dis. 2015.
23. Adams R, Appleton S, Gill T, Taylor A, Wilson D, Hill C. Cause for concern in the use of non-steroidal anti-inflammatory medications in the community - a population-based study. BMC Fam Pract. 2011;12(1):70.
24. Koffeman AR, Valkhoff VE, Çelik S, Jong GW, Sturkenboom MC, Bindels PJ, et al. High-risk use of over-the-counter non-steroidal anti-inflammatory drugs: a population-based cross-sectional study. Br J Gen Pract. 2014;64(621):e191–8.
25. Silvani MC, Motola D, Poluzzi E, Bottoni A, De Ponti F, Vaccheri A, et al. Gastro-intestinal problems and concomitant medication in NSAID users: additional findings from a questionnaire-based survey in Italy. Eur J Clin Pharmacol. 2006;62(3):235–41.
26. Stosic R, Dunagan F, Palmer H, Fowler T, Adams I. Responsible self-medication: perceived risks and benefits of over-the-counter analgesic use. Int J Pharm Pract. 2011;19(4):236–45.

27. Wilcox CM, Cryer B, Triadafilopoulos G. Patterns of use and public perception of over-the-counter pain relievers: focus on nonsteroidal antiinflammatory drugs. J Rheumatol. 2005;32(11):2218–24.

28. Jacobsen BK, Eggen AE, Mathiesen EB, Wilsgaard T, Njolstad I. Cohort profile: the Tromso study. Int J Epidemiol. 2012;41(4):961–7.

29. Eggen AE, Mathiesen EB, Wilsgaard T, Jacobsen BK, Njølstad I. The sixth survey of the Tromsø study (Tromsø 6) in 2007–08: collaborative research in the interface between clinical medicine and epidemiology: study objectives, design, data collection procedures, and attendance in a multipurpose population-based health survey. Scand J Public Health. 2013;41(1):65–80.

30. Hallan SI, Coresh J, Astor BC, Asberg A, Powe NR, Romundstad S, et al. International comparison of the relationship of chronic kidney disease prevalence and ESRD risk. J Am Soc Nephrol. 2006;17(8):2275–84.

31. Levey AS, Stevens LA, Schmid CH, Zhang Y, Castro IIIAF, Feldman HI, et al. A new equation to estimate glomerular filtration rate. Ann Intern Med. 2009;150(9):604–12.

32. Selmer R, Lindman AS, Tverdal A, Pedersen JI, Njolstad I, Veierod MB. Model for estimation of cardiovascular risk in Norway. Tidsskr Nor Laegeforen. 2008;128(3):286–90.

33. The Norwegian Directorate of Health. National guideline on individual primary prevention of cardiovascular disease. 2009. Available at: http://www.helsedirektoratet.no/.

34. Statistics Norway. Population, by sex and age (table 10211). Available at: http://www.ssb.no/.

35. Fredheim OM, Skurtveit S, Breivik H, Borchgrevink PC. Increasing use of opioids from 2004 to 2007 - pharmacoepidemiological data from a complete national prescription database in Norway. Eur J Pain. 2010;14(3):289–94.

36. Hamunen K, Paakkari P, Kalso E. Trends in opioid consumption in the Nordic countries 2002-2006. Eur J Pain. 2009;13(9):954–62.

37. Ruscitto A, Smith BH, Guthrie B. Changes in opioid and other analgesic use 1995–2010: Repeated cross-sectional analysis of dispensed prescribing for a large geographical population in Scotland. Eur J Pain. 2014.

38. Carlsten A, Wennberg M, Bergendal L. The influence of Rx-to-OTC changes on drug sales. Experiences from Sweden 1980–1994. J Clin Pharm Ther. 1996;21(6):423–30.

39. Plantinga L, Grubbs V, Sarkar U, Hsu CY, Hedgeman E, Robinson B, et al. Nonsteroidal anti-inflammatory drug use among persons with chronic kidney disease in the United States. Ann Fam Med. 2011;9(5):423–30.

40. Mellbye A, Svendsen K, Borchgrevink PC, Skurtveit S, Fredheim OMS. Concomitant medication among persistent opioid users with chronic non-malignant pain. Acta Anaesthesiol Scand. 2012;56(10):1267–76.

41. Nielsen MW, Søndergaard B, Kjøller M, Hansen EH. Agreement between self-reported data on medicine use and prescription records vary according to method of analysis and therapeutic group. J Clin Epidemiol. 2008;61(9):919–24.

42. Loo RL, Chan Q, Brown IJ, Robertson CE, Stamler J, Nicholson JK, et al. A comparison of self-reported analgesic use and detection of urinary ibuprofen and acetaminophen metabolites by means of metabonomics: The INTERMAP study. Am J Epidemiol. 2012;175(4):348–58.

43. Lewis JD, Strom BL, Kimmel SE, Farrar J, Metz DC, Brensinger C, et al. Predictors of recall of over-the-counter and prescription non-steroidal anti-inflammatory drug exposure. Pharmacoepidemiol Drug Saf. 2006;15(1):39–45.

Permissions

The contributors of this book come from diverse backgrounds, making this book a truly international effort. This book will bring forth new frontiers with its revolutionizing research information and detailed analysis of the nascent developments around the world.

We would like to thank all the contributing authors for lending their expertise to make the book truly unique. They have played a crucial role in the development of this book. Without their invaluable contributions this book wouldn't have been possible. They have made vital efforts to compile up to date information on the varied aspects of this subject to make this book a valuable addition to the collection of many professionals and students.

This book was conceptualized with the vision of imparting up-to-date information and advanced data in this field. To ensure the same, a matchless editorial board was set up. Every individual on the board went through rigorous rounds of assessment to prove their worth. After which they invested a large part of their time researching and compiling the most relevant data for our readers.

The editorial board has been involved in producing this book since its inception. They have spent rigorous hours researching and exploring the diverse topics which have resulted in the successful publishing of this book. They have passed on their knowledge of decades through this book. To expedite this challenging task, the publisher supported the team at every step. A small team of assistant editors was also appointed to further simplify the editing procedure and attain best results for the readers.

Apart from the editorial board, the designing team has also invested a significant amount of their time in understanding the subject and creating the most relevant covers. They scrutinized every image to scout for the most suitable representation of the subject and create an appropriate cover for the book.

The publishing team has been an ardent support to the editorial, designing and production team. Their endless efforts to recruit the best for this project, has resulted in the accomplishment of this book. They are a veteran in the field of academics and their pool of knowledge is as vast as their experience in printing. Their expertise and guidance has proved useful at every step. Their uncompromising quality standards have made this book an exceptional effort. Their encouragement from time to time has been an inspiration for everyone.

The publisher and the editorial board hope that this book will prove to be a valuable piece of knowledge for researchers, students, practitioners and scholars across the globe.

List of Contributors

Do Thi Thuy Nga
Wellcome Trust Major Overseas Programme, Oxford University Clinical Research Unit, Hanoi, Vietnam

Nguyen Thi Kim Chuc
Hanoi Medical University, Hanoi, Vietnam

Nguyen Phuong Hoa
Hanoi Medical University, Hanoi, Vietnam

Nguyen Quynh Hoa
Vietnam National Cancer Hospital, Hanoi, Vietnam

Nguyen Thi Thuy Nguyen
Hanoi Medical University, Hanoi, Vietnam

Hoang Thi Loan
Hanoi Medical University, Hanoi, Vietnam

Tran Khanh Toan
Hanoi Medical University, Hanoi, Vietnam

Ho Dang Phuc
Department of Probability and Statistics, Institute of Mathematics, VAST, Hanoi, Vietnam

Peter Horby
Wellcome Trust Major Overseas Programme, Oxford University Clinical Research Unit, Hanoi, Vietnam
Nuffield Department of Clinical Medicine, Centre for Tropical Diseases, Oxford, UK

Nguyen Van Yen
Hanoi Department of Health, Hanoi, Vietnam

Nguyen Van Kinh
National Hospital for Tropical Diseases, Hanoi, Vietnam

Heiman FL Wertheim
Wellcome Trust Major Overseas Programme, Oxford University Clinical Research Unit, Hanoi, Vietnam
Nuffield Department of Clinical Medicine, Centre for Tropical Diseases, Oxford, UK

Naoko Yoshida
Drug Management and Policy, Faculty of Pharmacy, Institute of Medical, Pharmaceutical and Health Sciences, Kanazawa University, Kakuma-machi, Kanazawa, Ishikawa 920-1192, Japan

Mohiuddin Hussain Khan
Drug Management and Policy, Faculty of Pharmacy, Institute of Medical, Pharmaceutical and Health Sciences, Kanazawa University, Kakuma-machi, Kanazawa, Ishikawa 920-1192, Japan

Hitomi Tabata
Drug Management and Policy, Faculty of Pharmacy, Institute of Medical, Pharmaceutical and Health Sciences, Kanazawa University, Kakuma-machi, Kanazawa, Ishikawa 920-1192, Japan

Eav Dararath
Department of Drugs and Food, Ministry of Health, 151-153, Kampuchea Krom St, Khan 7 Makara, Phnom Penh, Cambodia

Tey Sovannarith
National Health Product Quality Control Center, Ministry of Health, 151-153, Kampuchea Krom St, Khan 7 Makara, Phnom Penh, Cambodia

Heng Bun Kiet
Department of Drugs and Food, Ministry of Health, 151-153, Kampuchea Krom St, Khan 7 Makara, Phnom Penh, Cambodia

Nam Nivanna
National Health Product Quality Control Center, Ministry of Health, 151-153, Kampuchea Krom St, Khan 7 Makara, Phnom Penh, Cambodia

Manabu Akazawa
Department of Public Health and Epidemiology, Meiji Pharmaceutical University, 2-522-1 Noshio, Kiyose, Tokyo 204-8588, Japan

Hirohito Tsuboi
Drug Management and Policy, Faculty of Pharmacy, Institute of Medical, Pharmaceutical and Health Sciences, Kanazawa University, Kakuma-machi, Kanazawa, Ishikawa 920-1192, Japan

Tsuyoshi Tanimoto
Faculty of Pharmaceutical Sciences, Doshisha Women's University, Kodo, Kyotanabe, Kyoto 610-0395, Japan

Kazuko Kimura
Drug Management and Policy, Faculty of Pharmacy, Institute of Medical, Pharmaceutical and Health Sciences, Kanazawa University, Kakuma-machi, Kanazawa, Ishikawa 920-1192, Japan

Ping Song
Department of Pharmacy, the Second Affiliated Hospital, School of Medicine, Zhejiang University, Jiefang Road No. 88, Hangzhou, Zhejiang 310009, China

Wei Li
Division of Medical Affairs, the Second Affiliated Hospital, School of Medicine, Zhejiang University, Hangzhou, Zhejiang 310009, Province, China

Quan Zhou
Department of Pharmacy, the Second Affiliated Hospital, School of Medicine, Zhejiang University, Jiefang Road No. 88, Hangzhou, Zhejiang 310009, China

Bayeh Abera
Department of Microbiology, Parasitology and Immunology, College of Medicine and Health Sciences, Bahir Dar University, P.O. Box 79, Bahir Dar, Ethiopia

Mulugeta Kibret
Department of Biology, Science College, Bahir Dar University, P.O. Box 79, Bahir Dar, Ethiopia

Wondemagegn Mulu
Department of Microbiology, Parasitology and Immunology, College of Medicine and Health Sciences, Bahir Dar University, P.O. Box 79, Bahir Dar, Ethiopia

Pilar Carrasco-Garrido
Department of Preventive Medicine and Public Health, Rey Juan Carlos University, Avda. Atenas s/n., Alcorcón, Madrid, Spain

Ana López de Andrés
Department of Preventive Medicine and Public Health, Rey Juan Carlos University, Avda. Atenas s/n., Alcorcón, Madrid, Spain

Valentín Hernández Barrera
Department of Preventive Medicine and Public Health, Rey Juan Carlos University, Avda. Atenas s/n., Alcorcón, Madrid, Spain

Isabel Jiménez-Trujillo
Department of Preventive Medicine and Public Health, Rey Juan Carlos University, Avda. Atenas s/n., Alcorcón, Madrid, Spain

César Fernandez-de-las-Peñas
Department of Physical Therapy, Occupational Therapy, Rehabilitation and Physical Medicine, Rey Juan Carlos University, Alcorcón, Madrid, Spain

Domingo Palacios-Ceña
Department of Nursing, Rey Juan Carlos University, Alcorcón, Madrid, Spain

Soledad García-Gómez-Heras
Department of Human Histology and Pathological Anatomy, Rey Juan Carlos University, Alcorcón, Madrid, Spain

Rodrigo Jiménez-García
Department of Preventive Medicine and Public Health, Rey Juan Carlos University, Avda. Atenas s/n., Alcorcón, Madrid, Spain

Carolina Garcia-Canton
British American Tobacco, Group Research and Development, Regents Park Road, Southampton, Hampshire SO15 8TL, UK
Department of Toxicology and Pharmacology, Universidad Complutense de Madrid, Madrid, Spain

Graham Errington
British American Tobacco, Group Research and Development, Regents Park Road, Southampton, Hampshire SO15 8TL, UK

Arturo Anadon
Department of Toxicology and Pharmacology, Universidad Complutense de Madrid, Madrid, Spain

Clive Meredith
British American Tobacco, Group Research and Development, Regents Park Road, Southampton, Hampshire SO15 8TL, UK

Christian Wunderlich
University of Veterinary Medicine Hannover, Foundation, Institute of Pharmacology, Toxicology and Pharmacy, Bünteweg 17, Hannover 30559, Germany

Stephan Schumacher
University of Veterinary Medicine Hannover, Foundation, Institute of Pharmacology, Toxicology and Pharmacy, Bünteweg 17, Hannover 30559, Germany

Manfred Kietzmann
University of Veterinary Medicine Hannover, Foundation, Institute of Pharmacology, Toxicology and Pharmacy, Bünteweg 17, Hannover 30559, Germany

Getachew Tadesse
Department of Biomedical Sciences, College of Veterinary Medicine and Agriculture, Addis Ababa University, P.O. Box 34, Debre Zeit, Ethiopia

Øystein Kravdal
Norwegian Institute of Public Health, Oslo, Norway
Department of Economics, University of Oslo, Oslo, Norway
Postal address: Department of Economics, P.O. Box 1095 Blindern, 0317 Oslo, Norway

Emily Grundy
Department of Social Policy, London School of Economics and Political Science, London, UK

Michiel Haeseker
Department of Medical Microbiology, Maastricht University Medical Centre, Maastricht, the Netherlands Care and Public Health Research Institute (CAPHRI), Maastricht, the Netherlands
Present address: Maastricht University Medical Centre, P. Debyelaan 25, PO Box 58006202 AZ Maastricht, the Netherlands

Thomas Havenith
Department of Clinical Pharmacy, Maastricht University Medical Centre, Maastricht, the Netherlands

Leo Stolk
Department of Clinical Pharmacy, Maastricht University Medical Centre, Maastricht, the Netherlands

Cees Neef
Department of Clinical Pharmacy, Maastricht University Medical Centre, Maastricht, the Netherlands

Cathrien Bruggeman
Department of Medical Microbiology, Maastricht University Medical Centre, Maastricht, the Netherlands Care and Public Health Research Institute (CAPHRI), Maastricht, the Netherlands

Annelies Verbon
Department of Internal Medicine, Erasmus Medical Centre, Rotterdam, the Netherlands

Françoise Livio
Division of Clinical Pharmacology, Biomedicine, Department of Laboratories, Centre Hospitalier Universitaire Vaudois, Lausanne 1011, Switzerland

Peter Wahl
Department of Orthopedic Surgery, Cantonal Hospital, Fribourg, Switzerland

Chantal Csajka
Division of Clinical Pharmacology, Biomedicine, Department of Laboratories, Centre Hospitalier Universitaire Vaudois, Lausanne 1011, Switzerland
Department of Pharmaceutical Sciences, Clinical Pharmacy Unit, University of Geneva, Rue du Général- Dufour 24, Genève 4 1211, Switzerland

Emanuel Gautier
Department of Orthopedic Surgery, Cantonal Hospital, Fribourg, Switzerland

Thierry Buclin
Division of Clinical Pharmacology, Biomedicine, Department of Laboratories, Centre Hospitalier Universitaire Vaudois, Lausanne 1011, Switzerland

Helmut Ostermann
Medical Clinic III, Department of Haematology and Oncology, University Hospital Munich – Grosshadern, Munich, Germany

Carlos Solano
Haematology and Oncology Department, Hospital Clínico Universitario INCLIVA, University of Valencia, Valencia, Spain

Isidro Jarque
Haematology Service, Hospital Universitari i Politècnic La Fe, Valencia, Spain

Carolina Garcia-Vidal
Hospital Universitari de Bellvitge, Universitat de Barcelona, Barcelona, Spain

Xin Gao
Pharmerit International, Bethesda, MD, USA

Jon Andoni Barrueta
Medical Unit, Pfizer Spain, Madrid, Spain

Marina De Salas-Cansado
Health Economics and Outcomes Research Department, Pfizer Spain, Madrid, Spain

Jennifer Stephens
Pharmerit International, Bethesda, MD, USA

Mei Xue
Pharmerit International, Bethesda, MD, USA

Bertram Weber
Health Technology Assessment and Outcomes Research Department, Pfizer Germany, Berlin, Germany

Claudie Charbonneau
Health Economics and Outcomes Research Department, Pfizer International Operations, Paris, France

Robert J Brosnan
Department of Surgical and Radiological Sciences, School of Veterinary Medicine, University of California, Davis, CA 95616, USA

Trung L Pham
Department of Surgical and Radiological Sciences, School of Veterinary Medicine, University of California, Davis, CA 95616, USA

Emma Loveman
Southampton Health Technology Assessments Centre
(SHTAC), University of Southampton, Southampton, UK

Vicky R Copley
Southampton Health Technology Assessments Centre
(SHTAC), University of Southampton, Southampton, UK

Jill L Colquitt
Southampton Health Technology Assessments Centre
(SHTAC), University of Southampton, Southampton, UK

David A Scott
Icon PLC, Oxford, UK

Andy J Clegg
Southampton Health Technology Assessments Centre
(SHTAC), University of Southampton, Southampton, UK

Jeremy Jones
Southampton Health Technology Assessments Centre
(SHTAC), University of Southampton, Southampton, UK

Katherine MA O'Reilly
Mater Misericordiae University Hospital, Dublin, Ireland

Sally Singh
University Hospitals of Leicester NHS Trust, Leicester,
UK

Claudia Bausewein
Department of Palliative Medicine, University Hospital
of Munich, Munich, Germany

Athol Wells
Green Lane Hospital, London, UK

Olivier Michel
Clinic of Allergology and Immunology, CHU Brugmann
(Université Libre de Bruxelles - ULB), 4 pl Van Gehuchten,
B −1020, Brussels, Belgium

Phong Huy Duc Dinh
Department of Immunology, Pham Ngoc Thach University
of Medicine (PNTU), Ho Chi Minh, Vietnam

Virginie Doyen
Clinic of Allergology and Immunology, CHU Brugmann
(Université Libre de Bruxelles - ULB), 4 pl Van Gehuchten,
B −1020, Brussels, Belgium

Francis Corazza
Laboratory of Immunology, CHU Brugmann (Université
Libre de Bruxelles - ULB), Brussels, Belgium

Dieter Pullirsch
AGES - Austrian Agency for Health & Food Safety,
Austrian Medicines and Medical Devices Agency,
Traisengasse 5, Vienna AT-1200, Austria

Julie Bellemare
Health Canada, 1001 St-Laurent West, Longueuil, Qc J4K
1C7, Canada

Andreas Hackl
AGES - Austrian Agency for Health & Food Safety,
Austrian Medicines and Medical Devices Agency,
Traisengasse 5, Vienna AT-1200, Austria

Yvon-Louis Trottier
Health Canada, 1001 St-Laurent West, Longueuil, Qc J4K
1C7, Canada

Andreas Mayrhofer
AGES - Austrian Agency for Health & Food Safety,
Austrian Medicines and Medical Devices Agency,
Traisengasse 5, Vienna AT-1200, Austria

Heidemarie Schindl
AGES - Austrian Agency for Health & Food Safety,
Austrian Medicines and Medical Devices Agency,
Traisengasse 5, Vienna AT-1200, Austria

Christine Taillon
Health Canada, 1001 St-Laurent West, Longueuil, Qc J4K
1C7, Canada

Christian Gartner
AGES - Austrian Agency for Health & Food Safety,
Austrian Medicines and Medical Devices Agency,
Traisengasse 5, Vienna AT-1200, Austria

Brigitte Hottowy
AGES - Austrian Agency for Health & Food Safety,
Austrian Medicines and Medical Devices Agency,
Traisengasse 5, Vienna AT-1200, Austria

Gerhard Beck
AGES - Austrian Agency for Health & Food Safety,
Austrian Medicines and Medical Devices Agency,
Traisengasse 5, Vienna AT-1200, Austria

Jacques Gagnon
Health Canada, 1001 St-Laurent West, Longueuil, Qc J4K
1C7, Canada

Masahiro Inoue
Department of Clinical Oncology, Graduate School of
Medicine, Akita University, Akita, Japan
Division of Chemotherapy for Outpatient, Akita
University, Akita, Japan

Manabu Shoji
Division of Chemotherapy for Outpatient, Akita
University, Akita, Japan
Department of Pharmacy, Akita University, Akita, Japan

Naomi Shindo
Division of Chemotherapy for Outpatient, Akita University, Akita, Japan

Kazunori Otsuka
Department of Clinical Oncology, Graduate School of Medicine, Akita University, Akita, Japan
Division of Chemotherapy for Outpatient, Akita University, Akita, Japan

Masatomo Miura
Department of Pharmacy, Akita University, Akita, Japan

Hiroyuki Shibata
Department of Clinical Oncology, Graduate School of Medicine, Akita University, Akita, Japan
Division of Chemotherapy for Outpatient, Akita University, Akita, Japan

Syed Jawad Shah
Aga Khan University, Karachi, Pakistan

Hamna Ahmad
Aga Khan University, Karachi, Pakistan

Rija Binte Rehan
Aga Khan University, Karachi, Pakistan

Sidra Najeeb
Aga Khan University, Karachi, Pakistan

Mirrah Mumtaz
Aga Khan University, Karachi, Pakistan

Muhammad Hashim Jilani
Aga Khan University, Karachi, Pakistan

Muhammad Sharoz Rabbani
Aga Khan University, Karachi, Pakistan

Muhammad Zakariya Alam
Aga Khan University, Karachi, Pakistan

Saba Farooq
Aga Khan University, Karachi, Pakistan

M Masood Kadir
Department of Community Health Sciences, Aga Khan University, Karachi, Pakistan

Fabíola Giordani
Department of Epidemiology and Biostatistics, Institute of Community Health, Fluminense Federal University, Marquês de Paraná Street 303, Annex HUAP 3rd floor, Niterói, RJ 24033-900, Brazil

Suely Rozenfeld
Sérgio Arouca National School of Public Health, Oswaldo Cruz Foundation, Rio de Janeiro, Brazil

Mônica Martins
Sérgio Arouca National School of Public Health, Oswaldo Cruz Foundation, Rio de Janeiro, Brazil

Qin Ouyang
Department of Pharmaceutical Sciences, Computational Chemical Genomics Screening Center, School of Pharmacy, NIH National Center, of Excellence for Computational Drug Abuse Research, Drug Discovery Institute, College of Pharmacy, Third Military Medical University, Chongqing 400038, China

Lirong Wang
Department of Pharmaceutical Sciences, Computational Chemical Genomics Screening Center, School of Pharmacy, NIH National Center, of Excellence for Computational Drug Abuse Research, Drug Discovery Institute, Pittsburgh, PA 15261, USA

Ying Mu
Division of Biology, Office of Science and Engineering Laboratories, Center for Devices and Radiobiological Health, US Food and Drug Administration, Silver Spring, MD 20993, USA

Xiang-Qun Xie
Department of Pharmaceutical Sciences, Computational Chemical Genomics Screening Center, School of Pharmacy, NIH National Center, of Excellence for Computational Drug Abuse Research, Drug Discovery Institute, Pittsburgh, PA 15261, USA
Department of Computational and Systems Biology, University of Pittsburgh, Pittsburgh, PA 15261, USA

John N Kateregga
College of Veterinary Medicine, Animal Resources & Biosecurity, Makerere University, P.O Box 7062, Kampala, Uganda

Ronah Kantume
College of Veterinary Medicine, Animal Resources & Biosecurity, Makerere University, P.O Box 7062, Kampala, Uganda

Collins Atuhaire
College of Veterinary Medicine, Animal Resources & Biosecurity, Makerere University, P.O Box 7062, Kampala, Uganda

Musisi Nathan Lubowa
College of Veterinary Medicine, Animal Resources & Biosecurity, Makerere University, P.O Box 7062, Kampala, Uganda

James G Ndukui
College of Veterinary Medicine, Animal Resources & Biosecurity, Makerere University, P.O Box 7062, Kampala, Uganda

Brooke M Ramay
Department of Pharmaceutical Chemistry, Universidad del Valle de Guatemala, Guatemala City, Guatemala

Paola Lambour
Department of Pharmaceutical Chemistry, Universidad del Valle de Guatemala, Guatemala City, Guatemala

Alejandro Cerón
Department of Anthropology, University of Denver, Denver, Colorado, USA

Nicola Laurieri
Department of Pharmacology, University of Oxford, Oxford, UK

Akane Kawamura
Department of Chemistry, Chemistry Research Laboratory, University of Oxford, Oxford, UK

Isaac M Westwood
Current address: Divisions of Structural Biology and Cancer Therapeutics, The Institute of Cancer Research, Chester Beatty Laboratories, London, UK

Amy Varney
Department of Pharmacology, University of Oxford, Oxford, UK

Elizabeth Morris
Department of Pharmacology, University of Oxford, Oxford, UK

Angela J Russell
Department of Pharmacology, University of Oxford, Oxford, UK
Department of Chemistry, Chemistry Research Laboratory, University of Oxford, Oxford, UK

Lesley A Stanley
Consultant in Investigative Toxicology, Linlithgow, West Lothian, Scotland

Edith Sim
Department of Pharmacology, University of Oxford, Oxford, UK
Faculty of Science, Engineering and Computing, Kingston University, Kingston on Thames, UK

André S. Pollmann
Faculty of Medicine, Dalhousie University, Mail Box #259, 5849 University Avenue, Room C-125, PO Box 15000, Halifax, NS B3H 4R2, Canada

Andrea L. Murphy
College of Pharmacy and Department of Psychiatry, Dalhousie University, 5968 College St, PO Box 15000, Halifax, NS B3H 4R2, Canada

Joel C. Bergman
College of Pharmacy and Department of Psychiatry, Dalhousie University, 5968 College St, PO Box 15000, Halifax, NS B3H 4R2, Canada

David M. Gardner
Department of Psychiatry and College of Pharmacy, Dalhousie University, QEII HSC, AJLB 7517, 5909 Veterans' Memorial Lane, Halifax, NS B3H 2E2, Canada

Per-Jostein Samuelsen
Regional Medicines Information and Pharmacovigilance Center (RELIS), University Hospital of North Norway, N-9038 Tromsø, Norway
Department of Community Medicine, UiT-The Arctic University of Norway, Tromsø, Norway

Lars Slørdal
Department of Laboratory Medicine, Children's and Women's Health, Norwegian University of Science and Technology, Trondheim, Norway
Department of Clinical Pharmacology, St. Olav University Hospital, Trondheim, Norway

Ulla Dorte Mathisen
Section of Nephrology, University Hospital of North Norway, Tromsø, Norway

Anne Elise Eggen
Department of Community Medicine, UiT-The Arctic University of Norway, Tromsø, Norway

www.ingramcontent.com/pod-product-compliance
Lightning Source LLC
Chambersburg PA
CBHW080525200326
41458CB00012B/4341

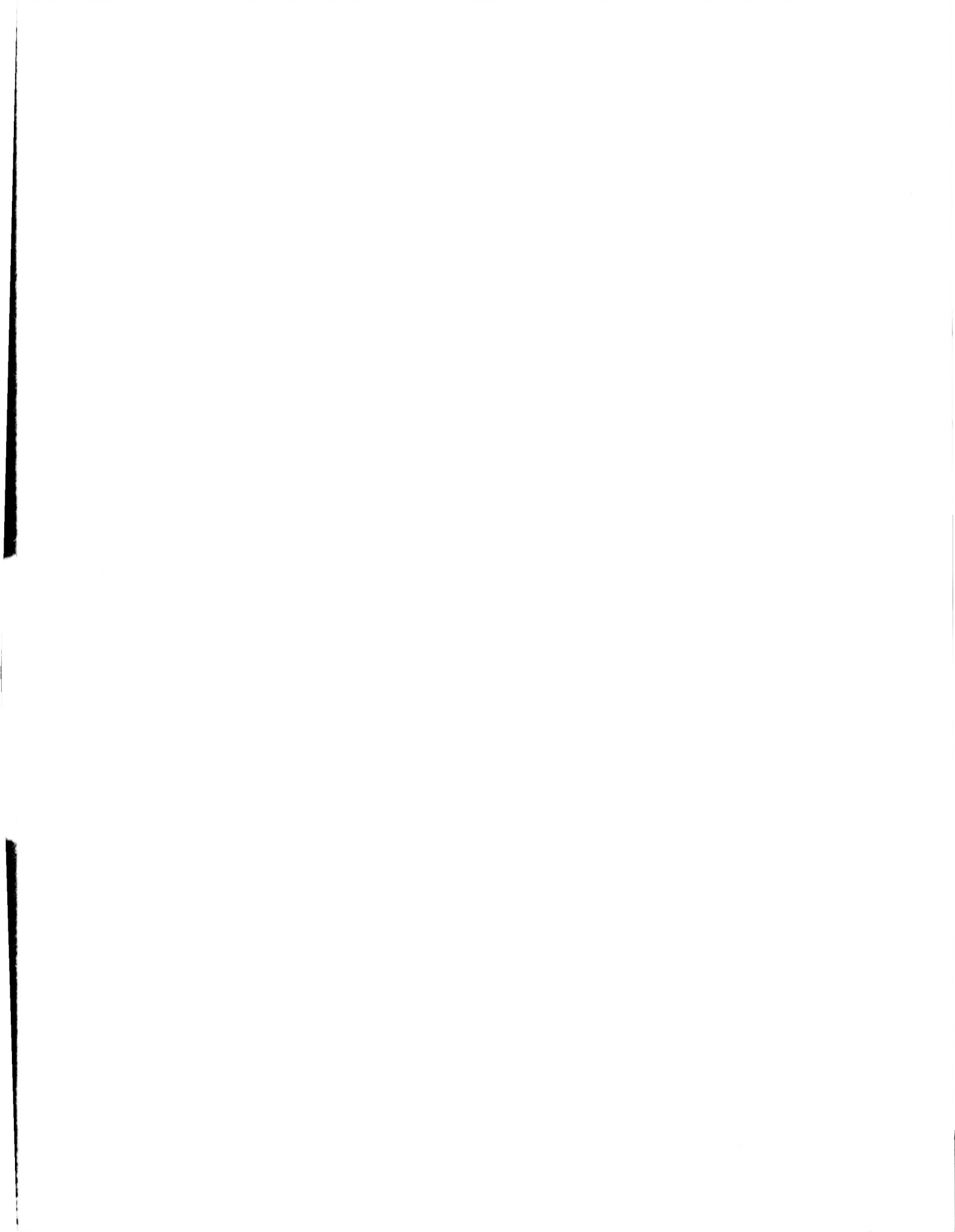